OCT and Imaging in Central Nervous System Diseases

Andrzej Grzybowski • Piero Barboni
Editors

OCT and Imaging in Central Nervous System Diseases

The Eye as a Window to the Brain

Second Edition

Springer

Editors
Andrzej Grzybowski
University of Warmia and Mazury
Olsztyn
Poland

Institute for Research in Ophthalmology
Poznań
Poland

Piero Barboni
Studio Oculistico d'Azeglio
Bologna
Italy

Scientific Institute San Raffaele
Milan
Italy

ISBN 978-3-030-26271-6 ISBN 978-3-030-26269-3 (eBook)
https://doi.org/10.1007/978-3-030-26269-3

This Springer imprint is published by the registered company Springer Nature Switzerland AG
The registered company address is: Gewerbestrasse 11, 6330 Cham, Switzerland

Contents

About the Editors

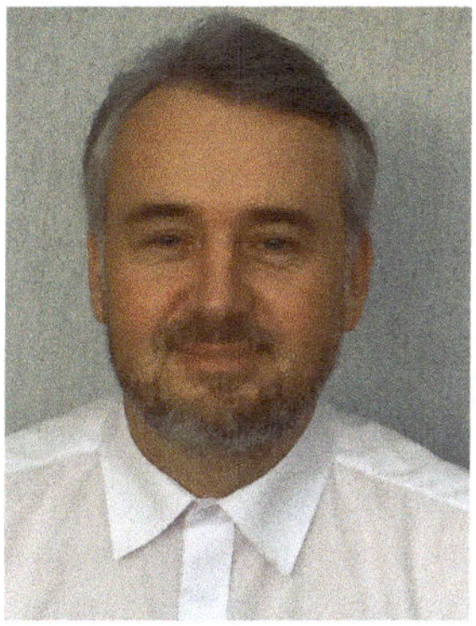

Andrzej Grzybowski MD, PhD, MBA, is a Professor of Ophthalmology and Chair of the Department of Ophthalmology, University of Warmia and Mazury, Olsztyn, Poland, and Head of the Institute for Research in Ophthalmology, Foundation for Ophthalmology Development, Poznan, Poland.

He is active in international scientific societies including EURETINA (Co-opted Board Member 2016–2018); Retina Society, AAO (International Fellow and Member of the Global ONE Advisory Board and Museum of Vision's Programme Committee); EVER (Board Member and Chair of Cataract Section); ESCRS (Curator of ESCRS Archive); ISRS (Member of the ISRS International Council); ISBCS, International Council of Ophthalmology (Programme Coordinator for the WCO in 2011–2018); and Cogan Society. He became Lifelong Member (Chair LIV) of the European Academy of Ophthalmology (http://www.eao.eu) and its Treasurer. He has been active contributor to major ophthalmic conferences worldwide, including AAO (Achievement Award 2017, International Scholar Award 2018), APAO (International Coordinator 2017, Achievement Award 2018), WCO (Programme Coordinator 2010–2018), EURETINA, ESCRS, EVER, ISOPT, etc.

He has been active Editor, Editor in Chief, and Author of more than 450 peer-reviewed international publications (total IF higher than 1000) and over 50 book chapters and Reviewer for more than 20 journals. He is a Member of editorial boards of *American Journal of Ophthalmology* (IF 4.795), *Acta Ophthalmologica* (IF 3.157), *PLOS One* (IF 2.806), *Graefe's Archive for Clinical and Experimental Ophthalmology* (IF 2.349),

Translational Vision Science & Technology (*TVST*, IF 2.221), *BMC Ophthalmology* (IF 1.586), *Clinics in Dermatology* (IF 2.253), *Clinical Medicine* (IF 5.8), *Frontiers in Neurology* (IF 3.5), *Journal of Neuro-Ophthalmology* (IF 0.2), *Saudi Journal of Ophthalmology*, and *Asia-Pacific Journal of Ophthalmology* and Editor in Chief of *Archives of History and Philosophy of Medicine* and *Historia Ophthalmologica Internationalis* (www.histoph.com).

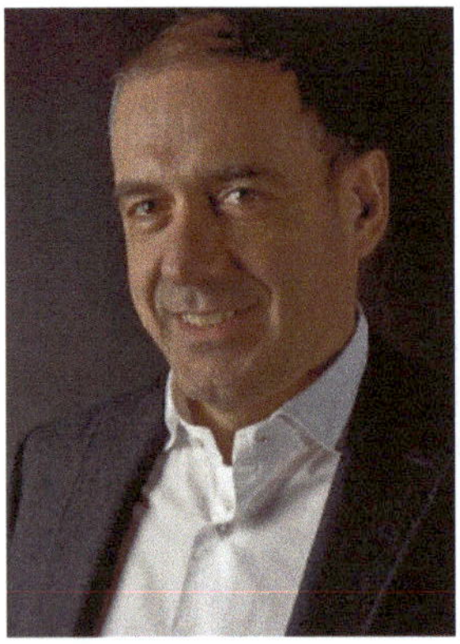

Piero Barboni received his undergraduate degree from the University of Bologna in 1986 and his medical and surgical training from the University of Bologna, Italy, in 1990. Since then, he has been working in private practice and appointed Professor at the Department of Neurological Science of Bologna University from 2007 to 2011. Currently, he is Consultant Neuro-ophthalmologist at Scientific Institute San Raffaele, University of Milan, since 2012. He is also devoted to the study of hereditary optic neuropathies, for which he collaborates with several university-based centres (Bologna, London, Los Angeles, Tubingen, São Paulo). This project includes the international research project on Leber's hereditary optic neuropathy in Brazil. He is also Sub-investigator in many clinical trials. He has authored more than 80 papers on international peer-reviewed journals and several books.

Introduction: Retina Imaging—Past and Present

1

Andrzej Grzybowski and Piero Barboni

The retina is a mysterious structure. The first use of the term comes, as to our present knowledge, from Herophilos (335–280 or 255 BC), Greek anatomist, one of founders of Greek school in Alexandria. He used two different words, arachnoeides and amfiblesteroides, for retina. For many years, both meanings were related to casting net, and retiform, a word which the modern "retina" is derived. However, as it was nicely shown recently, there might be another explanation of these original terms [1]. Amfiblesteroides meant at that time also anything that is thrown around and encircling walls. For many years it was believed, however, that the lens, not retina is the reception organ of the eye responsible for vision and there was even no agreement as to whether the eye emanated light (extramission theory) or received it (intromission theory) [2, 3]. Leonardo da Vinci (1452–1519) and Johannes Kepler (1571–1630) questioned the role of the lens in light reception. Felix Plater (1536–1614), attributed that role to the retina, what was further experimentally supported by Christopher Scheiner (1575–1650) who, by removing part of the sclera and choroids, was able to notice the reversed picture projected onto the bottom of the eye [3–6].

For the next two centuries, it was disputable weather retina or choroid was a precise structure responsible for vision reception [7]. This was finally settled by Herman von Helmholtz (1821–1894), who also constructed and popularized the first ophthalmoscope in 1851 [8]. This revolutionized the development of retinology.

A. Grzybowski (✉)
University of Warmia and Mazury, Olsztyn, Poland

Institute for Research in Ophthalmology, Poznań, Poland

P. Barboni
Studio Oculistico d'Azeglio, Bologna, Italy

Scientific Institute San Raffaele, Milan, Italy
e-mail: p.barboni@studiodazeglio.it

A. Grzybowski, P. Barboni (eds.), *OCT and Imaging in Central Nervous System Diseases*, https://doi.org/10.1007/978-3-030-26269-3_1

The first visualization of the eye fundus of the living animal, however, was conducted by Jean Mery (1654–1718) in 1704. By plunging the head of a cat in water, Mery was able to observe the retinal vessels, the optic nerve head and the choroid (Fig. 1.1) [9]. This was later confirmed by Adolf Kussmaul in 1845 [10], Johann Nepomuk Czermak in 1851 [11] and Adolf Ernst Coccius in 1852, who introduced a water-box named "orthoscope", to neutralize the corneal curvature [12, 13]. It was, however, Johannes Purkinje (1787–1869) in 1823 who described the basics of ophthalmoscopy based on his observations living animal and human eye [14]. One of the pioneers in the use of ophthalmoscopy for the diagnosis of central nervous system disorders was Xavier Galezowski (1832–1907), who published one of early textbooks on this subject and coined a term of cerebroscopy for this examination (Fig. 1.2) [15].

The microscopical structure of the retina was described in the nineteenth century, and by the end of the twentieth century it was believed that its histological and functional characteristics was largely recognized. Then, the discovery of intrinsically photosensitive ganglion cells, a novel class of retinal photoreceptors, which express melanopsin, are sensitive to short-wavelength blue light and project throughout the brain, have presented a completely unknown area of retina-brain possible interactions [16, 17]. It is quite clear today that other cellular components of the retina, namely amacrine cells, bipolar cells and microglial cells, although somehow

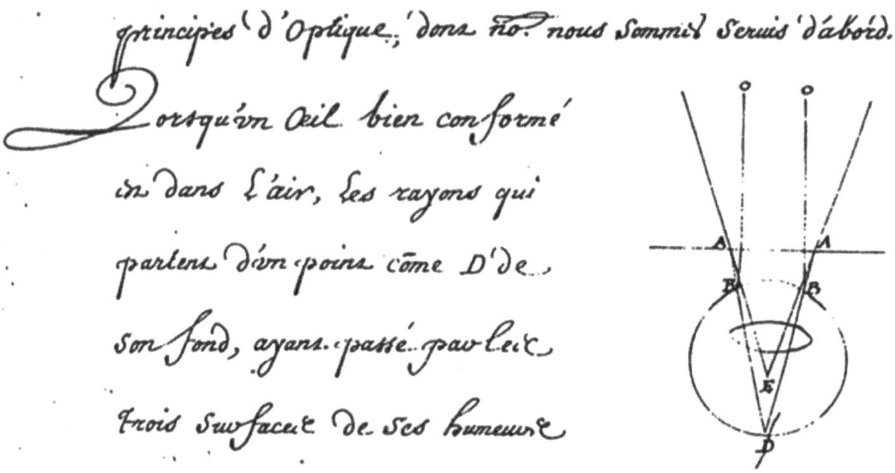

Fig. 1.1 Extract from the Proceedings of the Royal Academy of Sciences for the year 1709—Session of 20th March 1709. By this diagram, La Hire explains the visualization of the fundus of the submerged cat by the fact that the surface of the water having abolished the corneal dioptric power, the rays coming out of the eye would no longer be parallel, but would diverge and that would make the eye fundus visible to the observer. Source: Heitz RF. Earliest Visualizations of the Living Eye's Fundus by Immersion in Water. Archiwum Historii I Filozofii Medycyny 2012; 75: 11–15

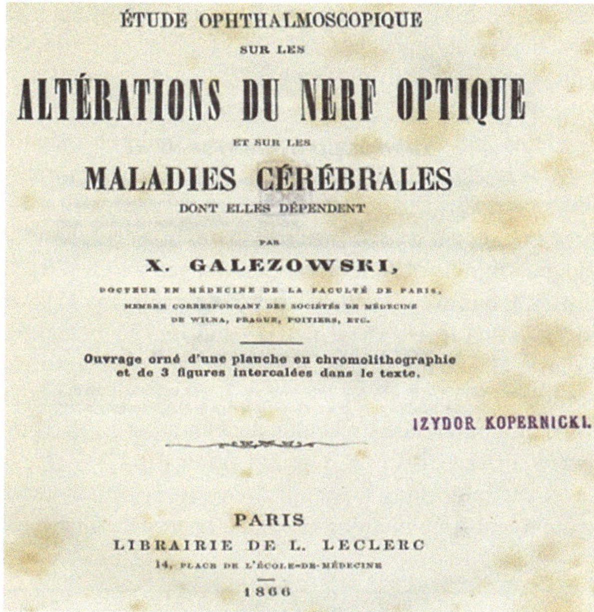

ÉTUDE OPHTHALMOSCOPIQUE

SUR LES

ALTÉRATIONS DU NERF OPTIQUE

ET SUR LES

MALADIES CÉRÉBRALES

DONT ELLES DÉPENDENT

PAR

X. GALEZOWSKI,

DOCTEUR EN MÉDECINE DE LA FACULTÉ DE PARIS,
MEMBRE CORRESPONDANT DES SOCIÉTÉS DE MÉDECINE
DE WILNA, PRAGUE, POITIERS, ETC.

Ouvrage orné d'une planche en chromolithographie
et de 3 figures intercalées dans le texte.

IZYDOR KOPERNICKI.

PARIS

LIBRAIRIE DE L. LECLERC

14, PLACE DE L'ÉCOLE-DE-MÉDECINE

1866

Fig. 1.2 Cover page of the book "Etude ophtalmoscopique sur les altérations du nerf optique et les maladies cérébrales dont elles dépenden" by Xavery Gałęzowski, Paris, 1866

neglected in the past, play important functions both in physiology and pathology of the retina. For example, it was proposed that microglia are involved in the pathogenesis of several degenerative conditions of the retina, including glaucoma, age-related macular degeneration, and inherited photoreceptor degeneration [18]. Moreover, recently the evidence of retinal astrocytopathy in neuromyelitis optica spectrum disorder was provided [19].

One of the major developments in recent years in retinal imaging was the introduction of optical coherence tomography (OCT). OCT was firstly reported by Huang et al. in 1991 [20]. In vivo studies were first reported in 1993 [21, 22], and in 1995 imaging of the normal retina [23] and macular pathology [24] was presented. OCT delivers high-resolution cross-sectional or 3-dimensional images of the retinal and choroid structures, which are generated by an optical beam scanned across the retina (and choroid). OCT testing is quick, easy and noninvasive, and pupil dilation is typically not required. Moreover, OCT yields quantitative anatomical data and is related with low variation for repeated measurements, low intra-individual and inter-individual variation and low variability across different centers using the same device.

Retinal ganglion cells axons are nonmyelinated within the retina, thus retinal nerve fiber layer (RNFL) is an optimal structure to visualize the process of neurodegeneration, neuro-protection and neuro-repair [25]. Moreover, OCT enables evaluation of retinal ganglion cells (RGC). For example, it was reported in patients with MS a dropout of RGC in 79% of eyes and inner nuclear layer atrophy (including amacrine cells and bipolar cells) in 40% of eyes [26]. It was also argued that OCT might reveal RNFL abnormalities in many patients with no clinical symptoms [27].

Retina and optic nerve originates from diencephalon, thus are a part of central nervous system (CNS). RGC present the typical morphology of CNS neurons. Optic nerve, like all fiber tracts in CNS, is covered with myelin and is unsheathed in all three meningeal layers. Insult to the optic nerve, similar to CNS, lead to retrograde and anterograde degeneration of damaged axons [28]. Because of these many similarities, it has not been very surprising that many CNS diseases can be also detected on the retina level. They include multiple sclerosis, Alzheimer disease, Parkinson disease, and many others. Moreover, it was shown that there are some common degenerative mechanisms between Alzheimer disease and eye diseases, like glaucoma and age-related macular degeneration [29]. Thus, the aim of this book is to review all aspects of OCT retina studies in CNS diseases, and present some other novel and interesting techniques, including retinal amyloid imaging, retinal oximetry, and real-time imaging of single neuronal cell apoptosis.

References

1. de Jong PT. From where does "rete" in retina originate? Graefes Arch Clin Exp Ophthalmol. 2014;252:1525–7.
2. Magnus H. Ophthalmology of the ancients, vol. 2 (Waugh RL, Translator). Oostende: Wayenborgh; 1999. p. 461–9.
3. Duke-Elder S, Wybar KC. The history of ophthalmic optics. In: Duke-Elder S, editor. System of ophthalmology, vol. 5. London: Henry Kimpton; 1970. p. 3–23.
4. Mark H. Johanees Kepler on the eye and vision. Am J Ophthalmol. 1971;72:869–78.
5. Daxecker F. Further studies by Christoph Scheiner concerning the optics of the eye. Doc Ophthalmol. 1994;86:153–61.
6. Daxecker F. Christoph Scheiner's eye studies. Doc Ophthalmol. 1992;81:27–35.
7. Grzybowski A, Aydin P. Edme Mariotte (1620-1684): pioneer of neurophysiology. Surv Ophthalmol. 2007;52:443–51.
8. Helmholtz HLFV. Beschreibung eines Augenspiegels zur Untersuchung der Netzhaut im lebenden Auge. Berlin: Forstner; 1851.
9. Heitz RF. Earliest visualizations of the living eye's fundus by immersion in water. Arch Hist Filoz Med. 2012;75:11–5.
10. Kussmaul A. Die Farben-Erscheinungen im Grunde des menschlichen Auges. Heidelberg: Groos; 1845.
11. Czermak JN. Ueber eine neue Methode zur genaueren Untersuchung des gesunden und kranken Auges. Vjschr prakt Heilk. 1851;8:154–65.
12. Coccius AE. Ueber die Ernährungsweise der Hornhaut und die Serum führenden Gefässe im menschlichen Körper. Leipzig: Muller; 1852.
13. Coccius AE. Ueber die Anwendung des Augen-Spiegels nebst Angabe eines neuen Instruments. Leipzig: Muller; 1853.
14. Reese PD. The neglect of Purkinje's technique of ophthalmoscopy prior to Helmholtz's invention of the ophthalmoscope. Ophthalmology. 1986;93:1457–60.
15. Gałęzowski X. Etude ophtalmoscopique sur les altérations du nerf optique et les maladies cérébrales dont elles dépendent. Paris: Librairie de L. Leclerc; 1866.

16. Lucas RJ, Freedman MS, Munoz M, Garcia-Fernandez JM, Foster RG. Regulation of the mammalian pineal by non-rod, non-cone, ocular photoreceptors. Science. 1999;284:505–7.
17. Schmidt TM, Chen SK, Hattar S. Intrinsically photosensitive retinal ganglion cells: many subtypes, diverse functions. Trends Neurosci. 2011;34:572–80.
18. Silverman SM, Wong WT. Microglia in the retina: roles in development, maturity, and disease. Annu Rev Vis Sci. 2018;4:45–77.
19. You Y, Zhu L, Zhang T, Shen T, Fontes A, Yiannikas C, Parratt J, Barton J, Schulz A, Gupta V, Barnett MH, Fraser CL, Gillies M, Graham SL, Klistorner A. Evidence of Müller glial dysfunction in patients with aquaporin-4 immunoglobulin G–positive neuromyelitis optica spectrum disorder. Ophthalmology. 2019; https://doi.org/10.1016/j.ophtha.2019.01.016.
20. Huang D, Swanson EZ, Lin CP, et al. Optical coherence tomography. Science. 1991;254:1178–81.
21. Swanson EA, Izatt JA, Hee MR, et al. In vivo retinal imaging by optical coherence tomography. Opt Lett. 1993;18:1864–6.
22. Fercher AF, Hitzenberger CK, Drexler W, et al. In vivo optical coherence tomography. Am J Ophthalmol. 1993;116:113–4.
23. Hee MR, Puliafito CA, Wong C, et al. Optical coherence tomography of the human retina. Arch Ophthalmol. 1995;113:325–32.
24. Puliafito CA, Hee MR, Lin CP, et al. Imaging of macular diseases with optical coherence tomography. Ophthalmology. 1995;102:217–29.
25. Galetta KM, Calabresi PA, Frohman EM, Balcer LJ. Optical coherence tomography (OCT): imaging the visual. Pathway as a model for neurodegeneration. Neurotherapeutics. 2011;8:117–32.
26. Green A, McQuaid S, Hauser SL, Allen IV, Lyness R. Ocular pathology in multiple sclerosis: retinal atrophy and inflammation irrespective of disease duration. Brain. 2010;133:1591–601.
27. Cettomai D, Hiremath G, Ratchford J, et al. Associations between retinal nerve fiber layer abnormalities and optic nerve examination. Neurology. 2010;75:1318–25.
28. London A, Benhar I, Schwartz M. The retina as a window to the brain-from eye research to CNS disorders. Nat Rev Neurol. 2013;9:44–53.
29. Sivak JM. The aging eye: common degenerative mechanisms between the Alzheimer's brain and retinal disease. Invest Ophthalmol Vis Sci. 2013;54:871–80.

OCT Technique: Past, Present and Future

2

Tigran Kostanyan, Maria de los Angeles Ramos-Cadena, Gadi Wollstein, and Joel S. Schuman

Abbreviations

2D	Two-dimensional
3D	Three-dimensional
AO	Adaptive optics
CCD	Charge-coupled device
EDI	Enhanced depth imaging
FD	Fourier domain
GCC	Ganglion cell complex
ILM	Internal limiting membrane
IPL	Inner plexiform layer
IS	Inner segment
LC	Lamina cribrosa
OCT	Optical coherence tomography
OCTA	Optical coherence tomography angiography
ONH	Optic nerve head
OS	Outer segment
PS	Polarization sensitive
RGC	Retinal ganglion cell
RNFL	Retinal nerve fiber layer
RPE	Retinal pigment epithelium
SD	Spectral domain

T. Kostanyan
Department of Ophthalmology, University of Pittsburgh School of Medicine, UPMC Eye Center, Eye and Ear Institute, Ophthalmology and Visual Sciences Research Center, Pittsburgh, PA, USA

M. de los Angeles Ramos-Cadena · G. Wollstein · J. S. Schuman (✉)
Department of Ophthalmology, NYU Langone Health, New York, NY, USA
e-mail: Joel.Schuman@med.nyu.edu

A. Grzybowski, P. Barboni (eds.), *OCT and Imaging in Central Nervous System Diseases*, https://doi.org/10.1007/978-3-030-26269-3_2

SS	Swept source
TD	Time-domain
Vis-OCT	Visible light optical coherence tomography

2.1 Introduction

Optical coherence tomography (OCT), first developed in the 1990s, is a diagnostic imaging technology that has gained a leading position in research and clinical practice due to its ability to obtain noncontact, in vivo, high-resolution, micron-scale images of tissue structures. OCT makes *in situ* imaging of tissue microstructure possible with a resolution approaching that of histology [1].

The technology uses the principle of low-coherence interferometry, which was originally applied to ophthalmology for in vivo measurements of the axial length of the eye [2].

At the time of introduction, the technology was used to acquire in vivo, cross-sectional images of the anterior segment [3], and retinal pathologies. Since then, OCT has evolved significantly, with improvements in both image acquisition methods and image analysis. The evolution of OCT began with the time domain (TD) technique, followed by spectral domain (SD) systems and later, newer iterations with faster acquisition speeds [4, 5] and improved axial resolution [6].

This chapter describes the basic principles of OCT techniques, its history, current status, major ophthalmic applications, and research that will determine the future of the technology.

2.2 Basic Principles

OCT provides cross-sectional and volumetric images of areas of interest by acquiring either the echo time delay or frequency information of back-reflected light. Differences in the optical properties of biological tissues allow the recognition of layered structures. The speed of light makes it impossible to analyze the acquired information directly, since it would be in the order of femtoseconds thus, OCT systems use the optical technique known as *interferometry*. Low-coherence interferometry enables the analysis of this information and the composition of a depth-resolved reflectivity profile (A-scan) of the scanned tissue by matching the light profiles from the scanning and reference arms.

Utilization of light provides OCT technology the ability to obtain images in a non-contact fashion and to achieve resolutions of 1–15 μm, which is 1–2 orders of magnitude finer than other conventional clinical imaging technologies such as ultrasound, computerized tomography, or magnetic resonance. Light is highly absorbed or scattered in most biological tissues, therefore the use of this technology is limited only to locations that are optically accessible or that can be imaged using devices such as endoscopes or catheters. The eye is the most optically accessible organ of the human body since the anterior and posterior segments can be visualized and imaged [7].

The key parameters that are typically used to characterize OCT technology are the wavelength of the light source, axial and transverse resolution, scanning speed, and imaging depth.

Axial resolution determines the smallest distance along the axial direction where two adjacent points are discernable, and it is inversely related to the bandwidth of the light source. Current commercial OCT devices achieve axial resolutions up to 4 μm, and research systems can achieve up to ~1 μm [8]. The penetration depth (in the axial direction) is approximately 2 mm in the various OCT iterations with the exception of Visible-light OCT that does not penetrate beyond the RPE layer.

Transverse resolution is determined by the spot size projected into the eye, which is limited by the optical properties of the eye. As such, the transverse resolution of OCT ranges between 15–20 μm among the different generations of the technology. Improving transverse resolution requires the correction of the optical aberrations of the eye using technologies such as adaptive optics.

Scanning speed is dictated by mechanical constrains and the sensitivity of the detector to the back-reflected light. As scanning speed increases, the time the detector remains in the same location is shorter, thus reducing the light that can be detected in each location. Since the power of the projected light is limited in order to be within safety limits, faster scans require a more sensitive detector that can function with a lower level of light.

The achievable imaging depth is related to the central wavelength of the light source, with longer wavelengths providing increased imaging depth [9, 10]. However, longer wavelengths are limited by the increased optical absorption of water [11].

Currently available OCT techniques are based on several iterations of the technology: spectral-domain (SD; also known as Fourier or frequency domain), swept-source (SS), and visible-light (Vis-OCT). The earliest iteration of the technology, time-domain (TD), is no longer manufactured for ophthalmic use and therefore will not be discussed.

SD-OCT uses a broad-bandwidth, low-coherence superluminescent diode laser light that is divided into two arms by a partially reflecting mirror (beam splitter). In the first arm light is projected toward the sampling location, while in the second arm light is projected toward a reference mirror. The backscattered light from both arms travels back to a spectrometer and recombines to form an interference pattern. Light frequency information is analyzed by Fourier transformation to encode distances within tissue microstructure [12]. SD technology allows the acquisition of information from all points along each axial scan (A-scan) simultaneously at a scanning speed of ~25,000–100,000 A-scans/s [13, 14] and up to 20 million A-scans/s in research devices [5]. A cross-sectional image, also known as a B-scan, is generated by performing fast, subsequent A-scans at different transverse positions. Combining rapidly acquired subsequent cross-sectional scans allows the creation of three-dimensional (3D) datasets, enabling advanced post-processing analysis. The wide bandwidth of the SD-OCT light source also facilitates an axial resolution of 3–6 μm in commercially available systems and up to 1 μm in research systems [15, 16].

SS-OCT uses a tunable laser light source that sweeps through different frequencies in rapid succession to cover the entire broad spectrum. The reflectance of the light from the scanned area is captured by a photodetector, which allows a substantially faster acquisition rate (up to 400,000 A-scans/s) than the spectrometry of SD-OCT [4, 17]. Another important advantage of SS-OCT is an improved signal-to-noise ratio and reduction in the depth dependent signal drop-off observed with SD-OCT technology [18]. Most SS-OCT devices operate with light sources centered at around 1050 nm (compared with 840 nm in the commercially available SD-OCT devices), which reduces the axial resolution to approximately 8 μm but allows for better penetration into the tissue. This combination of improved tissue penetration and reduced signal attenuation allows detailed scanning of structures such as the choroid and the lamina cribrosa (LC) within the ONH.

Vis-OCT. Unlike other OCT iterations that use near infrared light sources (~800 and 1000 nm), Vis-OCT utilizes a light source with a shorter center wavelength of ~550 nm resulting in an improved axial resolution of <1 μm but with reduced achievable imaging depth [19, 20]. Using spectroscopic analysis, it is possible to quantify chromophore concentration from Vis-OCT images [19]. Retinal oximetry is one of its first applications, providing objective, functional information about retinal vasculature. Light absorbance for oxygenated and de-oxygenated hemoglobin peaks in separate wavelengths, both of which are within the spectrum of Vis-OCT. Tissue oxygen consumption can be determined by extracting the venous de-oxygenated level from the arterial oxygenated level. The oximetry information can be aligned to the structural location observed in the same images, opening a new venue for global and local functional assessment.

The major characteristics of these 3 different OCT techniques are presented in Table 2.1.

2.3 The Past

OCT technology was first described by Huang and colleagues in 1991 [21]. The authors scanned human retinas and atherosclerotic plaques ex vivo with a prototype device using infrared light at a ~800 nm wavelength. The axial resolution of cross-sectional images of the retina, optic nerve, and coronary artery wall was 15 μm, which allowed the visualization of some retinal layers, optic nerve head structures, and the composition of the coronary artery. In vivo retinal scanning was conducted using a prototype device based on a slit-lamp biomicroscope that was modified to provide a view of the fundus while scanning with OCT. The development of scan patterns that enabled the acquisition of reproducible measurements [22] led to the use of the technology in clinical practice. The first commercially available OCT, called OCT 1000, was marketed in 1996 by Zeiss (Dublin, CA). The technology went through 2 iterations, resulting in OCT 2000 in the year 2000 and then OCT 3 (Stratus), which became commercially available in 2002. Stratus OCT had an axial

Table 2.1 Comparison of SD-OCT, SS-OCT, and Vis-OCT technologies

Technology	Light source	Primary advantages	Primary disadvantages
SD-OCT	Near infrared broadband width	High scanning speed (up to 100,000 A-scans/s in commercial ophthalmic systems); axial resolution 4–7 μm	Noticeable signal drop-off with depth
SS-OCT	Near infrared narrow bandwidth, swept through broad range	Very high scanning speeds (up to 400,000 A-scans/s in ophthalmic systems); minimal signal drop-off with depth; improved penetration into structures	Most ophthalmic systems operate at longer wavelengths (~1000 nm); with lower axial resolution than SD-OCT (7–8 μm)
Vis-OCT	Center wavelength of ~550 nm from incoherent light sources either spatially coherent or broadband	Highest axial resolution (<1 μm)	Limited penetration into deep tissues; slower scanning speed (up to 30,000 A-scans/s)

resolution of ~10 μm, a transverse resolution of 20 μm, and a scan speed of 400 A-scans/s [1, 23]. The typical cross-sectional scan was composed of 128–512 A-scans, comprising an image area of 4–6 mm.

Due to its ability to obtain quantitative and reproducible measurements of the macula [24, 25], retinal nerve fiber layer thickness [22, 26], and optic nerve head [27], OCT became the gold standard clinical imaging device for posterior segment pathologies in a relatively short period of time.

Early iterations of OCT had a relatively slow acquisition rate, and therefore the conventional scan patterns were comprised of 6 radial scans through the macula (6 mm diameter) or optic nerve (4 mm) with a circular 3.4 mm diameter scan centered on the ONH. Using automated segmentation, the total macular thickness (internal limiting membrane (ILM) to the photoreceptor inner segment-outer segment (IS–OS) junction), retinal nerve fiber layer (RNFL) thickness, and ONH structures were automatically quantified.

The introduction of SD-OCT added a dramatic increase in scanning speed and substantially extended the clinical utility of OCT. The faster scanning speed enabled new scanning patterns such as raster scans, where volumetric data is constructed with a rapidly acquired succession of adjacent B-scans. A 3D dataset allows a thorough sampling of the scanned region, advanced post-processing, and improved registration of consecutive scans. Another commonly used approach is the averaging of consecutive scans acquired at the same location that result in improved image quality.

The majority of commercial OCT systems applied SD technology for posterior eye imaging and visualization of the cross-sectional structures of the retina and optic disc [1] (Fig. 2.1). OCT has been used extensively in the diagnosis and management of a wide range of ocular pathologies including glaucoma, age-related macular degeneration, macular edema, macular holes, diabetic retinopathy,

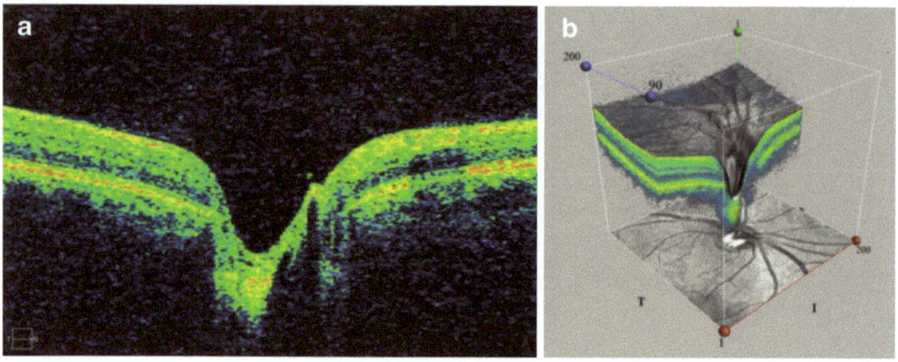

Fig. 2.1 OCT c ross-sectional image of a healthy optic disc (**a**) and a 3D volumetric scan (**b**)

alterations in the vitreoretinal interface, papilledema, and others. In addition to acquiring tissue structural information, OCT has been incorporated into multimodal imaging systems that provide further insight into the functional characteristics of tissue [28–30].

OCT has become a key ophthalmic diagnostic imaging tool due to its ability to provide information about tissue microstructure. Over the years, it has continuously evolved with improved visualization, new retinal imaging locations, increased reliability, and enhanced longitudinal analysis.

2.4 The Present

Since the advent of OCT, 25 years ago, countless improvements have been implemented in an effort to acquire quantitative data with high reliability and sensitivity for precise evaluation of the structure and function of ocular structures.

2.4.1 Spectral-Domain OCT

Since the first FDA-approved SD-OCT became available in 2006, numerous improvements have enriched the capabilities of OCT. One application of advanced processing is the OCT enface image generated by integrating the information from all A-scans into an image of the surface of the retina [31]. The enface image is identical to the retinal fundus view and it can be used for subjective assessment of image quality and eye motion detection, comparison with clinical findings, and further focus on specific location within the region of interest.

Various scan patterns are available for ONH imaging from the different commercially available SD-OCT devices. This includes raster (also known as 3D or volumetric) scans, radial scans, circular scans, and a combination of radial and concentric scans. All of the devices can automatically detect the optic disc boundary as the location at which the photoreceptor layer, retinal pigment epithelium (RPE), and choriocapillaries terminate. The machine provides quantification of ONH structures such as the disc area, cup-to-disc ratio, and others along with the circumpapillary RNFL thickness measurement reported as global, quadrant, and sectoral thicknesses. Evaluation of the ONH provides important clinical information in multiple ocular and central nervous system pathologies like glaucoma and papilledema.

One of the most useful measurements provided by OCT is the circumpapillary RNFL thickness. Because the axons from the retinal ganglion cells gather to form the optic nerve, a circular scan around the ONH allows sampling of the axons from the entire retina. The limitation of this approach is that the sampling of the tissue is performed only along the circle, therefore any misplacement of the circle during consecutive scanning will result in increased measurement variability [32]. Another option is to extract the RNFL thickness from the raster scan pattern. This method can ensure that the tissue sampling location is consistent through multiple scans, as the repositioning of the circle is possible if needed during post-processing. Several devices also report the RNFL thickness as a color-coded thickness map of the peripapillary region. This map provides additive information to the circumpapillary RNFL thickness measurement, as it can highlight small, localized thinning or defects outside the circumpapillary sampling location. Furthermore, in many devices, the RNFL thickness is compared to population-derived normative data to highlight locations deviating from normal.

Figure 2.2A shows a Cirrus HD-OCT (Zeiss, Dublin, CA) ONH scan printout that provides the RNFL thickness map (a) and cross-section (c). The deviation map (b) compares the RNFL measurements at each superpixel with an age-matched normative database, and locations thinner than the lowest 95% of the normal range are highlighted. In the center panel, quantitative parameters are provided for ONH structures, along with RNFL thickness presented as a thickness profile around the ONH, in quadrants and in clock hours. The background coloring reflects the comparison with the normative database, with green representing the normal range, yellow representing <5% of the normal population, and red representing <1% of the normal population. The right eye shows an example of eye within the normal limits while the left eye shows a glaucomatous eye with thin average RNFL, superior, inferior, and temporal thin RNFL, enlarged cup-to-disc ratio and an inferior notch. OptoVue Avanti (Optovue, Redmont, CA) peripapillary scan (Fig. 2.2B) is created from 13 circular scans with diameters of 1.3–4.9 mm centered on the ONH. Comparison with a normative database is performed in 16 sectors and presented as the deviation map that surrounds the RNFL thickness map. Figure 2.2C shows the circumpapillary RNFL scans obtained with the Spectralis OCT (Heidelberg Engineering, Heidelberg, Germany). A retinal cross section image with delineation of RNFL boundaries is shown in (a). Note the visualization of fine details that is accomplished by averaging repetitive scans acquired in the same location while engaging eye motion tracking systems to reduce motion artifacts. Thickness measurements and color-coded comparison with normative data are presented for global average thickness, quadrants, and in six sectors (b).

The improvements introduced in SD-OCT also have a substantial impact on macular imaging. Thorough sampling of the macula, the improved visualization of the retina and choroid, and the ability to automatically segment the various layers of the retina substantially impacted clinical management. The scan patterns that are

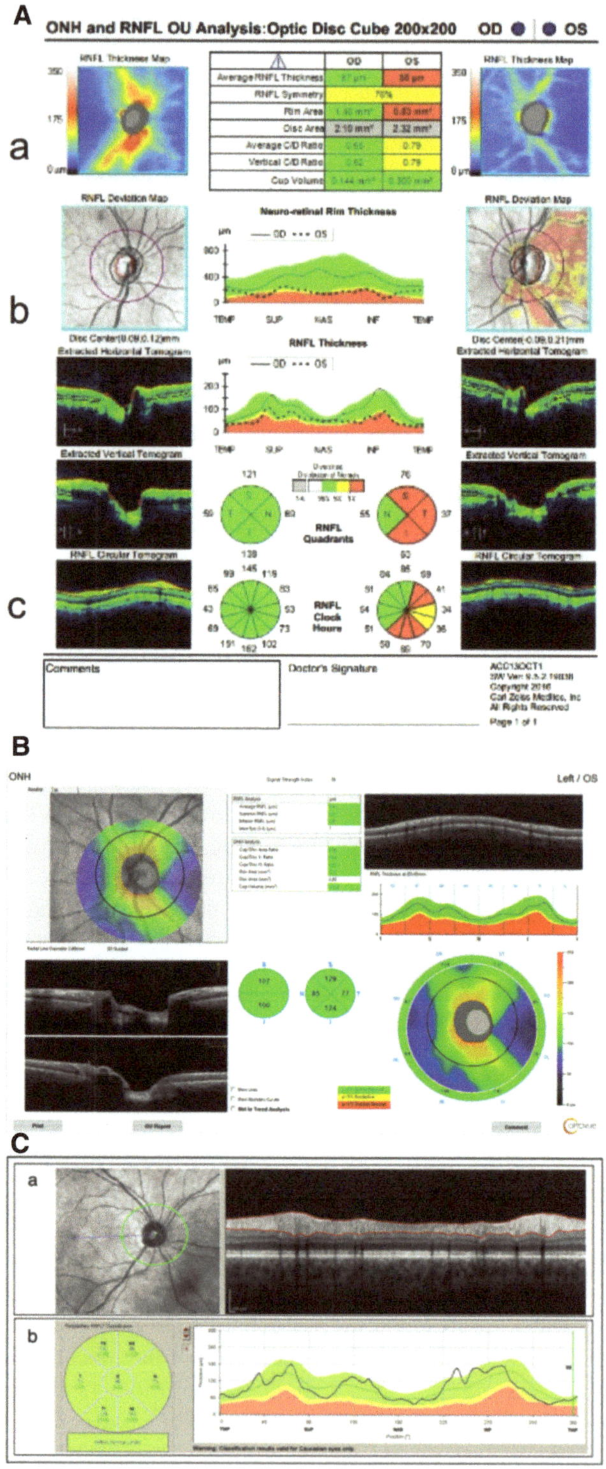

Fig. 2.2 SD-OCT optic nerve head and retinal nerve fiber layer analysis, (**A**) Cirrus, (**B**) Avanti, and (**C**) Spectralis OCT

often used to image the macula include line, cross-line, raster, mesh, and radial scan patterns. Line scans are typically composed from the averaging of multiple scans at the same location. This is typically performed at a single linear location (Fig. 2.3A) or along several parallel lines (Fig. 2.3B). Line scans are clinically useful for obtaining retinal images with the highest level of detail. The principle of the volumetric cube scan is similar to the 3D ONH scan patterns described above. Volumetric macular scans are very helpful in clinical management of macular pathologies, such as macular edema, age related macular degeneration, and macular holes.

Some SD-OCT systems are capable of acquiring scans in horizontal and vertical orientations to provide a mesh scan pattern. The logic behind this scan pattern is that even at a fast scanning rate there is a relatively long temporal gap between adjacent points that are perpendicular to the scan orientation. For example, in a horizontal raster scan, the time gap between adjacent points in the horizontal direction is much shorter than the gap between adjacent points vertically. This can lead to image distortion along the slow axis of the scan. Registering the horizontal and vertical scans together can reduce the distortion in the slow axis and improve scan quality. Figure 2.4 shows the macula thickness map acquired by a retina map scanning pattern (left side of the report) with the correspondent cross-sectional image (right side of the report) obtained with Optovue Avanti (Optovue, Redmont, CA). The pattern consists of an inner, dense grid and outer grid, visible as white grid lines.

Radial scan protocols acquire multiple evenly spaced linear scans that intersect at the fovea. This pattern provides information from the entire macular region, with dense coverage near the fovea where the lines intersect and sparse coverage at the macula periphery. Figure 2.5 demonstrates a radial scanning pattern of the macula from two different healthy subjects using different commercial SD-OCT systems.

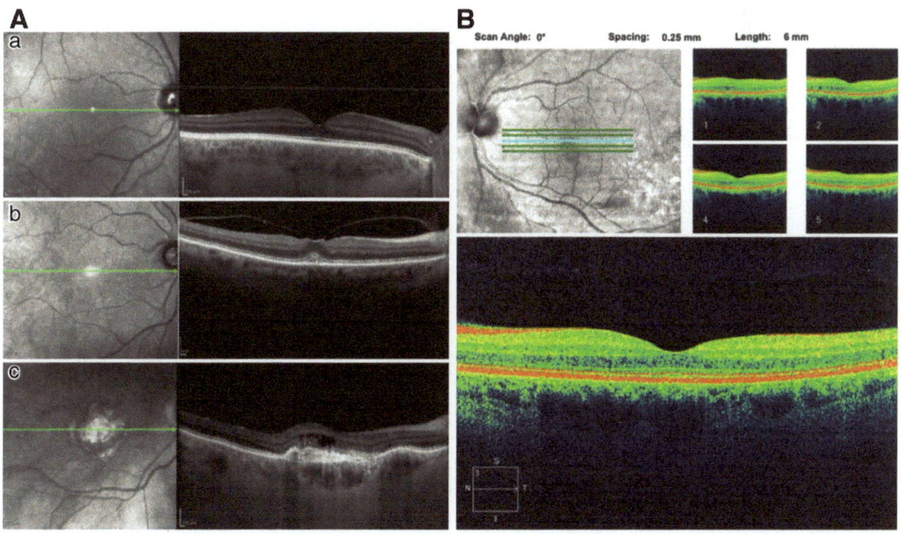

Fig. 2.3 (**A**) Line scans of the macular region obtained with Spectralis OCT from a healthy eye (a), an eye with vitreomacular traction (b), and wet age-related macular degeneration (c). (**B**) Macular five-line raster scan of a healthy eye obtained with Cirrus HD-OCT

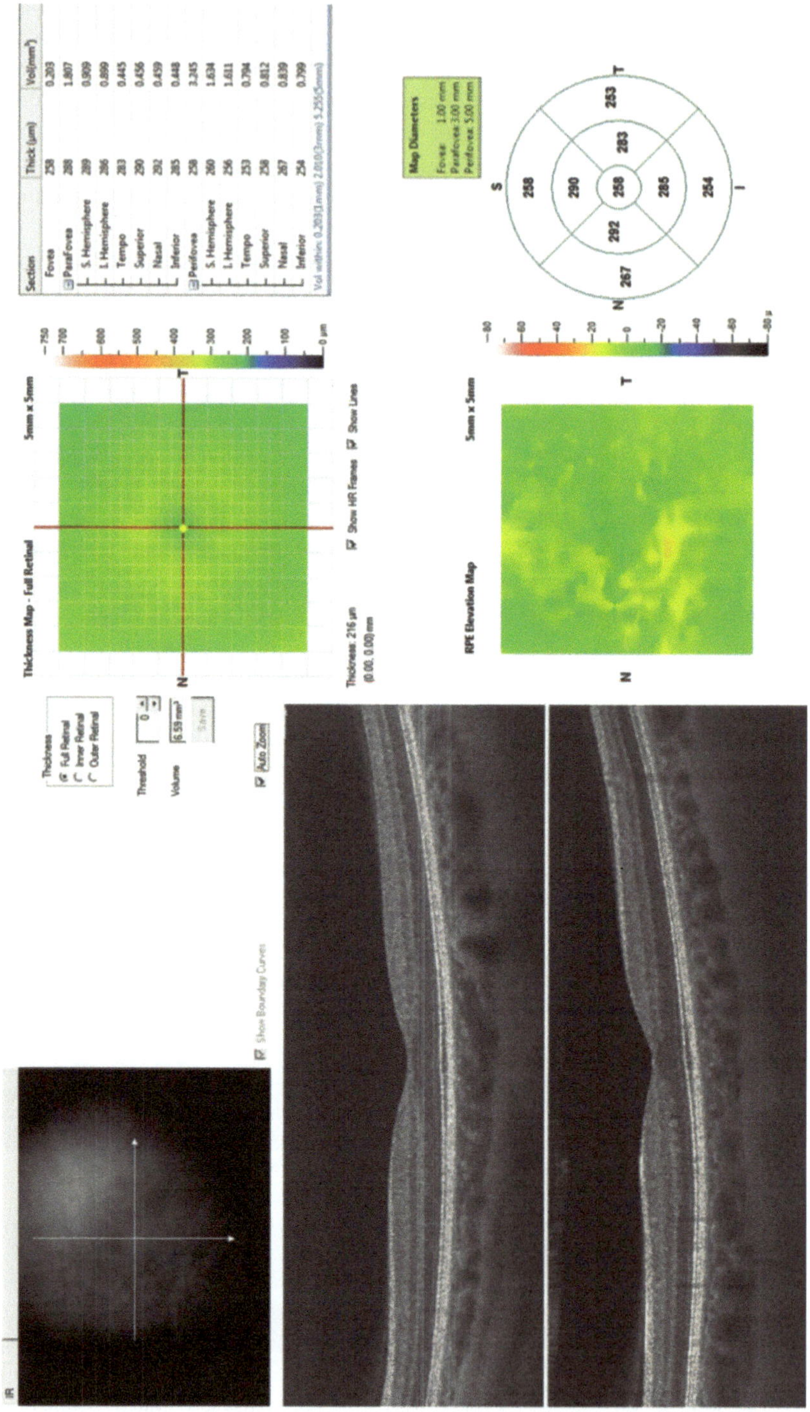

Fig. 2.4 Macular thickness with a retina map scanning pattern obtained with Optovue Avanti

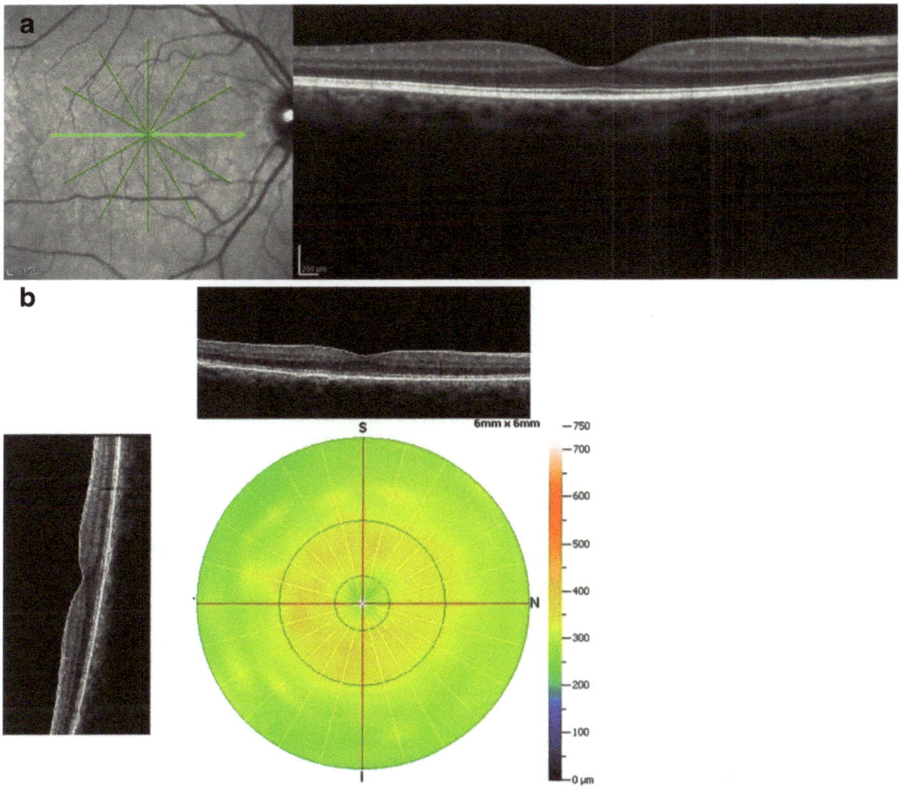

Fig. 2.5 Macular radial scanning pattern obtained with Spectralis OCT (**a**) and RTVue Premier (**b**)

The high resolution of SD-OCT enables automated segmentation and the analysis of individual macular layers that are of particular diagnostic interest in many ocular diseases including glaucoma and diabetic retinopathy [33–35]. Cirrus HD-OCT extracts the information from an ellipse (vertical radius of 2 mm, horizontal radius of 2.4 mm) centered on the fovea and provides a combined measurement of the retinal ganglion cell (RGC) layer and the inner plexiform layer (IPL), called the ganglion cell inner plexiform layer (GCIPL) analysis (Fig. 2.6). The macula protocol of RTVue Premier provides the ganglion cell complex (GCC), which includes the macular nerve fiber layer, RGC layer, and IPL. The data is captured from a 7 mm^2 area centered 1 mm temporal to the fovea.

2.4.2 Retinal and Macular Guided Progression Analysis

The ability of OCT to provide highly reproducible, quantitative, micron-scale measurements is useful in tracking small structural changes that occur over time due to disease deterioration. Several commercial SD-OCT devices include a progression analysis tool. Automatic progression algorithms utilize trend-based analysis

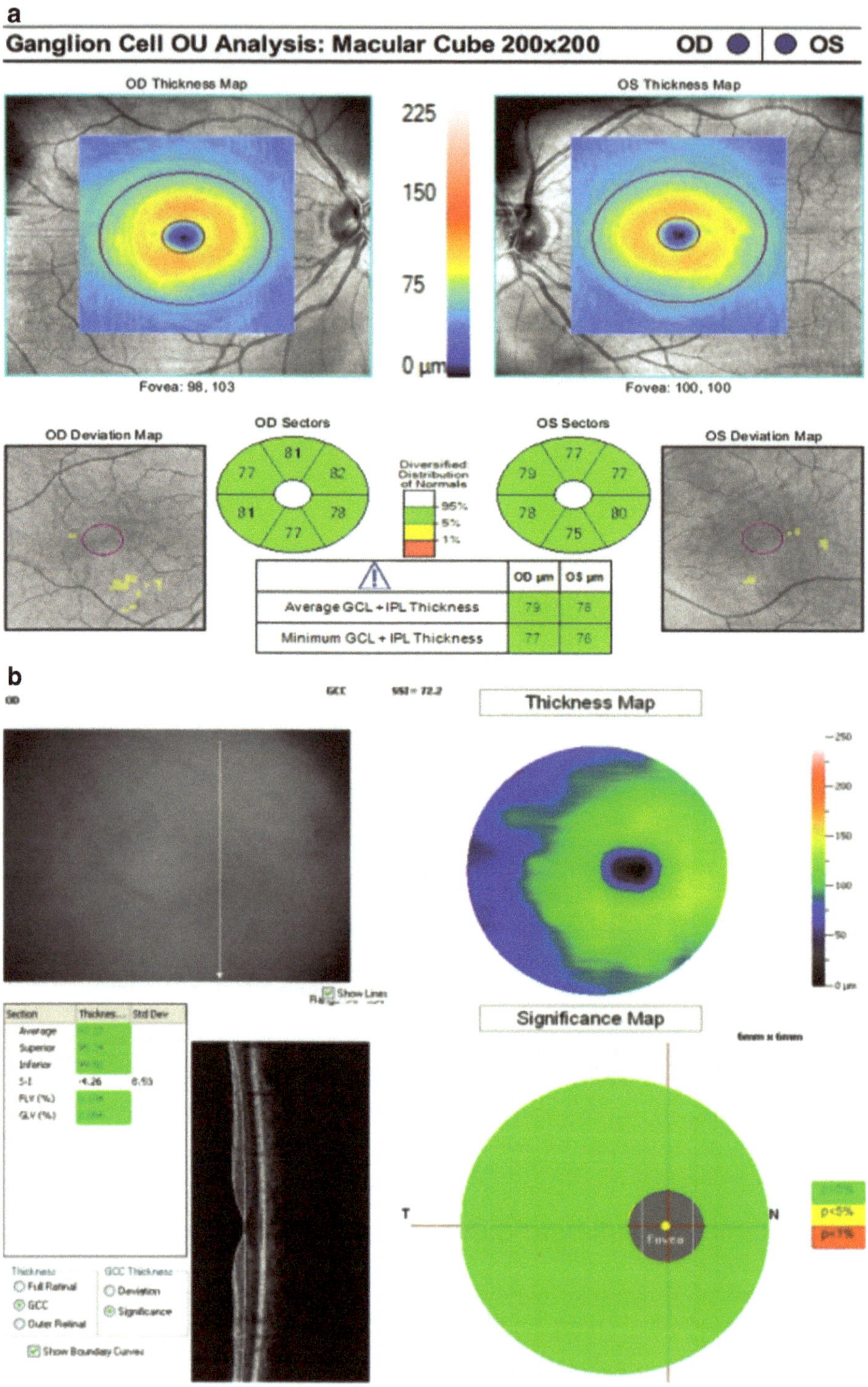

Fig. 2.6 Cirrus HD-OCT ganglion cell analysis (**a**) and RTVue Premier GCC analysis (**b**)

methods, primarily linear regression analysis, for computing the rate of change in structural parameters over time. The computed rate is compared to a no-change slope to determine if the rate is statistically significant. This rate of change is also used to predict future progression beyond the most recent visit. This prediction can be useful when discussing disease forecast with a patient or to assess the effect of treatment modification. Several commercial devices also provide event-based analysis, where a series of follow-up measurements are compared with baseline measurements and progression is defined as measurements changing by exceeding a predetermined threshold from baseline.

It has been described that the peripapillary and macular regions are both capable of detecting glaucoma progression. Glaucoma progression identification has only moderate agreement when looking at these two retinal locations, and different causal theories have been suggested, such as varying dynamic ranges of thickness measurements and minimal measurable thickness (floor effect) with different residual thickness composition (i.e., blood vessels and glial cells), or because one region is affected prior to the other [36–38] .

Figure 2.7 shows the Cirrus HD-OCT guided progression analysis (GPA) for RNFL (A) and GCIPL (B). It provides RNFL and GCIPL event and trend analyses showing a visual display of the location of structural change. In event analysis (a), baseline values are obtained by averaging the data from the first two exams. At least 20 adjacent superpixels must be flagged in the RNFL or GCIPL thickness change maps for a change to be classified as significant. If the difference from baseline is confirmed to be outside the range of test-retest variability, it is classified as "possible loss" and is color-coded in yellow; if the change is confirmed in the subsequent follow-up examination it is classified as "likely loss" and is marked in red. Trend analysis (b) evaluates the rate of change over time using linear regression in the GCIPL, RNFL, and ONH parameters (rim area, average cup-to-disc ratio, vertical cup-to-disc ratio, and cup volume) .

Lately, it was described that macular (GCIPL average, superior, and inferior) and ONH parameters (rim area, cup volume, and cup-to-disc ratio) are sensitive biomarkers to detect glaucoma progression, even in eyes with structural glaucomatous damage, that have reached the floor effect level of RNFL OCT parameters [39] .

2.4.3 Swept Source OCT

At the time of this writing, several SS-OCT devices have been recently approved for use in the USA and worldwide. The major advantages of this OCT iteration compared to earlier ones are the faster scanning speed, deeper penetration into the tissue, and reduced signal attenuation within the scanned window. The counter-effect is a reduced resolution. These properties improve visualization of choroid, sclera, and retinal sub-RPE pathologies such as central serous chorioretinopathy, AMD, choroidal tumors, and retinitis pigmentosa [40, 41]. Examination of the LC and posterior sclera will improve the understanding of the mechanical aspects of glaucoma pathogenesis. Significant differences were documented in the 3D LC

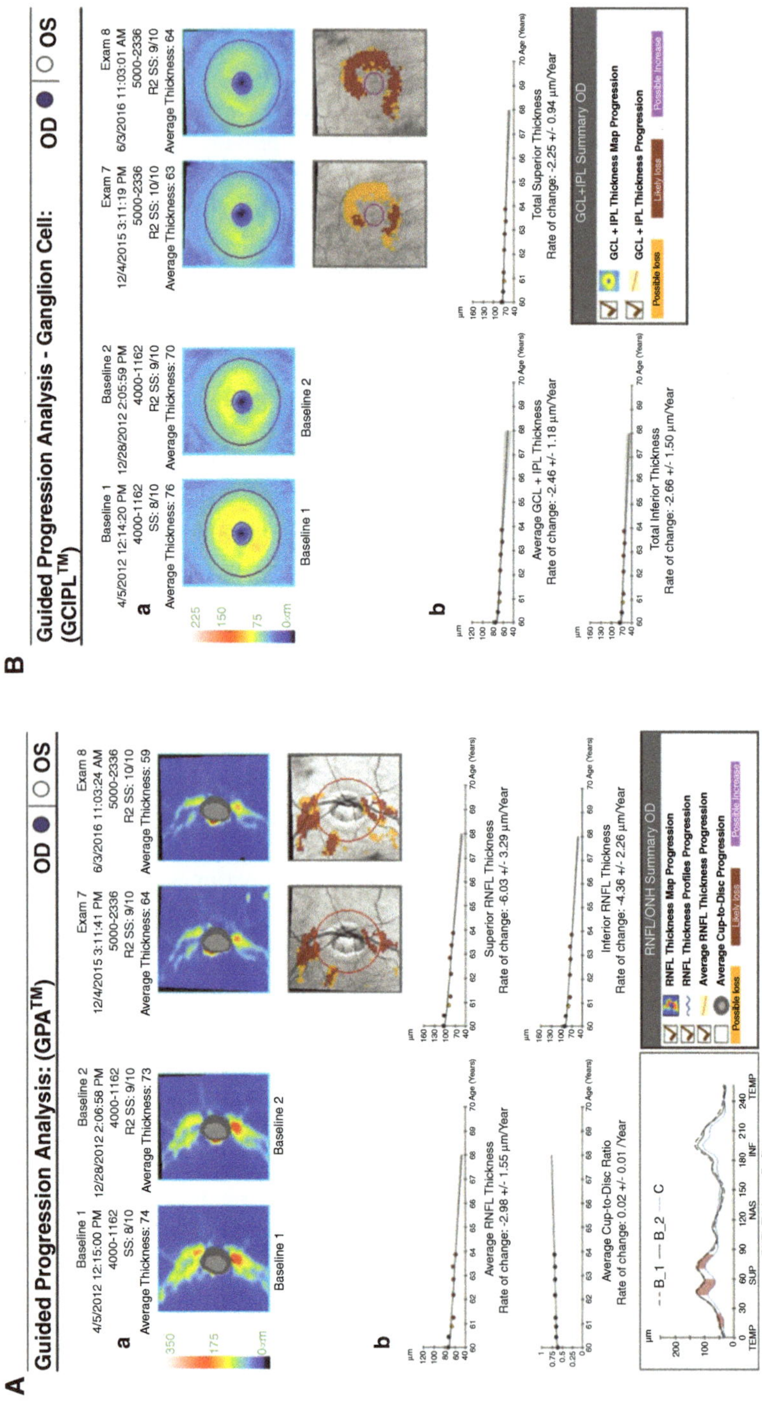

Fig. 2.7 RNFL (A) and GCIPL (B) guided progression analysis

microstructure between healthy and glaucomatous eyes [42, 43] as well as a more tortuous pathway of the pores in glaucomatous eyes as a potential mechanism for axonal flow obstruction and subsequent damage [44] (Figs. 2.8, 2.9, and 2.10).

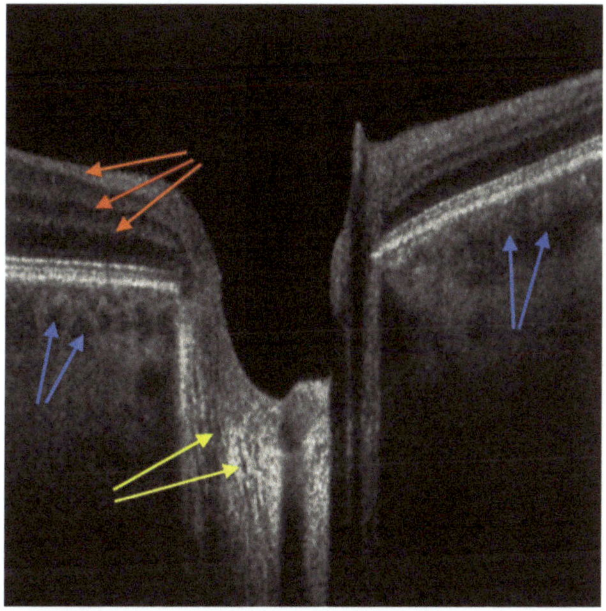

Fig. 2.8 SS-OCT cross section where retinal layers (red arrows), lamina cribrosa (yellow arrows), and choroidal vessels (blue arrows) are all captured in the same scan because this technology is less prone to signal drop-off in comparison with other OCT iterations

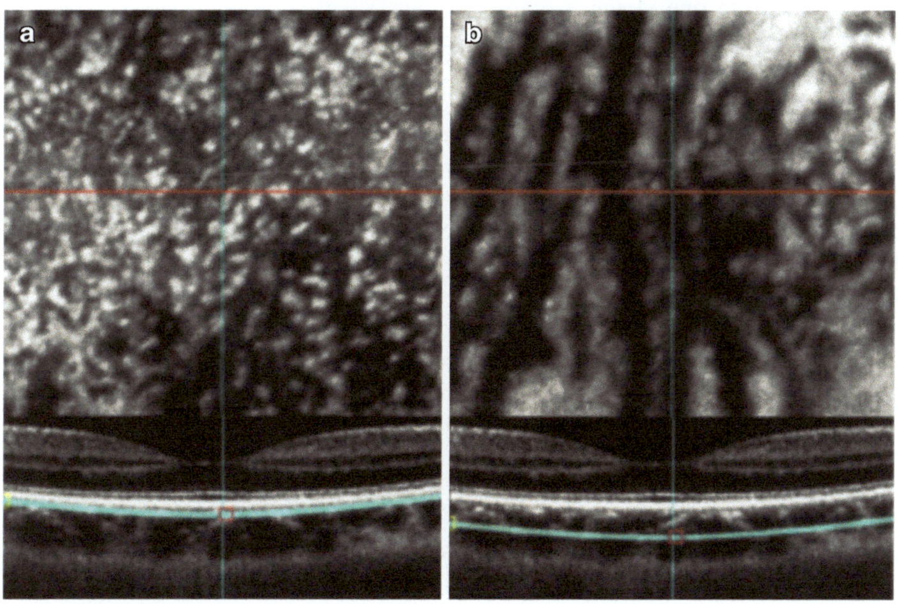

Fig. 2.9 Upper panel demonstrates enface images of SS-OCT of choriocapillaries (**a**) and the large vessels of the choroid (**b**). Bottom panel shows the corresponding cross-sectional scans with the turquoise lines marking the plane where the enface image was acquired

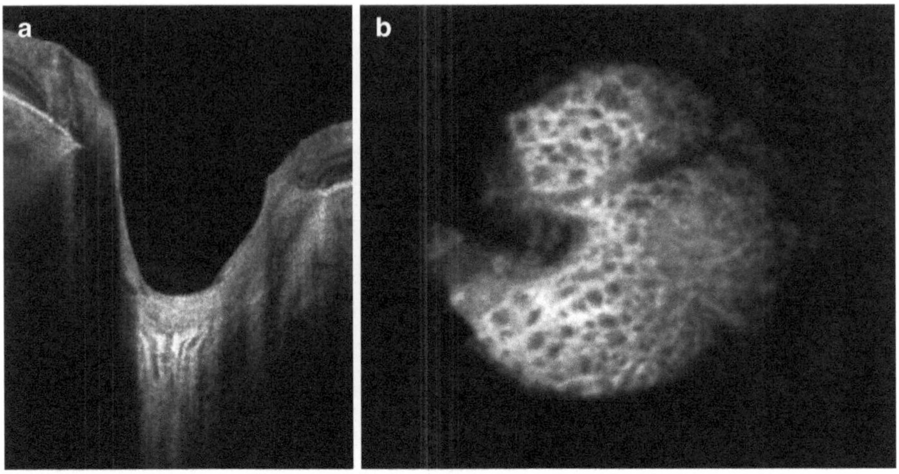

Fig. 2.10 Swept-source OCT cross-section image of the optic nerve head region (**a**). Enface image at the lamina cribrosa level demonstrating the intricate structure of the hyper-reflective beams (white) and hypo-reflective pores (black) (**b**)

2.4.4 Optical Coherence Tomography Angiography (OCTA)

OCTA is an in-vivo, non-invasive, dye-free OCT-based imaging of the blood vessels that provides volumetric vascular analysis [45]. Multiple sequential B-scans are acquired in rapid succession and then compared [41]. The dynamic motion of red blood cells from one image to the other causes a decorrelation signal which is detected by the machine to generate three-dimensional angiograms of the retinal, ONH and choroidal vasculature [41, 45]. It should be noted that this method only provides the anatomical location of blood vessels with flow within a predefined range. Vessels with fast or slow flow outside of this range will not be detected. Furthermore, the device does not report the actual flow within the vessels. The device provides the visualization of blood vessel networks and quantitative analysis of the blood vessel density in the scanned region. OCTA can be performed using both SD-OCT and SS-OCT technologies. At the time of this writing, a few different OCTA are commercially available.

Figure 2.11 shows the SD-OCTA Angioplex report of both ONH and macula angiography scans. The report includes the enface angiography images at different depths on the left, the superficial vascular network and cross-sectional scan overlaid with the location of detected vessels in the middle, and the vessel density analysis by region in the inferior right corner.

Figure 2.12 shows the ONH SS-OCT Triton angiography report. The top row of the report shows the angiography analysis in different depths starting with the innermost section closest to the ILM (labeled as the "nerve head"), followed by an intermediary depth (vitreous), then the analysis at the level of retinal photoreceptor cells (RPC), and ending closest to the choroid (choroid disc). The inferior row shows on the left a cross-sectional image of the optic nerve and in the middle a color-coded vessel density map.

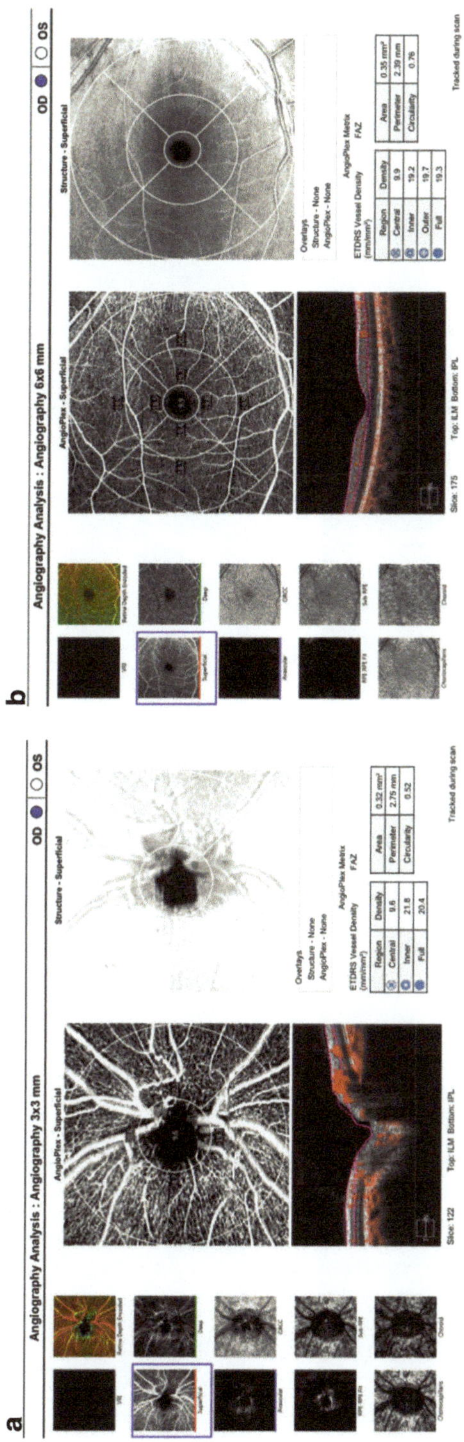

Fig. 2.11 Angioplex angiography with the 3 × 3 ONH (**a**) and 6 × 6 macula (**b**) report

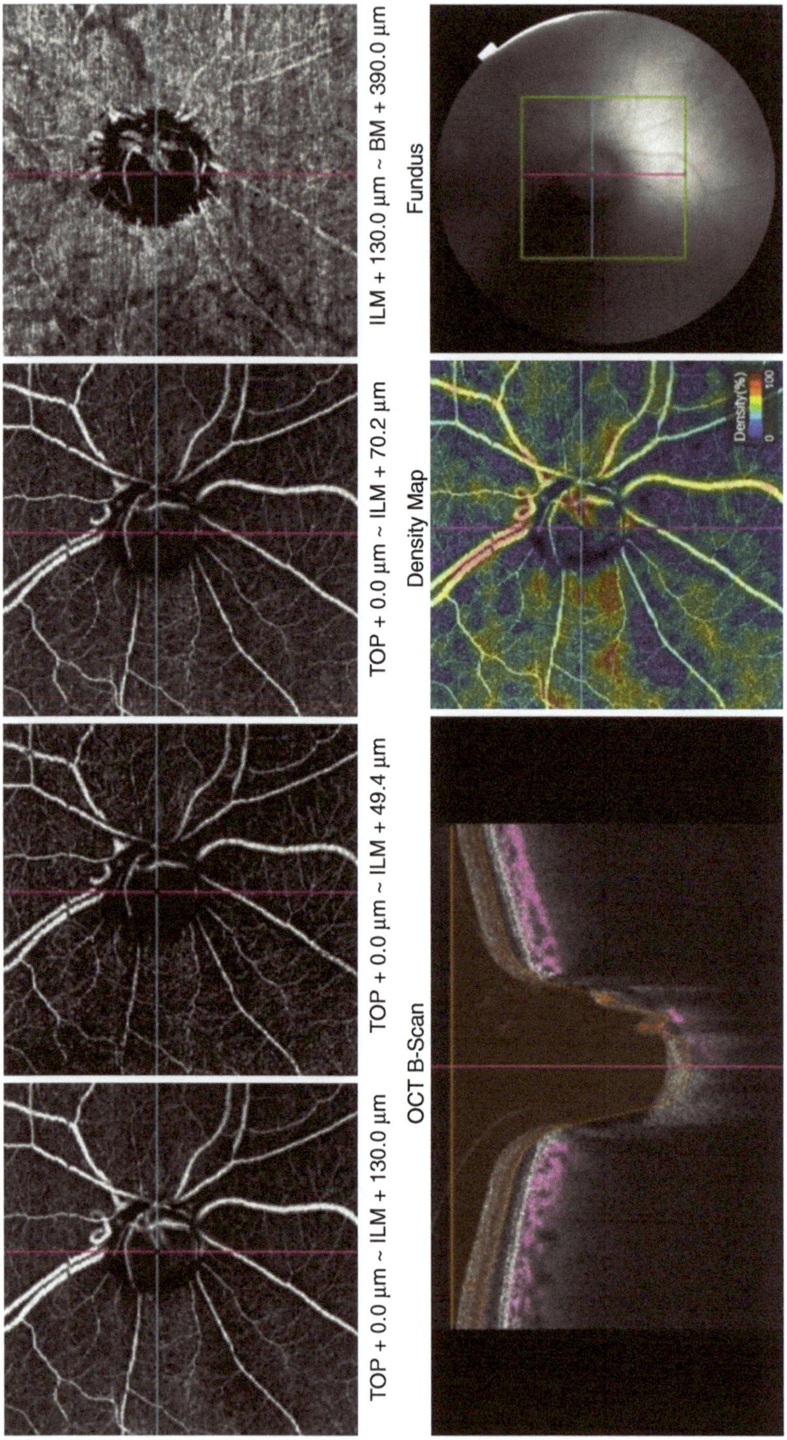

Fig. 2.12 Triton ONH angiography report

2.5 Doppler Optical Coherence Tomography

This technique allow determining arterial and venous blood flow through spectral-domain and swept-source based Doppler OCT [46]. Based on the Doppler shift detected in the OCT signal, this method can determine depth-resolved retinal vessels flow without the use if dye [47]. However, notable drawback of this method are that it cannot detect flow if the vessels are perpendicular to the incident OCT beam or in smaller size vessels [48]. While Doppler OCT retinal blood flow measurements showed good repeatability and excellent correlation with clinical presentations of retinal diseases, the role of this technique in disease detection and monitoring is yet to be determined [48].

2.6 The Future

As technology keeps evolving, several innovative OCT technologies are being tested. The following sections will provide a brief description of some of the most promising developments.

2.7 Adaptive Optics

Adaptive optics (AO) is an optical method designed to dynamically adjust monochromatic aberrations in optical systems. AO was initially used in astronomy for correcting distortions of light passing through the atmosphere. The first in vivo examination of the retina with an AO fundus camera using a wave front sensor and a deformable mirror was introduced in 1997 [49]. A few years later, AO was combined with scanning laser ophthalmoscope [50] and OCT systems [51]. As discussed above, the transverse resolution of all conventional OCT systems is limited to the range of 15–20 μm due to the optical aberrations of light beams when passing through various media in the eye. AO measures and corrects the optical aberrations, reduces the projected spot size, and improves the transverse resolution from 20 μm to the range of 5–10 μm [51]. This resolution allows the acquisition of highly detailed images, enabling the visualization of fine details such as the retinal microvasculature, photoreceptor mosaic [52], LC, and microstructures within the RNFL [6, 53] and ganglion cell layer. The ability to acquire highly detailed in vivo images of these structures allow further insight into ocular anatomy in health and disease, providing the opportunity to expand the understanding of pathologic processes in the eye.

The major limitation of the AO technique is the small field of view, which is restricted to approximately 1°–3°. The use of an eye-tracking system to acquire a series of neighboring scans to cover a larger volume can resolve this limitation, though the longer scanning time might prohibit large scale clinical use [54]. Similarly, the focusing depth of the AO technique is also limited, and therefore acquiring high quality images of thick structures such as the choroid and retina in the same image is difficult to obtain. It may be possible to address this limitation by varying the focal plane while scanning in depth [55]. The volume of data, needed for image processing, and advanced analysis requirements are also a limiting factors for commercialization of the technology. Datasets are 100 times larger than the conventional OCT counterparts, and therefore storage and accessibility of the information are challenging [56].

2.8 Visible-Light OCT

Switching to light sources in the visible light wavelength (~550 nm), instead of near infrared wavelengths, allows further improvement in axial resolution to the level of <1 μm and the extraction of spectroscopic information that is registered to the structural information. The higher scattering coefficients of biological tissue with visible light improves imaging contrast, but at the expense of reduced imaging depth (Fig. 2.13) [19]. Speckle noise reduction techniques can be applied to reduce background noise level and further improve image quality.

The evaluation of oxygen saturation through spectroscopy analysis is one of the most promising applications of the Vis-OCT system [19]. By taking advantage of the distinct light absorption of oxygenated and de-oxygenated hemoglobin within the visible spectral range it is possible to determine the oxygen consumption of tissue in a given region [20]. The role of oxygen saturation and consumption by the ocular tissue for diagnosing and monitoring various ophthalmic disease is currently being examined. Other chromatophores indicating metabolic and biochemical tissue activity are also being initially evaluated.

2.9 Polarization Sensitive OCT

Polarization sensitive OCT (PS-OCT) uses the polarization state of polarized light for the assessment of tissue function. Different ocular structures and tissues alter the polarization state of light in different ways, such as through birefringence (sclera, RNFL), polarization-preservation (photoreceptors), and depolarization (RPE) (Fig. 2.14). PS-OCT estimates these light state alterations by simultaneously

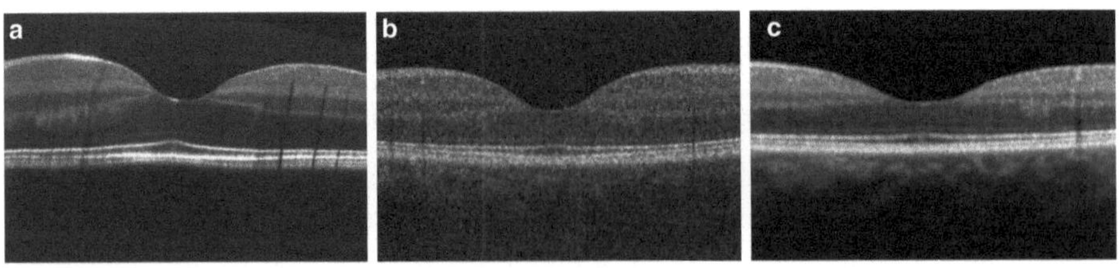

Fig. 2.13 Macula scan of the same subject with Vis-OCT with speckle reduction (**a**) Cirrus OCT (**b**), and Spectralis OCT (**c**). Note the improved visualization with the Vis-OCT and the distinct interface between retinal layers without the need of averaging of multiple images

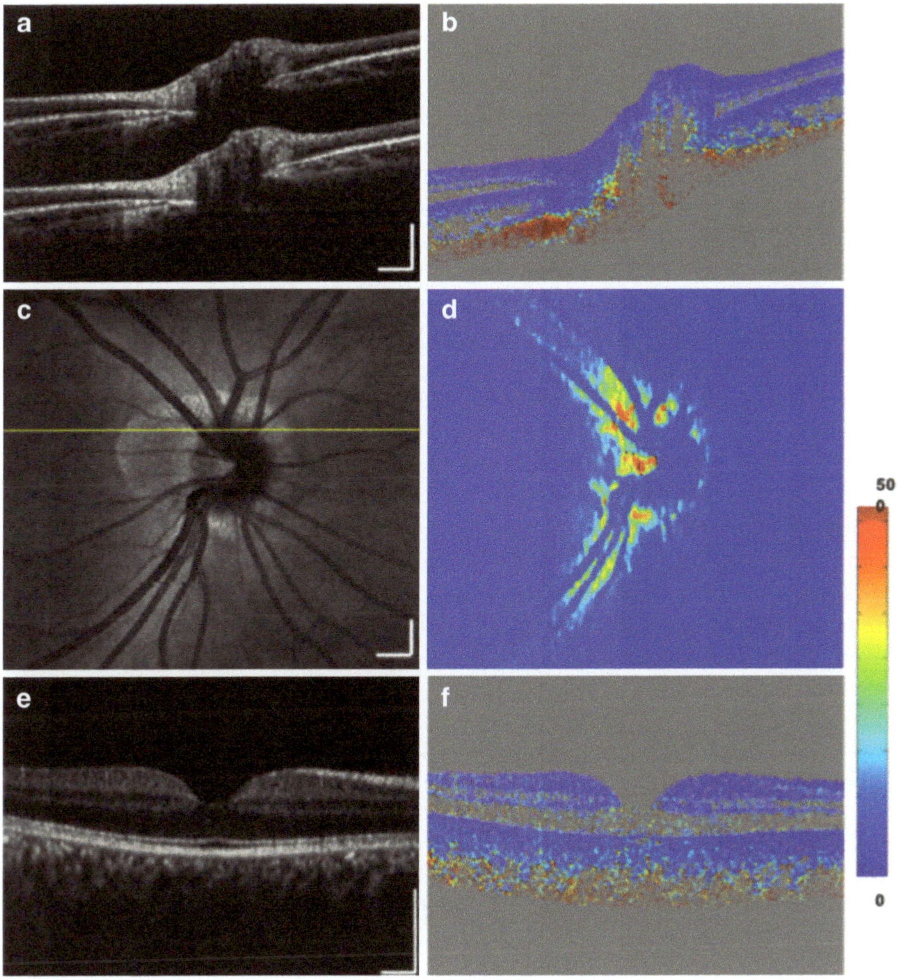

Fig. 2.14 PS-OCT optic nerve head and retinal imaging in healthy subjects. (**a**) A cross-sectional intensity image with two depth-encoded copies of the optic nerve head region. (**b**) Corresponding PS-OCT image shows high retardance in the RNFL and sclera. (**c**) OCT fundus image. (**d**) Corresponding PS-OCT map shows high retardance around the optic nerve head region. (**e**) A cross-sectional intensity image at the fovea region. (**f**) Corresponding PS-OCT image shows low retardance in the retinal layers

measuring intensity, retardation, and optic axis information, thus providing both tissue structural and functional information. The technology was initially incorporated into TD-OCT system, with subsequent introduction into all known OCT iterations such as SD-OCT [57], SS-OCT [30], and AO-OCT [58]. A few studies demonstrated that alteration in the polarization of ocular tissues might precede the occurrence of structural alteration, thus evaluation of the functional properties of the RNFL [59], sclera, and RPE [60] using PS-OCT technology could be an attractive candidate for improving the detection of ocular pathologies such as glaucoma and age-related macular degeneration.

2.10 Phase Sensitive OCT

The Phase Sensitive OCT technique is able to provide in vivo information on micron scale movements or vibrations within the tissue [61]. The technology analyzes the phase information of the back-reflected light beam, which is typically ignored in conventional OCT systems. OCT phase imaging has been demonstrated with SD-OCT [62] and SS-OCT [63] technologies. Phase sensitive OCT offers the advantage of simultaneously assessing both the structural and functional information of the scanned tissue. The device has been shown to capture the retinal pigment epithelium layer, Henle's loop of the macula and retinal nerve fiber layer [64–67]. PS-OCT might be clinically useful in the context of glaucoma, AMD and potentially multiple sclerosis [64, 66, 68], but the clinical application is challenging because it is very sensitive to eye motion.

In conclusion, OCT has an important clinical role in the diagnosis of ocular diseases and in tracking changes overtime, leading to improved clinical management and better insight into pathophysiology of diseases. The constant enhancement of this technology ensures that clinicians will have an indispensable diagnostic tool in their armament.

References

1. Fujimoto JG, Brezinski ME, Tearney GJ, Boppart SA, Bouma B, Hee MR, et al. Optical biopsy and imaging using optical coherence tomography. Nat Med. 1995;1(9):970–2.
2. Fercher AF, Mengedoht K, Werner W. Eye-length measurement by interferometry with partially coherent light. Opt Lett. 1988;13(3):186–8.
3. Izatt JA, Hee MR, Swanson EA, Lin CP, Huang D, Schuman JS, et al. Micrometer-scale resolution imaging of the anterior eye in vivo with optical coherence tomography. Arch Ophthalmol. 1994;112(12):1584–9.
4. Potsaid B, Baumann B, Huang D, Barry S, Cable AE, Schuman JS, et al. Ultrahigh speed 1050nm swept source/Fourier domain OCT retinal and anterior segment imaging at 100,000 to 400,000 axial scans per second. Opt Express. 2010;18(19):20029–48.
5. Wieser W, Biedermann BR, Klein T, Eigenwillig CM, Huber R. Multi-megahertz OCT: high quality 3D imaging at 20 million A-scans and 4.5 GVoxels per second. Opt Express. 2010;18(14):14685–704.
6. Kocaoglu OP, Cense B, Jonnal RS, Wang Q, Lee S, Gao W, et al. Imaging retinal nerve fiber bundles using optical coherence tomography with adaptive optics. Vis Res. 2011;51(16):1835–44.
7. Lavinsky F, Lavinsky D. Novel perspectives on swept-source optical coherence tomography. Int J Retina Vitreous. 2016;2:25.
8. Kuroda HBM, Suzuki M, Yoneya S. A high speed three-dimensional spectral domain optical coherence tomography with <2 mc axial resolution using wide bandwidth femtosecond mode-locked laser. Appl Phys Lett. 2013;102(25):251102.
9. Unterhuber A, Povazay B, Hermann B, Sattmann H, Chavez-Pirson A, Drexler W. In vivo retinal optical coherence tomography at 1040 nm - enhanced penetration into the choroid. Opt Express. 2005;13(9):3252–8.

10. Yasuno Y, Hong Y, Makita S, Yamanari M, Akiba M, Miura M, et al. In vivo high-contrast imaging of deep posterior eye by 1-microm swept source optical coherence tomography and scattering optical coherence angiography. Opt Express. 2007;15(10):6121–39.
11. Hale GM, Querry MR. Optical constants of water in the 200-nm to 200-microm wavelength region. Appl Opt. 1973;12(3):555–63.
12. Fercher AF, Hitzenberger CK, Drexler W, Kamp G, Sattmann H. In vivo optical coherence tomography. Am J Ophthalmol. 1993;116(1):113–4.
13. Ahlers C, Schmidt-Erfurth U. Three-dimensional high resolution OCT imaging of macular pathology. Opt Express. 2009;17(5):4037–45.
14. Kim JS, Ishikawa H, Sung KR, Xu J, Wollstein G, Bilonick RA, et al. Retinal nerve fibre layer thickness measurement reproducibility improved with spectral domain optical coherence tomography. Br J Ophthalmol. 2009;93(8):1057–63.
15. Drexler W, Morgner U, Kartner FX, Pitris C, Boppart SA, Li XD, et al. In vivo ultrahigh-resolution optical coherence tomography. Opt Lett. 1999;24(17):1221–3.
16. Lim H, Jiang Y, Wang Y, Huang YC, Chen Z, Wise FW. Ultrahigh-resolution optical coherence tomography with a fiber laser source at 1 microm. Opt Lett. 2005;30(10):1171–3.
17. Huber R, Adler DC, Fujimoto JG. Buffered Fourier domain mode locking: unidirectional swept laser sources for optical coherence tomography imaging at 370,000 lines/s. Opt Lett. 2006;31(20):2975–7.
18. Yaqoob Z, Wu J, Yang C. Spectral domain optical coherence tomography: a better OCT imaging strategy. BioTechniques. 2005;39(6 Suppl):S6–13.
19. Shu X, Beckmann L, Zhang H. Visible-light optical coherence tomography: a review. J Biomed Opt. 2017;22(12):1–14.
20. Yi J, Wei Q, Liu W, Backman V, Zhang HF. Visible-light optical coherence tomography for retinal oximetry. Opt Lett. 2013;38(11):1796–8.
21. Huang D, Swanson EA, Lin CP, Schuman JS, Stinson WG, Chang W, et al. Optical coherence tomography. Science. 1991;254(5035):1178–81.
22. Schuman JS, Pedut-Kloizman T, Hertzmark E, Hee MR, Wilkins JR, Coker JG, et al. Reproducibility of nerve fiber layer thickness measurements using optical coherence tomography. Ophthalmology. 1996;103(11):1889–98.
23. Hee MR, Izatt JA, Swanson EA, Huang D, Schuman JS, Lin CP, et al. Optical coherence tomography of the human retina. Arch Ophthalmol. 1995;113(3):325–32.
24. Otani T, Kishi S, Maruyama Y. Patterns of diabetic macular edema with optical coherence tomography. Am J Ophthalmol. 1999;127(6):688–93.
25. Sanchez-Tocino H, Alvarez-Vidal A, Maldonado MJ, Moreno-Montanes J, Garcia-Layana A. Retinal thickness study with optical coherence tomography in patients with diabetes. Invest Ophthalmol Vis Sci. 2002;43(5):1588–94.
26. Medeiros FA, Zangwill LM, Bowd C, Weinreb RN. Comparison of the GDx VCC scanning laser polarimeter, HRT II confocal scanning laser ophthalmoscope, and stratus OCT optical coherence tomograph for the detection of glaucoma. Arch Ophthalmol. 2004;122(6):827–37.
27. Paunescu LA, Schuman JS, Price LL, Stark PC, Beaton S, Ishikawa H, et al. Reproducibility of nerve fiber thickness, macular thickness, and optic nerve head measurements using StratusOCT. Invest Ophthalmol Vis Sci. 2004;45(6):1716–24.
28. Kagemann L, Wollstein G, Wojtkowski M, Ishikawa H, Townsend KA, Gabriele ML, et al. Spectral oximetry assessed with high-speed ultra-high-resolution optical coherence tomography. J Biomed Opt. 2007;12(4):041212.
29. Srinivasan VJ, Wojtkowski M, Fujimoto JG, Duker JS. In vivo measurement of retinal physiology with high-speed ultrahigh-resolution optical coherence tomography. Opt Lett. 2006;31(15):2308–10.
30. Yamanari M, Makita S, Lim Y, Yasuno Y. Full-range polarization-sensitive swept-source optical coherence tomography by simultaneous transversal and spectral modulation. Opt Express. 2010;18(13):13964–80.

31. Wojtkowski M, Srinivasan V, Fujimoto JG, Ko T, Schuman JS, Kowalczyk A, et al. Three-dimensional retinal imaging with high-speed ultrahigh-resolution optical coherence tomography. Ophthalmology. 2005;112(10):1734–46.
32. Leung CK, Cheung CY, Weinreb RN, Qiu Q, Liu S, Li H, et al. Retinal nerve fiber layer imaging with spectral-domain optical coherence tomography: a variability and diagnostic performance study. Ophthalmology. 2009;116(7):1257–63, 63e1–2.
33. Asrani S, Rosdahl JA, Allingham RR. Novel software strategy for glaucoma diagnosis: asymmetry analysis of retinal thickness. Arch Ophthalmol. 2011;129(9):1205–11.
34. Tan O, Chopra V, Lu AT, Schuman JS, Ishikawa H, Wollstein G, et al. Detection of macular ganglion cell loss in glaucoma by Fourier-domain optical coherence tomography. Ophthalmology. 2009;116(12):2305–14 e1–2.
35. Tan O, Li G, Lu AT, Varma R, Huang D, Advanced Imaging for Glaucoma Study G. Mapping of macular substructures with optical coherence tomography for glaucoma diagnosis. Ophthalmology. 2008;115(6):949–56.
36. Belghith A, Medeiros FA, Bowd C, Liebmann JM, Girkin CA, Weinreb RN, et al. Structural change can be detected in advanced-glaucoma eyes. Invest Ophthalmol Vis Sci. 2016;57(9):OCT511–8.
37. Bowd C, Zangwill LM, Weinreb RN, Medeiros FA, Belghith A. Estimating optical coherence tomography structural measurement floors to improve detection of progression in advanced glaucoma. Am J Ophthalmol. 2017;175:37–44.
38. Kim KE, Park KH, Jeoung JW, Kim SH, Kim DM. Severity-dependent association between ganglion cell inner plexiform layer thickness and macular mean sensitivity in open-angle glaucoma. Acta Ophthalmol. 2014;92(8):e650–6.
39. Lavinsky F, Wu M, Schuman JS, Lucy KA, Liu M, Song Y, et al. Can macula and optic nerve head parameters detect glaucoma progression in eyes with advanced circumpapillary retinal nerve fiber layer damage? Ophthalmology. 2018;125(12):1907–12.
40. Keane PA, Ruiz-Garcia H, Sadda SR. Clinical applications of long-wavelength (1,000-nm) optical coherence tomography. Ophthalmic Surg Lasers Imaging. 2011;42(Suppl):S67–74.
41. Yasin Alibhai A, Or C, Witkin AJ. Swept source optical coherence tomography: a review. Curr Ophthalmol Rep. 2018;6:7–16.
42. Wang B, Nevins JE, Nadler Z, Wollstein G, Ishikawa H, Bilonick RA, et al. In vivo lamina cribrosa micro-architecture in healthy and glaucomatous eyes as assessed by optical coherence tomography. Invest Ophthalmol Vis Sci. 2013;54(13):8270–4.
43. Omodaka K, Maekawa S, An G, Tsuda S, Shiga Y, Takada N, et al. Pilot study for three-dimensional assessment of laminar pore structure in patients with glaucoma, as measured with swept source optical coherence tomography. PLoS One. 2018;13(11):e0207600.
44. Wang B, Lucy KA, Schuman JS, Sigal IA, Bilonick RA, Lu C, et al. Tortuous pore path through the glaucomatous lamina cribrosa. Sci Rep. 2018;8(1):7281.
45. Hou H, Moghimi S, Zangwill LM, Shoji T, Ghahari E, Penteado RC, et al. Macula vessel density and thickness in early primary open-angle glaucoma. Am J Ophthalmol. 2019;199:120–32.
46. Leitgeb RA, Werkmeister RM, Blatter C, Schmetterer L. Doppler optical coherence tomography. Prog Retin Eye Res. 2014;41:26–43.
47. Werkmeister RM, Dragostinoff N, Pircher M, Gotzinger E, Hitzenberger CK, Leitgeb RA, et al. Bidirectional Doppler Fourier-domain optical coherence tomography for measurement of absolute flow velocities in human retinal vessels. Opt Lett. 2008;33(24):2967–9.
48. Wang Y, Fawzi AA, Varma R, Sadun AA, Zhang X, Tan O, et al. Pilot study of optical coherence tomography measurement of retinal blood flow in retinal and optic nerve diseases. Invest Ophthalmol Vis Sci. 2011;52(2):840–5.
49. Liang J, Williams DR, Miller DT. Supernormal vision and high-resolution retinal imaging through adaptive optics. J Opt Soc Am A Opt Image Sci Vis. 1997;14(11):2884–92.
50. Roorda A, Romero-Borja F, Donnelly Iii W, Queener H, Hebert T, Campbell M. Adaptive optics scanning laser ophthalmoscopy. Opt Express. 2002;10(9):405–12.
51. Hermann B, Fernandez EJ, Unterhuber A, Sattmann H, Fercher AF, Drexler W, et al. Adaptive-optics ultrahigh-resolution optical coherence tomography. Opt Lett. 2004;29(18):2142–4.

52. Kocaoglu OP, Lee S, Jonnal RS, Wang Q, Herde AE, Derby JC, et al. Imaging cone photoreceptors in three dimensions and in time using ultrahigh resolution optical coherence tomography with adaptive optics. Biomed Opt Express. 2011;2(4):748–63.
53. Takayama K, Ooto S, Hangai M, Ueda-Arakawa N, Yoshida S, Akagi T, et al. High-resolution imaging of retinal nerve fiber bundles in glaucoma using adaptive optics scanning laser ophthalmoscopy. Am J Ophthalmol. 2013;155(5):870–81.
54. Burns SA, Tumbar R, Elsner AE, Ferguson D, Hammer DX. Large-field-of-view, modular, stabilized, adaptive-optics-based scanning laser ophthalmoscope. J Opt Soc Am A Opt Image Sci Vis. 2007;24(5):1313–26.
55. Zawadzki RJ, Choi SS, Fuller AR, Evans JW, Hamann B, Werner JS. Cellular resolution volumetric in vivo retinal imaging with adaptive optics-optical coherence tomography. Opt Express. 2009;17(5):4084–94.
56. Jonnal RS, Kocaoglu OP, Zawadzki RJ, Liu Z, Miller DT, Werner JS. A review of adaptive optics optical coherence tomography: technical advances, scientific applications, and the future. Invest Ophthalmol Vis Sci. 2016;57(9):OCT51–68.
57. Gotzinger E, Pircher M, Baumann B, Ahlers C, Geitzenauer W, Schmidt-Erfurth U, et al. Three-dimensional polarization sensitive OCT imaging and interactive display of the human retina. Opt Express. 2009;17(5):4151–65.
58. Cense B, Gao W, Brown JM, Jones SM, Jonnal RS, Mujat M, et al. Retinal imaging with polarization-sensitive optical coherence tomography and adaptive optics. Opt Express. 2009;17(24):21634–51.
59. Liu S, Wang B, Yin B, Milner TE, Markey MK, McKinnon SJ, et al. Retinal nerve fiber layer reflectance for early glaucoma diagnosis. J Glaucoma. 2014;23(1):e45–52.
60. Michels S, Pircher M, Geitzenauer W, Simader C, Gotzinger E, Findl O, et al. Value of polarisation-sensitive optical coherence tomography in diseases affecting the retinal pigment epithelium. Br J Ophthalmol. 2008;92(2):204–9.
61. Choma MA, Ellerbee AK, Yang C, Creazzo TL, Izatt JA. Spectral-domain phase microscopy. Opt Lett. 2005;30(10):1162–4.
62. Joo C, Akkin T, Cense B, Park BH, de Boer JF. Spectral-domain optical coherence phase microscopy for quantitative phase-contrast imaging. Opt Lett. 2005;30(16):2131–3.
63. Sarunic MV, Weinberg S, Izatt JA. Full-field swept-source phase microscopy. Opt Lett. 2006;31(10):1462–4.
64. Ju MJ, Hong YJ, Makita S, Lim Y, Kurokawa K, Duan L, et al. Advanced multi-contrast Jones matrix optical coherence tomography for Doppler and polarization sensitive imaging. Opt Express. 2013;21(16):19412–36.
65. Cense B, Wang Q, Lee S, Zhao L, Elsner AE, Hitzenberger CK, et al. Henle fiber layer phase retardation measured with polarization-sensitive optical coherence tomography. Biomed Opt Express. 2013;4(11):2296–306.
66. Braaf B, Vermeer KA, de Groot M, Vienola KV, de Boer JF. Fiber-based polarization-sensitive OCT of the human retina with correction of system polarization distortions. Biomed Opt Express. 2014;5(8):2736–58.
67. Wang Z, Lee HC, Ahsen OO, Lee B, Choi W, Potsaid B, et al. Depth-encoded all-fiber swept source polarization sensitive OCT. Biomed Opt Express. 2014;5(9):2931–49.
68. Jiang H, Chen W, Delgado S, Liu Y, Lin Y, Wang J. Altered birefringence of peripapillary retinal nerve fiber layer in multiple sclerosis measured by polarization sensitive optical coherence tomography. Eye Vis (Lond). 2018;5:14.

The APOSTEL Recommendations

3

Aykut Aytulun, Andrés Cruz-Herranz, Lisanne Balk, Alexander U. Brandt, and Philipp Albrecht

As the number of quantitative OCT studies rapidly increases, there is an obvious need for standardization on how these studies should be performed and reported. Important steps for standardization were the development of quality control criteria and of a consensus on the nomenclature of retinal structures accessible to OCT imaging. The OSCAR-IB Consensus Criteria for Retinal OCT Quality Assessment [1] were developed to validate the accuracy and quality of peripapillary ring scans assessing the retinal nerve fiber layer (RNFL) in multiple sclerosis (MS). The majority of these criteria not only apply to imaging of the peripapillary RNFL in

A. Aytulun · P. Albrecht (✉)
Department of Neurology, Medical Faculty, Heinrich Heine University Düsseldorf, Düsseldorf, Germany
e-mail: ahmetaykut.aytulun@med.uni-duesseldorf.de; philipp.albrecht@med.uni-duesseldorf.de

A. Cruz-Herranz
Department of Neurology, University of California, San Francisco, CA, USA
e-mail: Andres.CruzHerranz@ucsf.edu

L. Balk
Departments of Neurology and Ophthalmology, VU University Medical Centre, Amsterdam, The Netherlands
e-mail: l.balk@vumc.nl

A. U. Brandt
NeuroCure Clinical Research Center, Berlin, Germany

Charité-Universitätsmedizin Berlin, Berlin, Germany

Freie Universität Berlin, Berlin, Germany

Humboldt-Universität zu Berlin, Berlin, Germany

Berlin Institute of Health, Berlin, Germany

Department of Neurology, University of California, Irvine, CA, USA
e-mail: alexander.brandt@charite.de

A. Grzybowski, P. Barboni (eds.), *OCT and Imaging in Central Nervous System Diseases*, https://doi.org/10.1007/978-3-030-26269-3_3

MS but can also be used to rate e.g. macular scans or be applied in other conditions associated with quantitative changes of retinal layers (e.g. neurodegenerative disorders). The International Nomenclature for Optical Coherence Tomography (INOCT) Panel has proposed a consensus nomenclature for the classification of retinal and choroidal layers and bands visible on spectral-domain optical coherence tomography (SD-OCT) images of a normal eye [2].

However, despite these recommendations, imprecise reporting of quantitative OCT studies has sometimes led to uncertainty about methodological aspects, such as scan protocols, analysis software, the use of quality control criteria and inclusion or exclusion of patients and/or eyes. This impacts the interpretability and generalizability of these reports. Therefore, a panel of experts from the International MS Visual (IMSVISUAL) consortium convened at two international meetings in 2015 to develop the Advised Protocol for OCT Study Terminology and Elements recommendations ("APOSTEL recommendations"). These recommendations include a checklist of nine items of particular relevance when reporting quantitative OCT studies.

In the following, a short overview of the nine items is provided:

3.1 Describe the Study Protocol

The study design should be reported in line with the applicable guidelines STROBE, CONSORT or CARE [3]. Additionally, for OCT studies, authors should define if inclusion and exclusion criteria were applied at the eye or patient level and if/how confounding ocular pathologies, e.g. as listed in the OSCAR-IB criteria [1], were ruled out. Reporting the history of and time span from events of particular relevance for the OCT outcomes at study, i.e. optic neuritis (ON) in neuroinflammatory diseases or first symptoms in Leber's hereditary optic neuropathy, is of major importance.

3.2 State the Acquisition Device Type, Name and Version

As OCT technology is continuously evolving, it is important to provide not only the specifications of the devices used (manufacturer, model, interferometric technique) but also the exact version of the software used for the acquisition.

3.3 Define the Acquisition Setting

The exact conditions, under which and how OCT measurements were performed, should be reported, including the use of methods to facilitate imaging such as the use of device-specific control for movement artifacts or pupil dilation.

3.4 Define the OCT Scanning Protocol

It is essential to report the target structures imaged and the exact acquisition parameters of the full measurement protocol, including a detailed description of all scan types employed in a study.

3.5 Define Fundoscopic Imaging

In case additional fundus imaging modalities such as confocal scanning laser ophthalmoscopy (cSLO), retinal angiography and auto-fluorescence imaging are reported, these should be described. Likewise, the acquisition protocol, including the excitation wavelength, filter sets and the number of frames averaged (if applicable), should be indicated.

3.6 Describe Post-acquisition Data Selection

A crucial point of all studies is the quality of the scans, which can have a major impact on the results and their interpretation. If strategies to select or exclude scans from analyses were applied, these should be described in detail. In order to ensure a high quality of scans and interpretability of the results, the use of quality control criteria is recommended. For example, an extensive set of quality control criteria has been published in the form of the OSCAR-IB criteria [1, 4].

3.7 Describe Post-acquisition Data Analysis

Authors should precisely report how the post-processing analysis (e.g. intraretinal layer segmentation) was performed (e.g. fully automated, semi-automated with manual correction of obvious errors or fully manual) [5].

To obtain thickness or volume data from volume scans, differently sized and/or shaped grids can be employed, such as the ring-shaped grid defined for the Early Treatment of Diabetic Retinopathy Study (ETDRS) [6]. Area shape and size of these analysis grids should be reported in addition to the size and location of the source scan (see scanning protocol) [7].

3.8 Use Common Nomenclature and Abbreviations

All structures analyzed should be precisely defined and described ideally using the recommended nomenclature proposed by the IN-OCT consortium (Fig. 3.1) [2]. If additional (composite) structures are reported, these should clearly be defined .

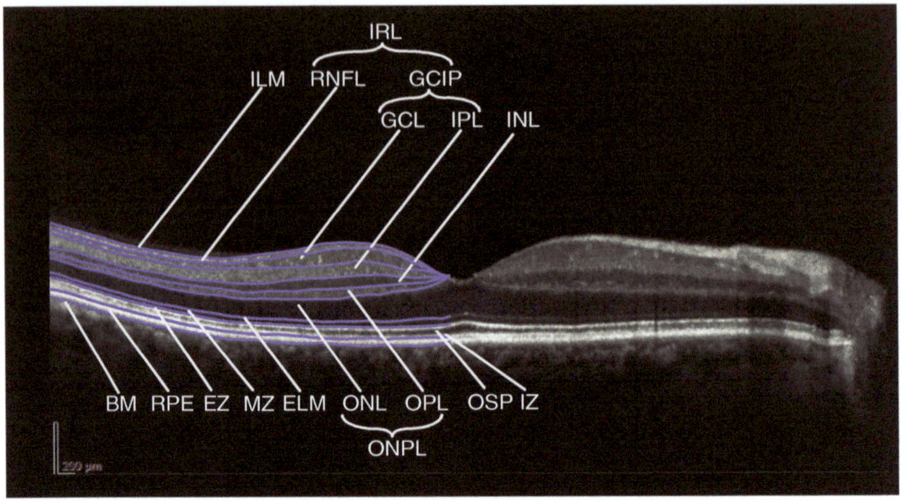

Fig. 3.1 The consensus nomenclature for retinal structures. The different layers (and their borders) are illustrated in a central vertical scan through the middle of the foveola. Abbreviations of retinal structures and layers: ILM (Inner limiting membrane), RNFL (Retinal nerve fiber layer), GCL (Ganglion cell layer), IPL (Inner plexiform layer), INL (Inner nuclear layer), OPL (Outer plexiform layer), ONL (Outer nuclear layer), ELM (External limiting membrane), MZ (Myoid Zone), EZ (Ellipsoid Zone) (Inner and Outer segment Junction), OSP (Outer segment of photoreceptors), IZ (Interdigitation zone), RPE (Retinal pigment epithelium), BM (Bruch's Membrane). Compound layers are Ganglion cell and inner plexiform layer (GCIP) composite of macular GCL and IPL, Inner retinal layers (IRL) composite of macular RNFL, GCL and IPL, and Outer nuclear and plexiform layer (ONPL) composite of ONL and OPL (Image courtesy of Philipp Albrecht and Aykut Aytulun)

3.9 Define the Statistical Approach with Exact Model Description

Reporting of statistical analyses should adhere to the applicable reporting guidelines [3]. As data for both eyes of each subject are usually available in OCT studies, it is important to describe how the inter-eye within-patient dependencies are accounted for. Strategies to deal with this include either randomly selecting one eye, calculating the mean of both eyes or applying statistical methods accounting for these dependencies, such as general mixed effects models or generalized estimating equation models (GEE). Specific questions may require different strategies [8] and advanced statistical models should be reported in sufficient detail.

3.10 Outlook/Future Development

Shortly after their publication, a letter to the editor by James Cameron has commented on the retinal layer nomenclature proposed by the APOSTEL recommendations. He pointed out that additional structures can be described below the external limiting membrane (ELM), which have been detailed in the International

Nomenclature for Optical Coherence Tomography (IN-OCT) consensus paper. Between the inner segment/outer segment junction (ISOS) and the ELM, a myoid zone can be defined; between the ISOS and the outer photoreceptor tips (OPT), an ellipsoid zone; and between the OPT and the retinal pigment epithelium (RPE), an interdigitation zone. These structures are already included in Fig. 3.1. The APOSTEL recommendations are currently being revised using the formalized consensus finding approach of a Delphi process involving a large public of neurologists and ophthalmologists. The nomenclature proposed by the revised recommendations will be harmonized with the IN-OCT consensus (Table 3.1).

Table 3.1 9-Point APOSTEL checklist (adapted from [9])

Item		Recommendation	
1	Study protocol	(a) Describe how many OCT operating sites and graders were included	❑
		(b) Report the timing of OCT compared to other measurements (same day, delayed)	❑
		(c) Describe the inclusion and exclusion criteria	❑
2	Acquisition device	For all OCT devices used, report data on:	
		(a) Manufacturer	❑
		(b) Model	❑
		(c) Version	❑
		(d) Software version	❑
3	Acquisition settings	Clearly describe the settings in which OCT scans were obtained:	
		(a) Room light conditions	❑
		(b) Pupils dilated before exam (y/n)	❑
		(c) Number of operators and devices	❑
4	Scanning protocol	Clearly describe the scanning protocol, including:	
		(a) Type of scan (circular, volume, star, line, other)	❑
		(b) Location (area of interest, macula, optic nerve head, papillo-macular bundle, other?)	❑
		(c) Scan parameters (with or without eye tracking) – *Volume scan: size of scan area (degrees or mm), number of B-scans, alignment of B-scans, number of A-scans per B-scan,* – *Radial scan: size of scan area (degrees or mm), number of B-scans, alignment of B-scans, number of A-scans per B-scan* – *Ring scan: diameter, A-scans/B-scan, manual or automatic placement of ring or method of centering, depth resolution* – *Line scan: angle, location, number of A-scans, depth resolution*	❑
5	Fundoscopic imaging	(a) Report other imaging modalities used in addition to OCT (fundoscopy, CSLO, retinal angiography, autofluorescence imaging, etc.)	❑
		(b) Describe acquisition protocol, including: 1. Excitation wavelength 2. Filter sets 3. Number of frames averaged (if applicable)	❑

(continued)

Table 3.1 (continued)

Item		Recommendation	
6	Post-acquisition data selection	Describe image selection process including:	
		(a) Quality control criteria (i.e. OSCAR-IB [1] or other criteria)	❑
		(b) Post-acquisition discard (number and criteria)	❑
		(c) Eye selection strategy (if applicable)	❑
7	Post-acquisition analysis	Describe all post-acquisition steps:	
		(a) Software used for processing scans and segmentation (may be different from acquisition software)	❑
		(b) Which individual retinal layers were segmented/included	❑
		(c) Method of segmentation (automated, semi-automated or manually)	❑
		(d) How potential bias was addressed in the case of manual segmentation (masking)	❑
		(e) Grid used for data-extraction (size, shape, selected sections)	❑
8	Nomenclature and abbreviations	Define:	
		(a) Anatomical structures analyzed	❑
		(b) Units of provided measurements (e.g. volume or thickness)	❑
9	Statistical approach	Describe:	
		(a) Statistical models used for the analyses of OCT data	❑
		(b) Whether data was analyzed by eye or by patient	❑

References

1. Tewarie P, Balk L, Costello F, Green A, Martin R, Schippling S, Petzold A. The OSCAR-IB consensus criteria for retinal OCT quality assessment. PLoS One. 2012;7:e34823. http://www.pubmedcentral.nih.gov/articlerender.fcgi?artid=3334941&tool=pmcentrez&rendertype=abstract. Accessed 20 May 2014.
2. Staurenghi G, Sadda S, Chakravarthy U, Spaide RF. Proposed lexicon for anatomic landmarks in normal posterior segment spectral-domain optical coherence tomography: the IN•OCT consensus. Ophthalmology. 2014;121:1572–8. https://doi.org/10.1016/j.ophtha.2014.02.023.
3. Pandis N, Fedorowicz Z. The international EQUATOR network: enhancing the quality and transparency of health care research. J Appl Oral Sci. 2011;19. http://www.ncbi.nlm.nih.gov/pubmed/21986662. Accessed 24 Nov 2018.
4. Schippling S, Balk L, Costello F, Albrecht P, Balcer L, Calabresi P, Frederiksen J, Frohman E, Green A, Klistorner A, Outteryck O, Paul F, Plant G, Traber G, Vermersch P, Villoslada P, Wolf S, Petzold A. Quality control for retinal OCT in multiple sclerosis: validation of the OSCAR-IB criteria. Mult Scler. 2014;21:163–70.
5. Oberwahrenbrock T, Traber GL, Lukas S, Gabilondo I, Nolan R, Songster C, Balk L, Petzold A, Paul F, Villoslada P, Brandt AU, Green AJ, Schippling S. Multicenter reliability of semiautomatic retinal layer segmentation using OCT. Neurol Neuroimmunol Neuroinflamm. 2018;5:e449. http://nn.neurology.org/lookup/doi/10.1212/NXI.0000000000000449.
6. Anon. Photocoagulation for diabetic macular edema. Early Treatment Diabetic Retinopathy Study report number 1. Early Treatment Diabetic Retinopathy Study research group. Arch Ophthalmol (Chicago, Ill 1960). 1985;103:1796–806.

7. Oberwahrenbrock T, Weinhold M, Mikolajczak J, Zimmermann H, Paul F, Beckers I, Brandt AU. Reliability of intra-retinal layer thickness estimates. PLoS One. 2015;10:e0137316.
8. Fan Q, Teo Y-Y, Saw S-M. Application of advanced statistics in ophthalmology. Invest Ophthalmol Vis Sci. 2011;52:6059–65. http://www.ncbi.nlm.nih.gov/pubmed/21807933. Accessed 5 Nov 2014.
9. Cruz-Herranz A, Balk LJ, Oberwahrenbrock T, Saidha S, Martinez-Lapiscina EH, Lagreze WA, Schuman JS, Villoslada P, Calabresi P, Balcer L, Petzold A, Green AJ, Paul F, Brandt AU, Albrecht P. The APOSTEL recommendations for reporting quantitative optical coherence tomography studies. Neurology. 2016;86:2303–9.

OCT Angiography: Guidelines for Analysis and Interpretation

4

Enrico Borrelli, Srinivas R. Sadda, Akihito Uji, and Giuseppe Querques

4.1 Introduction

Optical coherence tomography angiography (OCTA) is an emerging noninvasive imaging technique that rapidly produces three-dimensional angiographic images of the eye [1, 2]. The basic concept of OCTA is to detect the movement of erythrocytes within vasculature as an intrinsic contrast agent. To obtain this, several repeated OCT B-scans are performed in the same location and are compared in order to detect differences, or decorrelation, in the blood flow signal. Since repeated B-scans are executed at successively locations, this generates volumetric OCTA data.

OCTA has several potential advantages, including the absence of dye administration, a fast acquisition time, and the ability to perform depth-resolved analysis of the vasculature, with some devices providing automated quantitative data. Despite its many advantages, OCTA is not without limitation. Therefore, some issues should be considered during the analysis and interpretation of OCTA images, including lack of information on flow or filling speed, and different artifacts which may affect the images [1].

E. Borrelli (✉) · G. Querques
Ophthalmology Department, San Raffaele University Hospital, Milan, Italy

S. R. Sadda
Department of Ophthalmology, David Geffen School of Medicine at UCLA, Los Angeles, CA, USA

Doheny Image Reading Center, Doheny Eye Institute, Los Angeles, CA, USA
e-mail: ssadda@doheny.org

A. Uji
Department of Ophthalmology and Visual Sciences, Kyoto University Graduate School of Medicine, Kyoto, Japan
e-mail: akihito1@kuhp.kyoto-u.ac.jp

A. Grzybowski, P. Barboni (eds.), *OCT and Imaging in Central Nervous System Diseases*, https://doi.org/10.1007/978-3-030-26269-3_4

In this chapter, we will describe the basic principles of OCTA technology and the approaches to quantify OCTA variables. This chapter is thus intended to help better guide clinicians on how to interpret OCTA findings.

4.2 Ocular Vascularization

The ophthalmic artery provides the vascular supply to the eye. This artery arises, from the internal carotid artery and divides to give rise to the central retinal artery, the short and long posterior ciliary arteries (SPCAs and LPCAs, respectively), and the anterior ciliary arteries [3].

The central retinal artery is contained in the optic nerve and from the optic nerve head to the retinal periphery progressively branches into smaller retinal arterioles. These retinal arterioles supply the inner retina, while the outer retina is supplied by the choroid. The central retinal vein drains the retinal tissue and leaves the eye through the optic nerve. Importantly, histological studies of the human retina have demonstrated that retinal vessels constitute three distinct capillary layers: the superficial (SCP), middle (MCP), and deep capillary (DCP) plexuses [4, 5]. In addition, a fourth vascular layer, the radial peripapillary capillary plexus (RPCP) or nerve fiber plexus (NFP), is mainly located within the superficial nerve fiber layer (NFL) surrounding the optic disc [4, 5]. In the latter vascular plexus, long capillary segments are oriented parallel to the direction of retinal ganglion cell axons. It is worth noting that the retinal capillaries feature walls without fenestrations and endothelial cells with tight junctions constituting the inner blood-retinal barrier which is impermeable to even small molecules.

The choroid is supplied by the short and long posterior ciliary arteries. Some branches of the SPCAs also supply the optic disc via an anastomotic ring named the circle of Zinn-Haller. Histological studies have demonstrated that the choroid is constituted of five sublayers: Bruch's membrane, the choriocapillaris (CC), Haller's and Sattler's layers, and the suprachoroidal space [6]. The Haller's and Sattler's layers contain larger diameter vessels which are directly supplied by the SPCAs and LPCAs. Conversely, the choriocapillaris is a highly anastomosed network of capillaries arising from the arterioles in Sattler's layer and is located between Bruch's membrane and the medium-sized choroidal vessels. This vascular layer is organized into a series of hexagonal-shaped lobules, which were demonstrated to be progressively larger toward the periphery [6]. In contrast with the retinal vessels, the CC is unique in that it is fenestrated and this facilitates the movement of even large macromolecules into the extra-capillary compartment [7].

The LPCAs run anteriorly between the sclera and choroid and connect to the anterior ciliary arteries shaping the major arterial circle of the iris [3]. The anterior ciliary arteries reach the sclera near the limbus after travelling with the extraocular muscles [3].

4.3 Optical Coherence Tomography Angiography

4.3.1 Overview on Technical Aspects

Structural OCT can acquire volumetric images of the retina by executing successive single B-scans at different retinal locations. Conversely, OCTA devices perform several repeated B-scans at the same retinal location and the obtained structural information are compared to detect signal changes secondary to flowing erythrocytes (motion contrast). Furthermore, each B-scan is composed of several A scans that are acquired at sequential positions to generate the B-scan. The A-scan rate is dependent on the OCT instrument and is typically ranges between 70,000 A-scans per second (spectral domain devices) and 100,000 A-scans per second (swept source instruments) among commercially available devices. Of note, faster acquisition speeds are available in various research instruments.

The interscan time, which represents the delay between two B-scan repeated at the same retinal location, has a crucial role. Therefore, while a longer interscan time may increase sensitivity to motion, this also increase the occurrence of bulk eye motion which can confound the motion signal [8].

In order to detect the motion contrast, three different methodologies may be used by OCTA devices, as follows: (1) phase-based; (2) amplitude-based; and (3) complex amplitude-based, in which OCTA algorithm uses both phase and amplitude information. The OCTA signal is typically normalized between 0 and 1. The interscan time and the background noise determine the slowest detectable flow. Erythrocytes must move a sufficient distance within repeated B-scans to be detected. In addition, differences in signal must be higher than the background noise to be detected as flow. This causes an intrinsic limitation to current OCTA technology which may not be able to distinguish the absence of flow from slow flow below a detectable threshold range [8].

Optical coherence tomography angiography may be captured with spectral domain OCT (SD OCT), which in commercial devices employs a wavelength at around 840 nm, or with swept-source OCT (SS OCT), which uses a longer wavelength (~1050 nm).

4.3.2 Visualization of the OCTA Images

While OCT is considered a cross-sectional imaging modality, OCTA images are mainly displayed with *en face* visualization. The *en face* approach combines the 3-dimensional volumetric information obtained from previously established OCT techniques for the automated segmentation of anatomic reference planes, which allow the definition of "slabs" and the segmentation of the volumetric OCTA scans at specific depths (Fig. 4.1). Using this strategy, the flow data within any slab are summed or projected into a two-dimensional *en face* image that can be viewed and studied.

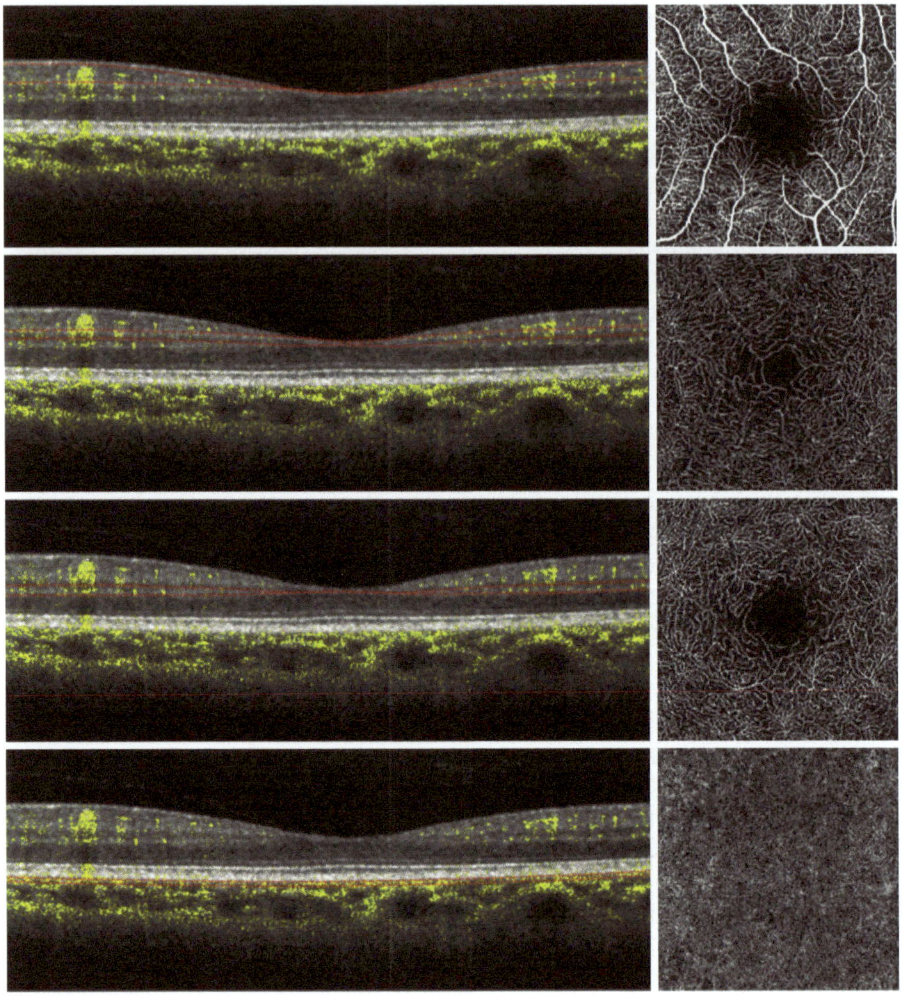

Fig. 4.1 Optical coherence tomographic angiographic image of the macula of a healthy subject. The retinal vascularization at the macula includes four different plexuses: the superficial (SCP—top line), middle (MCP—second from top), deep (DCP—third from top) retinal capillary plexuses, and choriocapillaris (CC—bottom). OCTA images are mainly displayed with *en face* visualization (images on the right) which is obtained by segmenting the volumetric OCTA scans at specific depths. Using this strategy, the flow data within any slab, whose boundaries are red in the left images, are summed or projected into a two-dimensional *en face* image that can be viewed and studied

The generation of 2-dimensional OCTA *en face* images can be performed with different methods. The "maximal intensity projection" approach projects the maximal intensity pixel from each column onto a flat two-dimensional summary. While the advantage of this strategy is that it has more sensitivity for detecting smaller vessels and subtle flow, it may also yield more noise. Another approach to obtain the

2-dimensional OCTA images is through the use of an "average intensity projection", which is less susceptible to noise but may be less sensitive for small vessels.

Notably, while most OCTA studies use the *en face* visualization of the images, this visualization is more susceptible to segmentation artifacts, especially in eyes with retinal and choroidal pathologies [9]. For this reason, cross-sectional OCTA scans may be helpful for studying these eyes. These OCTA B-scans typically depict flow as a pseudocolor overlay on the grayscale structural OCT image.

4.3.3 Comparison with Previous Dye-Based Imaging Techniques

Fluorescein angiography (FA) and indocyanine green angiography (ICGA) have traditionally been considered the gold standard for clinical assessment of the retinal and choroidal vasculature *in vivo*. Even though dye administration is generally safe in patients, serious allergic reactions may occur, and these techniques are considered invasive and require considerable patient cooperation. In contrast, OCTA provides non-invasive assessment of the retinal and choroidal vasculatures [10]. Moreover, OCTA has the additional advantage of depth-resolution with improved visualization of the deeper vascular plexuses. Despite these limitations, dye-based imaging provides other advantages including dynamic estimation of dye transit and dye leakage in diseases affecting the blood-retinal barrier (e.g. diabetic retinopathy).

In addition, FA has some limitations in the assessment of the retinal vessels, given that visibility of the capillaries is lower with increasing distance from the fovea and for smaller vessels [11]. Furthermore, FA has significant deficiencies in the visualization of the choroid, given that fluorescein is a small molecule which rapidly leaks from the choroidal vessels. In contrast to FA, ICGA grants an improved visualization of the choroid. ICGA employs an alternative dye that is significantly (99%) bound to plasma lipoproteins thus limiting CC leakage [12]. Furthermore, ICGA uses a longer excitation wavelength and emits fluorescence in the 800–860 nm range, allowing a more efficient penetration through RPE and other ocular pigments [13].

4.3.4 Limitations and Artifacts

Imaging the vascular plexuses with OCTA may also be challenging because of different artifacts which may alter their visualization.

Low signal strength may significantly affect the quality of the OCTA images. The ratio between the signal (signal to noise ratio), which is the information component dependent on the imaged tissue, and the non-signal component (or noise), is a mathematical relationship which may influence the image quality. As an example, media opacities may reduce the signal to noise ratio by decreasing the OCT signal. A decreased signal to noise ratio leads to an adjustment of the grayscale range with a consequent increase in image noise and artifactitious OCTA signal. Averaging of multiple *en face* OCTA images may reduce noise and improve vessels' continuity, as well as significantly improve qualitative and quantitative measurements [14, 15].

False OCTA signals may be also generated by movement of the eye, head, or body [16]. Recent advancements in eye tracking systems have significantly decreased the impact of these artifacts in OCTA imaging. Using eye tracking, the retina position is rapidly tracked and corrective movements are applied.

Segmentation error represents a significant and recurring OCTA artifact [9, 16]. As discussed above, *en face* OCTA images are displayed by locating two boundaries throughout the retinal and/or choroidal structure and vessels are therefore visualized using different available processes. These boundaries may be set by selecting pre-defined layers which can be differentiated on the basis of reflectivity, texture, or other attributes. The main problem with this strategy is that these parameters used to differentiate retinal and choroidal layers may be significantly modified in pathological conditions [9]. As an example, the automatic segmentation of vascular layers may be challenging in eyes with myopia, even in the absence of chorioretinal complications. Of note, many OCTA devices employ software enabling manual correction of segmentation errors and propagation of corrections throughout multiple B-scans, but this process may result extremely time-consuming.

Projection artifacts, also known as decorrelation tails, may affect the visualization of the deeper vascular layers (ICP, DCP, and CC). In order to image the deeper structures, the OCT beam passes through the retinal layers, and vessels included in these layers may be falsely detected in the deeper layers, even in the absence of real flow in these slabs. Since the transmitted light diffuses through flowing blood, the deeper layers are thus reached by fluctuating light which can create a decorrelation between two successive B-scans at the same location. The projection artifact may be more prominent at high reflective layers, such as the RPE. In addition, projection artifacts from the retina are attenuated by the RPE, thereby limiting this confounding problem in the superficial choroid, at the expense of overall loss of signal. Several strategies have been evolved to limit projection artifacts [17, 18]. One of the easiest strategies is to subtract the SCP OCTA *en face* image from the deeper layers. Using this strategy, the bright projections from the superficial retinal vessels are replaced with dark versions of the vessels. However, unintentional removal of real blood flow from the resultant images can represent a relevant limit of this strategy.

Shadowing artifact represents another important artifact in the visualization of the deeper vascular layers. This artifact occurs when the OCT beam is attenuated or blocked thereby impeding its passage to the deeper layers of the retina/choroid. This may occur due to the presence of different structures, including vitreous opacities, hemorrhage, and drusen. SS-OCTA systems have partially overcome this limitation, since a longer wavelength limits attenuation from media opacities and improves penetration into the deeper retinal and choroidal layers. However, this light is known to be more scattered by water absorption in the vitreous [19–21].

OCTA is still limited in the visualization of the larger vessels of the choroid. This limitation is secondary to the signal attenuation due to scattering by the RPE and by the CC vessels [2]. As a result, choroidal vessels are typically displayed as silhouettes with complete loss of signal at greater depths. These limitations have been partially resolved with ultrahigh-speed SS OCTA instruments [22]. A novel research device with a Fourier-domain mode-locked laser system operating with a 1.7-MHz sweep rate (1.7 million A-scans/s), at a 1065-nm center wavelength, has recently been used to image the choroid [23]. This instrument was demonstrated to obtain an improved visualization of the medium and larger-sized choroidal vessels. Of note, this device was demonstrated to be even better than ICGA in the visualization of the medium-sized choroidal vessels. An improved visualization of medium-sized choroidal vessels may also be obtained in highly myopic eyes using the projection artifacts in the sclera [24].

4.3.5 OCTA Quantitative Metrics

Various different commercial devices use different algorithms to obtain OCTA images and quantifiable metrics applied to these images were demonstrated to be not comparable between devices [25]. However, a number studies have used quantitative variables to quantify the retinal and choroidal vasculature with OCTA.

OCTA *en face* images are composed of pixels which may be in a grayscale range of possible values from 0 to 255, where typically 0 is taken to be black, and 255 is taken to be white. In order to obtain quantitative analysis, a threshold may be applied to these images. Thresholding is used to create binary images (in which pixels over the applied threshold are displayed as white and pixels falling under the threshold are shown as black) from grayscale images. Moreover, thresholding may be obtained using different methodologies that can significantly influence the final quantification [26]. The binarized OCTA images may be also skeletonized, in order to obtain an image in which vessels are visualized as tracings of 1 pixel in width [27].

Remarkably, Rabiolo et al. demonstrated that the quantification of retinal perfusion is strictly dependent on the OCTA *en face* image's size [28].

Binarized and skeletonized OCTA images may be used to provide different quantitative metrics (Fig. 4.2):

- The *perfusion density* can be calculated as a unitless proportion of the number of pixels over the threshold divided by the total number of pixels in the analyzed area on the binarized image.
- The *vessel length density* is defined as the total length of the perfused vasculature divided by the total number of pixels in the analyzed area on the skeletonized image.
- The *vessel diameter index*, which represents the average vessel caliber, may be calculated by dividing the total vessel area in the binarized image by the total vessel length in the skeletonized image [29].
- The *fractal dimension*, which is a mathematical parameter that describes the complexity of a biological structure [30].

Previous studies on the CC have investigated the distribution, size and percentage of flow voids (also called signal voids), which are small dark regions that

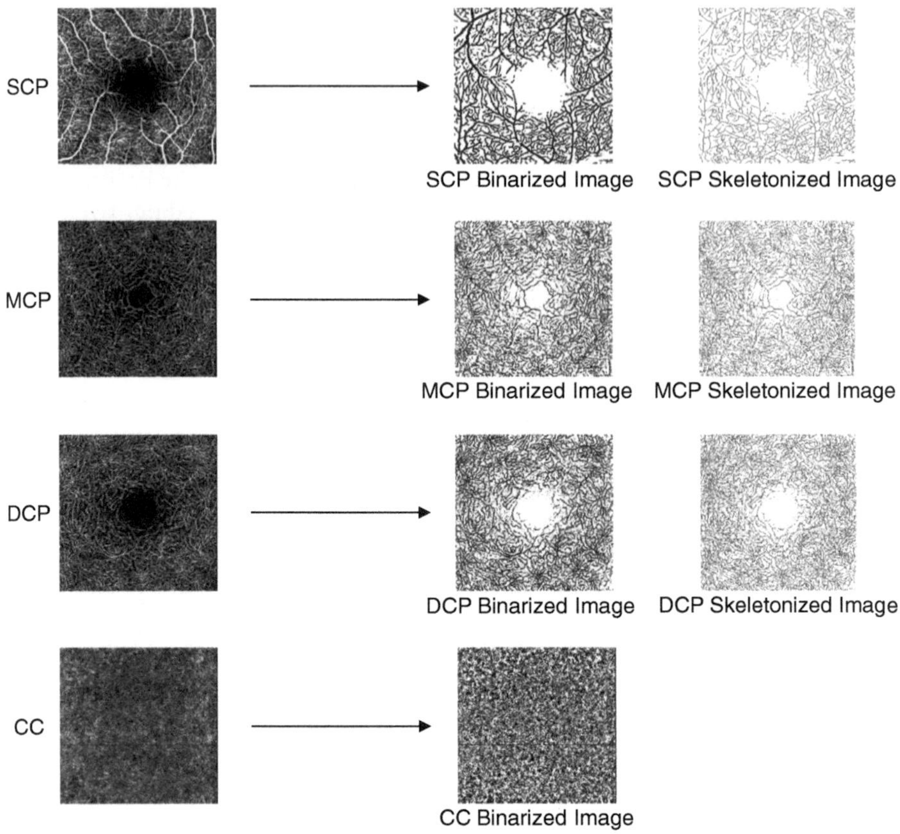

Fig. 4.2 Main OCTA metrics to quantify the retinal and choroidal vasculature. The OCTA images can be thresholded to obtain binarized and skeletonized images which are utilized to provide a quantitative analysis

alternate with granular bright areas, the latter thought to represent CC flow, and the former more likely to be secondary to CC vascular dropout or flow reduction [2, 31, 32].

4.4 Evaluation of the Vascular Layers with OCTA

4.4.1 The Retinal Vessels

OCTA has significantly improved our knowledge on the organization of the retinal vessels. The retinal vascularization may be separated into the following plexuses: the superficial capillary plexus, the middle capillary plexus, the deep capillary plexus, and the radial peripapillary capillary plexus (Fig. 4.1) [33–36]. The RPCP is unique in that it is mainly located within the superficial nerve fiber layer surrounding the optic disc and is therefore discussed separately.

Since the introduction of OCTA, a number of models have been proposed regarding connections among the retinal vascular plexuses [35–38].

The SCP is a dense meshwork of vessels accommodated in the retinal ganglion cell layer (GCL) [24]. The small capillaries arise from SCP arterioles and drain into SCP venules. The GCL slab enhanced visualization of the capillary-free zones around the arteries and arterioles and helped to differentiate arterial and venous systems [38]. Using OCTA, SCP arterioles were demonstrated to be located more superficially than SCP venules [36]. The SCP capillaries were shown to be arranged in a centripetal pattern in the macula and to converge on the parafoveal capillary ring [35]. In the periphery, the superior and inferior circulations converge in an interlaced comb pattern [35].

The SCP capillaries are connected with the other two layers of vessels at the inner plexiform layer/inner nuclear layer (IPL/INL) border (MCP) and inner nuclear layer/outer plexiform layer (INL/OPL) border (DCP). While the MCP colocalizes with the bipolar cell processes and amacrine cells, the DCP colocalizes with horizontal cells. These two plexuses are thus close to the high oxygen demand synapses of the IPL and OPL, respectively. The capillaries of the MCP and DCP have a lobular configuration without directional preference within their laminar planes [35]. Because the middle and deep capillary plexuses consist of capillaries of uniform size and are separated by only a small distance, they are often grouped together as the deep vascular complex (DVC).

Around the foveal avascular zone (FAZ), these three retinal capillary plexuses converge to form a single parafoveal capillary loop and collectively define the borders of the FAZ [35].

Recently, using higher axial resolution OCTA technology, Nesper and Fawzi [36] identified distinct vascular connections from large-caliber arterioles and venules in the SCP to each of the three retinal capillary plexuses in healthy subjects. This organization accounts for the high oxygen demand of the plexiform layers that need highly oxygenated (arteriolar) blood in the MCP and DCP. Furthermore, they provided further evidence for the presence of vortices in the DCP, these draining into conduits which are straightly connected to venules in the SCP. Interestingly, collateral vessels crossing the horizontal raphe were identified at the DCP level. These crossing vessels were speculated to represent an alternative pathway of least resistance in the event of occlusive diseases. Nesper and Fawzi's observations would appear to support the theory that each of the three plexuses has its own arteriolar supply and venular drainage, which would theoretically allow each neurovascular unit to have independent control of its vascular supply under physiologic conditions.

This parallel organization of the retinal circulation suggested by Nesper and Fawzi has been challenged by Freund and Sarraf [37] who have suggested a predominantly series-based arrangement of the retinal circulation, with the bulk of the venous drainage of the retina originating at the level of the DCP. The presence of collateral vessels in the setting of retinal venous occlusive disease at the level of the DCP, but not at the SCP, would appear to support this contention.

Recently, using a full-spectrum probabilistic OCTA with a novel algorithm for 3-D projection artifact removal (PAR), Hirano and colleagues [39] investigated the retinal microcirculation. Since full-spectrum OCTA algorithms improve axial resolution, the authors provided important insights into the 3-D architecture of the retinal vasculature. Remarkably, unlike the MCP and DCP, the location of the SVP significantly varied among retinal regions. In all parafoveal regions tested, the SVP was featured by a small peak at the NFL-GCL junction and a larger, broader peak within the GCL. Conversely, the perifovea had only a single SVP peak. Furthermore, this peak was closer to the ILM in the perifoveal nasal, superior, and inferior quadrants. The authors presumed that this displacement was secondary to the thicker NFL associated with the arcuate and papillo-macular bundles in these regions.

4.4.2 The Radial Peripapillary Capillary Plexus

The nerve fibers in the retina are unmyelinated and they thus require large amounts of energy to maintain ion concentration gradients [40]. The retinal nerve fiber layer contains the radial peripapillary capillary network to supply oxygen and metabolites to the optic nerve axons. The RPCP is composed of long, straight vessels with few apparent feed points and anastomoses [38]. These capillaries arise from peripapillary retinal arterioles, extend radially from the optic disc in parallel with the nerve fiber axons, farthest along the temporal arcades [41].

Since OCTA provides a reliable visualization of the capillaries in the optic nerve head and peripapillary regions, OCTA has been extensively used to characterize the RPCP in healthy eyes and to assess microvascular changes occurring in various optic nerve and neurological disorders. Using widefield OCTA, Jia and colleagues [42] examined the RPCP flow characteristics in 10 eyes of 10 healthy patients and illustrated an association between perfusion in this vascular network and nerve fiber layer thickness. The perfusion of these regions may thus serve as a surrogate measure for the metabolic activity of the ganglion cell axons. RPCP measurements have the potential of providing key functional information in disease processes such as glaucoma and other optic neuropathies.

4.4.3 The Choriocapillaris

Given that previous imaging techniques have significant limitations for the evaluation of the CC, OCTA has evolved into a key technology for investigation of the CC [2, 31, 32].

En face OCTA images of the CC are generated by segmenting a thin slab with a thickness of 10–30-μm starting at Bruch's membrane. In these OCTA CC *en face* images, small dark regions (called flow voids or signal voids) [43, 44] alternate with granular bright areas, the latter thought to represent CC flow, and the former more likely to be secondary to CC vascular dropout or flow reduction [44]. Signal voids seem to represent the inter-capillary spaces which have been characterized in histological studies on the CC [45].

However, histological images of the CC are slightly similar to the OCTA versions. With more advancing OCTA technology, we expect to have an improved and more truthful visualization of the CC. However, an enhanced visualization of the CC network may be even obtained with commercially available devices using multiple *en face* image averaging [46]. The registration and averaging of sequential *en face* OCTA images was shown to transform the poorly defined granular appearance of the CC displayed with OCTA to a morphologic pattern that more closely represented the meshwork pattern observed on histology. Notably, not only did averaging improve CC visualization, but more precise quantitative measures of the CC were obtained.

In the CC OCTA images, the number and size of the signal voids have been shown to follow a mathematical relationship of a power law: log [number of signal voids] equals a scaling factor times the log [size of signal voids] plus a constant [47]. The presence of a power law relationship presumes that the CC is characterized by a propensity for capillary segments to be affected in the vicinity of an already nonfunctional segment.

4.5 Conclusions

OCTA is an evolving technology that has significantly enhanced the visualization of the retinal and choroidal vessels. However, major limitations still affect its widespread application. The employment of OCTA to study ocular and systemic diseases, along with advancements of this technology, will certainly expand our knowledge of optic nerve and neurological disorders.

Acknowledgements None.

References

1. Spaide RF, Fujimoto JG, Waheed NK, Sadda SR, Staurenghi G. Optical coherence tomography angiography. Prog Retin Eye Res. 2018;64:1–55. https://doi.org/10.1016/j.preteyeres.2017.11.003.
2. Borrelli E, Sarraf D, Freund KB, Sadda SR. OCT angiography and evaluation of the choroid and choroidal vascular disorders. Prog Retin Eye Res. 2018; https://doi.org/10.1016/j.preteyeres.2018.07.002.
3. Kiel JW. The ocular circulation. Colloq Ser Integr Syst Physiol Mol Funct. 2011; https://doi.org/10.4199/C00024ED1V01Y201012ISP012.
4. Tan PEZ, Yu PK, Balaratnasingam C, et al. Quantitative confocal imaging of the retinal microvasculature in the human retina. Investig Ophthalmol Vis Sci. 2012; https://doi.org/10.1167/iovs.12-10017.
5. Chan G, Balaratnasingam C, Yu PK, et al. Quantitative morphometry of perifoveal capillary networks in the human retina. Investig Ophthalmol Vis Sci. 2012; https://doi.org/10.1167/iovs.12-10265.

6. Olver JM. Functional anatomy of the choroidal circulation: methyl methacrylate casting of human choroid. Eye. 1990;4(2):262–72. https://doi.org/10.1038/eye.1990.38.
7. De Stefano ME, Mugnaini E. Fine structure of the choroidal coat of the avian eye. Vascularization, supporting tissue and innervation. Anat Embryol (Berl). 1997;195(5):393–418. https://doi.org/10.1007/s004290050060.
8. Spaide R, Fujimoto JG, Waheed NK, Sadda SR, Staurenghi G. Optical coherence tomography angiography. Prog Retin Eye Res. 2017; https://doi.org/10.1016/j.preteyeres.2017.11.003.
9. Ghasemi Falavarjani K, Al-Sheikh M, Akil H, Sadda SR, et al. Br J Ophthalmol. 2016; https://doi.org/10.1136/bjophthalmol-2016-309104.
10. Jia Y, Tan O, Tokayer J, et al. Split-spectrum amplitude-decorrelation angiography with optical coherence tomography. Opt Express. 2012;20(4):4710–25. http://www.pubmedcentral.nih.gov/articlerender.fcgi?artid=3381646&tool=pmcentrez&rendertype=abstract. Accessed 12 Mar 2016.
11. Weinhaus RS, Burke JM, Delori FC, Snodderly DM. Comparison of fluorescein angiography with microvascular anatomy of macaque retinas. Exp Eye Res. 1995; https://doi.org/10.1016/S0014-4835(95)80053-0.
12. Mames RN, Shady-McCoy L, Guy J. Central retinal and posterior ciliary artery occlusion after particle embolization of the external carotid artery system. Ophthalmology. 1991;98(4):527–31. https://doi.org/10.1016/S0161-6420(91)32261-9.
13. Ozawa G. Fundus fluorescein and indocyanine green angiography: a textbook and atlas, vol. 86. 2009. https://doi.org/10.1097/OPX.0b013e3181b31a29.
14. Uji A, Balasubramanian S, Lei J, Baghdasaryan E, Al-Sheikh M, Sadda SR. Impact of multiple en face image averaging on quantitative assessment from optical coherence tomography angiography images. Ophthalmology. 2017; https://doi.org/10.1016/j.ophtha.2017.02.006.
15. Uji A, Balasubramanian S, Lei J, et al. Multiple enface image averaging for enhanced optical coherence tomography angiography imaging. Acta Ophthalmol. 2018; https://doi.org/10.1111/aos.13740.
16. Spaide RF, Fujimoto JG, Waheed NK. Image artifacts in optical coherence tomography angiography. Retina. 2015;35(11):2163–80. https://doi.org/10.1097/IAE.0000000000000765.
17. Long AW, Zhang J, Granick S, Ferguson AL. Machine learning assembly landscapes from particle tracking data. Soft Matter. 2015;11(41):8141–53. https://doi.org/10.1039/C5SM01981H.
18. Zhang M, Hwang TS, Campbell JP, et al. Projection-resolved optical coherence tomographic angiography. Biomed Opt Express. 2016;7(3):816. https://doi.org/10.1364/BOE.7.000816.
19. Povazay B, Bizheva K, Hermann B, et al. Enhanced visualization of choroidal vessels using ultrahigh resolution ophthalmic OCT at 1050 nm. Opt Express. 2003;11(17):1980–6. https://doi.org/10.1364/OE.11.001980.
20. Považay B, Hermann B, Unterhuber A, et al. Three-dimensional optical coherence tomography at 1050 nm versus 800 nm in retinal pathologies: enhanced performance and choroidal penetration in cataract patients. J Biomed Opt. 2007;12(4):041211. https://doi.org/10.1117/1.2773728.
21. Unterhuber A, Povazay B, Hermann B, Sattmann H, Chavez-Pirson A, Drexler W. In vivo retinal optical coherence tomography at 1040 nm - enhanced penetration into the choroid. Opt Express. 2005;13(9):3252. https://doi.org/10.1364/OPEX.13.003252.
22. Choi W, Mohler KJ, Potsaid B, et al. Choriocapillaris and choroidal microvasculature imaging with ultrahigh speed OCT angiography. PLoS One. 2013;8(12):e81499. https://doi.org/10.1371/journal.pone.0081499.
23. Poddar R, Migacz JV, Schwartz DM, Werner JS, Gorczynska I. Challenges and advantages in widefield optical coherence tomography angiography imaging of the human retinal and choroidal vasculature at 1.7-MHz A-scan rate. J Biomed Opt. 2017;20(10):1–14. https://doi.org/10.1117/1.JBO.22.10.106018.
24. Maruko I, Kawano T, Arakawa H, Hasegawa T, Iida T. Visualizing large choroidal blood flow by subtraction of the choriocapillaris projection artifacts in swept source optical coherence tomography angiography in normal eyes. Sci Rep. 2018;8(1):15694. https://doi.org/10.1038/s41598-018-34102-6.

25. Corvi F, Pellegrini M, Erba S, Cozzi M, Staurenghi G, Giani A. Reproducibility of vessel density, fractal dimension, and foveal avascular zone using 7 different optical coherence tomography angiography devices. Am J Ophthalmol. 2018; https://doi.org/10.1016/j.ajo.2017.11.011.
26. Rabiolo A, Gelormini F, Sacconi R, et al. Comparison of methods to quantify macular and peripapillary vessel density in optical coherence tomography angiography. PLoS One. 2018;13(10):e0205773. https://doi.org/10.1371/journal.pone.0205773.
27. Durbin MK, An L, Shemonski ND, et al. Quantification of retinal microvascular density in optical coherence tomographic angiography images in diabetic retinopathy. JAMA Ophthalmol. 2017;135(4):370. https://doi.org/10.1001/jamaophthalmol.2017.0080.
28. Rabiolo A, Gelormini F, Marchese A, et al. Macular perfusion parameters in different angiocube sizes: does the size matter in quantitative optical coherence tomography angiography? Investig Ophthalmol Vis Sci. 2018; https://doi.org/10.1167/iovs.17-22359.
29. Borrelli E, Balasubramanian S, Triolo G, Barboni P, Sadda SR, Sadun AA. Topographic macular microvascular changes and correlation with visual loss in chronic Leber hereditary optic neuropathy. Am J Ophthalmol. 2018;192:217–28. https://doi.org/10.1016/j.ajo.2018.05.029.
30. Zahid S, Dolz-Marco R, Freund KB, et al. Fractal dimensional analysis of optical coherence tomography angiography in eyes with diabetic retinopathy. Investig Ophthalmol Vis Sci. 2016; https://doi.org/10.1167/iovs.16-19656.
31. Sacconi R, Borrelli E, Corbelli E, et al. Quantitative changes in the ageing choriocapillaris as measured by swept source optical coherence tomography angiography. Br J Ophthalmol. 2018; https://doi.org/10.1136/bjophthalmol-2018-313004.
32. Nassisi M, Baghdasaryan E, Tepelus T, Asanad S, Borrelli E, Sadda SR. Topographic distribution of choriocapillaris flow deficits in healthy eyes. PLoS One. 2018;13(11):e0207638. https://doi.org/10.1371/journal.pone.0207638.
33. Savastano MC, Lumbroso B, Rispoli M. In vivo characterization of retinal vascularization morphology using optical coherence tomography angiography. Retina. 2015; https://doi.org/10.1097/IAE.0000000000000635.
34. Garrity ST, Paques M, Gaudric A, Freund KB, Sarraf D. Considerations in the understanding of venous outflow in the retinal capillary plexus. Retina. 2017; https://doi.org/10.1097/IAE.0000000000001784.
35. Campbell JP, Zhang M, Hwang TS, et al. Detailed vascular anatomy of the human retina by projection-resolved optical coherence tomography angiography. Sci Rep. 2017; https://doi.org/10.1038/srep42201.
36. Nesper PL, Fawzi AA. Human parafoveal capillary vascular anatomy and connectivity revealed by optical coherence tomography angiography. Investig Ophthalmol Vis Sci. 2018; https://doi.org/10.1167/iovs.18-24710.
37. Freund KB, Sarraf D, Leong BCS, Garrity ST, Vupparaboina KK, Dansingani KK. Association of optical coherence tomography angiography of collaterals in retinal vein occlusion with major venous outflow through the deep vascular complex. JAMA Ophthalmol. 2018; https://doi.org/10.1001/jamaophthalmol.2018.3586.
38. Muraoka Y, Uji A, Ishikura M, Iida Y, Ooto S, Tsujikawa A. Segmentation of the four-layered retinal vasculature using high-resolution optical coherence tomography angiography reveals the microcirculation unit. Invest Opthalmol Vis Sci. 2018;59(15):5847. https://doi.org/10.1167/iovs.18-25301.
39. Hirano T, Chanwimol K, Weichsel J, Tepelus T, Sadda S. Distinct retinal capillary plexuses in normal eyes as observed in optical coherence tomography angiography axial profile analysis. Sci Rep. 2018; https://doi.org/10.1038/s41598-018-27536-5.
40. Carelli V, La Morgia C, Sadun AA. Mitochondrial dysfunction in optic neuropathies: animal models and therapeutic options. Curr Opin Neurol. 2013; https://doi.org/10.1097/WCO.0b013e32835c5f0b.
41. Henkind P. Radial peripapillary capillaries of the retina. I. Anatomy: human and comparative. Br J Ophthalmol. 1967; https://doi.org/10.1136/bjo.51.2.115.

42. Jia Y, Simonett JM, Wang J, et al. Wide-field OCT angiography investigation of the relationship between radial peripapillary capillary plexus density and nerve fiber layer thickness. Investig Ophthalmol Vis Sci. 2017; https://doi.org/10.1167/iovs.17-22593.
43. Choi W, Moult EM, Waheed NK, et al. Ultrahigh-speed, swept-source optical coherence tomography angiography in nonexudative age-related macular degeneration with geographic atrophy. Ophthalmology. 2015;122(12):2532–44. https://doi.org/10.1016/j.ophtha.2015.08.029.
44. Spaide RF. Choriocapillaris signal voids in maternally inherited diabetes and deafness and in pseudoxanthoma elasticum. Retina. 2017;1 https://doi.org/10.1097/IAE.0000000000001497.
45. Seddon JM, McLeod DS, Bhutto IA, et al. Histopathological insights into choroidal vascular loss in clinically documented cases of age-related macular degeneration. JAMA Ophthalmol. 2016; https://doi.org/10.1001/jamaophthalmol.2016.3519.
46. Uji A, Balasubramanian S, Lei J, Baghdasaryan E, Al-Sheikh M, Sadda SR. Choriocapillaris imaging using multiple en face optical coherence tomography angiography image averaging. JAMA Ophthalmol. 2017; https://doi.org/10.1001/jamaophthalmol.2017.3904.
47. Spaide RF. Choriocapillaris flow features follow a power law distribution: implications for characterization and mechanisms of disease progression. Am J Ophthalmol. 2016;170:58–67. https://doi.org/10.1016/j.ajo.2016.07.023.

Seeing the Brain Through the Eye: What Is Next for Neuroimaging and Neurology Applications

5

Delia Cabrera DeBuc, Gábor Márk Somfai, Gabriella Szatmáry, Edmund Arthur, Jorge A. Jimenez, Carlos Mendoza-Santiesteban, and Andrzej Grzybowski

5.1 Introduction

"*We can only see what we expect to see*", or "*the eyes see what the mind knows*" by Johann Wolfgang von Goethe. These sayings highlight the fundamental challenge that we face in exploring the function of the mind while also confined by the limitations of the mind, through its major sensory input, vision. Increasing evidence suggests that the conditions of retinal morphology and microvascular network are indicators to a variety of cerebrovascular, neurodegenerative, psychiatric, and developmental diseases [1]. Visual function is indeed often affected in subjects with cerebrovascular and neurodegenerative diseases, including ocular motility abnormalities, visual loss, contrast sensitivity changes, and defects in color vision [1].

The changes of the retinal structure and microvasculature are seemingly correlated with neurodegenerative and cerebrovascular lesions, which in turn supports

D. Cabrera DeBuc (✉) · E. Arthur · C. Mendoza-Santiesteban
Bascom Palmer Eye Institute, University of Miami Miller School of Medicine, Miami, FL, USA
e-mail: dcabrera2@med.miami.edu; exa647@med.miami.edu; cxm1244@med.miami.edu

G. M. Somfai
Retinology Unit, Augenzentrum, Pallas Kliniken, Olten, Switzerland

Department of Ophthalmology, Semmelweis University, Budapest, Hungary

G. Szatmáry
Hattiesburg Clinic, Hattiesburg, MS, USA

J. A. Jimenez
University of Mississippi School of Medicine, Jackson, MS, USA
e-mail: jjimenez@umc.edu

A. Grzybowski
University of Warmia and Mazury, Olsztyn, Poland

Institute for Research in Ophthalmology, Poznań, Poland

A. Grzybowski, P. Barboni (eds.), *OCT and Imaging in Central Nervous System Diseases*, https://doi.org/10.1007/978-3-030-26269-3_5

the view that the retina may serve as a window to the brain. It can be postulated that retinal microvascular structure could be mirroring that of the brain while the substructure of the retina may be like the structure of the brain. Both features of the central nervous system (CNS) are difficult and costly to assess, whereas retinal imaging could provide a meaningful and low-cost means to provide surrogate markers for disease detection and disease management that could be valuable assets for the neurologists and general doctors at primary clinical care settings. In the long run, retinal imaging could replace or complement neuroimaging techniques and could contribute to a better understanding of disease etiology of cerebrovascular and neurodegenerative disorders.

The area of optical imaging of the retina is progressing rapidly, enabling the noninvasive quantitative and qualitative assessment and follow-up of the retina and its changes. Optical coherence tomography (OCT) is a noninvasive imaging technique routinely used in ophthalmology to visualize and quantify eye structures (e.g., retinal and corneal tissue). Considering the pathophysiological complexity of cerebrovascular and neurodegenerative diseases, the targets for surrogate markers should come from combined diagnostic modalities that could even facilitate the early screening efforts or the prediction of prognosis. Once these ophthalmic biomarkers are combined with the standard clinical toolkit used for the clinical workup of neurological changes in various CNS pathologies, a powerful clinical tool could be developed to reduce the otherwise heavy burden of these diseases.

In this chapter, we will give an overview of OCT as an emerging technology in neurology applications and express our view about how retinal imaging could serve the above goals and open a window, which could serve as a direct view to the brain.

5.2 Eye-Brain Connectome

Investigating the eye-brain connections may unravel the relationship between the connecting pathways of neurons in the brain and eye. This undertaking may help us to determine how vision impairment affects the brain, and facilitate a better explanation about how changes in the brain might influence the outcome of potential therapeutic approaches targeting vision restoration. Connectomics is the science to map out connections, extensively used in brain research to obtain its wiring diagram to better understand patterns in brain connectivity (Fig. 5.1) [2]. Interestingly, determining the circuit diagram of the retina, considering that a little piece of neural tissue such as the photoreceptor segments sense light and sends visual information to the brain, will be valuable to help to decode novel medical treatments yet undiscovered. Therefore, the idea that patients may respond to treatment differently based on how their eye-brain connections are wired and not only on the specific conditions of the eye disease is provocative and deserves attention.

Our understanding of the path the retinal neurons take to the primary visual cortex (V1) and the extrastriate areas has come a long way from early human cadaver and staining studies to a much sophisticated and audacious approach of tracing the path of each specific retinal location in the brain termed the human connectome project [3–6]. The audacious goal of these projects is to find the precise mapping of

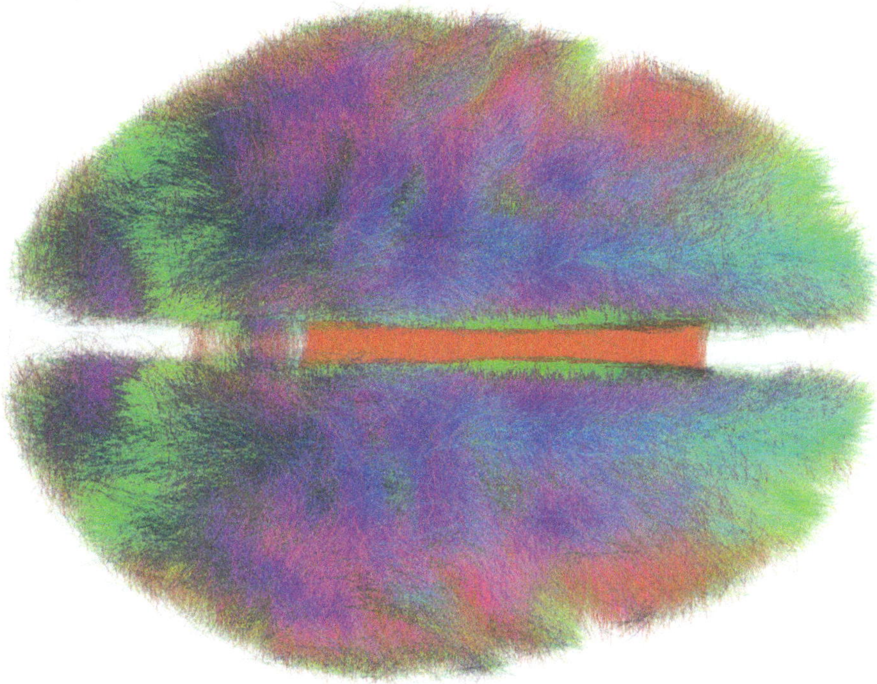

Fig. 5.1 Typical wiring diagram used in connectomics to better understand patterns in the brain connectivity (*image source labeled for reuse*: https://hu.wikipedia.org/wiki/Konnektom)

the retinal neural fibers in the brain that may help us to identify the corresponding brain locations of specific retinal locations with pathology in the eye. This mapping could be useful to investigate whether treatment of a specific retinal disease influences their unique brain locations [3–6]. For example, the connection between the eye and the brain is evident in parts of V1 not developed in amblyopia during the critical period of the infant eye development as certain parts of the retina are not stimulated by light (e.g., in deprivational amblyopia) and hence the corresponding points in the brain are not developed. The question of whether the visual areas in the brain are rewired and developed during vision therapy or when the cause of amblyopia such as refractive error, strabismus, and cataract is removed has been the focus of many researchers for decades [7]. The more peculiar question in this perspective is whether there is rewiring of the neurons in V1 and the extrastriate areas of the brain beyond the critical period of the infant eye development. The above questions are bolstered by the fact there is evidence in the literature that wearing customized therapeutic eyeglasses in a participant with refractive error reduces the deviations in the electroencephalogram (EEG) and the quantitative EEG recordings towards normative values [8]. Perhaps, this evidence may point researchers in the right direction of how the decline in vision affects the brain and how the changes in the brain may eventually affect the outcome of treatments aimed at restoring vision.

The human connectome project which also revolves around the eye-brain connectome has been the major focus of many researchers [4–6]. The audacious goal is to link every diseased point in the retina to a corresponding point in the brain, and this may be possible using advanced brain imaging modalities such as the Siemens 3T Prism Scanner, which is the most preferred MRI scanner for the human connectome project [4]. The idea is that these fine eye-brain connections will help optimize vision restoration treatments such as the Argus II implants for patients with Retinitis Pigmentosa (RP) and to investigate the effect of stem cell treatment for age-related macular degeneration (AMD) [4]. Both RP and AMD have been extensively investigated using OCT technology which may enrich the eye-brain connectome research quest by providing additional information on the retinal neural layers involved in such pathological eye conditions [9–12].

Also, it is well established in the literature that the mapping of the brain neurons (brain connectome) is disrupted in Alzheimer's disease (AD) [13]. Alzheimer's disease is the most common form of dementia and a public health burden as the life expectancy of the aged is increased. Although there are no current drugs to completely treat AD, there are anti-amyloid drugs that can slow the progression of the disease and hence the early detection of the disease is imperative. Classically AD is diagnosed when amyloid plaques and Tau proteins are seen in the brain and the cerebrospinal fluid respectively using expensive and invasive methods such as Positron Emission Tomography (PET) and spinal tap, respectively. The retina of the human eye thus offers a potential window to study AD as it can be imaged with noninvasive imaging modalities and hence aid in the early detection of the disease. Peripheral drusen are observed in the eyes of AD patients and may serve as a potential retinal biomarker for AD (Fig. 5.2) [14–21]. AD is classified by 3 stages including the preclinical, mild cognitive impairment (MCI, prodromal), and the cognitive impairment stages. Much research aimed towards detecting the disease in the MCI and preclinical stages is based on the idea that there is ongoing neurodegeneration occurring in the brain; however, there are no active corresponding symptoms. Perhaps, the human connectome project aimed at mapping the retina and brain will elucidate much better the potential of retinal biomarkers for early detection of AD.

As the human connectome project progresses with the advent of sophisticated brain mapping and imaging techniques, the specific location of each retinal pathology may be traced to a corresponding location in the brain. This project may improve our understanding of the effect of the use of therapeutic glasses on neural activities in the brain and help elucidate whether vision therapy treatment aid in the rewiring of brain neurons not developed during the critical period of the infant eye development. It may also help optimize current and future vision restoration treatments and improve our understanding of whether treatment modalities for eye diseases such as stem cell treatment has any effect on rewiring of the brain neurons in the visual cortex. It may also help improve our understanding of potential retinal biomarkers for the detection of AD and other neurodegenerative diseases such as PD and multiple sclerosis (MS). Perhaps; the next decade holds much excitement for our understanding of the above eye-brain connections as the human connectome project progresses.

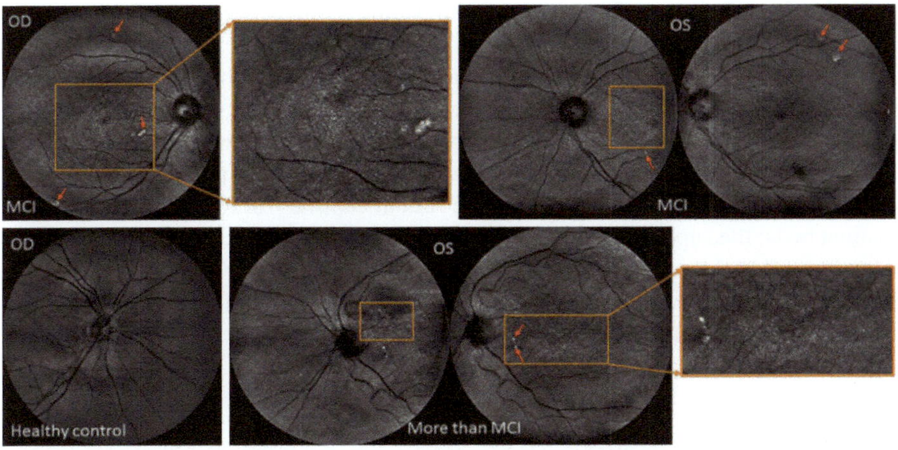

Fig. 5.2 Retinal topographical features observed in individuals with mild cognitive impairment. *Top row*: Central and nasal infrared light-images obtained from a female subject (79 years old) with MCI showing extramacular features such as drusen-like regions depicted by irregularly shaped bright spots in the periphery of the superior quadrant as well as with pigment dispersion in both eyes. *Bottom image*: *Right*—Central and nasal infrared light-images obtained from a female subject (81 years old) with MCI showing tortuous vessels, extramacular features such as drusen-like regions along with pigment dispersion in the left eye. *Left*—Nasal infrared-light image obtained from a healthy control (71 years old). All images were acquired with the EasyScan Unit (i-Optics Corporation, The Netherlands). The EasyScan camera is a dual color confocal SLO: Infrared (785 nm) and pure green (532 nm). The different colors are related to different penetration depth. The red arrows indicate the location of the drusen and white spots observed at extramacular locations. The ROIs enclosed by the orange rectangles indicate the locations where pigment dispersion was observed. The green light-image is reflected at the retinal nerve fiber layer (RNFL) showing the vascular structure up to the 4th bifurcation. The infrared light-image is reaching the choroidal vessel layer (*Image Courtesy of Delia Cabrera DeBuc, Ph.D.*)

5.3 Homology Between the Eye and Brain

The retina and optic nerve extend from the diencephalon during their embryonic development. Thus, both are part of the central nervous system (CNS). The retina contains various neural elements, which are interconnected with each other and play a crucial role in visual processing, beginning already at the retinal level [22]. The final processing stage occurs at the level of the retinal ganglion cells (RGCs), and the axons of many RGCs are collected in a bundle to form the optic nerve. The optic nerve, similarly to all fiber tracts in the CNS, is covered with oligodendrocyte-produced myelin and is being sheathed by all three meningeal layers.

However, it is not only the neural structure that shares similarities with the CNS [23, 24]. Like the CNS, the eye, and the retina has a unique relationship with the immune system that involves specialized barriers, such as the inner blood-retinal barrier, the retinal analog of the blood-brain barrier (BBB) [25]. This analogy is in great part due to the same radial pattern of vascularization during development that is driven in part by the expression of vascular endothelial growth factors (VEGFs) and other growth factors [25–28]. Accordingly, the retinal vasculature shares certain features with the vasculature of the brain because both networks must provide sufficient levels of oxygen and substrates to the large demand of the tissues supplied. It is known that cerebral capillary density mirrors the metabolic demand and activity of the given brain regions [29, 30]. Accordingly, retinal capillary density is greatest in the central, macular area, whereas the peripheral retina is practically avascular (Fig. 5.3). It is important to note that the retinal capillary networks consist of two distinct beds: the superficial capillary layer in the ganglion cell layer (GCL), and the deeper capillary layer at the level of the outer plexiform layer (OPL) (Fig. 5.3) [31]. Interestingly, these capillaries are smaller than cerebral capillaries, with a diameter of approximately 5 μm [32, 33].

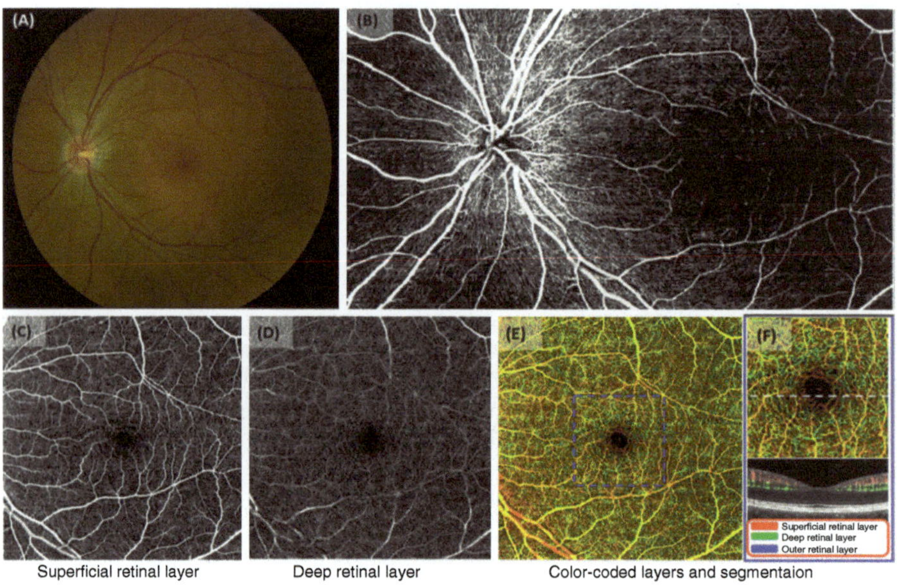

Fig. 5.3 Details of the retinal microvasculature. (**a**) Fundus photograph of a healthy eye allowing visualization of the entire posterior pole of the ocular fundus, including the optic nerve, the macula, and the major retinal vessels. (**b**) Montage of images of the nerve fiber layer obtained by wide-field optical coherence tomography based microangiography (OMAG) for the same eye. Note the radial pericapillary network within the RNFL. (**c**) The superficial retinal layer slab contains the vascular network within the ganglion cell layer (GCL) and the outer plexiform layer (OPL). Both the arcade vessels and the fine capillaries are shown. (**d**) The deep retinal layer demonstrates deeper capillary network. (**e**) The whole retinal layer slab composed of the superficial retinal layer, the deep retinal layer, and the outer retinal layer allows visualization of the shallow, intermediate, and deep retinal capillary plexuses. Different colors identify various levels of the retina. (**f**) The magnified image of the central macula (identified as in the blue box from (**e**)). The cross-sectional flow image of the area marked with a white dashed line on the magnified OMAG image. Blood flow detected in the superficial retinal layer, the deep retinal layer, and the outer retinal layer (ORL) in red, green, blue; respectively. Note that flow can be detected in the ORL (*Images adapted with permission from Scientific Reports 6, Article number: 22017 (2016)*)

It is noteworthy that retinal blood vessels are so-called end arteries and arterioles having no anastomotic connections, and thus occlusion of these vessels leads to infarction and atrophy of the inner retina [34]. In contrast, cerebral microvasculature, similarly to most human organs (except the heart), has enough collateral vessels [32]. Also, unlike cerebral arterioles, retinal arterioles often show sharp, 90° branching patterns allowing substantial plasma skimming, i.e. separation of plasma and cellular elements of blood, providing flow-perfusion through the smaller size of capillaries in the retina [32].

As mentioned above, the blood-retina barrier (BRB) is very similar to its cerebral counterpart, protecting the neural tissue of the retina from various large molecules and hematogenous cells. The BRB consists of both mechanical (tight junctional complexes) and metabolic components (metabolic transport acting as a metabolic barrier), similarly to the BBB [35, 36]. Early ultrastructural studies in both brain and retinal vessels showed the presence of caveolae (also called plasmalemma vesicles) and specific membrane enzymes at the abluminal plasma membrane of endothelial cells. These vesicles are static structures, facilitating the transport of small ions and solutes across the BRB and BBB. The number of vesicles and their polarity are similar in retinal and cerebral microvessels and likely contribute to their barriers, further supporting the idea that the two systems resemble each other [37].

The micro-vessels of the retina contain non-fenestrated endothelial cells and pericytes, both playing an important role in the maintenance of the BRB [31]. Also, the retinal microvasculature includes many perivascular end-feet (also called astrocytic processes) that are actively involved in the regulation of barrier properties and the release of various pericyte-derived factors, which also influence angiogenesis, stabilize micro-vessels and contribute to vasomotor control and neurovascular coupling [31, 38–40].

Finally, because both organs are enclosed in hard capsules, both cerebral and the retinal microcirculation have mechanisms to control vascular resistance in the face of changing systemic blood pressure (and flow) to maintain a relatively constant blood flow called autoregulation [41]. Like the brain, in the eye, the autoregulation is supported by the retinal pericytes and the vascular smooth muscles, in part by the myogenic and perhaps flow sensitive mechanisms [42, 43]. Nevertheless, locally there is still sufficient room for metabolic factors to couple regulation of blood flow to regional neuronal activity—neurovascular coupling [44, 45]. Indeed, the temporal retina that contains the macula has a greater blood flow compared to the nasal retina, reflecting the differences in metabolic activity [46]. It is worth noting that both the retina and the brain are non-homogeneous organs frequently exhibiting similar microvascular pathology suggesting that both bodies undergo similar disease developments.

Although there is no clear evidence regarding a neurogenic control of blood flow in the retina, there are data on the neurogenic control of cerebral blood flow (CBF). Under normal physiological conditions gas, chemical and metabolic vasomotor controls are dominant in the brain; whereas in severely challenging circumstances, such as delayed cerebral ischemia following subarachnoidal hemorrhage, these local mechanisms are suppressed, increasing the relative importance of neurogenic, sympathetic control of CBF [47].

5.4 OCT Challenges in Neuroimaging

The importance and challenges of exploring the function of the brain is highlighted by the concerted efforts of scientists around the world and huge financial investments like the Human Connectome Project and Allen Brain Atlas [48, 49]. It is of utmost importance to be mindful of the major technical and clinical limitations of OCT and to use OCT-based imaging judiciously, correlating it continuously with the clinical findings. Therefore, it is helpful to consider its challenges by comparing it to the most frequently used neuro-imaging modality, MRI. As future technological advances translate from bench to bedside, it is critical to bear in mind the limitations of these tools.

5.4.1 Challenges of OCT as a Neuro-Imaging Tool Using the MRI Simile

Challenges of optical coherence tomography-based imaging can be divided into technical and clinical (Table 5.1). The technical aspect is defined by the laws of physics and this has been reviewed by several excellent publications [50–53]. Therefore, this will only be reviewed briefly here and the emphasis will be placed on the clinical scenarios where expectations from OCT-based imaging are reasonable but still pending.

The first challenge is to become more familiar with the wide spectrum of pre-disease neuro-retinal findings that potentially affect OCT measurements after disease onset, so as not to label a "normal variant" as abnormal. Secondly, to understand the relevance of eye structural and functional findings in both health and disease of the brain. Because understanding the normal spectrum is a prerequisite to disentangle disease states, we must first better define the former to tackle the latter.

Presently, there are several unknown physiological variables that limit understanding cause and effect relationships between retinal measurements and brain states. For example, inability to determine the translaminar gradient across the lamina cribrosa due to the invasiveness of intracranial pressure (ICP) measurements results in uncertainty of its direct and indirect effect on OCT measurements [54]. Recently, promising MRI-based techniques in patients with idiopathic intracranial hypertension (IIH) have been described for indirect measurement of ICP [55, 56]. Additionally, another mechanical factor that likely affects RNFL, and perhaps ganglion cell complex (GCC: GCL-IPL) thickness, is repetitive traction at the optic nerve head during eye movements, which has been implicated to cause peripapillary temporal choroidal atrophy and possibly normal tension glaucoma [57].

Furthermore, there is lack of information on *anatomical* variables due to great inter-individual variability in the number of retinal ganglion cells, which is estimated to vary between 0.7 to 1.5 million in the human retina [58]. Moreover, there could be structure and function discrepancy in the spectrum of normality, exemplified by the so-called normal neuroanatomical variants or incidentalomas on MRI brain scan, such as pineal cysts or enlarged cisterna magna that are often clinically

Table 5.1 Challenges of OCT: technical and clinical with risk of misinterpretation

Technical challenges	Comments
Reduced signal strength due to media opacity and operator dependence	Example: dry eyes, cataracts
Truncation due to decentering scan in the z-axis	RNFL thickness can only drop to about 30–40 μm
Effects of refractive error	Need to adjust for ocular magnification
Effects of eye's axial length	• Longer associated with thinner RNFL • Manufacturers normal population database excludes subjects with high refractive error
Effects of cyclotorsion	Shift in the RNFL-TSNIT profile on OCT
Segmentation algorithm failure of RNFL in disease states	• In peripapillary atrophy (e.g. glaucoma, myopia) • In optic disc edema (e.g., papilledema)
Segmentation algorithm failure of GCC (GCL + IPL)	GCC more prone to segmentation failure than RNFL
Artificial increase in RNFL thickness	In gliosis, myelinated nerve fibers, optic disc edema
Structural abnormalities of the outer retina affect segmentation of the inner retinal layers	Outer retina not routinely segmented
Different algorithms used by different vendors	Data is not comparable between OCT brands, even between same brand but different software
Effects of the scanning distance	Boundary detection errors predominant in the peripheral regions of the macula
Suboptimal repeatability	To improve implement gaze tracker, faster scanning

Clinical challenges	Comments
Non-specific findings	• Differential diagnosis of incidental optic neuropathy • Similar findings in neurodegenerative disorders: • AD, MS, NMO, MOG, PD
Non-localizing	ON reflects pathology of the entire retina, thus RNFL is less localizing than GCC
Unable to differentiate antegrade from retrograde degeneration	RNFL and GCC affected by antegrade and retrograde degeneration, even trans-synaptic retrograde degeneration from retro-chiasmal lesion can develop even in few months
Unable to differentiate congenital versus acquired abnormality	Unable to assess acquired on the top of congenital variant, an example: myelinated nerve fiber layer and papilledema

insignificant [59]. Therefore, in the era of personalized, so-called precision medicine, ophthalmo-anatomical variants must be defined. Although, some findings that were previously considered to be incidental on brain MRI, such as so-called Virchow-Robin or enlarged perivascular spaces, have later been implicated as pathological and possibly indicative of mild cognitive impairment [60]. Therefore, the most important challenge is to determine if a finding is clinically significant (contributory or relevant to the present clinical complaint and examination findings) or incidental. This is exemplified in considering patients who have an empty sella on brain MRI. An empty sella can represent a secondary finding, an epiphenomenon, as in the case of IIH or it can be a normal variant, as in the case of patients with normal ICP [61]. Ultimately, this neuro-imaging finding must be interpreted within the clinical context, such as cases of normal opening pressure on lumbar puncture in patients with typical phenotypes and clinical history for the disease and who also have optic nerve head (ONH) swelling on fundus examination. Thus, in this example, the neuro-imaging information adds to the diagnosis of probable IIH (see Chap. 7: OCT and Optic disc edema). Another frequently encountered example of this non-specificity of neuro-imaging on brain MRI is the so-called non-specific white matter disease (WMD) [62]. Often, this finding does not correlate with the patient's symptoms but rather represents a wide differential diagnosis that ranges in severity from the more "severe" demyelinating or microvascular etiologies to the more "benign" etiologies such as migraine. Therefore, having the knowledge of patient specific symptoms and physical examination findings in combination with multimodal imaging offers the best available option to address the underlying pathophysiology. Analogy between OCT and MRI, particularly in the use of CNS disorders is helpful to address the need for OCT as a neuroimaging tool. For example, perhaps the microvascular rarefaction seen on OCTA in several neurodegenerative disorders is the retinal correlate of brain WMD [63–65].

In determining clinical significance, OCT findings are confounded by intra-individual (inter-eye) structural variability in the number of ganglion cells and their axons that make up the optic nerve and their correlation to the approximately 10,000 times more brain neurons [66]. In addition, the optic nerve is not only made of ganglion cell axons but are outnumbered by glial cells, similar to the brain where it is estimated that the ratio of glial cells to neurons is 10 to 1 [48].

5.4.2 Multimodal Imaging Advantage

One way to partially overcome some of these shortcomings of OCT-based imaging is to follow a multimodal approach, with the aim of subtracting complementary information about the clinical problem [67, 68]. However, the imaging-based information will need to be integrated with neuro-ophthalmic history and physical examination findings to decide whether it is relevant to the presenting complaint.

While deciphering the eye and brain connections (structure) and visual perception (function), we rely on a growing number of sophisticated imaging technologies such as adaptive optics, computer tomography, fundus imaging (including autofluorescence, infrared reflectance, hyperspectral cameras), MRI, OCT, optogenetics, calcium imaging with the utilization of 3D-photon imaging of neuronal and dendritic spine assemblies of the visual cortex, scanning laser ophthalmoscopy, ultrasonography, and/or a combination of these tools [67–78]. These methods rely on the function of our own visual system; therefore, they are subject to its limitations. However, when we combine ophthalmic and neuro-imaging structural with functional tools, such as electrophysiology (electroretinography, pupillometry, visual evoked potentials) [79], functional MRI (fMRI), OCTA, and visual field testing, there is a higher likelihood that the limitations of each of these methods are overcome, or at least decreased. Therefore, both the neurology and the ophthalmology community has been using some combination of complementary technologies.

A frequent but difficult neuro-ophthalmic complaint is monocular transient visual loss [80], when evaluation of orbital vascular supply is of interest but is a particularly difficult area to assess. The use of OCT and OCTA is limited in this area secondary to its poor penetrance. Ultrasonography has better penetrance but limited field of view. Traditional magnetic resonance angiography (MRA), like 2D-and 3D time-of-flight sequences are limited by suboptimal resolution and the fact that orbital adipose tissue, in which the vasculature is buried, has short T1 and long T2 relaxation times and therefore appears bright (hyperintense) on both T1- and T2 weighted sequences. Moreover, the usually applied fat suppression methods have significant artifacts that make them suboptimal for the assessment of small vessels such as the central retinal and medial and lateral posterior ciliary arteries that supply the retina and optic nerve, as well as having great inter-individual variability (see Sect. 5.3 above). Therefore, to achieve maximal MRA contrast between arteries and fat in retrobulbar space, the ideal way is to completely suppress fat signal while leaving blood signal high. Moreover, high resolution imaging is needed to reduce partial volume effects on small branches of the vessels [81]. MRA, even with the above limitations, complements OCTA in the visualization of the vascular network of the eye, especially with the use of contrast agents that improve vessel signals.

In daily clinical practice, there is also lack of sensitivity of these methods compared to the ideal research environment due to subject-based technical limitations, such as degraded quality due to inability to cooperate resulting in poor fixation and motion-induced artifacts, which is a major issue in patients with neurodegenerative disorders and visual fixation instability due to underlying disease such as optic neuropathy [82].

Also, a major drawback of OCT-based neuroimaging is lack of specificity for not only a particular disorder but even for underlying pathophysiology such as compressive–infiltrative, hereditary, degenerative, inflammatory-infectious, traumatic, and vascular etiologies [83, 84].

Moreover, another defy is associated to normal changes in the anatomy of the retina and optic nerve due to aging, and that the retina might not entirely reveal the extent of neurological damage because of the characteristic diffuse manner in which typically neurodegenerative diseases occur in the CNS.

Other major clinical disadvantages of OCT are that it is likely to miss early changes [85], thereby limiting its role in determining the time course of disease, and that it provides non-localizing information (e.g., symptoms and signs suggestive of orbital disease: localizing versus non-localizing) [86–88]. Therefore, correlation with other structural and functional studies, such as visual field testing, is needed to localize and determine etiology [89, 90]. When evaluating complex neurodegenerative disorders, it is important to segment the entire retina and not only the neuroretina, as outer retinal changes have already been described [91]. Also, subtracting additional information from the available datasets, such as shape, texture, and other voxel-based morphometry is necessary due to the limited information thickness provides [92].

5.4.3 OCT Challenges in the Brain

Regarding the cerebral cortex, OCT-based imaging has the capability to visualize cortical neurons and microvasculature, especially of the deeper layers that are presently inaccessible by existing methods such as MRA and fMRI. Cortical neurons are assembled into functional units consisting of horizontal layers and vertical columns, an example of such architecture is the interdigitated column system of the V1 (see Sect. 5.3 above). The superficial cortical layers are supplied by the so-called microvascular lobules [93]. Horton et al. raised the question as to how the so-called cytochrome oxidase (CO) patches that define the metabolic activity of neurons areable to maintain a 49% higher mean firing rate without having a richer microcirculation. The answer is not yet known but it is hypothesized that it is secondary to faster blood flow and/or a higher oxygen extraction ratio compared to other areas. Because of this discrepancy, fMRI findings may not necessarily correlate with increased neuronal activity. Perhaps this question is best addressed in humans through multimodal manners, such as by combining in vivo non-invasive fMRI, 3D-photon microscopy, and even OCT and OCT-angiography (OCTA) [94–96].

A major advantage of OCT and OCTA over MRI is lower cost and therefore easier accessibility, and as such would be an ideal screening tool in neurodegenerative disorders. However, presently, high cost is still a limiting factor to academic research centers in some of the newer methods, such as OCTA (Fig. 5.4).

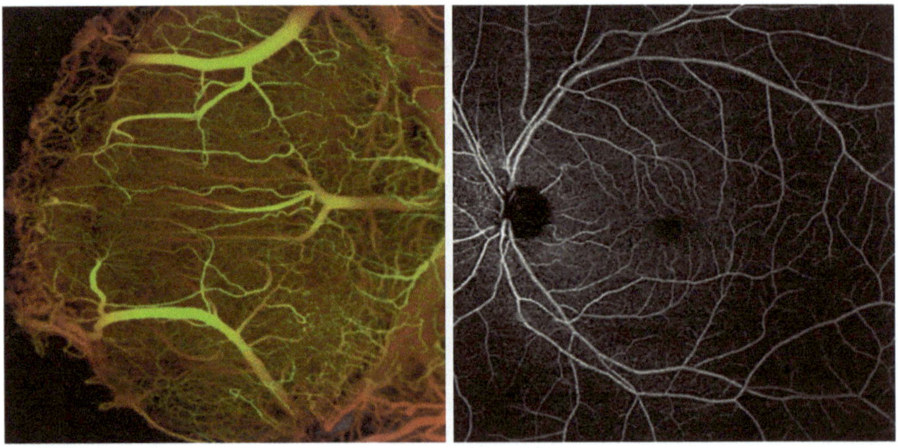

Fig. 5.4 OCT-angiography images. (**Left**) Three-dimensional cerebral vascular map (mouse, *image courtesy of Nishan Mohan, Ph.D., Wasatch Photonics, Inc.*). The depth location of the vessels is color-coded from superficial green to deepest red colors. (**Right**) OCTA image form a glaucomatous' patients (*image courtesy of Luis Vazques, MD*)

5.5 Emerging Applications of OCT in Neurology

Imaging of the eye is increasingly investigated as a potential tool for discovering ocular biomarkers of primarily non-ophthalmic disorders, ranging from neurovascular and neurodegenerative diseases to cardiovascular disease [17]. As reported by the World Health Organization, millions of individuals around the world have various types of neurological disorders, including 326 million who suffer from migraines and 24 million that suffer from AD [97]. These neurological diseases affect vision and originate eye complaints characterized by ocular symptoms that can range from double vision to dry eye to legal blindness. The eye complaints related to neurologic disorders include primary glaucomatous optic nerve disease, ischemic optic neuropathy and optic neuritis, whereas those related to systemic neurologic diseases such as Alzheimer's and Parkinson's diseases have ocular signs associated to decline of the brain' function. Also, visual problems are often reported in patients after stroke due to the associated neurologic damage. Numerous studies have revealed that many brain diseases like AD could be reflected in retinal alterations, and therefore could also be correlated with structural changes in the retinal neural layers and [17]. For example, it has been hypothesized that if an association can be made between the amyloid in the brain and the amyloid in the eye, then it would be feasible to diagnose AD by looking into the eye. This evidence has progressively accumulated, supporting the hypothesis that the retina may be a window to the brain [1, 17, 18].

Various publications using OCT suggest that several neurologic ailments have pathologic changes in the RNFL of the eye, proposing that the RNFL thickness could be a potential surrogate marker for neurodegeneration [17]. For example, Fig. 5.5 shows the exponential loss of the RNFL in the affected eye of a subject with acute ON. Also, several studies have reported the atrophy of the RNFL around the optic disc in patients with MS with and even without optic neuritis (ON) in medical history [98–103]. The mean overall circumpapillary RNFL (cpRNFL) thickness and the cpRNFL thickness in each quadrant has been found significantly lower in the eyes of MS patients with a history of ON compared to the non-ON-affected eyes and in comparison, with healthy eyes except for the nasal quadrant [104]. However, the cpRNFL thickness is decreased only in the temporal quadrant of the non-affected eyes of MS patients compared to healthy eyes [104]. A strong correlation with disease severity measured by the EDSS score was also obtained in the case of the GCC thickness which implies that this parameter might also be useful in the estimation of disease progression as a surrogate marker. Similarly, the most pronounced reduction in the thickness of cpRNFL (27% and 17% in the ON-affected and non-affected eyes, respectively) was also observed in the temporal quadrant [104]. These findings agree with previous OCT studies confirming that the fibers of the papillomacular bundle are the most susceptible to damage in ON [101, 105]. One important aspect of this fact, as it has been widely reported in glaucomatous damage, is that the evaluation of the sectoral thickness values could provide the possibility to discriminate the RNFL atrophy caused by glaucomatous damage and other disorders affecting the optic nerve, such as MS [98].

Also, OCT has been very useful in identifying maculopathy that mimics optic neuropathy in the neuro-ophthalmic practice (Fig. 5.5). As a matter of fact, OCT

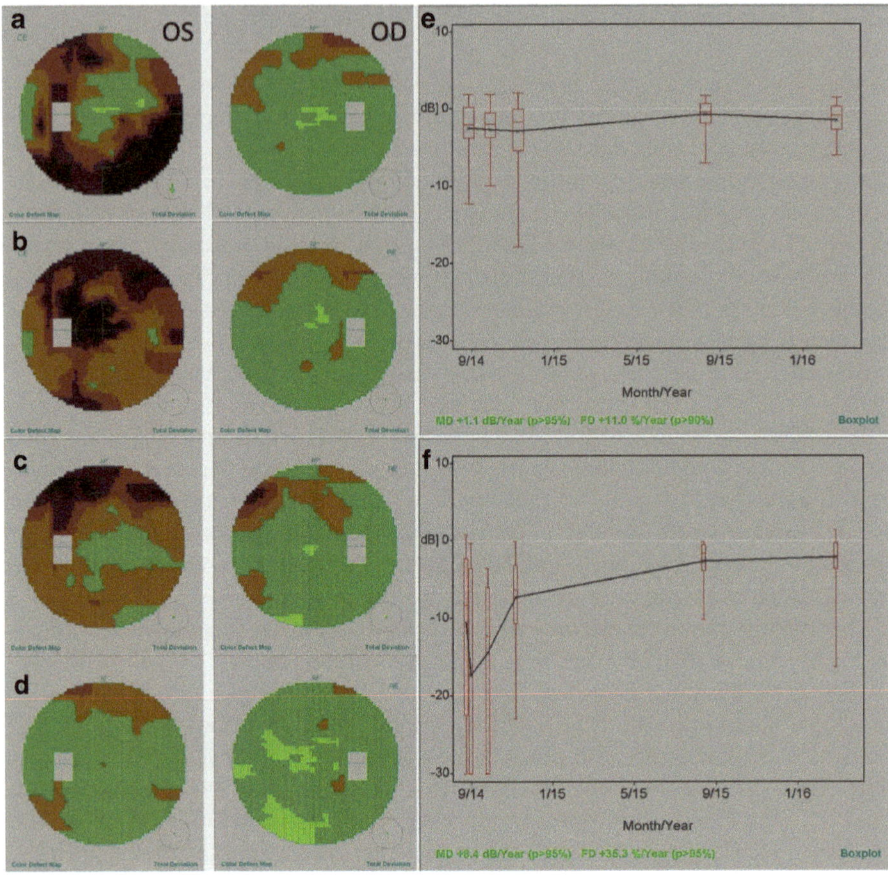

Fig. 5.5 Follow-up of a 38-year old female patient with acute optic neuritis (ON) in the left eye. The patient presented with mild visual symptoms in the left eye with a VA of 0.6 and a visual field seen on (**a**). The ON that progressed within 2 weeks to a total loss of the visual field with VA 0.1 left (**b**). Three months after presentation her visual acuity and visual field began to improve (**c**, VA 0.8), whereas 1 year after the onset of symptoms her visual field was almost preserved with full visual function (**d**, VA 1.0). Figures (**e**) and (**f**) are showing the changes in the MD (mean defect) value in the right and left eye, respectively. Figures (**g**) and (**h**) are showing the circumpapillary RNFL measurements obtained during follow-up. In the right eye (**g**) the values are unchanged, in the affected left eye (**h**) there is an exponential decrease in the amount of nerve fibers. Please note that the baseline values are similar in both eyes. Figures (**i**–**k**) are showing images from the 1-year follow-up of the patient. (Please note that for the easier reading of the figure we are showing the two eyes similarly to the visual field data, with the left eye being on the left, unlike the way OCT readings are presented.) In the right eye there is a marked, diffuse reduction of RNFL thickness (**i**), with all sectors being markedly reduced as compared to the right eye but still within normal limits, except for the global thickness values. Figure (**k**) is showing the global and fine structural changes of the inner retina in both eyes. In the right eye there is a marked, diffuse thinning of the macula, reflected in the macular volume; also, the RNFL, the GCL and the IPL layers are similarly diffusely thinner in the affected left eye (see also the layer volume data in red) indicating the neurodegenerative changes in the inner retina. It is of note that despite the observed changes the visual field is showing only minimal changes and the visual function is also full. (The reason for the latter is that visual acuity is routinely assessed by full acuity and not contrast sensitivity tests that would be more sensitive for such changes.) The patient had relapsing-remitting MS for which the findings of relatively mild changes after one ON episode are quite typical (*Image courtesy of Gabor Mark Somfai, M.D., Ph.D.*)

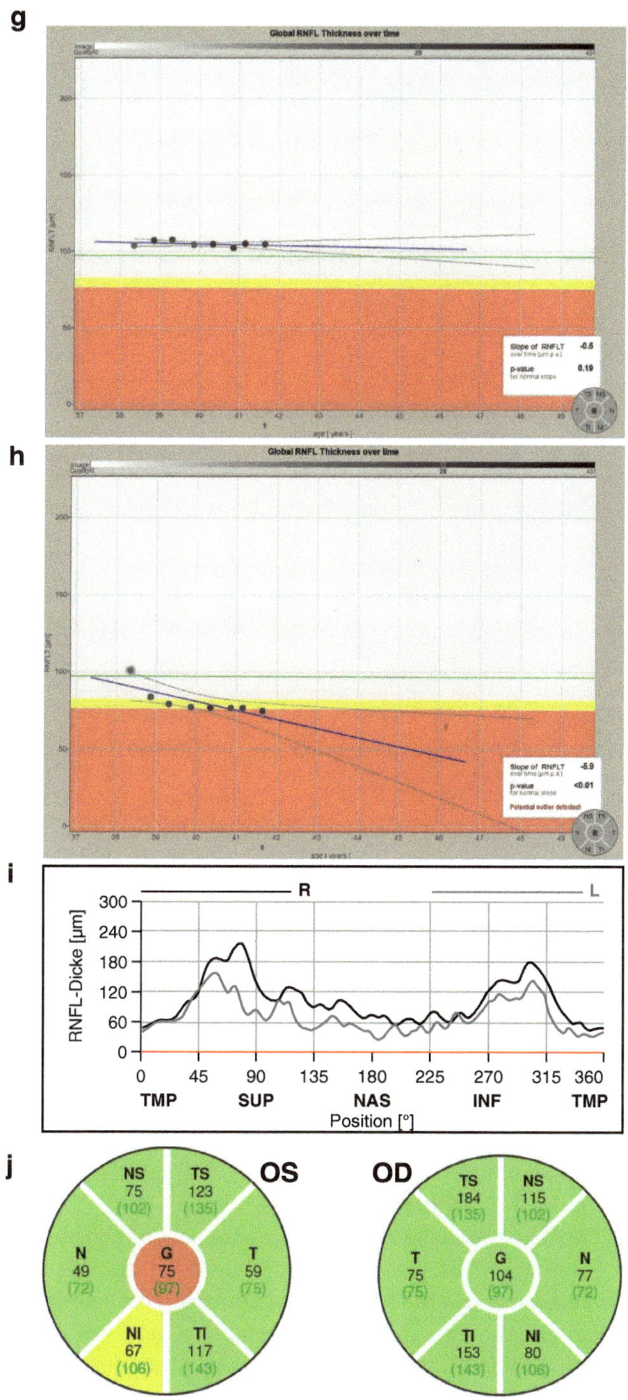

Fig. 5.5 (continued)

k

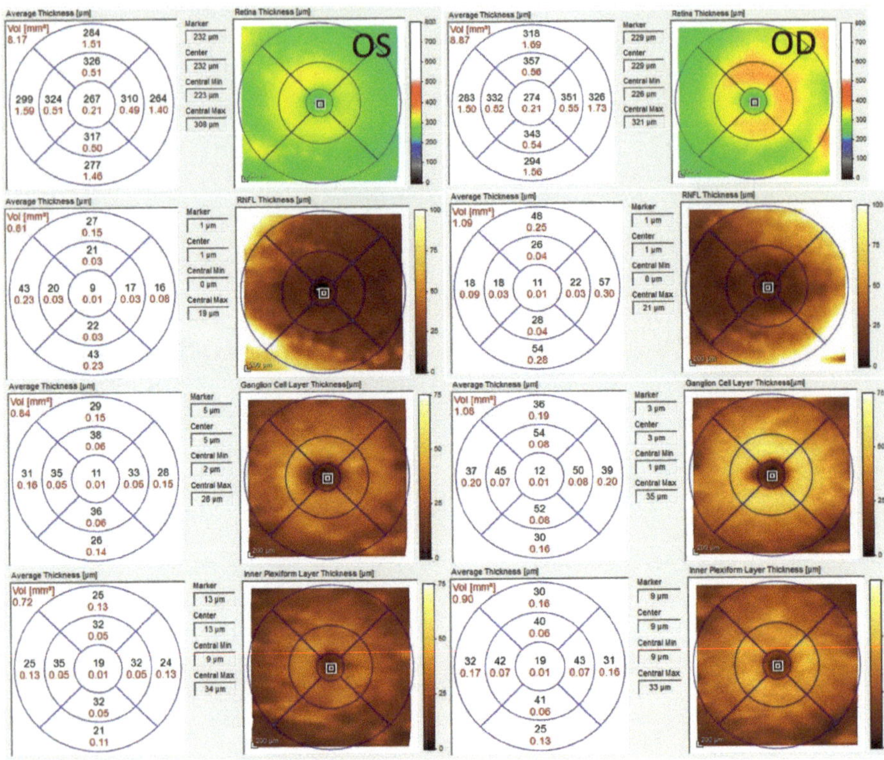

Fig. 5.5 (continued)

offers evidence of normality in the retinal structure when there may be functional or fictitious loss of vision and may be relied upon when there has been long-standing functional loss of vision [106–111]. Moreover, OCT has been useful in dealing with a range of conditions related with optic disc swelling, including papilledema, pseudopapilledema, and anterior ischemic optic neuropathy (AION). OCT can also be useful in toxic, hereditary and nutritional neuropathy as well as in many cases of optic atrophy, including optic neuritis and optic nerve compression [106–115]. It has been also noted that OCT may not always reflect the overall degree of demyelination occurring in individuals with ON, although OCT can serve as a biomarker for the progression of demyelinating disease [116–118].

Recent studies of the retina using OCT have also being helpful in revealing atrophy of the peripapillary RNFL and to a lesser extent the macular GCL in patients with multiple system atrophy (MSA) which rarely have visual complaints (Fig. 5.6) [119]. OCT imaging in this rare, adult-onset, rapidly progressive fatal synucleinopathy that primarily affects oligodendroglial cells in the brain, has shown that the retinal damage in patients with MSA appears to follow a different pattern to that observed in those with Parkinson's disease (PD) (Fig. 5.7). Whereas in individuals with PD the atrophy of temporal RNFL sectors and internal retinal layers (i.e., GCC) at the parafoveal region are prominent, in subjects with MSA the inferior, superior and nasal RNFL sectors are more affected than in PD.

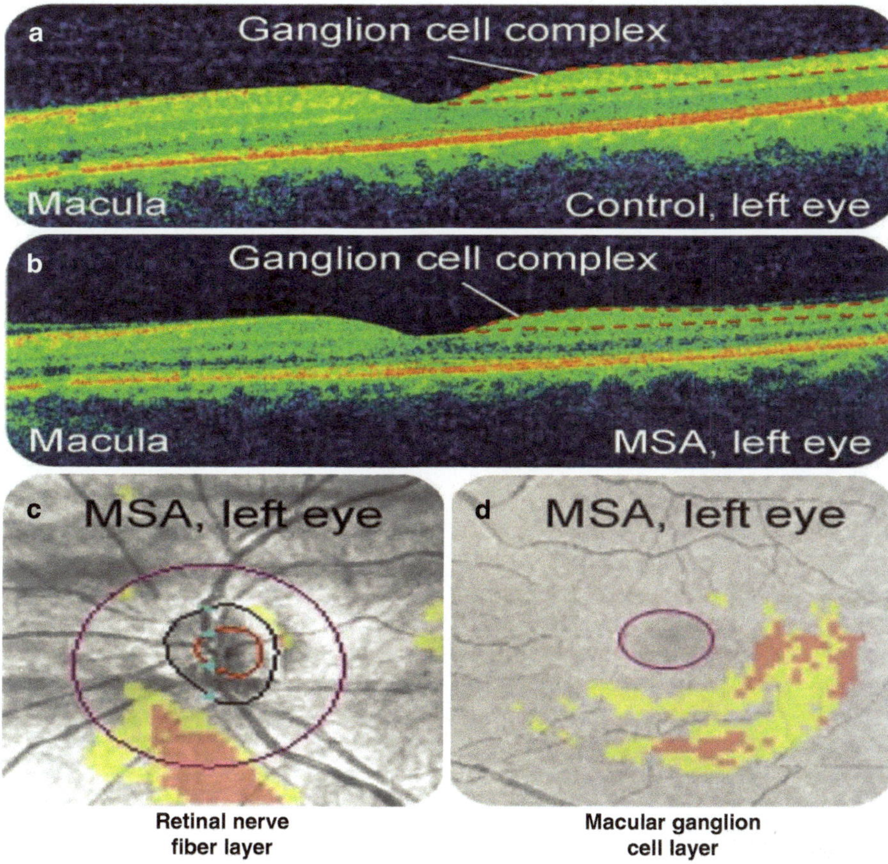

Fig. 5.6 OCT imaging in a control eye and a patient with MSA showing OCT macular sections where the different layers of the retina can be appreciated. The ganglion cell layer (GCL) complex (delimited with a dashed red line) is thinner in a patient with MSA (**b**) compared to an age-matched normal control (**a**). In the same patient with MSA, the thickness of the inferior quadrant of the retinal nerve fiber layer (**c**) and the macular ganglion cell complex layer (**d**), measured by OCT, are substantially reduced (reduced thickness identified in yellow and red) (*Image courtesy of Carlos Mendoza-Santiesteban, M.D.*)

The differences in the preferential damage of parvocellular pathway (P-cells) versus magnocellular pathway (M-cells) could explain dissimilarities between PD and MSA patients at the clinical and retinal level [120]. Axons from M-cells (with cell bodies situated in peripheral macula and retina) are in the superior, nasal, and inferior regions around the optic nerve (where the RNFL is measured). On the other side, P-cells predominate in the central macular region (where the macular GCC is measured), their axons project to the temporal portion of the RNFL and they are highly related to color discrimination, visual acuity, central visual field sensitivity, and contrast sensitivity for high spatial frequencies. These M-cells relay information about achromatic vision, motion detection, peripheral visual field sensitivity and contrast sensitivity for low spatial frequencies.

The fact that MSA patients typically have normal visual acuity and color vision in combination with inferior RNFL atrophy may indicate that, in MSA, M-cells

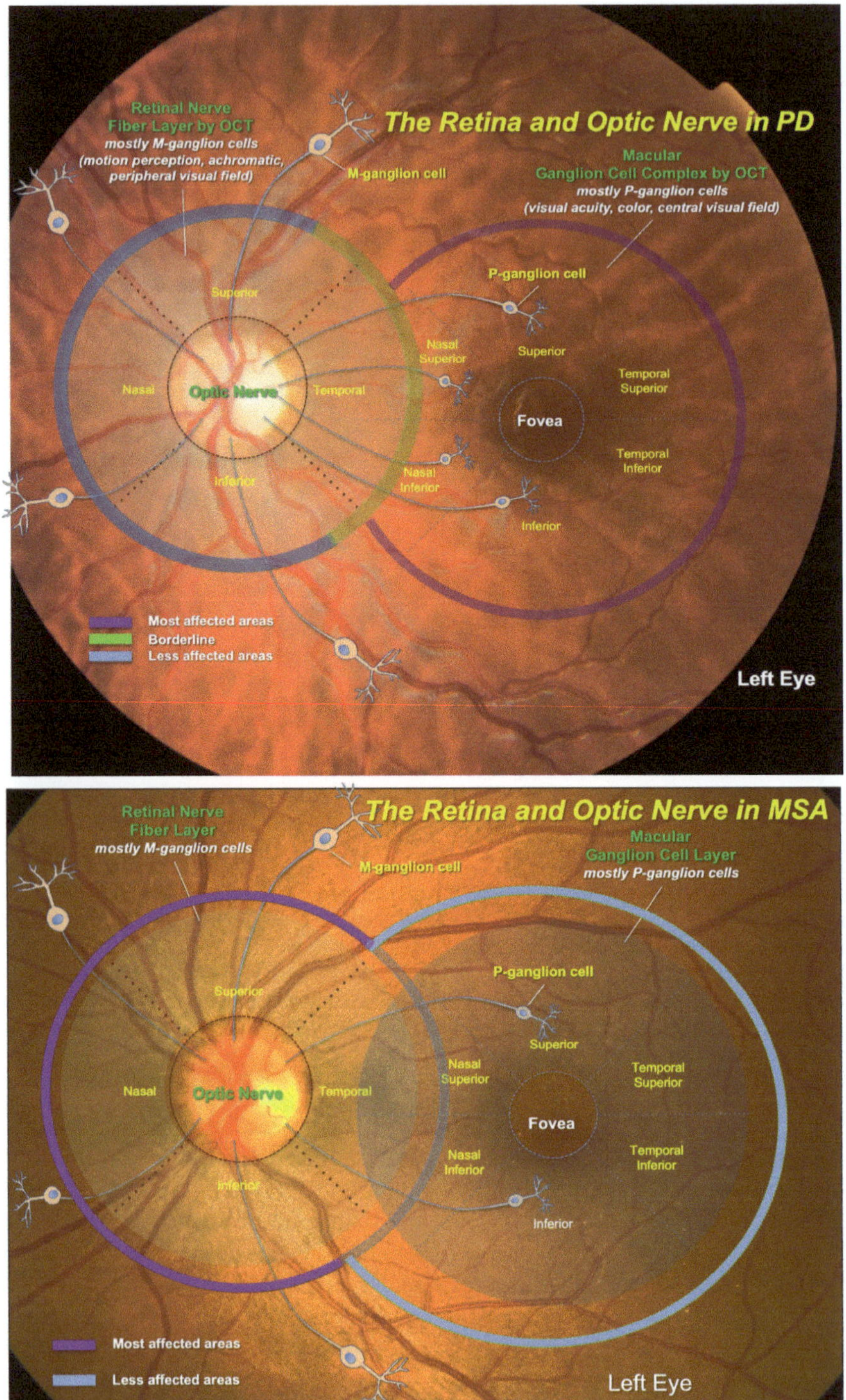

Fig. 5.7 Differences in the preferential damage of parvocellular pathway (P-cells) versus magnocellular pathway (M-cells) in PD and MSA (*Image courtesy of Carlos Mendoza-Santiesteban, M.D.*)

are more affected than P-cells. This contrasts with PD patients, who have preferential atrophy of temporal RNFL sectors and higher central macular GCC atrophy (compared to MSA), and is in keeping with their relatively frequent complains of visual problems, such as decreased visual acuity, impaired color discrimination, defective motion perception, and visual hallucinations. The hypothesis of a preferential injury of P-cells in PD and M-cells in MSA is still unproven, but it may be related to a predominant damage of optic nerve axons in MSA that being especially coarse and myelinated (like those from M-cells) require high support from oligodendrocytes.

The link between retina pathology and a variety of neurodegenerative and cerebrovascular diseases has been established in various OCT studies which are also well detailed in different chapters of this book [17, 121, 122]. Particularly, this link reinforces the use of retinal microvasculature and neural layers as biomarkers to assess the condition of the cerebral vessels supplying the neurons in the brain. Therefore, examining pathologic alterations of the retinal tissue using OCT technology may be valuable for understanding the etiology of brain disorders.

5.6 Controversies and Challenges in Neurology

A great challenge exists to understanding how changes in the retinal neurovascular unit reflect neurovascular pathology in the brain, which seems to play a critical role to understand cerebral neurovascular pathogenesis. Another challenge is the variations in retinal structural and vascular features between individuals due to aging along with the existing confounding variables that may also result in retinal changes. Also, in the case of AD, it has been reported that amyloid deposition can be identified among cognitively normal elderly persons during life and the prevalence of asymptomatic amyloid deposition may be like that of symptomatic amyloid deposition. An early study has shown that in a group of participants without clinically significant impairment, amyloid deposition was not associated with worse cognitive function, suggesting that an elderly person with a significant amyloid burden can remain cognitively normal [123]. Therefore, OCT algorithms and potential OCT-base biomarkers should carefully consider potential pitfalls related to both confounding factors and asymptomatic amyloid deposition features.

The use of different OCT instruments or technologies to collect imaging data for neurologic applications is another major limitation affecting the integration and correlation of ocular and brain data [124, 125]. Therefore, improved software analysis considering different OCT imaging technologies and magnification correction factors would allow for better data structure and standardization once an efficient strategy is in place for better comparability between different imaging instruments. The quality assurance of the data and algorithms precision to extract image-based features are additional important factors to consider when using OCT imaging in neurologic applications.

Another imperative consideration is to carefully collect OCT imaging data from healthy subjects without subtle brain abnormalities. In general, it is unknown whether healthy subjects included in normative databases of OCT imaging devices may have focal discrete lesions (i.e. mild signs) in the brain without visible or detectable ocular manifestations. Thus, caution should be exercised when considering normative data from OCT imaging, particularly if considering them for OCT applications of neurologic conditions with complications in the eye. Also, it is important to consider the variance of normal healthy OCT findings because there is anatomical variability between normal healthy eyes of different people as well as differences between the normal healthy findings between the right and left eyes of everyone. This consideration may be useful to better demarcate pathological asymmetry. A valid example of this respect being the OCT recent findings revealing that thinning of the foveal region was more prominent in the eye opposite the side of the body extremely affected by tremor in patients with PD as well as subjects with essential tremor [122].

Additional aspects to be considered in the detection and evaluation of features for OCT imaging in neurology are the differences in phenotyping, the velocity of disease development in patients, the disease duration and impact of age, the subclinical retinal damage, and the practicality of features to be confirmed in independent populations. Also, we note that the OCT biomarkers at the population level may not apply to all individuals and that large-scale studies are frequently needed. Although OCT imaging has expanded our understanding of the pathology of numerous diseases of the retina and optic nerve, differential diagnosis and cellular distinction-based pathology are still needed to determine the role that OCT may play in the diagnosis and monitoring of neurological diseases in the future.

5.7 Advantages in Seeing the Brain Through the Eye

The use of OCT technology as a non-invasive technique to extract important information from the brain in certain neurological conditions has gained much attention recently. Current procedures, such as neuroimaging methods (e.g. MRI and PET) are very high-priced, extremely invasive, lacking in specificity and not readily accessible to most clinicians and affected individuals. The average cost of an MRI exam is about $2175 and a PET scan can cost up to $4000 depending of the scan type needed. Particularly, for a new, state-of-the-art 3 T MRI machine the price can reach $3 million. The room that houses the machine can cost hundreds of thousands more because safety features must be built in to protect the outside personnel from the magnetic field. Add in patient support areas and installation costs, and a suite with just one machine can cost anywhere from $3 million to $5 million. In contrast, OCT imaging is a low-cost and user-friendly approach that can advance research in many brain disorders and eye diseases as well as enhance healthcare even at points of care representing a significant cost reduction when compared to the current standard care in brain diseases. This simplified yet effective technique has the potential to change the way we diagnose certain neurological conditions. But more importantly perhaps, this could possibly be done at the level of geriatric clinics and primary health care facilities, such as day hospitals and community clinics. In this perspective, OCT imaging can possibly provide an affordable and faster option, potentially replacing or complementing the current expensive neuroimaging methods.

5.8 Final Remarks and Future Directions

In summary, OCT has already proven to offer invaluable information in several retinal and optic nerve head disorders that is not available by any other method to date and has improved patient management and outcomes [123]. Also, OCT might facilitate earlier detection of axonal loss than visual field testing or funduscopic examination, and could be used to monitor patients with optic neuropathies as well as neurologic disorders affecting the anterior visual pathways. However, OCT-based imaging in the realm of complex brain anatomy, physiology, and pathophysiology, presently offers non-specific, non-localizing, and sometimes contradictory information emphasizing its limitations by only offering one piece of the puzzle.

In the era of precision medicine, future well-designed, prospective, controlled, and longitudinal studies with homogeneous populations are needed in both health and disease to be able to answer patient specific questions while filling out the current gaps of knowledge by utilizing high quality standardized scanning protocols and reporting [123, 124]. The future is bright as pieces of the brain-eye connection puzzle are falling into place through technologies such as OCT-based neuro-imaging and minimally invasive theranostics [124–127]. Keeping in mind though that the usefulness of these tools in clinical practice requires familiarity with detailed anatomy and physiology and pathophysiology of the entire visual system. Moreover, the acquired high quality OCT data to be clinically useful (establish cause and effect relationship, provide prognostic value, follow treatment effect) needs to be scrutinized and correlated with clinical findings [128–130]. Accordingly, it is important to note the following future directions needed to improve the use of the OCT technology as a neuroimaging tool:

- The manufacturer's normative database needs to be routinely corrected for refractive errors, AL, and ophthalmo-anatomical variants
- Individual eye and brain layers should not be looked at in isolation
- To assess the past, present and predict the future of eye and brain states by OCT, longitudinal studies and correlation with histopathology and in vivo multimodal imaging is needed
- Disease process specific and localizing neuro-imaging markers are needed

Ultimately, the continuous improvement and development of novel applications of the OCT technology could allow us to further characterize eye-brain signatures that may facilitate a more comprehensive assessment of the effect of both age-decline and impairment ailments on ocular and cerebral function at the early stage.

References

1. London A, Benhar I, Schwartz M. The retina as a window to the brain-from eye research to CNS disorders. Nat Rev Neurol. 2013;9:44–53. https://doi.org/10.1038/nrneurol.2012.227.
2. Seung S. Tracing the wires of the brain. In: Connectomics. 2018. http://dana.org/Cerebrum/2008/Connectomics__Tracing_the_Wires_of_the_Brain/. Accessed 6 Dec 2018.

3. Schmolesky M. The primary visual cortex. In: The organization of the retina and visual system. 2018. https://webvision.med.utah.edu/book/part-ix-psychophysics-of-vision/the-primary-visual-cortex/. Accessed 6 Dec 2018.
4. USC Eye Institute. USC Eye Institute researchers use Human Connectome Project brain mapping techniques to unlock mysteries that can lead to vision-restoring therapies. 2018. https://www.prnewswire.com/news-releases/usc-eye-institute-researchers-use-human-connectome-project-brain-mapping-techniques-to-unlock-mysteries-that-can-lead-to-vision-restoring-therapies-300226553.html. Accessed 6 Dec 2018.
5. Chen C, Bickford ME, Hirsch JA. Untangling the web between eye and brain. Cell. 2016;165:20–1. https://doi.org/10.1016/j.cell.2016.03.010.
6. Seung S. Connectome: how the brain's wiring makes us who we are. Boston: HMH; 2012.
7. Joly O, Frankó E. Neuroimaging of amblyopia and binocular vision: a review. Front Integr Neurosci. 2014;8:62. https://doi.org/10.3389/fnint.2014.00062.
8. Zelinsky D, Feinberg C. Quantitative electroencephalograms and neuro-optometry: a case study that explores changes in electrophysiology while wearing therapeutic eyeglasses. Neurophotonics. 2017;4:011013. https://doi.org/10.1117/1.NPh.4.1.011013.
9. Vámos R, Tátrai E, Németh J, Holder GE, DeBuc DC, Somfai GM. The structure and function of the macula in patients with advanced retinitis pigmentosa. Invest Ophthalmol Vis Sci. 2011;52:8425–32. https://doi.org/10.1167/iovs.11-7780.
10. Liu G, Liu X, Li H, Du Q, Wang F. Optical coherence tomographic analysis of retina in retinitis pigmentosa patients. Ophthalmic Res. 2016;56:111–22. https://doi.org/10.1159/000445063.
11. Bhende M, Shetty S, Parthasarathy MK, Ramya S. Optical coherence tomography: a guide to interpretation of common macular diseases. Indian J Ophthalmol. 2018;66:20–35. https://doi.org/10.4103/ijo.IJO_902_17.
12. Garcia-Layana A, Ciuffo G, Zarranz-Ventura J, Alvarez-Vidal A. Optical coherence tomography in age-related macular degeneration. 2018. http://amdbook.org/content/optical-coherence-tomography-age-related-macular-degeneration. Accessed 10 Dec 2018.
13. Wang J, Zuo X, Dai Z, Xia M, Zhao Z, Zhao X, et al. Disrupted functional brain connectome in individuals at risk for Alzheimer's disease. Biol Psychiatry. 2013;73:472–81. https://doi.org/10.1016/j.biopsych.2012.03.026.
14. Duke Science Review. 2018. http://dukesciencereview.com/content/2-issues/4-issue-4/issue4.pdf. Accessed 6 Dec 2018.
15. Cabrera DeBuc D, Somfai GM, Arthur E, Kostic M, Oropesa S, Mendoza-Santiesteban C. Investigating multimodal diagnostic eye biomarkers of cognitive impairment by measuring vascular and neurogenic changes in the retina. Front Physiol. 2018;9:1721. https://doi.org/10.3389/fphys.2018.01721.
16. Berisha F, Feke GT, Trempe CL, Mcmeel JW, Schepens CL. Retinal abnormalities in early Alzheimer's disease. Invest Ophthalmol Vis Sci. 2007;48:2285–9. https://doi.org/10.1167/iovs.06-1029.
17. Cabrera DeBuc D, Somfai GM, Koller A. Retinal microvascular network alterations: potential biomarkers of cerebrovascular and neural diseases. Am J Physiol Heart Circ Physiol. 2017;312:H201–12. https://doi.org/10.1152/ajpheart.00201.2016.
18. Cheung CY, Ong YT, Ikram MK, Ong SY, Li X, Hilal S, et al. Microvascular network alterations in the retina of patients with Alzheimer's disease. Alzheimers Dement. 2014;10:135–42. https://doi.org/10.1016/j.jalz.2013.06.009.
19. Koronyo Y, Biggs D, Barron E, Boyer DS, Pearlman JA, Au WJ, et al. Retinal amyloid pathology and proof-of-concept imaging trial in Alzheimer's disease. JCI Insight. 2017;2:pii: 93621. https://doi.org/10.1172/jci.insight.93621.
20. Koronyo Y, Salumbides BC, Black KL, Koronyo-Hamaoui M. Alzheimer's disease in the retina: imaging retinal abeta plaques for early diagnosis and therapy assessment. Neurodegener Dis. 2012;10:285–93. https://doi.org/10.1159/000335154.
21. Koronyo-Hamaoui M, Koronyo Y, Ljubimov AV, Miller CA, Ko MK, Black KL, et al. Identification of amyloid plaques in retinas from Alzheimer's patients and noninvasive

in vivo optical imaging of retinal plaques in a mouse model. NeuroImage. 2011;54:S204–17. https://doi.org/10.1016/j.neuroimage.2010.06.020.
22. Patton N, Aslam T, Macgillivray T, Pattie A, Deary IJ, Dhillon B. Retinal vascular image analysis as a potential screening tool for cerebrovascular disease: a rationale based on homology between cerebral and retinal microvasculatures. J Anat. 2005;206:319–48. https://doi.org/10.1111/j.1469-7580.2005.00395.x.
23. Murray CD. The physiological principle of minimum work: I. The vascular system and the cost of blood volume. Proc Natl Acad Sci U S A. 1926;12:207–14.
24. Zamboni P, Galeotti R, Menegatti E, Malagoni AM, Tacconi G, Dall'Ara S, et al. Chronic cerebrospinal venous insufficiency in patients with multiple sclerosis. J Neurol Neurosurg Psychiatry. 2009;80:392–9. https://doi.org/10.1136/jnnp.2008.157164.
25. Gariano RF, Gardner TW. Retinal angiogenesis in development and disease. Nature. 2005;438:960–6. https://doi.org/10.1038/nature04482.
26. Haigh JJ, Morelli PI, Gerhardt H, Haigh K, Tsien J, Damert A, et al. Cortical and retinal defects caused by dosage-dependent reductions in VEGF-A paracrine signaling. Dev Biol. 2003;262:225–41.
27. Hughes S, Yang H, Chan-Ling T. Vascularization of the human fetal retina: roles of vasculogenesis and angiogenesis. Invest Ophthalmol Vis Sci. 1997;41:1217–28.
28. Risau W. Mechanisms of angiogenesis. Nature. 1997;386:671–4.
29. Gjedde A, Diemer NH. Double-tracer study of the fine regional blood-brain glucose transfer in the rat by computer-assisted autoradiography. J Cereb Blood Flow Metab. 1985;5:282–9. https://doi.org/10.1038/2Fjcbfm.1985.36.
30. Klein B, Kuschinsky W, Schrock H, Vetterlein F. Interdependency of local capillary density, blood flow, and metabolism in rat brains. Am J Phys. 1986;251:H1333–40. https://doi.org/10.1152/ajpheart.1986.251.6.H1333.
31. Toussaint D, Kuwabara T, Cogan DG. Retinal vascular patterns. II. Human retinal vessels studied in three dimensions. Arch Ophthalmol. 1961;65:575–81.
32. Cogan DG, Kuwabara T. Comparison of retinal and cerebral vasculature in trypsin digest preparations. Br J Ophthalmol. 1984;68:10–2.
33. Zirkulations TL. Ernahrungsverhaltnisse des Auges. In: Graefe AST, editor. Handbuch der Gesamten Augenheilkunde. Leipzig: Springer-Verlag; 1903.
34. Wong TY, Klein R, Sharrett AR, Couper DJ, Klein BE, Liao DP, et al. Cerebral white matter lesions, retinopathy, and incident clinical stroke. JAMA. 2002;288:67–74.
35. Neuwelt EA. Implications of the blood-brain barrier and its manipulation. New York: Plenum; 1989.
36. Tornquist P, Alm A. Carrier-mediated transport of amino acids through the blood-retinal and the blood-brain barriers. Graefes Arch Clin Exp Ophthalmol. 1986;224:21–5.
37. Sagaties MJ, Raviola G, Schaeffer S, Miller C. The structural basis of the inner blood-retina barrier in the eye of Macaca mulatta. Invest Ophthalmol Vis Sci. 1987;28:2000–14.
38. Zhang Y, Stone J. Role of astrocytes in the control of developing retinal vessels. Invest Ophthalmol Vis Sci. 1997;38:1653–66.
39. Janzer RC. The blood-brain barrier: cellular basis. J Inherit Metab Dis. 1993;16:639–47.
40. Abbott NJ, Revest PA, Romero IA. Astrocyte-endothelial interaction: physiology and pathology. Neuropathol Appl Neurobiol. 1992;18:424–33.
41. Koller A, Toth P. Contribution of flow-dependent vasomotor mechanisms to the autoregulation of cerebral blood flow. J Vasc Res. 2012;49:375–89. https://doi.org/10.1159/000338747.
42. Wallis SJ, Firth J, Dunn WR. Pressure-induced myogenic responses in human isolated cerebral resistance arteries. Stroke. 1996;27:2287–90. Discussion 2291.
43. Yu DY, Su EN, Cringle SJ, Yu PK. Isolated preparations of ocular vasculature and their applications in ophthalmic research. Prog Retin Eye Res. 2003;22:135–69.
44. Leenders KL, Perani D, Lammertsma AA, Heather JD, Buckingham P, Healy MJ, et al. Cerebral blood flow, blood volume and oxygen utilization. Normal values and effect of age. Brain. 1990;113:27–47.

45. Hoge RD, Atkinson J, Gill B, Crelier GR, Marrett S, Pike GB. Linear coupling between cerebral blood flow and oxygen consumption in activated human cortex. Proc Natl Acad Sci U S A. 1999;96:9403–8.
46. Rassam SM, Patel V, Chen HC, Kohner EM. Regional retinal blood flow and vascular autoregulation. Eye. 1996;10:331–7.
47. ter Laan M, van Dijk JM, Elting JW, Staal MJ, Absalom AR. Sympathetic regulation of cerebral blood flow in humans: a review. Br J Anaesth. 2013;111:361–7. https://doi.org/10.1093/bja/aet122.
48. Fields RD. Map the other brain. Nature. 2013;501:25–7.
49. Gilbert TL. The Allen brain atlas as a resource for teaching undergraduate neuroscience. J Undergrad Neurosci Educ. 2018;16:A261–7.
50. Chen JJ, Kardon RH. Avoiding clinical misinterpretation and artifacts of optical coherence tomography analysis of the optic nerve, retinal nerve fiber layer, and ganglion cell layer. J Neuroophthalmol. 2016;364:417–38. https://doi.org/10.1097/WNO.0000000000000422.
51. Coric D, Petzold A, Uitdehaag BMJ, Balk LJ. Software updates of OCT segmentation algorithms influence longitudinal assessment of retinal atrophy. J Neurol Sci. 2018;387:16–20. https://doi.org/10.1016/j.jns.2018.01.020.
52. Lang A, Carass A, Al-Louzi O, Bhargava P, Solomon SD, Calabresi PA, et al. Combined registration and motion correction of longitudinal retinal OCT data. Proc SPIE Int Soc Opt Eng. 2016;9784:97840X. https://doi.org/10.1117/12.2217157.
53. Watson GM, Keltner JL, Chin EK. Comparison of retinal nerve fiber layer and central macular thickness measurements among five different optical coherence tomography instruments in patients with multiple sclerosis and optic neuritis. J Neuroophthalmol. 2011;31:110–6. https://doi.org/10.1097/WNO.0b013e3181facbbd.
54. Lee SH, Kim TW, Lee EJ, Girard MJ, Mari JM, Ritch R. Ocular and clinical characteristics associated with the extent of posterior lamina cribrosa curve in normal tension glaucoma. Sci Rep. 2018;8:961. https://doi.org/10.1038/s41598-018-19321-1.
55. Hu R, Holbrook J, Newman NJ, Biousse V, Bruce BB, Qiu D, et al. Cerebrospinal fluid pressure reduction results in dynamic changes in optic nerve angle on magnetic resonance imaging. J Neuroophthalmol. 2018; https://doi.org/10.1097/WNO.0000000000000643.
56. Saindane AM, Qiu D, Oshinski JN, Newman NJ, Biousse V, Bruce BB, et al. Noninvasive assessment of intracranial pressure status in idiopathic intracranial hypertension using displacement encoding with stimulated echoes (DENSE) MRI: a prospective patient study with contemporaneous CSF pressure correlation. Am J Neuroradiol. 2018;392:311–6. https://doi.org/10.3174/ajnr.A5486.
57. Suh SY, Le A, Shin A, Park J, Demer JL. Progressive deformation of the optic nerve head and peripapillary structures by graded horizontal duction. Invest Ophthalmol Vis Sci. 2017;58:5015–21. https://doi.org/10.1167/iovs.17-22596.
58. Kolb H, Fernandez E, Nelson R. The Organization of the Retina and Visual System. Salt Lake City: University of Utah Health Sciences Center; 2018. https://webvision.med.utah.edu. Accessed 11 Dec 2018.
59. Ramji S, Touska P, Rich P, MacKinnon AD. Normal neuroanatomical variants that may be misinterpreted as disease entities. Clin Radiol. 2017;72:810–25. https://doi.org/10.1016/j.crad.2017.06.118.
60. Niazi M, Karaman M, Das S, Zhou XJ, Yushkevich P, Cai K. Quantitative MRI of perivascular spaces at 3T for early diagnosis of mild cognitive impairment. Am J Neuroradiol. 2018;39:1622–8. https://doi.org/10.3174/ajnr.A5734.
61. Saindane AM, Bruce BB, Riggeal BD, Newman NJ, Biousse V. Association of MRI findings and visual outcome in idiopathic intracranial hypertension. Am J Roentgenol. 2013;201:412–8. https://doi.org/10.2214/AJR.12.9638.
62. Habes M, Erus G, Toledo JB, Zhang T, Bryan N, Launer LJ, et al. White matter hyperintensities and imaging patterns of brain ageing in the general population. Brain. 2016;139:1164–79. https://doi.org/10.1093/brain/aww008.

63. Wang L, Murphy O, Caldito NG, Calabresi PA, Saidha S. Emerging applications of optical coherence tomography angiography (OCTA) in neurological research. Eye Vis (Lond). 2018;5:11. https://doi.org/10.1186/s40662-018-0104-3.
64. Lanzillo R, Cennamo G, Criscuolo C, Carotenuto A, Velotti N, Sparnelli F, et al. Optical coherence tomography angiography retinal vascular network assessment in multiple sclerosis. Mult Scler. 2018;24:1706–14. https://doi.org/10.1177/1352458517729463.
65. Spain RI, Liu L, Zhang X, Jia Y, Tan O, Bourdette D, et al. Optical coherence tomography angiography enhances the detection of optic nerve damage in multiple sclerosis. Br J Ophthalmol. 2018;102:520–4. https://doi.org/10.1136/bjophthalmol-2017-310477.
66. Herculano-Houzel S. The human brain in numbers: a linearly scaled-up primate brain. Front Hum Neurosci. 2009;3:31. https://doi.org/10.3389/neuro.09.031.2009.
67. Saidha S, Al-Louzi O, Ratchford JN, Bhargava P, Oh J, Newsome SD, et al. Optical coherence tomography reflects brain atrophy in multiple sclerosis: a four-year study. Ann Neurol. 2015;78:801–13. https://doi.org/10.1002/ana.24487.
68. Kuo AN, Verkicharla PK, McNabb RP, Cheung CY, Hilal S, Farsiu S, et al. Posterior eye shape measurement with retinal OCT compared to MRI. Invest Ophthalmol Vis Sci. 2016;57:OCT196–203. https://doi.org/10.1167/iovs.15-18886.
69. Meixner E, Michelson G. Measurement of retinal wall-to-lumen ratio by adaptive optics retinal camera: a clinical research. Graefes Arch Clin Exp Ophthalmol. 2015;253:1985–95. https://doi.org/10.1007/s00417-015-3115-y.
70. Zwillinger S, Paques M, Safran B. In vivo characterization of lamina cribrosa pore morphology in primary open-angle glaucoma. J Fr Ophtalmol. 2016;39:265–71. https://doi.org/10.1016/j.jfo.2015.11.006.
71. Szatmáry G. Imaging of the orbit. Neurol Clin. 2009;27:251–84. https://doi.org/10.1016/j.ncl.2008.09.008.
72. More SS, Beach JM, Vince R. Early detection of amyloidopathy in Alzheimer's mice by hyperspectral endoscopy. Invest Ophthalmol Vis Sci. 2016;57:3231–8. https://doi.org/10.1167/iovs.15-17406.
73. Szatmáry G. Imaging in patients with visual symptoms. Continuum (Minneap Minn). 2016;22:1499–528. https://doi.org/10.1212/CON.0000000000000375.
74. Mokbul MI. Optical coherence tomography: basic concepts and applications in neuroscience research. J Med Eng. 2017;2017:3409327. https://doi.org/10.1155/2017/3409327.
75. Oberwahrenbrock T, Traber GL, Lukas S, Gabilondo I, Nolan R, Songster C, et al. Multicenter reliability of semiautomatic retinal layer segmentation using OCT. Neurol Neuroimmunol Neuroinflamm. 2018;5:e449. https://doi.org/10.1212/NXI.0000000000000449.
76. Roska B, Sahel JA. Restoring vision. Nature. 2018;557:359–67. https://doi.org/10.1038/s41586-018-0076-4.
77. Hillier D, Fiscella M, Drinnenberg A, Trenholm S, Rompani SB, Raics Z, et al. Causal evidence for retina-dependent and -independent visual motion computations in mouse cortex. Nat Neurosci. 2017;20:960–8. https://doi.org/10.1038/nn.4566.
78. Mallery RM, Poolman P, Thurtell MJ, Full JM, Ledolter J, Kimbrough D, et al. Visual fixation instability in multiple sclerosis measured using SLO-OCT. Invest Ophthalmol Vis Sci. 2018;59:196–201. https://doi.org/10.1167/iovs.17-22391.
79. Meltzer E, Sguigna PV, Subei A, Beh S, Kildebeck E, Conger D, et al. Retinal architecture and melanopsin-mediated pupillary response characteristics: a putative pathophysiologic signature for the retino-hypothalamic tract in multiple sclerosis. JAMA Neurol. 2017;74:574–82. https://doi.org/10.1001/jamaneurol.2016.5131.
80. Biousse V, Nahab F, Newman NJ. Management of acute retinal ischemia: follow the guidelines! Ophthalmology. 2018;125:1597–607. https://doi.org/10.1016/j.ophtha.2018.03.054.
81. Graessl A, Muhle M, Schwerter M, Rieger J, Oezerdem C, Santoro D, et al. Ophthalmic magnetic resonance imaging at 7 T using a 6-channel transceiver radiofrequency coil array in healthy subjects and patients with intraocular masses. Investig Radiol. 2014;49:260–70. https://doi.org/10.1097/RLI.0000000000000049.

82. Mallery RM, Poolman P, Thurtell MJ, Wang JK, Garvin MK, Ledolter J, et al. The pattern of visual fixation eccentricity and instability in optic neuropathy and its spatial relationship to retinal ganglion cell layer thickness. Invest Ophthalmol Vis Sci. 2016;57:OCT429–37. https://doi.org/10.1167/iovs.15-18916.
83. Szatmáry G. Neuroimaging in the diagnostic evaluation of eye pain. Curr Pain Headache Rep. 2016;20:52. https://doi.org/10.1007/s11916-016-0582-8.
84. Chen JJ, AbouChehade JE, Iezzi R Jr, Leavitt JA, Kardon RH, et al. Optical coherence angiographic demonstration of retinal changes from chronic optic neuropathies. Neuroophthalmology. 2017;4:76–83. https://doi.org/10.1080/01658107.2016.1275703.
85. Kupersmith MJ, Garvin MK, Wang JK, Durbin M, Kardon R. Retinal ganglion cell layer thinning within one month of presentation for optic neuritis. Mult Scler. 2016;22:641–8. https://doi.org/10.1177/1352458515598020.
86. Al-Louzi O, Button J, Newsome SD, Calabresi PA, Saidha S. Retrograde trans-synaptic visual pathway degeneration in multiple sclerosis: a case series. Mult Scler. 2017;23:1035–9. https://doi.org/10.1177/1352458516679035.
87. Vislisel JM, Chen JJ, Kardon RH. Localizing the lesion in Foster Kennedy syndrome from hemiretinal atrophy at the macula. J Neuroophthalmol. 2014;34:422–5. https://doi.org/10.1097/WNO.0000000000000168.
88. Zehnder S, Wildberger H, Hanson JV, Lukas S, Pelz S, Landau K, et al. Retinal ganglion cell topography in patients with visual pathway pathology. J Neuroophthalmol. 2018;38:172–8. https://doi.org/10.1097/WNO.0000000000000589.
89. Blanch RJ, Micieli JA, Oyesiku NM, Newman NJ, Biousse V. Optical coherence tomography retinal ganglion cell complex analysis for the detection of early chiasmal compression. Pituitary. 2018;21:515–23. https://doi.org/10.1007/s11102-018-0906-2.
90. Micieli JA, Newman NJ, Biousse V. Retinal imaging of an optic tract lesion: OCT angiography of structural and functional defects. Ophthalmology. 2018;125:756. https://doi.org/10.1016/j.ophtha.2018.01.027.
91. Al-Louzi OA, Bhargava P, Newsome SD, Balcer LJ, Frohman EM, Crainiceanu C, et al. Outer retinal changes following acute optic neuritis. Mult Scler. 2016;22:362–72. https://doi.org/10.1177/1352458515590646.
92. Wang JK, Kardon RH, Ledolter J, Sibony PA, Kupersmith MJ, Garvin MK. Peripapillary retinal pigment epithelium layer shape changes from acetazolamide treatment in the idiopathic intracranial hypertension treatment trial. Invest Ophthalmol Vis Sci. 2017;58:2554–65. https://doi.org/10.1167/iovs.16-21089.
93. Adams DL, Piserchia V, Economides JR, Horton JC. Vascular supply of the cerebral cortex is specialized for cell layers but not columns. Cereb Cortex. 2015;25:3673–81. https://doi.org/10.1093/cercor/bhu221.
94. Chen W, You J, Gu X, Du C, Pan Y. High-speed swept source optical coherence Doppler tomography for deep brain microvascular imaging. Sci Rep. 2016;6:38786. https://doi.org/10.1038/srep38786.
95. Merkle CW, Srinivasan VJ. Laminar microvascular transit time distribution in the mouse somatosensory cortex revealed by dynamic contrast optical coherence tomography. NeuroImage. 2016;125:350–62. https://doi.org/10.1016/j.neuroimage.2015.10.017.
96. Drexler W, Liu M, Kumar A, Kamali T, Unterhuber A, Leitgeb RA. Optical coherence tomography today: speed, contrast, and multimodality. J Biomed Opt. 2014;19:071412.
97. World Health Organization. Neurological disorders: public health challenges. 2018. https://www.who.int/mental_health/neurology/neurological_disorders_report_web.pdf. Accessed 12 Dec 2018.
98. Bock M, Brandt AU, Dorr J, Kraft H, Weinges-Evers N, Gaede G, et al. Patterns of retinal nerve fiber layer loss in multiple sclerosis patients with or without optic neuritis and glaucoma patients. Clin Neurol Neurosurg. 2010;112:647–52. https://doi.org/10.1016/j.clineuro.2010.04.014.

99. Fjeldstad C, Bemben M, Pardo G. Reduced retinal nerve fiber layer and macular thickness in patients with multiple sclerosis with no history of optic neuritis identified by the use of spectral domain high-definition optical coherence tomography. J Clin Neurosci. 2011;18:1469–72. https://doi.org/10.1016/j.jocn.2011.04.008.
100. Parisi V, Manni G, Spadaro M, Colacino G, Restuccia R, Marchi S, et al. Correlation between morphological and functional retinal impairment in multiple sclerosis patients. Invest Ophthalmol Vis Sci. 1999;40:2520–7.
101. Pueyo V, Martin J, Fernandez J, Almarcegui C, Ara J, Egea C, et al. Axonal loss in the retinal nerve fiber layer in patients with multiple sclerosis. Mult Scler. 2018;14:609–14. https://doi.org/10.1177/1352458507087326.
102. Sepulcre J, Murie-Fernandez M, Salinas-Alaman A, García-Layana A, Bejarano B, Villoslada P. Diagnostic accuracy of retinal abnormalities in predicting disease activity in MS. Neurology. 2007;68:1488–94. https://doi.org/10.1212/01.wnl.0000260612.51849.ed.
103. Tegetmeyer H, Kuhn E. Quantitative analysis of changes in macular layers following optic neuritis. Neuro-Ophthalmology. 2011;35:101–7.
104. Tatrai E, Simo M, Iljicsov A, Nemeth J, Debuc DC, Somfai GM. In vivo evaluation of retinal neurodegeneration in patients with multiple sclerosis. PLoS One. 2012;7:e30922. https://doi.org/10.1371/journal.pone.0030922.
105. Klistorner A, Arvind H, Nguyen T, Garrick R, Paine M, Graham S, et al. Multifocal VEP and OCT in optic neuritis: a topographical study of the structure-function relationship. Doc Ophthalmol. 2009;118:129–37. https://doi.org/10.1007/s10633-008-9147-4.
106. Johnson LN, Diehl ML, Hamm CW, Sommerville DN, Petroski GF. Differentiating optic disc edema from optic nerve head drusen on optical coherence tomography. Arch Ophthalmol. 2009;127:45–9. https://doi.org/10.1001/archophthalmol.2008.524.
107. Hoye VJ, Berrocal AM, Hedges TR, Amaro-Quireza ML. Optical coherence tomography demonstrates subretinal macular edema from papilledema. Arch Ophthalmol. 2001;119:1287–90.
108. Hedges TR, Vuong LN, Gonzalez-Garcia AO, Mendoza-Santiesteban CE, Amaro-Quiereza AL. Subretinal fluid from anterior ischemic optic neuropathy demonstrated by optical coherence tomography. Arch Ophthalmol. 2008;126:812–5. https://doi.org/10.1001/archopht.126.6.812.
109. Hedges TR, Flattem NL, Bagga A. Vitreopapillary traction confirmed by optical coherence tomography. Arch Ophthalmol. 2006;124:279–81. https://doi.org/10.1001/archopht.124.2.279.
110. Kanamori A, Nakamura M, Matsui N, Nagai A, Nakanishi Y, Kusuhara S, et al. Optical coherence tomography detects characteristic retinal nerve fiber layer thickness corresponding to band atrophy of the optic discs. Ophthalmology. 2004;111:2278–83. https://doi.org/10.1016/j.ophtha.2004.05.035.
111. Monteiro MLR, Leal BC, Rosa AAM, Bronstein MD. Optical coherence tomography analysis of axonal loss in band atrophy of the optic nerve. Br J Ophthalmol. 2004;88:896–9. https://doi.org/10.1136/bjo.2003.038489.
112. Barboni P, Savini G, Valentino ML, Montagna P, Cortelli P, De Negri AM, et al. Retinal nerve fiber layer evaluation by optical coherence tomography in Leber's hereditary optic neuropathy. Ophthalmology. 2005;112:120–6. https://doi.org/10.1016/j.ophtha.2004.06.034.
113. Barboni P, Carbonelli M, Savini G, Ramos CVF, Carta A, Berezovsky A, et al. Natural history of Leber's hereditary optic neuropathy: longitudinal analysis of the retinal nerve fiber layer by optical coherence tomography. Ophthalmology. 2010;113:623–7. https://doi.org/10.1016/j.ophtha.2009.07.026.
114. Savini G, Barboni P, Valentino ML, Montagna P, Cortelli P, De Negri AM, et al. Retinal nerve fiber layer evaluation by optical coherence tomography in unaffected carriers with Leber hereditary optic neuropathy mutations. Ophthalmology. 2005;112:127–31. https://doi.org/10.1016/j.ophtha.2004.09.033.

115. Chicani CM, Carelli V, Berezovsky A. Leber's hereditary optic neuropathy: Project Brazil/LHON - 8 year summary. Vision Panamericana. 2009:170–7.
116. Zaveri MS, Conger A, Salter A, Frohman TC, Galetta SL, Markowitz CE, et al. Retinal imaging by laser polarimetry and optical coherence tomography evidence of axonal degeneration in multiple sclerosis. Arch Neurol. 2008;65:924–8. https://doi.org/10.1001/archneur.65.7.924.
117. Frohman EM, Dwyer MG, Frohman T, Cox JL, Salter A, Greenberg BM, et al. Relationship of optic nerve and brain conventional and non-conventional MRI measures and retinal nerve fiber layer thickness, as assessed by OCT and GDx: a pilot study. J Neurol Sci. 2009;282:96–105. https://doi.org/10.1001/archneur.65.7.924.
118. Costello F, Hodge W, Pan YI, Eggenberger E, Coupland S, Kardon RH. Tracking retinal nerve fiber layer loss after optic neuritis: a prospective study using optical coherence tomography. Mult Scler. 2008;14:893–905. https://doi.org/10.1177/1352458508091367.
119. Mendoza-Santiesteban CE, Gabilondo I, Palma JA, Norcliffe-Kaufmann L, Kaufmann H. The retina in multiple system atrophy: systematic review and meta-analysis. Front Neurol. 2017;8:206. https://doi.org/10.3389/fneur.2017.00206.
120. Mendoza-Santiesteban CE, Palma JA, Martinez J, Norcliffe-Kaufmann L, Hedges TR III, Kaufmann H. Progressive retinal structure abnormalities in multiple system atrophy. Mov Disord. 2015;30:1944–53. https://doi.org/10.1002/mds.26360.
121. Greenberg BM, Frohman E. Optical coherence tomography as a potential readout in clinical trials. Ther Adv Neurol Disord. 2010;3:153–60. https://doi.org/10.1177/1756285610368890.
122. Bodis-Wollner I, Miri S, Glazman S. Venturing into the no-man's land of the retina in Parkinson's disease. Mov Disord. 2014;29:15–22. https://doi.org/10.1002/mds.25741.
123. Malmqvist L, Sibony PA, Fraser CL, Wegener M, Heegaard S, Skougaard M, et al. Peripapillary ovoid hyperreflectivity in optic disc edema and pseudopapilledema. Ophthalmology. 2018;125:1662–4. https://doi.org/10.1016/j.ophtha.2018.04.036.
124. Cruz-Herranz A, Balk LJ, Oberwahrenbrock T, Saidha S, Martinez-Lapiscina EH, Lagreze WA, et al. The APOSTEL recommendations for reporting quantitative optical coherence tomography studies. Neurology. 2016;86:2303–9. https://doi.org/10.1212/WNL.0000000000002774.
125. Baran U, Wang RK. Review of optical coherence tomography based angiography in neuroscience. Neurophotonics. 2016;3:010902. https://doi.org/10.1117/1.NPh.3.1.010902.
126. Kut C, Chaichana KL, Xi J, Raza SM, Ye X, McVeigh ER, et al. Detection of human brain cancer infiltration ex vivo and in vivo using quantitative optical coherence tomography. Sci Transl Med. 2015;7:292ra100. https://doi.org/10.1126/scitranslmed.3010611.
127. Fan Y, Zhang B, Chang W, Zhang X, Liao H. A novel integration of spectral-domain optical-coherence tomography and laser-ablation system for precision treatment. Int J Comput Assist Radiol Surg. 2018;13(3):411–23. https://doi.org/10.1007/s11548-017-1664-8.
128. Chen JJ, Thurtell MJ, Longmuir RA, Garvin MK, Wang JK, Wall M, et al. Causes and prognosis of visual acuity loss at the time of initial presentation in idiopathic intracranial hypertension. Invest Ophthalmol Vis Sci. 2015;56:3850–9. https://doi.org/10.1167/iovs.15-16450.
129. Button J, Al-Louzi O, Lang A, Bhargava P, Newsome SD, Frohman T, et al. Disease-modifying therapies modulate retinal atrophy in multiple sclerosis: a retrospective study. Neurology. 2017;88:525–32. https://doi.org/10.1212/WNL.0000000000003582.
130. Feucht N, Maier M, Lepennetier G, Pettenkofer M, Wetzlmair C, Daltrozzo T, et al. Optical coherence tomography angiography indicates associations of the retinal vascular network and disease activity in multiple sclerosis. Mult Scler. 2018; https://doi.org/10.1177/1352458517750009.

Advances in Retinal Imaging: Retinal Amyloid Imaging

6

Maya Koronyo-Hamaoui, Jonah Doustar, Mia Oviatt, Keith L. Black, and Yosef Koronyo

6.1 Introduction

Alzheimer's Disease (AD) is an invariably fatal neurodegenerative disorder and the leading cause of senile dementia [1]. There is no cure and limited ability for early unequivocal diagnosis. Those afflicted experience cognitive decline such as short-term memory loss, confusion, disorientation and socio-behavioral abnormalities, as well as visual dysfunctions including impaired contrast and color recognition, narrowing of the visual field, and circadian rhythm disruptions [2, 3].

The pathological hallmarks of AD are amyloid β-protein (Aβ) plaques and neurofibrillary tangles (NFTs) comprised of hyperphosphorylated (p)tau protein, which have long been established in the brain [2, 4–9]. Progressive accumulation of Aβ pathology occurs as early as 20 years before the onset of clinical dementia, an insidious phase denoted as prodromal AD [2, 10, 11]. Aβ pathology is thought to drive tauopathy and inflammation [12, 13], co-contributing to synaptic and neuronal loss and eventually dementia [14]. A new NIA-AA research framework describes disease stage based on molecular biomarkers in living patients, specified as Aβ deposition (A), pathologic tau (T), and neurodegeneration [AT(N)], with AD treated as a continuum beginning with mild cognitive impairment (MCI) and progressing to full AD [15]. This research framework publication, together with other genetic, longitudinal brain imaging, physiological, and pathological studies, underline that Aβ deposits are essential to define Alzheimer's pathological changes, among other non-AD neuropathology that can lead to dementia. With the development of promising

M. Koronyo-Hamaoui (✉)
Department of Neurosurgery, Cedars-Sinai Medical Center, Los Angeles, CA, USA

Department of Biomedical Sciences, Cedars-Sinai Medical Center, Los Angeles, CA, USA
e-mail: maya.koronyo@csmc.edu

J. Doustar · M. Oviatt · K. L. Black · Y. Koronyo
Department of Neurosurgery, Cedars-Sinai Medical Center, Los Angeles, CA, USA

A. Grzybowski, P. Barboni (eds.), *OCT and Imaging in Central Nervous System Diseases*, https://doi.org/10.1007/978-3-030-26269-3_6

disease-modifying therapies for AD, intervention during the prodromal phase, when damage to synapses and neuronal tissue is minimal, should offer increased treatment efficacy.

In addition to the above, studies of postmortem brains from AD patients have demonstrated the presence of extra- and intracellular highly synaptotoxic soluble Aβ oligomers [5, 16] and pathogenic assemblies of (p)tau, which self-propagate into synaptically dense brain regions [17, 18]. The pathological signs of AD further include the effects of neuroinflammation and cerebral amyloid angiopathy (CAA), a vascular feature that occurs in 80–90% of all AD patients [19], with moderate to severe forms affecting cortical vessels in roughly 25% [20]. A low-grade chronic inflammation in the brain typically involves molecular mediators and cellular processes like astrogliosis, microgliosis, and infiltration of immune cells [21]. Studies in brains of AD patients have suggested that pathological hallmarks in conjunction with vascular pathology or inflammation may lead to tissue atrophy, and that their coexistence may synergistically drive conversion from prodromal AD to the clinical disease [22]. Further, although inflammation in AD is perceived as detrimental, there is growing evidence demonstrating that peripheral immune cells, such as monocytes, are recruited to the diseased brain and may provide neuroprotection by clearing cerebral Aβ, regulating local inflammation, and enhancing tissue regeneration [23–31].

Current brain imaging technologies are invaluable research tools, as measurements of cerebral atrophy using magnetic resonance imaging (MRI) and functional metabolic changes (e.g. ^{18}F-FDG-PET) can differentiate neuropathological conditions from normal aging [32–34]. However, due to their low specificity, these techniques cannot definitively diagnose AD; the tissue alterations, including degeneration, vascular abnormalities, and glucose metabolism changes are shared with other forms of dementia [2, 35]. Brain imaging of AD hallmarks amyloid and tau pathologies is possible using advanced positron emission tomography (PET) and various radioactive tracers (^{11}C-Pittsburgh compound B, PiB, ^{18}F-florbetapir, ^{18}F-flutemetamol, ^{18}F-florbetaben, ^{18}F-TKH5105 and ^{18}F-T807) [36–40]. However, for screening of large populations, these techniques are expensive, not widely accessible, have some technical limitations, and entail exposure to ionizing radiation [41, 42]. Furthermore, they do not provide sufficient detail about subtle changes in early amyloid build-up [41, 43, 44]. Cerebrospinal fluid (CSF) biomarkers have been widely studied, yet their detection necessitates a highly invasive procedure [45]. The inherent limitations of these methods present major challenges for screening large populations, monitoring response to therapy, and risk management applications [41]; therefore, another CNS tissue may provide a more accessible window through which to diagnose and track AD disease progression.

Growing evidence indicates that the brain is not the only CNS tissue affected by AD—the neurosensory retina is also massively impacted by this disease. The pathologies detected in the brain of MCI and AD patients have also been found in the retina [46–67]. These include a wide spectrum of retinal abnormalities, such as nerve fiber layer thinning, retinal ganglion cell (RGC) degeneration, and vascular abnormalities (reviewed in [46, 68]), and moreover the pathological hallmarks of AD, Aβ deposits and tauopathy [46, 69–75]. Figure 6.1 illustrates the anatomical

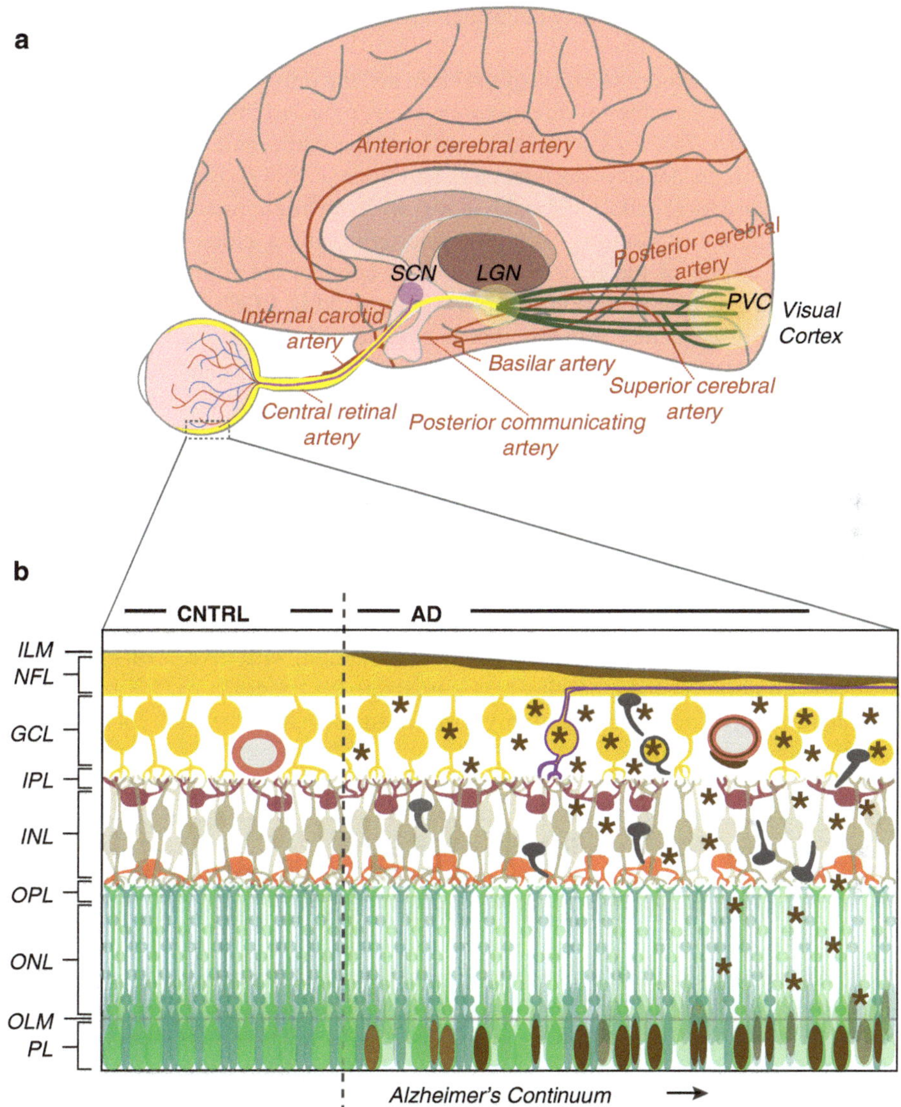

Fig. 6.1 Retinal projections into the brain and AD pathological progression in retinal tissue. (**a**) An illustration of the primary visual pathway with axonal projections to the lateral geniculate nucleus (LGN; yellow) proceeding to the primary visual cortex (PVC; green). Photosensitive retinal ganglion cells (RGCs), such as melanopsin (m)RGCs, form the retinohypothalamic tract (purple) and synapse to three other locations in the brain for specific visual regulations: pretectal nucleus, midbrain nuclei, and suprachiasmatic nucleus (SCN). (**b**) Schematic representation of healthy control (CNTRL) retinal layers and AD-associated progression in disease. Aβ aggregates (brown) appear in the nerve fiber layer (NFL) and ganglion cell layer (GCL) as well as the outer layers of the retina. mRGC (dark purple outline) degeneration associated with Aβ deposits is shown. AD tauopathy (dark grey) is found in the INL and GCL, and cellular atrophy is displayed in all retinal layers

brain-retina connections and key pathological signs of AD extending to the neurosensory retina.

The retina is a sensory extension of the brain and the only CNS tissue not shielded by bone, making it feasible for direct, noninvasive, repeated imaging with high spatial resolution [76–78]. As a tissue derived from the embryonic diencephalon, the retina contains high-density neuronal cells and fibers [77, 79]. Fittingly, it shares a multitude of structural and functional features with the brain, including but not limited to populations of neurons, astroglia, microglia, and a blood barrier [77–80]. Furthermore, axons of the optic nerve directly connect the retina and brain and facilitate vesicular transportation of AβPP synthesized in RGCs [80]. Retinal neurons and glia also secrete proteins that are related to the amyloid cascade (e.g. BACE1, γ-secretase, ApoE and clusterin) [81–84]. In retinas isolated from MCI and AD cases, the optic nerve and RGCs have been shown to undergo neurodegenerative changes, including consistent thinning of the nerve fiber layer (NFL) and macular volume changes [47, 49, 54, 57–60, 63, 73, 85–103]. Moreover, retinal and cerebral microvasculatures share many morphological and physiological properties and are tightly connected [104]. Recent studies suggest that vascular abnormalities are amongst the earliest to occur during AD continuum [105], providing a strong rationale to explore retinal vascular Aβ deposits in combination with vascular abnormalities and their relationship with cerebral Aβ and CAA in AD. This chapter highlights findings related to AD pathology in the retina, with a focus on characteristic Aβ accumulation and emerging new retinal amyloid imaging modalities, which provide new hope for advancing highly specific and sensitive methods for early AD detection and monitoring.

6.2 Amyloid-β Pathology in the Retina

6.2.1 In Alzheimer's Disease Patients

While AD is most commonly understood as a disease of cognition and behavior, a number of visual dysfunctions have become well-established symptoms, including narrowed visual field, loss of color sensitivity, motion and contrast recognition, and sleep cycle disturbances [2, 3, 44, 106–113]. Additionally, various regions of the retina and optic nerve have been implicated as the sites of severe deterioration in AD, perhaps leading to the above-mentioned visual dysfunction [97, 99–103]. These clinical symptoms and neuropathological changes have provoked researchers to assess whether AD-hallmark protein pathologies may extend beyond the brain and into the retina.

Koronyo-Hamaoui et al. first identified the presence of AD-characteristic Aβ deposits in all retinal tissues extracted from patients with definite or probable AD diagnoses. These human samples were characterized by both pre-mortem cognitive evaluations and extensive post-mortem neuropathological analyses [69].

Comparisons against a cohort of age- and gender-matched cognitively normal controls revealed a drastic separation in the observed Aβ pathology between the two diagnostic groups [69]. Since then, a number of studies have corroborated the findings by demonstrating the accumulation of $A\beta_{40}$ and $A\beta_{42}$ peptides [114], plaque aggregates [70, 72, 73], and additionally the presence of hyperphosphorylated (p) tau [71] in postmortem retinae of AD patients. A recent study validated the early studies in postmortem retinas of AD patients, detecting $A\beta^{+}$ immunoreactivity and deposits in various retinal layers, particularly INL, with intracellular deposits localized within amacrine, horizontal, and Müller cells [115]. Extracellular and vascular deposits were also found preferentially in the superior retina [115]. These reports led to further understanding of the spatial distribution and subtypes of Aβ aggregates in the human retina (Figs. 6.2, 6.3, 6.4, 6.5, and 6.6).

Retinal Aβ deposits were also identified in a number of early-stage cases of AD, including MCI (Fig. 6.6a–d) [69]. Large regions of flatmount retinae, after a thorough removal of the vitreous, choroid, and sclera (Fig. 6.2a, b), and extended retinal cross-sections were analyzed utilizing various Aβ-specific monoclonal antibodies (i.e. 12F4, 11A5-B10, 6E10, 4G8), anti-Aβ dyes (i.e. Curcumin, Thioflavin-S, Congo-Red), and Gallyas silver stain [69, 72, 73] (Figs. 6.2d–i, 6.3a–c, f–h, 6.4d, e, and 6.5a–i). These studies revealed that Aβ deposits were non-uniformly manifesting across the retina (Fig. 6.2j). They often appeared in clusters; this irregular pattern seemed to demonstrate a preferential accumulation in the mid- and far-periphery of the retina in AD patients [72, 73]. These areas were previously overlooked due to the difficulties in live acquisition and postmortem processing of entire human retinal whole-mounts, as well as the alleged focus on retinal regions relevant for visual acuity and other retinopathies (e.g. age-dependent macular degeneration and glaucoma).

In a quantitative histological study, definite AD patients presented with a 4.7-fold higher retinal $A\beta_{42}$-containing deposit burden ($12F4^{+}$ area) when compared with age- and sex-matched cognitively normal controls (Fig. 6.2k), indicating that while amyloid proteins may normally be present in the aged human retina, the extent of accumulation may be indicative of AD [72]. Overall, classical and neuritic-like plaques (Fig. 6.3f, g), albeit smaller in size compared to brain plaques, NFTs, $A\beta_{42}$ fibrils, protofibrils, and structures resembling oligomers (Figs. 6.2i and 6.5h, i) were observed in AD patient retinae—AD signs commonly seen in the brain [69, 72, 73, 115].

Before amyloid-related aggregation was shown in the human AD retinae, the presence of Aβ immunoreactivity in the sub-retinal pigment epithelium (RPE) was found in normal aged eyes [116]. In addition, a number of reports have described the presence of fibrillar and non-fibrillar toxic Aβ oligomers in hard and soft drusen in the macular RPE of aged and AMD patients [84, 117, 118]. Aβ assemblies were found to be a common component of drusen in the RPE outer retina, and the percentage of donor eyes with evidence of Aβ in drusen substantially increased with aging [118].

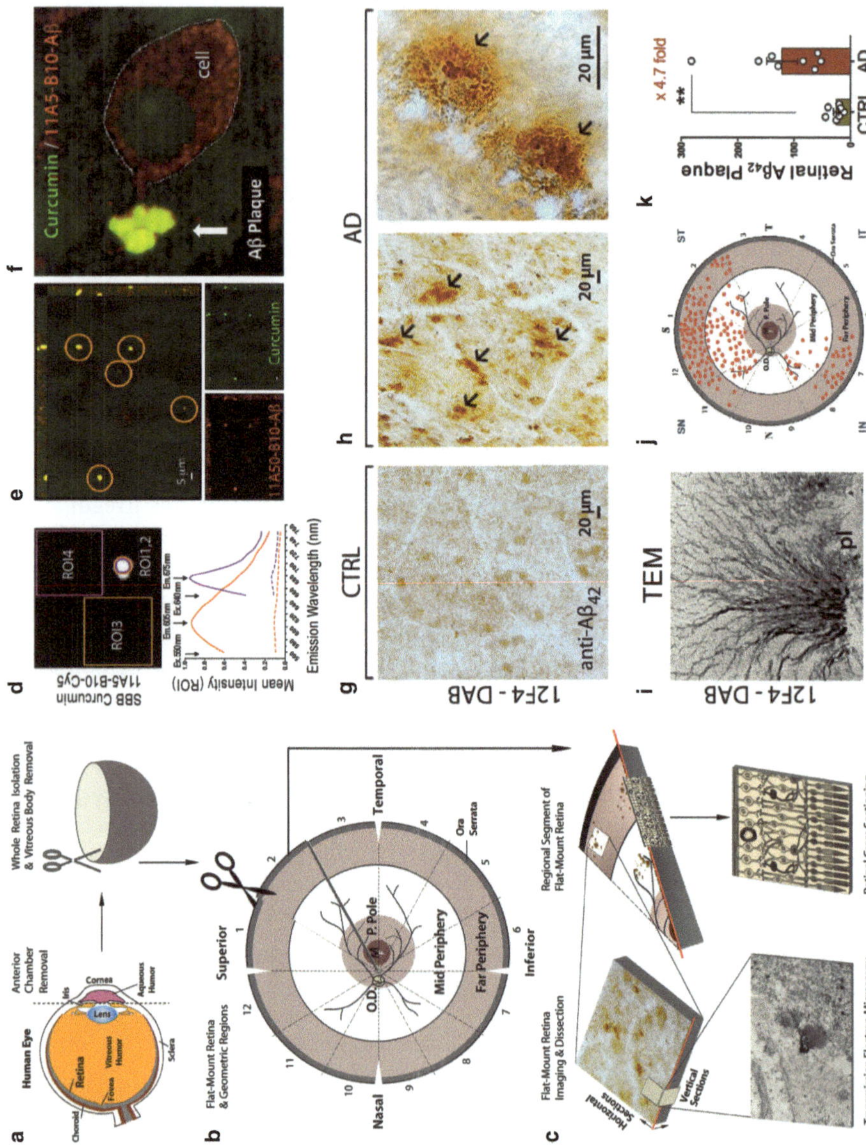
a
Human Eye
Anterior Chamber Removal
Whole Retina Isolation & Vitreous Body Removal
b
Flat-Mount Retina & Geometric Regions
Superior
Temporal
Inferior
Nasal
P. Pole
Mid Periphery
Far Periphery
O.D.
Ora Serrata
c
Flat-Mount Retina Imaging & Dissection
Regional Segment of Flat-Mount Retina
Transmission Electron Microscopy Cross Sectioning & Imaging
Retinal Cross Sectioning & Imaging
d
SBB Curcumin
11A5-B10-Cy5
ROI1,2
ROI3
ROI4
Mean Intensity (ROI)
Emission Wavelength (nm)
e
11A50-B10-Aβ
Curcumin
f
Curcumin / 11A5-B10-Aβ
cell
Aβ Plaque
g
CTRL
AD
h
12F4 - DAB
anti-Aβ42
20 µm
i
TEM
pl
j
k
Retinal Aβ42 Plaque
x 4.7 fold
**
CTRL
AD

Fig. 6.2 Identification of Aβ deposits in the retina of Alzheimer's disease patients. (**a–c**) Protocol for retinal extraction and preparations for flatmount and cross-sectional analyses. (**a**) Whole retinal isolation from donated human eyeballs following separation from the anterior chamber and removal of vitreous humor. (**b**) Sectioning of retinal flatmounts into 12 geometric regions. (**c**) Representative segmentation of retina stained for Aβ for flatmount, cross section, and transmission electron microscopy (TEM) imaging and analyses. (**d–f**) Specificity of curcumin Aβ plaque labeling. (**d**) Retinal Aβ plaque representative image (top panel) and emission spectra (bottom panel). Double-labeled retinal Aβ deposit shown under curcumin (ROI1; orange line) and Cy5-antibody 11A5-B10 conjugate (ROI2; purple line) staining with background areas (ROI3 and ROI4; dashed lines). Curcumin and Cy5-antibody express distinct and separable peak wavelengths in the same individual Aβ plaque. (**e**) Curcumin and 11A5-B10 staining of AD patient retina. (**f**) Distinction between compact extracellular plaque (indicated by arrow) and intracellular Aβ (demarcated by dotted line). (**g, h**) Representative retinal images displaying (**g**) minimal to no Aβ immunoreactivity in a healthy control and (**h**) substantial Aβ plaque pathology in AD. (**i**) 12F4-DAB$^+$ plaque TEM image demonstrating retinal Aβ plaque radial fibrillar arms found in the innermost retinal layers. (**j**) Regional distribution of retinal Aβ deposits analyzed from postmortem retinal flat mounts. (**k**) Quantification of 12F4+ area within ST1-3 regions in a subset of definite AD patients and age- and sex-matched controls (n = 7–8/group). Group mean and SEM are shown. $**P < 0.01$, unpaired 2-tailed Student's *t* test. Images and data of panels (**a–c**) and (**i–k**) are reproduced from Koronyo et al. [72] with permission of ASCI via Copyright Clearance Center. Images and data of panels (**d–f**) are reprinted from, Neuroimage, 54S1, Koronyo-Hamaoui M. et al., Identification of Amyloid Plaques in Retinas from Alzheimer's Patients and Noninvasive In Vivo Optical Imaging of Retinal Plaques in a Mouse Model, S204–S217, Copyright 2011, with permission from Elsevier [69]. Images and data of panels (**g, h**) are adapted from La Morgia et al. [73]

In AD patients, Aβ deposits were identified in the inner retina, and particularly concentrated in the ganglion cell layer (GCL)-NFL innermost layers (Figs. 6.3f, g, 6.4d, e, and 6.5d–g) [72, 115]. The presence of fibrillar and proto-fibrillar forms of $A\beta_{42}$ was confirmed with Birefringence (apple-green) of Congo red-stained retinas under polarized light (Fig. 6.5c) and transmission electron microscopy (TEM) (Figs. 6.2i and 6.5h, h'). Moreover, in a small cohort of aged and AD patients, strong direct correlations between $A\beta_{42}$-specific deposits (12F4$^+$ area) in retinal suprotemporal and cerebral Thioflavin-S and Gallyas silver stainings were detected in various functional and disease-associated regions of the brain (Fig. 6.3d). The primary visual cortex and entorhinal cortex displayed a highly significant and strong correlation with retinal amyloid deposition [72], further shedding light on pathological similarities and the relationship between the retina and brain. In order for retinal amyloid levels to be utilized as a diagnostic tool for AD, their association with cerebral Aβ burden must be further examined and established in future studies.

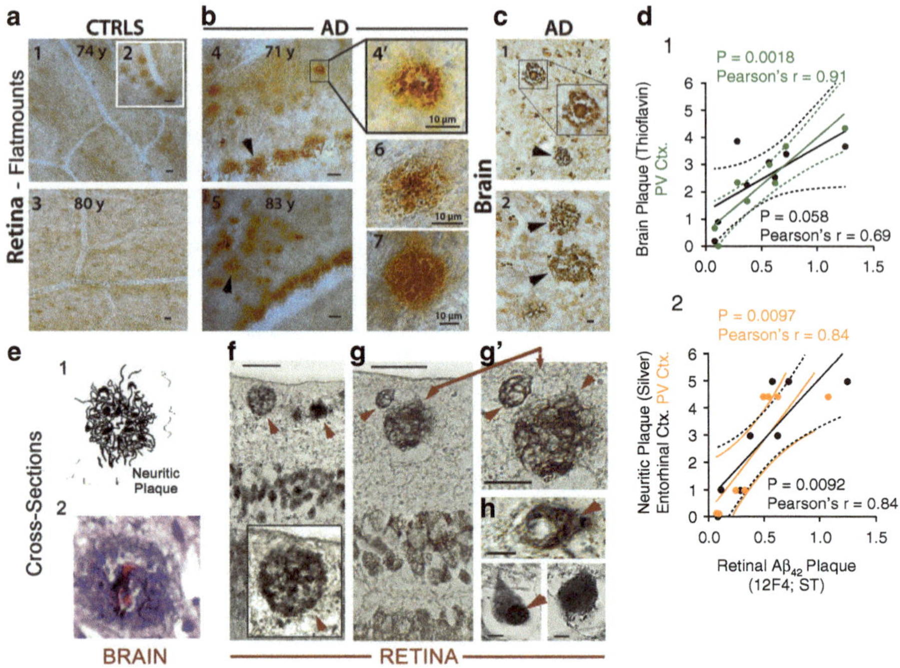

Fig. 6.3 Morphological similarities and quantitative correlations between brain and retinal Aβ plaques in human subjects. (**a–c**) 12F4 anti-$A\beta_{42}$ micrographs of (**a**) non-AD control retinas, (**b**) age- and sex-matched definite AD-patient retinas, along with high magnification images of diffuse, compact, and "classical" mature plaques, and (**c**) AD patient brain sections displaying similar plaque morphologies to retinal Aβ deposits. (**d1**) Pearson's *r* correlation analysis between retinal 12F4$^+$-plaque burden and cerebral plaques (Thioflavin-S) in a subset of AD patients and healthy controls (n = 8); including mean plaque burden from 7 brain regions (black) and the primary visual cortex (PV Ctx; green) and (**d2**) Pearson's *r* correlation analysis between retinal 12F4$^+$-plaque burden and cerebral neuritic plaque (Gallyas silver) in a subset of AD patients and healthy controls (n = 8), including mean plaque burden from the entorhinal cortex (Entorhinal Ctx.; black) and the primary visual cortex (PV Ctx; orange).(**e1**) Illustration of cerebral senile/neuritic plaque and (**e2**) Gallyas silver stain with subsequent immunochemistry of neuritic plaque in the hippocampus of an AD patient. (**f–h**) AD-associated protein aggregates in the retina of AD patients. (**f**) A classic Aβ plaque and compact deposits, along with high magnification image (insert). (**g, g'**) Neuritic senile plaque in the GCL. (**h**) Intracellular and nuclear dominant silver stain aggregates observed in the GCL and INL. Images and data of panels (**a–d**) and (**f–i**) are reproduced from Koronyo et al. [72] with permission of ASCI via Copyright Clearance Center. Image (**e1**) is reprinted from International Encyclopedia of the Social and Behavioral Sciences, Second edition number, Braak et al., Alzheimer's Disease, Neural Basis of, Pages 591–596, Copyright 2015, with permission from Elsevier. Image (**e2**) is reprinted from PNAS, Rajendran et al., Alzheimer's disease beta-amyloid peptides are released in association with exosomes, Copyright 2006 National Academy of Sciences

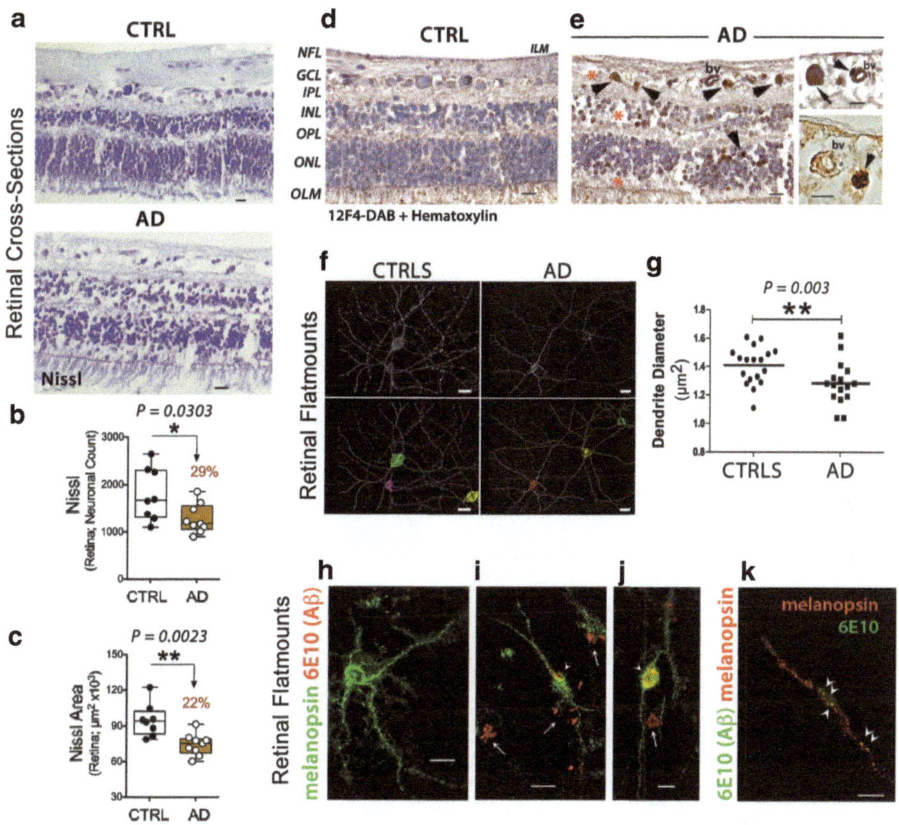

Fig. 6.4 Retinal neuronal loss including of melanopsin Retinal Ganglion Cells (mRGCs) implicated in circadian rhythms, along with retinal Aβ pathology in AD patients. (**a**) Nissl staining of retinal cross sections from a definite AD patient and matched control (CTRL). Changes in cytoplasmic staining patterns (chromatolysis) that could associate with neuronal loss are observed in AD patient. Scale bar: 20 μm. (**b**, **c**) Quantitative Nissl neuronal count and total area in a subset of AD patients and matched CTRLs. Percentage change compared with CTRLs is in red. Group mean and SEM are shown. $*P < 0.05$, $**P < 0.01$, unpaired 2-tailed Student's *t* test. (**d**, **e**) Retinal cross sections from superior quadrants of AD patient and matched healthy CTRL. AD retina contains a multitude of Aβ deposits (arrowheads), especially in the GCL. Marked loss of retinal cells is apparent in the GCL, INL, and ONL; areas of nuclei loss are indicated by red asterisks. Scale bars = 20 μm. Higher magnification images (right panels) show Aβ deposits near and inside blood vessel walls (bv; arrowheads) and inside ganglion cell soma (arrow). Scale bars = 10 μm. (**f**) Morphological analysis of control and AD mRGCs. 3 cells from a control (green, purple, and yellow; left panels) and 3 cells from an AD patient (right panels) as well as their dendritic processes are visualized. Scale bars: left panels, 25 μm; right panels, 24 μm. (**g**) The results of the total analysis of 18 cells from 3 controls and 16 cells from 4 AD patients are shown, demonstrating a significant reduction of dendrite diameter in AD patients. $*P = 0.003$. (**h**–**k**) Colocalization of Aβ deposition and mRGCs visualized via fluorescent immunohistochemistry analysis of flatmount retinas isolated from AD patients and matched control. (**h**) Representative micrograph from control individual demonstrates an intact melanopsin-containing RGC having long dendrites without presence of Aβ. (**i**, **j**) Representative micrographs from AD patients demonstrating intracellular Aβ deposition in mRGCs (arrowheads) as well as extracellular Aβ (arrows). Scale bars = 20 μm. (**k**) An example of an mRGC neurite from AD retina showing colocalization with Aβ (arrowheads). Scale bar = 20 μm. Images and data of panels (**a**–**e**) are reproduced from Koronyo et al. [72] with permission of ASCI via Copyright Clearance Center. Images and data of panels (**f**–**k**) are adapted from La Morgia et al. [73]

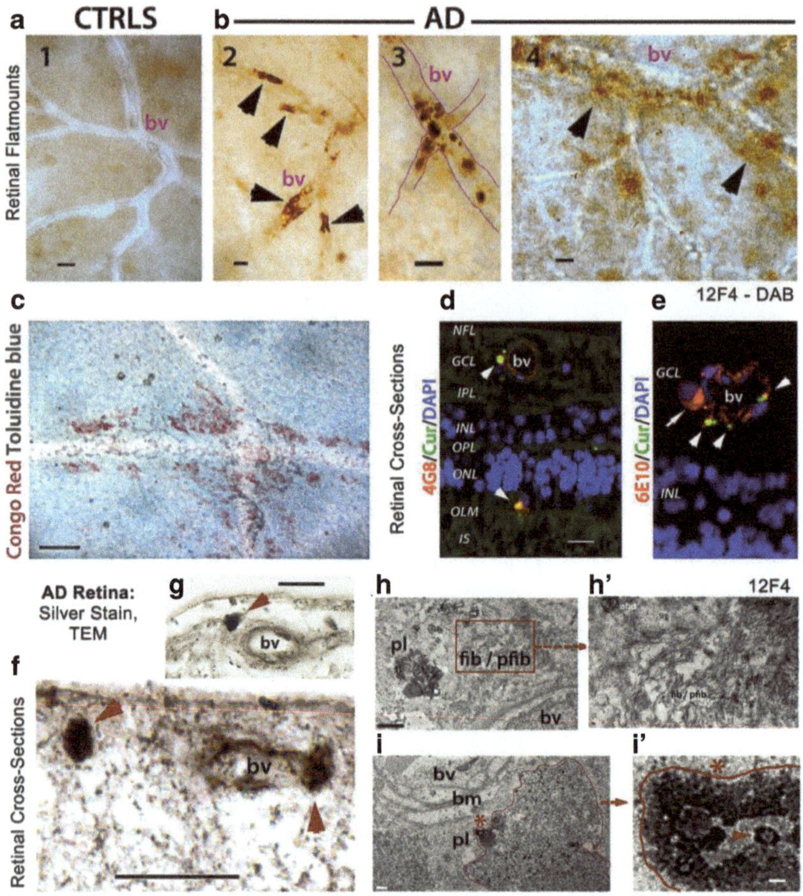

Fig. 6.5 Retinal vascular Aβ deposits in AD patients. (**a**, **b**) Representative micrographs from flatmount retinas of (**a**) definite non-AD control (CTRLS) and (**b**) AD patients. Retinal Aβ deposits are apparent inside blood vessels (bv), perivascular, and along the vessel walls (purple arrowheads). Scale bar = 20 μm. (**c**) Amyloid plaques in AD patient retina. Scale bar: 100 μm. (**d**, **e**) Fluorescent images from AD patient retinas showing curcumin-positive Aβ deposits colocalized with various anti-Aβ mAbs (arrowheads). (**d**) Aβ deposits detected in the outer nuclear layer (ONL), above the outer limiting membrane (OLM), and in the ganglion cell layer (GCL) near and inside blood vessel walls (arrowheads; Scale Bar = 20 μm). (**e**) Intracellular/somatic Aβ immunoreactivity (arrow) and colocalization of 6E10 with curcumin (arrowheads; Scale bar = 10 μm). (**f**) Retinal deposits in GCL near and surrounding a blood vessel. (**g**) AD-associated neuropathologies in the retina (red arrowhead). A compact plaque near a blood vessel (bv). (**h**, **i'**) Transmission electron microscopy (TEM) analyses of vertical (cross) retinal sections from definite AD patients. (**h**) TEM image showing ultrastructure of Aβ plaque (pl), fibrils (fib), and protofibrils (pfib) near a blood vessel (bv), in vertical sections. Scale bar = 1 μm. (**h'**) Higher magnification image indicating presence of 10–15 nm-wide Aβ fibrils, as well as protofibrils and Aβ deposits (abd; Scale bar = 50 nm). (**i**) Aβ plaque-like structure, marked by asterisk and bordering red line, in close proximity to basement membrane (bm) of a blood vessel (Scale bar = 0.5 μm). (**i'**) Higher magnification image of Aβ plaque-like area showing structures resembling paranuclei containing annular oligomers (arrowhead; Scale bar = 40 nm). Images and data are reproduced from Koronyo et al. [72] with permission of ASCI via Copyright Clearance Center

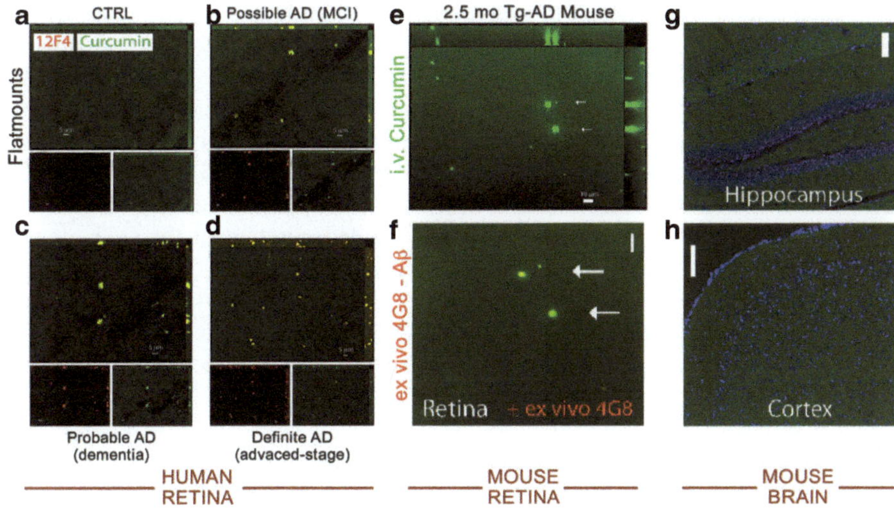

Fig. 6.6 Early signs of Aβ deposits in the retina of early-stage AD cases and murine models. (**a**–**d**) Representative whole-mount retinas from normal individuals (CTRL) and from possible/probable AD patients, stained with curcumin and anti-Aβ_{42} mAb. Separate channels for each staining shown below each image. (**a**) In the retina from cognitively normal individual with no AD pathology, Aβ plaques could not be detected. (**b**) In a patient with possible AD diagnosis, clusters of Aβ plaques were observed, and (**c**) in retina from patient with several years of dementia and postmortem diagnosis of probable AD, Aβ plaques were more common throughout the retina. (**d**) Abundant Aβ plaques were observed in the retina from severe-stage AD definite patient. (**e**–**h**) Bioavailability of systemically administered curcumin to the mouse eye: accumulation of curcumin-labeled retinal Aβ plaques with disease progression and detection at early pre-symptomatic stage. Representative z-axis projection images of whole-mount retinas and brain coronal cryosections from AD-Tg and non-Tg (wt) mice following i.v. curcumin injections. (**e**, **f**) Retinal curcumin-labeled Aβ plaques (green) were visible in vivo, with further (**f**) validation of Aβ plaque identity in the same retinal location (arrows) by staining ex vivo with anti-human Aβ mAb. Co-localization of curcumin and Aβ antibody in yellow pseudocolor. Scale bar = 10 μm. (**g**, **h**) No plaques were detected in the brain hippocampus and cortex of AD-Tg mice. Scale bars = 100 μm. Images and data are reprinted from Neuroimage, 54S1, Koronyo-Hamaoui M. et al., Identification of Amyloid Plaques in Retinas from Alzheimer's Patients and Noninvasive In Vivo Optical Imaging of Retinal Plaques in a Mouse Model, S204–S217, Copyright 2011, with permission from Elsevier [69]

6.2.2 Retinal Aβ Is Associated with Neuronal Degeneration in AD Patients

The described distribution of retinal Aβ deposits in AD patients indicating high frequency in the superior quadrants aligns with previous reports showing NFL thinning and RGC degeneration in the GCL primarily within these regions [58, 73, 86, 119]. Importantly, in a clinical study published by La Morgia et al. [73], AD patients displayed degeneration in a number of retinal layers, assessed with in vivo OCT imaging. This study further revealed a significant degeneration of melanopsin-containing retinal ganglion cells (mRGC), in both cell number and dendritic density (Fig. 6.4f, g). The mRGCs are photoreceptors known to drive circadian photoentrainment and believed to have a key role in circadian rhythms in humans [120]. Importantly, mRGC cell death and dendrite loss was tightly associated with Aβ deposition labeled with 6E10⁺ (Fig. 6.4h–k). The vulnerability of mRGCs in AD patients may indicate that Aβ is more detrimental to certain retinal cells and provides the first potential retina-based mechanistic explanation for the sleep disturbances seen in AD patients [73]. A more recent study showed that, along with accumulation of Aβ deposits, a marked loss of retinal cells was detected (Fig. 6.4d, e). Nissl staining demonstrated retinal neuronal degeneration in the GCL, inner nuclear layer (INL), and outer nuclear layer (ONL) in retinas from AD patients compared to age-matched cognitively normal controls (Fig. 6.4a–c). AD retinas showed a 29% reduction in Nissl⁺ neuronal number and a 22% reduction in Nissl⁺ area (Fig. 6.4a–c) [72].

6.2.3 Retinal Vascular Aβ in Alzheimer's Disease

Retinal Aβ deposits are frequently found along, around, and within blood vessel walls, as recently demonstrated in a subset of CAA-positive AD patients (Fig. 6.5), which was consistent with respective cerebral vascular pathology [72, 73]. Retinal and cerebral microvasculatures share many morphological and physiological properties [104]. This retinal vascular amyloidosis may provide an explanation for the well-documented narrowing of venous blood column diameter and reduced blood flow in the AD retina [52, 73, 86, 121–124], similar to findings in the brain [125–127]. The mechanism for this phenomenon was recently proposed in AD murine models, by demonstrating that vascular amyloid can cause rigidity in blood vessel walls and decrease blood flow [127]. Moreover, Koronyo et al. [72] data showed evidence of many forms of vascular-related retinal Aβ deposits in AD patients, inside epithelium, within Tunica media and outside the basement membrane (Figs. 6.4e and 6.5a–i). Both retinal flatmounts and cross sections with various anti-Aβ antibodies (12F4, 11A50-B10, 6E10, 4G8) and staining methods (Congo-Red, Thioflavin-S, curcumin, Gallyas silver stain) were used to identify vascular Aβ deposits [69, 72, 73, 115]. Together with a recent clinical study pointing to cerebral vascular pathologies as, perhaps, the earliest changes in AD [105], these data provide a strong rationale to explore in future studies how retinal Aβ deposits may affect or be affected by changes in retinal veins, arteries, and capillaries. Such an investigation could provide a fundamental understanding of how Aβ accumulation in the retina occurs and may affect or reflect neurodegeneration processes driving the clinical manifestation of cognitive impairment and eventually dementia.

It has been previously shown that the central retinal artery that originates in the optic nerve head branches into capillary networks that nourish the inner retinal layers. The choroidal blood vessels, which receive 65–85% of the blood flow, are vital for the maintenance of the outer retina (especially the photoreceptors). Thus, pathological changes within these arteries could detrimentally affect the retinal cell layers that they support. A key physiological mechanism of cerebral Aβ clearance is the efflux of Aβ to the peripheral blood through the blood-brain barrier [128–133]. Precapillary venules in the retina drain into the central retinal vein through local venules. In the retina of AD patients, perivascular Aβ surrounding probable veins are commonly seen (Figs. 6.4 and 6.5b2 arrowheads and Fig. 6.5d). This vascular Aβ pathology could reduce the efficiency of Aβ removal through the blood-retina barrier or limit accessibility of circulating and infiltrating Aβ-clearing monocytes and macrophages [23, 25, 134].

As mentioned above, to further study the ultrastructure of Aβ deposits in the retina, a recent study included a TEM analysis of vertical and *en face* retinal sections from a subset of AD patients that had been pre-labeled with 12F4 mAbs (anti-$A\beta_{42}$ alloforms) (Figs. 6.2i and 6.5h, i). This analysis revealed the ultrastructures of retinal Aβ plaques, fibrils, protofibrils, and other types of Aβ assemblies [72]. Similar to those in the brain [135], retinal Aβ fibrils were found to be 10–15 nm wide with anti-parallel β-sheets (Fig. 6.5h). Fibrils with parallel β-sheets were often found adjacent to basement membrane of blood vessels (Fig. 6.5h, i); TEM images of *en face* retinal sections indicated the presence of retinal Aβ plaques with radial fibrillar arms emanating from central cores (Fig. 6.2i: dark black lines indicating the core). Another example for retinal Aβ deposition associated with blood vessels in AD patients came from a recent report using flatmount AD retinas after Congo-red staining [72]. In this experiment, researchers visualized a patient's retina with two intersecting blood vessels that were surrounded by extensive Congo red–positive staining of Aβ deposition, while the background blue counterstain was of Toluidine blue (Fig. 6.5c). In the same experiment, birefringence (apple-green) of Congo red-stained retinas under polarized light confirmed the presence of amyloid fibrils [72]. A summary of AD-associated pathology in retinae and other ocular tissues of AD patients is presented in Table 6.1.

6.2.4 In Animal Models of Alzheimer's Disease

In line with findings in human cases, numerous studies examining the retinae of sporadic and transgenic animal models have reported soluble and insoluble Aβ deposition, often associated with local inflammation, ganglion cell degeneration, and functional deficits such as light response/electroretinogram amplitude. Interestingly, these retinal plaque formations were also detected prior to corresponding brain burden in a number of studies [69, 70, 73, 74, 155–158]. Furthermore, reports on the positive effects of therapy on cerebral Aβ burden of AD transgenic animal models also described similar responses observed in the respective retinas [69, 74, 156, 159–162]. These findings have not only been invaluable in our understanding of disease characteristics and progression but have also provided the foundation for the potential role of the retina as a measure of therapeutic efficacy.

The transmembrane amyloid precursor protein (APP), source of the toxic Aβ protein, has been identified in the retinas of numerous animal models for AD (ADtg), including transgenic drosophila, various transgenic mouse models (Tg2576, hTgAPP$^{tg/tg}$, $APP_{SWE}/PS1_{\Delta E9}$, and $APP_{SWE}/PS1_{M146L/L286V}$), and the non-transgenic, sporadic rodent strain *Octodon degus* (*O. degus*) [155, 156, 158, 163, 164]. Analysis of cytoplasmic APP levels in retinal layers revealed a marked increase in transgenic models [155, 164], while the sporadic *O. degus* shows reduction with age [158].

Table 6.1 Abnormalities observed in CNS and non-CNS ocular tissues of AD patients

Tissue		Pathology	Findings	References
CNS	Retina	Amyloid-β	• Elevated AβPP expression	[114, 136]
			• Increased $A\beta_{40}$ and $A\beta_{42}$ peptide levels	[114]
			• Classical and diffuse extracellular Aβ deposits, neuritic-like plaques, intracellular Aβ, and intranuclear Aβ, superior temporal	[69, 70, 72, 73, 115, 137]
			• Ultrastructure of $A\beta_{42}$ proto-fibrils and fibrils	[72]
			• Substantial increase in retinal $A\beta_{42}$ plaque area in AD patients compared to age- and gender-matched cognitively normal individuals	[72]
			• Correlation with cerebral amyloid burden, especially in PVC[a] and EC[b]	[72]
			• Aβ deposits inside and around degenerating melanopsin RGCs[c] and Aβ deposits colocalized with neuronal loss	[72, 73]
		Tau	• NFT[d]-like and pTau positive in GCL[e], IPL[f], INL[g], ONL[h], OPL[i]	[71, 72, 115, 138]
		Neuronal degeneration	• NFL[j] thinning and macular volume loss in all quadrants; mostly in superior and inferior quadrants; diffuse dropout; NFL thickness correlated with MMSE[k] score, NFL abnormalities	[47, 49, 52, 57–60, 63, 73, 86–97, 99, 138–142]
			• GCL degeneration from mild to severe; RGC swelling; loss of mRGC and dendritic arborization	[72, 73, 97, 99]
			• Neuronal loss in RGC, IPL, ONL	[72]
			• Reduced foveal thickness in CSF-$A\beta42^+$ vs. CSF-$A\beta42^-$	[143]
			• Decreased retinal thickness in AD and MCI patients	[51]
			• Reduced thickness in global and temporal superior quadrants in pRNFL[l] and in superior pericentral and peripheral sectors of RT[m]	[144]
			• Reduced GC-IPL and NFL thickness increases risk for dementia	[145]
		Inflammation	• Extensive cell processes suggesting gliosis from ILM[n] near GCL	[99]
		Vascular	• Perivascular and vascular Aβ deposits	[72, 73]
			• Reduction of venous blood flow, column diameter, speed, arteriolar and venular fractal dimensions, branching complexity and geometric optimality; changes to arteriolar and venular tortuosity; increased width variation; blood flow corr. with NFL thickness	[52, 86, 121, 122, 124]
			• Elevated oxygen saturation	[146]
			• Enlarged FAZ[o] in cerebral amyloid-PET[p]+ vs. amyloid-PET$^-$ early AD	[143]
		Other	• Intermediate hard drusen more common in the temporal region in AD; significant correlation with CAA[q] severity	[147]
	Optic nerve	Structural	• Large caliber fiber loss, superior and nasal quadrant axonal loss, overall reduction	[73, 97, 103]
			• Cup-to-disc ratio increase, intraocular pressure susceptibility increased, optic disc paleness, suggested link to glaucoma	[91, 103, 140, 141, 148–150]

Non-CNS	Lens	Amyloid	• Elevated AβPP expression	[136]
			• Cytosolic electron-dense Aβ nanodeposits in supranuclear, cortical regions and in anterior epithelial subregion in DS[r] lens	[91, 136, 151]
		Other	• Supranuclear cataracts, opacity[s], PS1[t] expressed in DS lens	[146, 152, 153]
	Cornea	Other	• PS1 expressed in the DS cornea	[153]
	Aq. Humor	Amyloid	• Increased $A\beta_{40}$ levels	[136]
	Choroid	Structural	• Thickness reduction	[70, 154]

[a]Primary visual cortex
[b]Entorhinal cortex
[c]Retinal ganglion cell
[d]Neurofibrillary tangles
[e]Ganglion cell layer
[f]Inner plexiform layer
[g]Inner nuclear layer
[h]Outer nuclear layer
[i]Outer plexiform layer
[j]Nerve fiber layer
[k]Mini-mental state examination
[l]Peripapillary retinal nerve fiber layer
[m]Retinal thickness
[n]Inner limiting membrane
[o]Foveal avascular zone
[p]Positron emission tomography
[q]Cerebral amyloid angiopathy
[r]Down's syndrome
[s]Opacity difference not statistically significant
[t]Presenilin-1 protein

A study by Ning et al. in 2008 identified APP immunoreactivity within cells of the GCL and INL but not the ONL. Additionally, the neuropil of the IPL and outer plexiform layer (OPL) as well as the OS and RPE displayed elevated APP levels. These regions exhibited elevated immunoreactivity with age [155].

These animal models have been reported to present with increases in soluble and insoluble forms of Aβ accumulating in an age-dependent manner and corresponding to AD-like progression. Such findings have been reported in a large group of ADtg rodent models, including Tg2576, APP/PS1, 3xTg, 5xFAD mice, the TgF344-AD rat, and *O. degus* [69, 70, 114, 156–158, 161, 164–169] (Fig. 6.7a–d). Studies on forms of Aβ most pathognomonic to AD—$A\beta_{40}$ and particularly $A\beta_{42}$—reported an elevation of these proteins in the retina of AD rodent models [70, 114, 156, 158, 161, 164, 167, 169] and even in ADtg drosophila [170, 171].

Insoluble Aβ formations and plaque deposits have been observed in the retinas of Tg2576, $APP_{SWE}/PS1_{\Delta E9}$, $APP_{SWE}/PS1_{M146L/L286V}$, 3xTg, and 5xFAD mice, as well as *O. degus* [69, 74, 114, 155–159, 164–166, 169, 172]. Cross sectional analysis of Tg2576 mouse retinas identified plaque pathology in ~85% of transgenic mice, as opposed to a consistent absence in WT controls. These plaques were primarily reported in the various nuclear retinal layers (GCL, INL and ONL) [156, 169]. However, one study reported minimal to no detection of retinal Aβ pathology in a Tg2576 mouse positive for cerebral amyloid burden under enzyme-linked immunosorbent assay (ELISA) and western blot [164]. Studies on 5xFAD mice, transgenic mice expressing both amyloid and tau associated pathologies, showed detectable levels of $A\beta_{42}$ in a number of ocular tissues, including the retina, and revealed notable increases in $A\beta_{40}$ in the non-neural RPE [161, 167]. The sporadic, naturally occurring *O. degus* model of AD appears to display a progressive abundance of Aβ deposition, initially arising in the NFL, GCL, and photoreceptors, then spreading to the remaining retinal layers. Histological examination of whole retinas showed the greatest plaque burden in the central regions, determined via a number of Aβ-specific stainings, except Congo red [158, 173].

Perhaps one of the more commonly studied ADtg models is the double transgenic $APP_{SWE}/PS1_{\Delta E9}$ mouse. A study by Koronyo-Hamaoui et al. utilized curcumin-specific staining of Aβ to visualize retinal plaque distribution [69]. This highly specific protocol for both human and mouse tissue interestingly revealed Aβ accumulation in whole-mount retinas prior to its deposition in the corresponding cerebral tissue (Fig. 6.6e–h). 2.5-month-old mice were intravenously injected with curcumin and examination of isolated retinal flatmounts revealed curcumin-positive deposits, further confirmed as Aβ-specific deposits by ex vivo 4G8 monoclonal antibody staining, detected prior to their appearance in the respective brains (Fig. 6.6e, f vs. Fig. 6.6g, h). Retinal cross section analysis demonstrated the presence of Aβ deposits from the innermost retinal layers of adult APP/PS1 Tg-AD mice, but also in the choroid and surrounding scleral tissue, with minimal to no fluorescence in non-transgenic controls (Fig. 6.7c, d) [69]. Similar findings were reported in a number of studies using the same mouse model and Tg344F-AD rats, which share the same double transgenes [70, 155–157]. In agreement with the above-mentioned studies, a recent study has detected the presence of retinal Aβ plaques and tau tangles in the RGC layer of young, pre-symptomatic 3xTg mice [174]. Table 6.2 summarizes AD hallmark pathology in various animal models of AD.

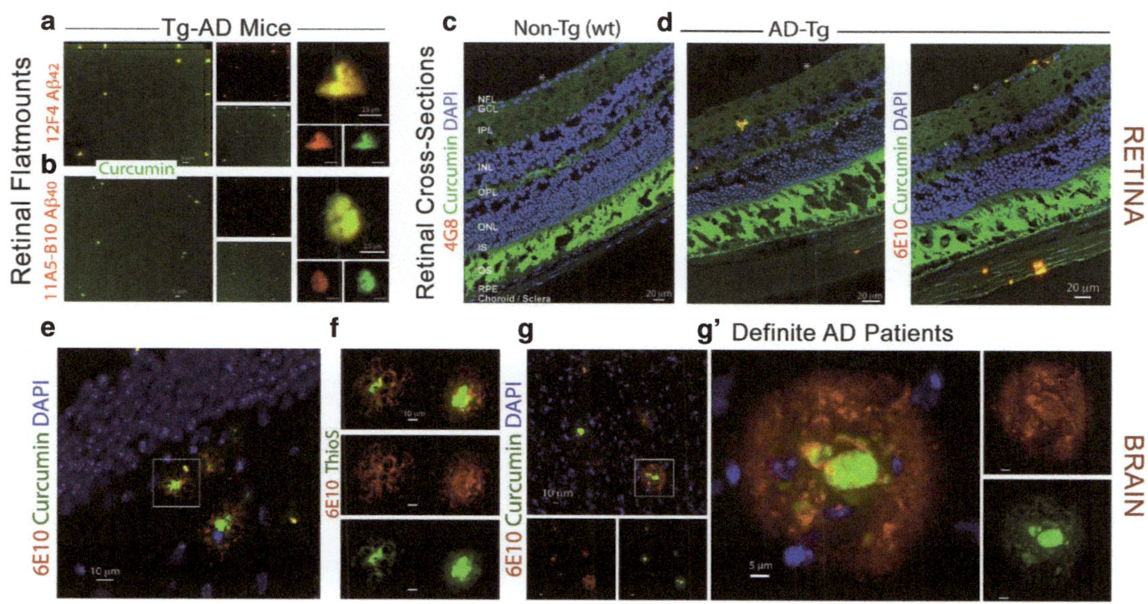

Fig. 6.7 Retinal Aβ deposits are associated with retinal neuronal loss and can be reliably labeled with curcumin in AD patients and transgenic murine models. (**a**, **b**) Representative whole mount retinas from a transgenic AD mouse model (ADtg) double stained with curcumin and either (**a**) 12F4$^+$ Aβ_{42} or (**b**) 11A5-B10$^+$ Aβ_{40}, alongside each respective channel displayed separately and in high magnification. (**c**, **d**) Non-transgenic wild-type (WT) and ADtg whole eyes cross-sectioned and stained with anti-Aβ mAbs (4G8 or 6E10), curcumin and DAPI-nuclei. (**c**) Absence of double-positive curcumin and 4G8$^+$ Aβ in WT mouse eye, compared to (**d**) co-labeled Aβ plaque (curcumin and 4G8/6E10) identified in various retinal layers of ADtg mice, in addition to the sclera. White asterisks indicate DAPI nuclei staining in the GCL: ADtg mice display a deficiency in this region. (**e**–**g'**) Curcumin and Aβ (6E10 and ThioS) ex vivo labelling patterns in (**e**, **f**) ADtg and (**g**, **g'**) definite AD patient brain cryosections with a preferential staining of curcumin on central core Aβ plaques. Higher magnification image demonstrating the fine structure of Aβ plaque and its specific staining pattern by curcumin and 6E10 mAb. Images and data are reprinted from Neuroimage, 54S1, Koronyo-Hamaoui M. et al., Identification of Amyloid Plaques in Retinas from Alzheimer's Patients and Noninvasive In Vivo Optical Imaging of Retinal Plaques in a Mouse Model, S204–S217, Copyright 2011, with permission from Elsevier [69]

Table 6.2 AD-specific ocular biomarkers in animal models

AD pathology		Species	Model	Findings	References
Amyloid-related	AβPP expression	Drosophila	AβPP[a]/dBACE[b]/dPsn[c]	Expression in fly eye; over-expression in all murine retinal layers, optic nerve, cornea, lens	[155, 156, 158, 164, 171, 172, 175]
		Mouse	Tg2576[d], APP/PS1[e]		
		O. degus[f]	Sporadic AD (aged)		
	Aβ peptides	Drosophila	pGMR-$A\beta_{42}$[g], dBACE-AβPPL[h]	Increased levels in retinal extracts from fly; NFL, GCL, IPL, INL, OPL, OS[i], RPE (extra- and intracellular), choroid, cornea, lens, vitreous humor, including oligomeric Aβ species and Aβ engulfed by astrocytes; in *O. degus*, more peptides and oligomers detected in central retina	[69, 114, 155, 156, 158, 161, 165–171, 176–178]
		Mouse	Tg2576, APP/PS1, 3xTg[j], 5xFAD[k]		
		O. degus	Sporadic AD (aged)		
	Aβ deposits	Drosophila	AβPP, dBACE-AβPPL, pGMR-$A\beta_{42}$	Retinal extracts from fly; deposits and/or plaques in most retinal layers (strongest in GCL and central retinal region), mostly in the inner retinal layer, optic nerve, sclera; endogenous dAβ[l] deposits; age-related increase	[69, 70, 114, 155–159, 164, 165, 170, 171, 174, 178]
		Mouse	Tg2576, APP/PS1, 3xTg, 5xFAD		
		O. degus	Sporadic AD (aged)		
		Rat	TgF344-AD[m]		
	Vascular Aβ	Mouse	Tg2576, APP/PS1	Vascular-associated deposition in GCL, IPL, INL, OPL, choroid in rodents	[69, 155, 156, 164]
		Rat	TgF344-AD		

Tau-related	pTau	Drosophila	hTau[n]	Differential cell type-specific pTau variants in fly eye; increased in most retinal layers, strongest in GCL, none in NFL, RPE; NFL, GCL, AT8[o] reactivity in *O. degus*; (p)tau were highly expressed in inner retinal neurons; age-related increase; early as 3 months of age and preceded tau aggregation in the brain	[156, 158, 172, 179–181]
		Mouse	Tg2576, APP/PS1, HTau[p], 3xTg		
		O. degus	Sporadic AD (aged)		
	NFT[q]	Mouse	APP/PS1, 3xTg	Immunoreactivity in murine retina, particularly in GCL, RPE, mostly in the inner retinal layer, age-related increase	[159, 160, 172, 174]

[a]Drosophila expressing amyloid-β protein precursor
[b]Drosophila expressing beta-secretase 1
[c]Model expressing drosophila presenilin-1 protein
[d]Mouse overexpressing APP isoform 695 bearing Swedish double mutations K670M/N671L
[e]Mouse overexpressing $APP_{SWE}/PS1_{\Delta E9}$ or $APP_{SWE}/PS1_{M146L}$
[f]*Octodon degus*, WT rodent native to Chile showing symptoms of sporadic AD
[g]Glass multiple reporter drosophila model expressing $A\beta_{42}$
[h]Drosophila expressing AβPP-like protein
[i]Outer segment of photoreceptors
[j]Mouse overexpressing $APP_{SWE}/PS1/TAU_{P301L}$
[k]Mouse overexpressing $APP_{SWE/FL/LON}/PS1_{M146L/L286V}$
[l]Drosophila amyloid-β protein
[m]$APP_{SWE}/PS1_{\Delta E9}$ rat model
[n]Drosophila expressing human Tau protein
[o]Antibody binding pTau phosphorylated at Ser202 and Thr205
[p]A transgenic murine model expressing human tau
[q]Neurofibrillary tangle

Noninvasive in vivo retinal imaging has provided the opportunity to monitor alterations in amyloid burden following therapeutic intervention. Studies aimed at determining co-reactions between retinal and cerebral amyloid burden in response to therapies provide valuable insight into the applicability of retinal imaging as a tool for measuring therapeutic efficacy. In 2009, Liu et al. reported his findings on the Tg2576 retinal response to subcutaneous vaccinations of amyloid-associated proteins. Namely, islet amyloid polypeptide (IAPP) and Aβ oligomer (AO) immunizations resulted in significant reductions in histological examinations of retinal amyloid burden. Interestingly, retinal amyloid angiopathy was markedly increased with these treatments, along with microglial and astroglial reactivity. Retinal thickness was greater with treatment compared to sham-PBS injected controls, but still displayed thinning compared to non-treated WT [156].

One of these therapies includes an FDA-approved drug currently deployed for multiple sclerosis and repurposed for studies on the effects of immunomodulation in AD. Over the past few years, the Koronyo-Hamaoui group has published their findings on the beneficial effects of the FDA-approved glatiramer acetate (GA) and a similar myelin-derived therapy, modified myelin oligodendrocyte glycoprotein-derived peptide (MOG45D), which was loaded onto dendritic cells (DC-45D) [69, 74]. Their initial investigation of MOG45D treatment on APP/PS1 mice in 2010 reported a remarkable 69% reduction of curcumin- and 4G8-positive retinal Aβ area assessed ex vivo (Fig. 6.10a–c). Importantly, this retinal response was comparable to the attenuation of the corresponding cerebral burden (Fig. 6.10c, d) [69]. Subsequent studies utilizing GA produced the first in vivo assessment of retinal Aβ deposition, revealing decreased deposition following 1- and 2-month regimens (Fig. 6.10e–h) [74]. An additional study by Yang et al. on bone marrow transplantation (BMT) in APP/PS1 mice showed significant reductions in both retinal and cerebral amyloid plaque burden when compared to non-treated controls [159].

Collectively, the abundant studies published in the past decade strongly support the retina as an extension of the brain in disease and in health: it may faithfully act as a reliable tool for measurements of disease progression and therapeutic response. Table 6.2 summarizes findings on retinal AD characteristic pathology in various animal models.

6.3 Other Alzheimer's-Associated Pathology in the Retina

6.3.1 In Alzheimer's Disease Patients

In addition to the hallmark signs of AD, amyloid-associated pathology has also been described in the patient retina, including but not limited to angiopathy, nerve fiber layer (NFL) thinning, RGC degeneration, macular volume changes, synaptic loss, and tauopathy [46, 49, 52, 54, 60, 63, 73, 88, 89, 92–94, 100, 102, 103, 112, 122, 124, 182, 183].

Hinton and colleagues first reported optic nerve degeneration, decreased ganglion cell numbers, and thinning of the NFL in AD patients [103]. Further reports of GCL pathology described severe degeneration of RGCs, including a phenotype of vacuolated mitochondria and nerve fiber cell degeneration. Evidence of AD-related GCL degeneration has been accumulating since then, including a report of 25% neuronal loss in the GCL, with the greatest losses noted in the superior and inferior retinal quadrants [99–102]. A recent report by Koronyo et al. [72] found a significant 22% retinal neuronal loss, as measured by Nissl stain, across retinal layers including RGC, INL, ONL in definite AD patients as compared to age- and gender-matched controls (Fig. 6.4a–c) [72]. In 1996, Blanks et al. further detected astrogliosis with neuronal loss in the retina of AD patients [100]. Structural changes in inner retinal layers were also found in these patients [57, 139], as well as alterations in cup-to-disc ratio, macular volume, blood flow, and vasculature density [46, 106, 122–124, 140, 146, 184]. Further, retinal angiopathy and vascular-related changes mirroring the brain were described, including narrowed veins, reduction of blood flow, elevated blood oxygen saturation, and increased tortuosity [52, 86, 121, 122, 124, 146].

The majority of studies investigating the NFL in AD patients reported significant thinning occurring nonuniformly [47, 49, 54, 57, 60, 63, 73, 85–88, 90, 92, 93, 95, 96], although some findings did not reach significance [52, 63, 89, 114, 138, 139, 185]. Thus, there is general agreement, including from large meta-analysis studies, that significant thinning of the superior quadrant of the NFL occurs in the retina of AD patients [49, 54, 57–60, 73, 86, 87, 89, 91, 94–97, 139, 140], even in early prodromal stages and correlating with cognitive status [143, 145]. It is important to note that these retinal structural and vascular differences are not considered specific to AD but are shared among other neurodegenerative diseases. Yet, they reflect functional changes in the retina of patients that may lead to some of the clinical manifestations in AD patients.

Another key hallmark pathology of AD, beyond Aβ deposits which were described in the retina of AD patients, is pTau [71] (Fig. 6.8a, b). A recent study by

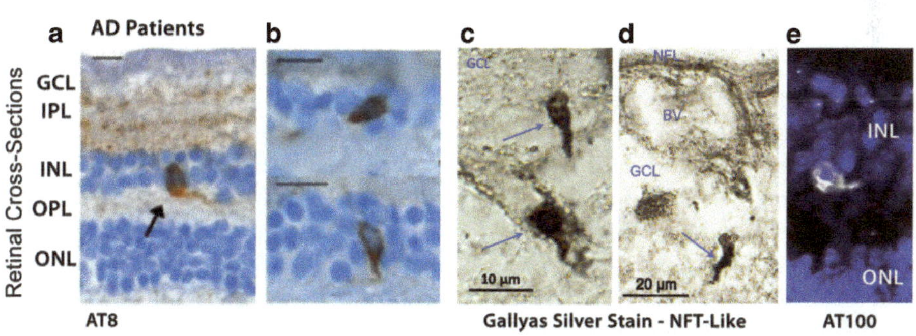

Fig. 6.8 Tauopathy in postmortem retinae of AD patients. (**a, b**) Postmortem retinas of AD patients showing (p)tau (AT8)-positive cells in the inner nuclear layer (INL; arrow) and stainings of the plexiform layers and ganglion cell layer (GCL). (**b**) Higher magnification images of individual AT8-positive cells in the INL. Scale bars: 10 μm. (**c, d**) Neurofibrillary tangles (NFTs)-like structures in retinal cross sections of definite AD patients. Gallyas silver staining shows intraneuronal positive staining resembling NFTs, especially in the retinal ganglion cell layer (marked in blue arrows). (**e**) A (p)tau (AT100)-positive cell in retinal INL from an AD patient [Koronyo-Hamaoui Lab, Unpublished Data]. Images and data of panels (**a, b**) are adapted from Schön et al. [71]. Images and data of panels (**c, d**) are reproduced from Koronyo et al. [72] with permission of ASCI via Copyright Clearance Center

Koronyo et al. further reported the presence of retinal NFT-like structures, especially in the innermost layers (Fig. 6.8c, d) [72]. Unpublished data show the existence of AT100-positive pTau/PHF cells in the INL of AD patients (Fig. 6.8e). Recently, tau and its phosphorylated isoforms were found to be increased in inner and outer plexiform layers of the retina in AD patients versus controls without CAA [115]. Another study reported correlations between changes in retinal fluorescent lifetime imaging ophthalmoscopy and total Tau and pTau-181 concentration in the CSF [138]. Importantly, eight independent groups studying AD patient eyes consistently found retinal tauopathy and Aβ deposits in retinas and lenses [69–71, 73, 91, 114, 136, 151, 186]. Table 6.1 summarizes AD-associated pathology in the retina and other ocular tissues of AD patients.

6.3.2 In Animal Models of Alzheimer's Disease

Aβ-associated pathology has also been reported in AD animal models, similar to the changes seen in AD patients [70, 155–157, 165, 167–171, 175–177, 187–189].

Many studies report degeneration in animal models of disease with elevated neurotoxic Aβ peptide as compared to control animals [70, 159, 167, 175]. Markers of degeneration vary by animal model: cellular swelling, nuclear disorganization, shape irregularity, and organelle loss in cortical fiber cells were reported in the lens of the $hTgAPP^{tg/tg}$ mouse [175]. In the 5xFAD mouse, the retinal pigment epithelium showed hypopigmentation, large vacuoles, and Bruch membrane thickening with Drusen-like deposits [167]. In the TgF344-AD rat, hypertrophy was reported [70]. In the $APP_{SWE}/PS1_{\Delta E9}$ mouse, RGCs density was decreased compared to matched WT controls [162, 178] and amacrine cell apoptosis was also observed [162]. Recently, in 3xTg mice, retinal tau tangles and Aβ plaques colocalized with neurodegeneration in the GCL [174]. Another recent study described tau accumulation associated with neural dysfunction in the retina of 3xTg mice [179]. In addition, in a mouse model expressing human tau (hTau), pTau was detected in the retina with aging but it did not induce retinal neurodegeneration [180].

As in patients, inflammatory responses in the retina were tightly associated with Aβ accumulation in animal models. Ning et al. were the first to report association of neurodegeneration and inflammation with Aβ in the retina of Tg mice [155]. Other studies have shown increased microgliosis, GFAP-reactive astrocytes (astrocytosis), as well as infiltration of lymphocytes and monocytes and upregulation of MCP-1 in multiple layers of the retina and choroid [70, 155–157, 159, 162, 165, 168, 188].

Structural changes in the retinas of AD animal models were also reported, including variations in vascular branching and budding, tight junction attenuation, and decreases in complexity, field area, and length of RGC dendrites [167, 169, 187–189]. Further, synaptic loss and impairment was described in the ApoE4 mouse retina [187, 188]. Changes in protein expression levels and mRNA transcripts required for normal cell function were also found, including increased ATP release in the retina of an APP/PS1 mouse model [190]. Taken together, the findings summarized above indicate that in addition to the Aβ hallmark pathology, Aβ-associated changes present in the brain also afflict the retina of animal models.

6.4 Non-invasive Retinal Amyloid Imaging in Alzheimer's Disease

The growing evidence for retinal abnormalities in AD motivated investigators to develop new retinal imaging approaches with the ability to noninvasively detect pathology in live animal models and living patients. An initial attempt by Tsai et al. using blue-light high-resolution photography, albeit non-amyloid imaging, revealed a correlation among optic nerve head changes and Alzheimer's Disease Assessment Scale (ADAS) scores in patients with Alzheimer's disease [140].

Later, cross-sectional imaging by OCT was explored [50, 53, 89, 96, 191, 192]. OCT is an in vivo technique capable of revealing retinal structural abnormalities and cell neurodegeneration. While there are some concerns for the ability to differentiate between healthy controls, AD patients, and other neurodegenerative diseases, the quantification of RNFL thinning, especially in the superior and inferior quadrants, has been very helpful to detect consistent pathology in the retina of MCI and AD patients. However, definitive diagnoses of AD can only be achieved by specific hallmark identification of Aβ and NFTs.

Recently, researchers used a modified scanning laser ophthalmoscope, fundus autofluorescence imaging (FAF) and/or OCT to detect retinal amyloid deposits, inclusion bodies, and auto-fluorescent spots in living MCI and AD patients [72, 137]. In a 2014 study, researchers examined 30 MCI patients via OCT and detected abnormal deposits, mostly in the outer plexiform, ganglion, and nerve fiber layers of the retina [137]. In a subset of 20 randomly selected patients and 20 matched controls following curcumin administration, FAF detected hyperintense dots, with OCT indicating more prominence in patients [137]. OCT examination of retinae in pre-clinical patients and comparison between neocortical amyloid aggregation via florbetapir PET imaging and various retinal sd-OCT markers of possible disease burden revealed a significant increase in retinal inclusion bodies as a function of cortical amyloid burden [64].

Koronyo-Hamaoui and colleagues modified a confocal scanning laser ophthalmoscope to capture curcumin fluorescence bound to amyloid plaques in a wide-field retinal image, and paired it with highly bioavailable and purified Longvida curcumin, a natural and safe phytopolylphenol flourochrome (Figs. 6.9, 6.10, and 6.11) [72, 193]. Curcumin has been found to cross the blood-retina and blood-brain barriers and label Aβ fibrils and oligomers with high affinity and specificity in vivo in mouse models and ex vivo in human brains and retinas [69, 74, 194]. In this manner, the group successfully developed a novel noninvasive retinal amyloid imaging method with high sensitivity, specificity, and repeatability. The method allowed for visualization of retinal Aβ pathology initially in live animal models following intravenous injection or oral administration of curcumin (Fig. 6.9) [69]. In a subsequent study, the Koronyo-Hamaoui team has demonstrated the feasibility to longitudinally monitor individual Aβ deposits, their appearance during disease progression, and their clearance following immunomodulation therapy in murine Tg-AD models (Fig. 6.10e–h) [69, 72, 74, 195–200].

In a proof-of-concept clinical study, Koronyo and colleagues established the feasibility to detect and quantify 2.1-fold greater retinal amyloid burden (termed retinal amyloid index or RAI score) in a cohort of ten AD patients versus six matched

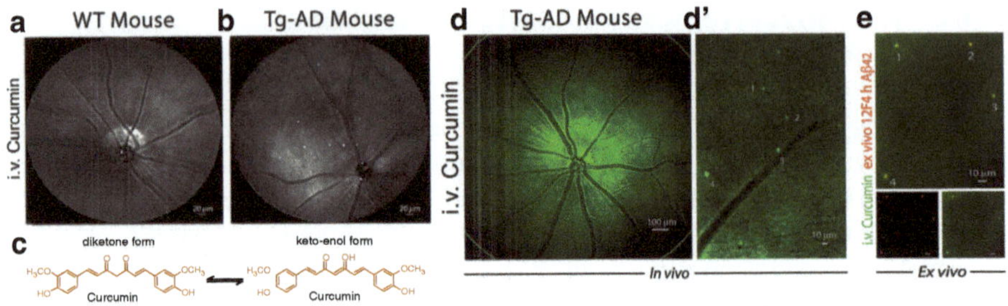

f

Effect of different commercial sources of curcumin on blood and brain levels in mice fed curcumin in chow for 2 weeks

Curcumin Source	RBC Curc (μM)	Brain Curc (μg/g t)	Brain Curc (μM)	Brain/RBC ratio
Vehicle	ND	ND	ND	N/A
Longvida	0.803 ± 0.429*	12.120 ± 7.847*	32.940 ± 19.014	41.02
Sabinsa	0.190 ± 0.167	1.114 ± 0.242*	3.028 ± 0.631	15.93
Acros	0.110 ± 0.052	0.382 ± 0.028*	1.039 ± 0.095	9.44

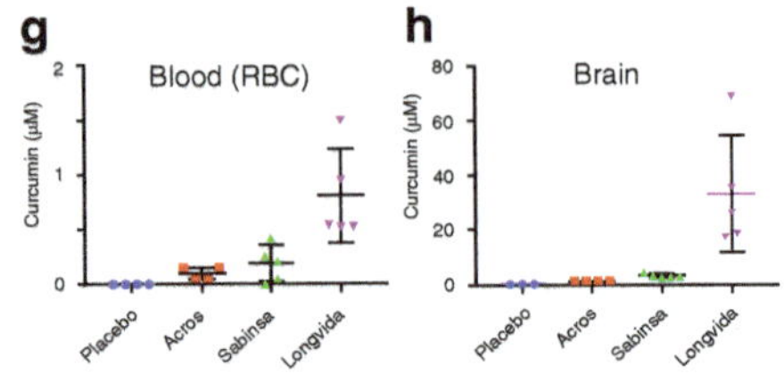

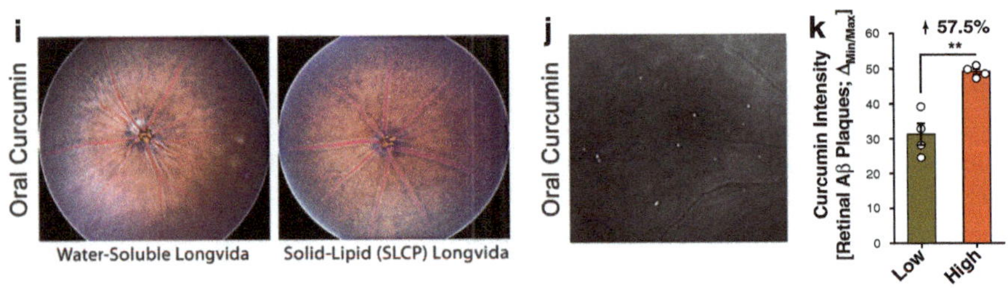

Fig. 6.9 Development of the first in vivo retinal Aβ imaging technique, using curcumin as a labeling compound and a noninvasive retinal optical microscope, shown in live murine models of AD. (**a, b**) Representative fundus retinal images capturing specific curcumin fluorescence bound to Aβ deposits following an intravenous (i.v.) injection of curcumin. (**c**) Curcumin tautomeric forms. (**d, d'**) Representative images demonstrate in vivo detection of curcumin-labeled plaques in the retinas of AD-Tg mice. (**d'**) Enlarged image shows individual plaques at high spatial resolution. (**e**) Whole-mount retina prepared from the same in vivo imaged mouse eye as in (**d**), following perfusion, stained with anti-human $A\beta_{42}$ mAb. Bottom panels show separate channels for each staining. A similar pattern of curcumin-positive plaques imaged in vivo was identified ex vivo following antibody labeling (indicated by the numbers 1–4). (**f–h**) Differences in bioavailability between commercial formulations in adult mice fed equivalent amounts of curcumin. (**f**) Group means and standard deviations of red blood cell (RBC) and brain levels [grams wet tissue (gt) or mM]. *ND* not detectable, *N/A* not applicable. Asterisks signify differences between source curcumin (within tissue compartment). $*p < 0.05$, one-way ANOVA. Note that concentrations in the brain are at least 9 times higher than in the blood. (**g, h**) The scattergram plots show individual values, means and standard deviation in RBC (**g**) and brain tissue (**h**). (**i**) Fundus bright-field images of live ADtg mouse retinas after oral administration of water soluble or non-water soluble proprietary SLCP (Solid lipid curcumin particle) Longvida (optimized curcumin). (**j**) Increased fluorescent signal of retinal Aβ deposits following high-dose SLCP Longvida. (**k**) Quantitative analysis showing increased mean curcumin-labeled plaque intensity fluorescent signals following high- vs. low-dose curcumin oral administration. Five plaques per image were analyzed for each mouse. Mean ± SEM are shown. $***\ P = 0.0014$ by two-tailed unpaired t-test. Images and data of panels (**a–c**) and (**f–k**) are reproduced from Koronyo et al. [72] with permission of ASCI via Copyright Clearance Center. Images and data of panels (**d, e**) are reprinted from Neuroimage, 54S1, Koronyo-Hamaoui M. et al., Identification of Amyloid Plaques in Retinas from Alzheimer's Patients and Noninvasive In Vivo Optical Imaging of Retinal Plaques in a Mouse Model, S204–S217, Copyright 2011, with permission from Elsevier [69]

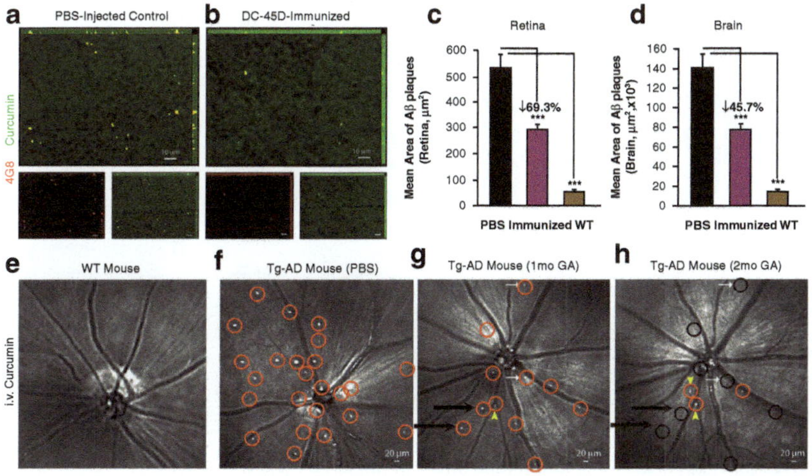

Fig. 6.10 Response to immunotherapy: similar reduction in retinal and brain Aβ deposits following DC-45D immunization and feasibility of monitoring response to GA-immunization via noninvasive retinal amyloid optical imaging in murine models. (**a–d**) Reduced Aβ-plaque burden in retinas from AD-Tg mice following MOG45D-loaded dendritic cells immunization. Representative z-axis projection images of whole-mount retinas from (**a**) PBS-treated control and (**b**) MOG45D-immunized AD-Tg mice, stained ex vivo with curcumin and anti-human Aβ mAb. (**c**) Following MOG45D-loaded DCs immunization, a significant reduction in mean curcumin-positive plaque area was observed in retinas from immunized AD-Tg mice as compared to PBS-treated controls and non-Tg (wt) mice. (**d**) A significant decrease in total area covered by plaques was detected in brain hippocampus and cortex from the same mice following immunotherapy. Curcumin staining revealed the same decrease in plaque burden following immunization in the retina and in the brain. Error bars represent SEM. Asterisks indicate statistical significance: ∗∗∗$P < 0.0001$; ∗∗$P < 0.005$, analyzed by one-way ANOVA followed by Bonferroni multiple comparison post-test. (**e, f**) Real-time monitoring of retinal Aβ plaque dynamics in ADtg mice following GA immunotherapy. (**e**) PBS-treated control wild-type (WT) and (**f**) Tg-AD mouse, (**g**) GA-immunized mouse after 1 month of treatment, and (**h**) the same GA-immunized mouse after 2 months of treatment. Representative appearance and clearance of retinal Aβ plaques: arrows indicate existence and removal of the same Aβ plaques, while arrowheads indicate a newly formed Aβ plaque. Images and data of panels (**a–d**) are reprinted from Neuroimage, 54S1, Koronyo-Hamaoui M. et al., Identification of Amyloid Plaques in Retinas from Alzheimer's Patients and Noninvasive In Vivo Optical Imaging of Retinal Plaques in a Mouse Model, S204–S217, Copyright 2011, with permission from Elsevier [69]. Images and data of panels (**e–h**) are adapted from Koronyo et al. [74], Copyright 2012 Karger Publishers, Basel, Switzerland

healthy controls [72]. This in vivo curcumin-based fundus imaging of AD patients and cognitively normal controls further expanded on the anatomical distribution of plaque pathology and illustrated the feasibility of retinal Aβ-specific imaging techniques. Similar to the findings from retinal histological samples, this study revealed that retinal Aβ aggregates appear in clusters with a large concentration located in the superior and inferior peripheral regions [72]. Two AMD patients that underwent curcumin oral uptake and modified confocal SLO imaging showed diffused curcumin fluorescence signals in the central retina that were different than that found in AD patients [72]. In contrast to AMD patients, focal scanning by OCT revealed amyloid deposits localized above the retinal pigment epithelium and in the outer

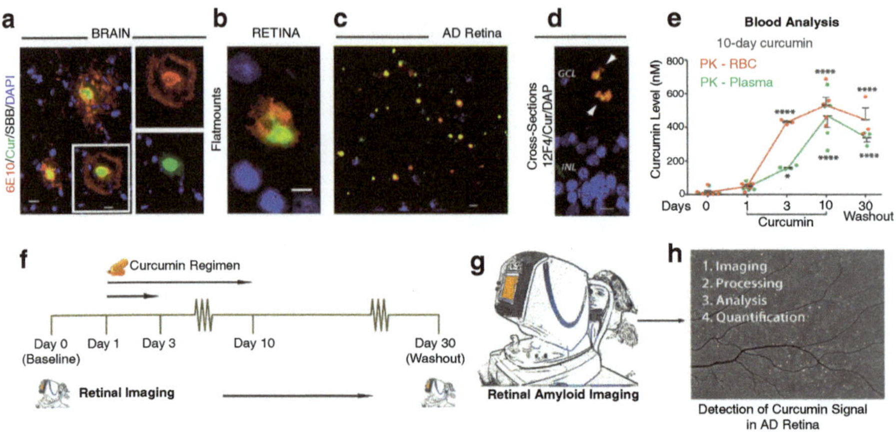

Fig. 6.11 Development of the first retinal amyloid imaging method, using curcumin labeling and a noninvasive, high-resolution ophthalmic imaging device: proof-of-concept trial for detecting and quantifying sub-cellular size retinal amyloid deposits in living patients. (**a, b**) Brain and retinal tissue taken from the same subset of AD patients stained with fluorescent 6E10 antibody for Aβ and Longvida curcumin (Cur) after treatment with Sudan Black B (SBB) to minimize autofluoresence. Colocalization of 6E10 and curcumin in both tissues. Staining portrays colabeling but with unique patterns between methods. Scale bar: 10 μm (brain); 5 μm (retina). (**c, d**) Distribution of Aβ deposition in (**c**) large retinal whole-mount region and (**d**) cross section retinal layers. (**e**) Pharmacokinetic (PK) analyses of Longvida curcumin plasma and red blood cell (RBC) levels in living healthy controls (CTRL; n = 6) during 10-day trial administration. Peak plasma and RBC levels reached at 10 days prior to wash out. Group mean and SEM are shown. $*P < 0.05$, $****P < 0.0001$ by 1-way ANOVA and Tukey's post hoc test. (**f, g**) Administration timeline of oral Longvida curcumin intake (2 or 10 days) and retinal imaging via modified retinal ophthalmoscope. (**h**) Representative retinal image and curcumin Aβ fluorescence in an AD patient. (**i, j**) Representative detection of retinal curcumin$^+$ spots in (**i**) an AD patient and (**j**) a healthy CTRL patient given curcumin under the same regimen. Scale bar: 400 μm. Curcumin fluorescence fundography of the superior temporal region (ST) reveals preferential Aβ deposition in the periphery. High magnification images displaying regions of interest determined by white square and further postprocessing of curcumin fluorescence with respective spot count and area (μm^2). Scale bar: 400 μm. (**k**) Quantitative longitudinal assessment of retinal curcumin fluorescent intensity in a CTRL and mild AD patient following a 2-day curcumin regimen. Exponential decay of integrated fluorescent intensity after day 2. Decay rate = 10.4% per day, half-life = 6.3 days, offset IFI = 21.5. (**l, l'**) Tracing certain retinal amyloid plaque, indicated by red arrow, under curcumin fluorescence fundography and OCT segmentation. Retinal cross section imaging by OCT reveals Aβ plaque in the outer retinal layers above the retinal pigment epithelium (RPE). (**m, n**) Threshold defining increased curcumin fluorescent signal in left eye superior hemisphere (LS) of a representative mild AD patient and an age-matched CTRL. Blue lines indicate 1:1 reference, and green lines represent the threshold level with red spots denoting above threshold. (**o, p**) Color-coded spot overlay images determined by threshold established in (**m, n**). Red spots are above threshold and considered curcumin-positive amyloid deposits. (**q–t**) Heatmap images with high fluorescence red spot centroids (left side). Overlay images of heatmap and regional fundus imaging displaying overlap with regions high in above threshold spots (right side) in a mild AD patient (top) and healthy CTRL (bottom). The same automated image processing and analysis was applied on all human subjects. (**u**) Pearson's r correlation between RAI scores and retinal spot number in all data set ($n = 16$ living subjects). (**v, w**) Comparison between RAI scores of AD patients ($n = 10$) and non-age-matched CTRLs ($n = 6$) (left) and between a subgroup of AD patients ($n = 6$) age-matched against CTRLs ($n = 5$) (right). Group mean and SEM are shown. $**P < 0.005$, $***P < 0.0005$, unpaired 2-tailed Student's t test. Adopted from JCI Insight 2017. Images and data are reproduced from Koronyo et al. [72] with permission of ASCI via Copyright Clearance Center

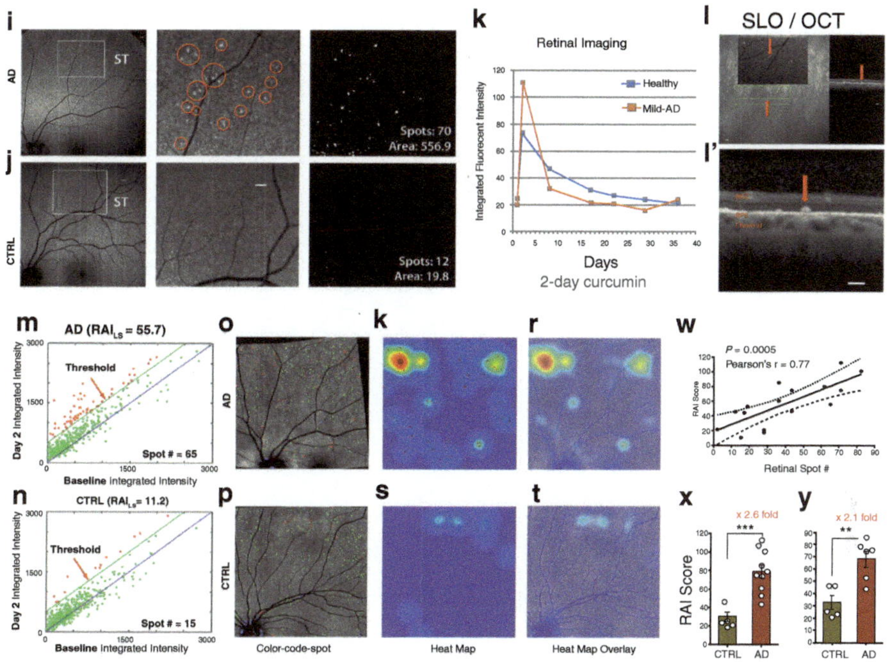

Fig. 6.11 (continued)

layers of the retina, with a stark absence of maculopathy (Fig. 6.11l, l'). This observation was consistent with histological examinations of Aβ pathology, which were concentrated in the mid- and far-periphery of the superior hemisphere, where RNFL thinning in AD patients is often detected via OCT studies (Fig. 6.11i, o, k, r) [72]. Thus, OCT could provide a noninvasive imaging method of layer localization to identify plaques, although current OCT methods are limited to the central retina.

A more recent study in 69 cognitively impaired subjects demonstrated multimodal retinal markers including advanced retinal imaging, full-field electroretinogram (ERG), and visual performance exams sensitive to cognitive decline [201]. Although the sample size was small, the findings add to evidence that retinal geometric vascular and functional parameters could be associated with physiological changes in the retina stemming from cognitive impairment [201]. These advancements are significant to the field and should be combined with specific retinal amyloid imaging.

Notably, in an earlier study published 2015, Rafii and colleagues demonstrated the feasibility to detect retinal amyloid deposits in patients with Down Syndrome (DS) [202]. This study utilized the developed NeuroVision/Koronyo et al. [72] imaging technology to detect curcumin-positive amyloid plaques in the retina [202]. DS patients have an additional copy of the APP gene and thus produce higher levels of amyloidogenic Aβ with age [203]. Strikingly, retinal amyloid plaques were detected in all 12 DS patients that were imaged and their plaques were tightly associated along and around blood vessels. Another group utilized hyperspectral-imaging technique to further demonstrate in living mice the ability to detect optical changes consistent with an increase in Rayleigh light scattering in neural retina due to soluble $A\beta_{1-42}$ aggregates [204]. Table 6.3 outlines studies that detected amyloid

Table 6.3 Retinal amyloid imaging in human subjects and animal models

	Retinal imaging modality	Contrast agent	Ophthalmic device	Resolution/specificity	Findings	Ref.
Human studies	Wide-field Fundus Optical Imaging: Confocal SLO and Narrow-field OCT	Oral, SLCP Longvida Curcumin	Mod. Topcon 50DXi, Heidelberg Spectralis HRA, Optos Optomap Tx, and Nidek F10, and HD-OCT (Heidelberg Spectralis)	High/high	Proof-of-concept: feasibility of detecting retinal Aβ deposits in AD (n=16 subjects) Aβ deposits found above the RPE in few AD patients	[72]
	Wide-field Fundus Optical Imaging: Confocal SLO	Oral, SLCP Longvida Curcumin	Mod. non-mydriatic Nidek F10	High/high	Increased RAI scores in AD patients vs matched controls	[72]
	Narrow-field OCT, Wide-field FAF	Oral, Curcumin (Turmeric Phytosome-Meriva)	OCT and SLO-FAF (Heidelberg Spectralis)	High/low	Autofluorescent drusen/plaque-like lesions detected in 26/30 MCI AD patients	[137]
	Wide-field Fundus Optical Imaging: Confocal SLO	Oral, Curcumin	NeuroVision Retina HD (Mod. Nidek F10)	High/high	Retinal Aβ deposits in all DS patients, in the vicinity of blood vessels (n = 12)	[202]
	30°-angle Fluorescence Lifetime Imaging Ophthalmoscopy	None	Heidelberg Spectralis HRA2, OCT	Low/low	Retinal Autofluorescence correlated with MMSE and CSF-Tau	[138]
	45°-angle Fundus Optic Imaging: Confocal SLO	None	EasyScan iOptics non-mydriatic camera	High/low	Drusen-like deposits in the peripheral retina of the cognitively impaired	[201]

Animal models	Retinal Imaging Microscope for Rodents	Oral or i.v., Sigma-Aldrich and Longvida Curcumin	Mod. Micron II and III (Phoenix Research Laboratories)	High/high	Detection of retinal Aβ deposits in Tg-AD mice. Validated via ex-vivo analysis	[69, 72, 74]
	Retinal Imaging Microscope for Rodents	I.v., Sigma-Aldrich Curcumin	Mod. Micron II and III (Phoenix Research Laboratories)	High/high	Longitudinal imaging of retinal Aβ deposits after immunotherapy in Tg-AD mice	[74]
	Near-Infrared Fluorescence Ocular Imaging (NIRFOI)	I.v., CRANAD-2, -3, -58, and -102 Curcumin	IVIS Spectrum In Vivo Imaging System	Low/high	Longitudinal monitoring of soluble and insoluble ocular Aβ signal after BACE-1-inhibitor treatment in Tg-AD	[205]
	Hyperspectral Fundus Imaging	None	CytoViva and Karl Storz Hyperspectral Endoscopy System	High/low	Short-wavelength reflectance from AD mice retinae significantly reduced compared to WT mice, consistent with increase in Rayleigh light scattering due to soluble $A\beta_{1-42}$ aggregates	[204]

SLO scanning laser ophthalmoscope, *SLCP* solid lipid-based, *RAI* retinal amyloid index, *OCT* optical coherence tomography, *HD-OCT* high definition OCT, *FAF* fundus autofluorescence, *DS* Down syndrome, *CSF-Tau* cerebral spinal fluid-tau, *Mod.* modified, *BACE-1* beta-secretase 1, *I.v.* intravenous deposits or amyloid signal in the retina of living human subjects or animal models via noninvasive retinal imaging methods.

6.5 Conclusion

Mounting evidence indicating the presence of AD hallmark pathology and associated degeneration and inflammation in the retina, mirroring that seen in the brain, as described here, is under intense investigation. With the number of individuals suffering from AD currently above 45 million and rising quickly—expected to more than double by 2040 [1, 206]—a noninvasive, affordable, and accurate method of diagnosis and disease monitoring is an urgent unmet need.

The previously demonstrated capacity to detect and quantify Aβ deposits, and perhaps vascular Aβ pathology in the future, using noninvasive retinal amyloid imaging may present an exceptional modality for early diagnosis and monitoring of AD therapies. There is currently no clinical method for noninvasive imaging of the CNS with such high resolution and specificity; the studies discussed here and related future work may pave the way towards translation.

Acknowledgments This work was funded by NIH/NIA R01AG056478 (MKH), NIH/NIA R01AG055865 (MKH), NIH/NIA R41AG044897 (MKH), The Saban Family Foundation (MKH), and The Maurice Marciano Family Foundation (MKH). This article is dedicated to the memories of Dr. Salomon Moni Hamaoui and Lillian Jones Black, both of whom died from Alzheimer's disease.

References

1. Alzheimer's A. 2016 Alzheimer's disease facts and figures. Alzheimers Dement. 2016;12(4):459–509.
2. Perrin RJ, Fagan AM, Holtzman DM. Multimodal techniques for diagnosis and prognosis of Alzheimer's disease. Nature. 2009;461(7266):916–22.
3. Petersen RC, Smith GE, Waring SC, Ivnik RJ, Tangalos EG, Kokmen E. Mild cognitive impairment: clinical characterization and outcome. Arch Neurol. 1999;56(3):303–8.
4. Hardy J, Selkoe DJ. The amyloid hypothesis of Alzheimer's disease: progress and problems on the road to therapeutics. Science (New York, NY). 2002;297(5580):353–6.
5. Selkoe DJ. Soluble oligomers of the amyloid beta-protein impair synaptic plasticity and behavior. Behav Brain Res. 2008;192(1):106–13.
6. Selkoe DJ. Cell biology of protein misfolding: the examples of Alzheimer's and Parkinson's diseases. Nat Cell Biol. 2004;6(11):1054–61.
7. Avila J, Pallas N, Bolos M, Sayas CL, Hernandez F. Intracellular and extracellular microtubule associated protein tau as a therapeutic target in Alzheimer disease and other tauopathies. Expert Opin Ther Targets. 2016;20(6):653–61.
8. Goedert M. NEURODEGENERATION. Alzheimer's and Parkinson's diseases: the prion concept in relation to assembled Abeta, tau, and alpha-synuclein. Science (New York, NY). 2015;349(6248):1255555.
9. Goedert M, Spillantini MG, Jakes R, Rutherford D, Crowther RA. Multiple isoforms of human microtubule-associated protein tau: sequences and localization in neurofibrillary tangles of Alzheimer's disease. Neuron. 1989;3(4):519–26.

10. Bateman RJ, Xiong C, Benzinger TL, Fagan AM, Goate A, Fox NC, et al. Clinical and biomarker changes in dominantly inherited Alzheimer's disease. N Engl J Med. 2012;367(9):795–804.
11. Bilgel M, An Y, Zhou Y, Wong DF, Prince JL, Ferrucci L, et al. Individual estimates of age at detectable amyloid onset for risk factor assessment. Alzheimers Dement. 2016;12(4):373–9.
12. Choi SH, Kim YH, Hebisch M, Sliwinski C, Lee S, D'Avanzo C, et al. A three-dimensional human neural cell culture model of Alzheimer's disease. Nature. 2014;515(7526):274–8.
13. Ontiveros-Torres MA, Labra-Barrios ML, Diaz-Cintra S, Aguilar-Vazquez AR, Moreno-Campuzano S, Flores-Rodriguez P, et al. Fibrillar amyloid-beta accumulation triggers an inflammatory mechanism leading to hyperphosphorylation of the carboxyl-terminal end of tau polypeptide in the hippocampal formation of the 3xTg-AD transgenic mouse. J Alzheimers Dis. 2016;52(1):243–69.
14. De Strooper B, Karran E. The cellular phase of Alzheimer's disease. Cell. 2016;164(4):603–15.
15. Jack CR Jr, Bennett DA, Blennow K, Carrillo MC, Dunn B, Haeberlein SB, et al. NIA-AA Research Framework: toward a biological definition of Alzheimer's disease. Alzheimers Dement. 2018;14(4):535–62.
16. Meli G, Lecci A, Manca A, Krako N, Albertini V, Benussi L, et al. Conformational targeting of intracellular Abeta oligomers demonstrates their pathological oligomerization inside the endoplasmic reticulum. Nat Commun. 2014;5:3867.
17. Takeda S, Wegmann S, Cho H, DeVos SL, Commins C, Roe AD, et al. Neuronal uptake and propagation of a rare phosphorylated high-molecular-weight tau derived from Alzheimer's disease brain. Nat Commun. 2015;6:8490.
18. Klein H-U, McCabe C, Gjoneska E, Sullivan SE, Kaskow BJ, Tang A, et al. Epigenome-wide study uncovers large-scale changes in histone acetylation driven by tau pathology in aging and Alzheimer's human brains. Nat Neurosci. 2019;22(1):37–46.
19. Vinters HV. Cerebral amyloid angiopathy. A critical review. Stroke. 1987;18(2):311–24.
20. Ellis RJ, Olichney JM, Thal LJ, Mirra SS, Morris JC, Beekly D, et al. Cerebral amyloid angiopathy in the brains of patients with Alzheimer's disease: the CERAD experience, Part XV. Neurology. 1996;46(6):1592–6.
21. Wyss-Coray T. Inflammation in Alzheimer disease: driving force, bystander or beneficial response? Nat Med. 2006;12(9):1005–15.
22. Montine TJ, Phelps CH, Beach TG, Bigio EH, Cairns NJ, Dickson DW, et al. National Institute on Aging-Alzheimer's Association guidelines for the neuropathologic assessment of Alzheimer's disease: a practical approach. Acta Neuropathol. 2012;123(1):1–11.
23. Koronyo Y, Salumbides BC, Sheyn J, Pelissier L, Li S, Ljubimov V, et al. Therapeutic effects of glatiramer acetate and grafted CD115(+) monocytes in a mouse model of Alzheimer's disease. Brain. 2015;138(Pt 8):2399–422.
24. Zuroff L, Daley D, Black KL, Koronyo-Hamaoui M. Clearance of cerebral Abeta in Alzheimer's disease: reassessing the role of microglia and monocytes. Cell Mol Life Sci. 2017;74(12):2167–201.
25. Rentsendorj A, Sheyn J, Fuchs DT, Daley D, Salumbides BC, Schubloom HE, et al. A novel role for osteopontin in macrophage-mediated amyloid-beta clearance in Alzheimer's models. Brain Behav Immun. 2018;67:163–80.
26. Butovsky O, Koronyo-Hamaoui M, Kunis G, Ophir E, Landa G, Cohen H, et al. Glatiramer acetate fights against Alzheimer's disease by inducing dendritic-like microglia expressing insulin-like growth factor 1. Proc Natl Acad Sci U S A. 2006;103(31):11784–9.
27. Butovsky O, Kunis G, Koronyo-Hamaoui M, Schwartz M. Selective ablation of bone marrow-derived dendritic cells increases amyloid plaques in a mouse Alzheimer's disease model. Eur J Neurosci. 2007;26(2):413–6.
28. Koronyo-Hamaoui M, Ko MK, Koronyo Y, Azoulay D, Seksenyan A, Kunis G, et al. Attenuation of AD-like neuropathology by harnessing peripheral immune cells: local elevation of IL-10 and MMP-9. J Neurochem. 2009;111(6):1409–24.
29. Lebson L, Nash K, Kamath S, Herber D, Carty N, Lee DC, et al. Trafficking CD11b-positive blood cells deliver therapeutic genes to the brain of amyloid-depositing transgenic mice. J Neurosci. 2010;30(29):9651–8.

30. Bakalash S, Pham M, Koronyo Y, Salumbides BC, Kramerov A, Seidenberg H, et al. Egr1 expression is induced following glatiramer acetate immunotherapy in rodent models of glaucoma and Alzheimer's disease. Invest Ophthalmol Vis Sci. 2011;52(12):9033–46.
31. Bernstein KE, Koronyo Y, Salumbides BC, Sheyn J, Pelissier L, Lopes DH, et al. Angiotensin-converting enzyme overexpression in myelomonocytes prevents Alzheimer's-like cognitive decline. J Clin Invest. 2014;124(3):1000–12.
32. Fox NC, Warrington EK, Rossor MN. Serial magnetic resonance imaging of cerebral atrophy in preclinical Alzheimer's disease. Lancet. 1999;353(9170):2125.
33. Carlson NE, Moore MM, Dame A, Howieson D, Silbert LC, Quinn JF, et al. Trajectories of brain loss in aging and the development of cognitive impairment. Neurology. 2008;70(11):828–33.
34. Devanand DP, Pradhaban G, Liu X, Khandji A, De Santi S, Segal S, et al. Hippocampal and entorhinal atrophy in mild cognitive impairment: prediction of Alzheimer disease. Neurology. 2007;68(11):828–36.
35. Kalia LV, Lang AE. Parkinson's disease. Lancet. 2015;386(9996):896–912.
36. Mathis CA, Mason NS, Lopresti BJ, Klunk WE. Development of positron emission tomography beta-amyloid plaque imaging agents. Semin Nucl Med. 2012;42(6):423–32.
37. Doraiswamy PM, Sperling RA, Johnson K, Reiman EM, Wong TZ, Sabbagh MN, et al. Florbetapir F 18 amyloid PET and 36-month cognitive decline: a prospective multicenter study. Mol Psychiatry. 2014;19(9):1044–51.
38. Heurling K, Leuzy A, Zimmer ER, Lubberink M, Nordberg A. Imaging beta-amyloid using [(18)F]flutemetamol positron emission tomography: from dosimetry to clinical diagnosis. Eur J Nucl Med Mol Imaging. 2016;43(2):362–73.
39. Tiepolt S, Hesse S, Patt M, Luthardt J, Schroeter ML, Hoffmann KT, et al. Early [F]florbetaben and [C]PiB PET images are a surrogate biomarker of neuronal injury in Alzheimer's disease. Eur J Nucl Med Mol Imaging. 2016;43:1700–9.
40. James OG, Doraiswamy PM, Borges-Neto S. PET imaging of tau pathology in Alzheimer's disease and tauopathies. Front Neurol. 2015;6:38.
41. Johnson KA, Fox NC, Sperling RA, Klunk WE. Brain imaging in Alzheimer disease. Cold Spring Harb Perspect Med. 2012;2(4):a006213.
42. Ono M, Saji H. SPECT imaging agents for detecting cerebral beta-amyloid plaques. Int J Mol Imaging. 2011;2011:543267.
43. Lockhart A, Lamb JR, Osredkar T, Sue LI, Joyce JN, Ye L, et al. PIB is a non-specific imaging marker of amyloid-beta (Abeta) peptide-related cerebral amyloidosis. Brain. 2007;130(Pt 10):2607–15.
44. Ng S, Villemagne VL, Berlangieri S, Lee ST, Cherk M, Gong SJ, et al. Visual assessment versus quantitative assessment of 11C-PIB PET and 18F-FDG PET for detection of Alzheimer's disease. J Nucl Med. 2007;48(4):547–52.
45. Humpel C. Identifying and validating biomarkers for Alzheimer's disease. Trends Biotechnol. 2011;29(1):26–32.
46. Hart NJ, Koronyo Y, Black KL, Koronyo-Hamaoui M. Ocular indicators of Alzheimer's: exploring disease in the retina. Acta Neuropathol. 2016;132(6):767–87.
47. Ascaso FJ, Cruz N, Modrego PJ, Lopez-Anton R, Santabarbara J, Pascual LF, et al. Retinal alterations in mild cognitive impairment and Alzheimer's disease: an optical coherence tomography study. J Neurol. 2014;261(8):1522–30.
48. Cheung CY, Ong YT, Hilal S, Ikram MK, Low S, Ong YL, et al. Retinal ganglion cell analysis using high-definition optical coherence tomography in patients with mild cognitive impairment and Alzheimer's disease. J Alzheimers Dis. 2015;45(1):45–56.
49. Coppola G, Di Renzo A, Ziccardi L, Martelli F, Fadda A, Manni G, et al. Optical coherence tomography in Alzheimer's disease: a meta-analysis. PLoS One. 2015;10(8):e0134750.
50. Cunha LP, Almeida AL, Costa-Cunha LV, Costa CF, Monteiro ML. The role of optical coherence tomography in Alzheimer's disease. Int J Retina Vitreous. 2016;2:24.
51. den Haan J, Verbraak FD, Visser PJ, Bouwman FH. Retinal thickness in Alzheimer's disease: a systematic review and meta-analysis. Alzheimers Dement (Amst). 2017;6:162–70.

52. Feke G, Hyman B, Stern R, Pasquale L. Retinal blood flow in mild cognitive impairment and Alzheimer's disease. Alzheimers Dement. 2015;1:144–51.
53. Ferrari L, Huang SC, Magnani G, Ambrosi A, Comi G, Leocani L. Optical coherence tomography reveals retinal neuroaxonal thinning in frontotemporal dementia as in Alzheimer's disease. J Alzheimers Dis. 2017;56(3):1101–7.
54. Gao L, Liu Y, Li X, Bai Q, Liu P. Abnormal retinal nerve fiber layer thickness and macula lutea in patients with mild cognitive impairment and Alzheimer's disease. Arch Gerontol Geriatr. 2015;60(1):162–7.
55. Goozee KG, Shah TM, Sohrabi HR, Rainey-Smith SR, Brown B, Verdile G, et al. Examining the potential clinical value of curcumin in the prevention and diagnosis of Alzheimer's disease. Br J Nutr. 2016;115(3):449–65.
56. Ikram MK, Cheung CY, Wong TY, Chen CP. Retinal pathology as biomarker for cognitive impairment and Alzheimer's disease. J Neurol Neurosurg Psychiatry. 2012;83(9):917–22.
57. Kesler A, Vakhapova V, Korczyn AD, Naftaliev E, Neudorfer M. Retinal thickness in patients with mild cognitive impairment and Alzheimer's disease. Clin Neurol Neurosurg. 2011;113(7):523–6.
58. Liu D, Zhang L, Li Z, Zhang X, Wu Y, Yang H, et al. Thinner changes of the retinal nerve fiber layer in patients with mild cognitive impairment and Alzheimer's disease. BMC Neurol. 2015;15:14.
59. Oktem EO, Derle E, Kibaroglu S, Oktem C, Akkoyun I, Can U. The relationship between the degree of cognitive impairment and retinal nerve fiber layer thickness. Neurol Sci. 2015;36(7):1141–6.
60. Paquet C, Boissonnot M, Roger F, Dighiero P, Gil R, Hugon J. Abnormal retinal thickness in patients with mild cognitive impairment and Alzheimer's disease. Neurosci Lett. 2007;420(2):97–9.
61. Pillai JA, Bermel R, Bonner-Jackson A, Rae-Grant A, Fernandez H, Bena J, et al. Retinal nerve fiber layer thinning in Alzheimer's disease: a case-control study in comparison to normal aging, Parkinson's disease, and non-Alzheimer's dementia. Am J Alzheimers Dis Other Dement. 2016;31(5):430–6.
62. Shen Y, Liu L, Cheng Y, Feng W, Shi Z, Zhu Y, et al. Retinal nerve fiber layer thickness is associated with episodic memory deficit in mild cognitive impairment patients. Curr Alzheimer Res. 2014;11(3):259–66.
63. Shi Z, Wu Y, Wang M, Cao J, Feng W, Cheng Y, et al. Greater attenuation of retinal nerve fiber layer thickness in Alzheimer's disease patients. J Alzheimers Dis. 2014;40(2):277–83.
64. Snyder PJ, Johnson LN, Lim YY, Santos CY, Alber J, Maruff P, et al. Nonvascular retinal imaging markers of preclinical Alzheimer's disease. Alzheimers Dement (Amst). 2016;4:169–78.
65. Thomson KL, Yeo JM, Waddell B, Cameron JR, Pal S. A systematic review and meta-analysis of retinal nerve fiber layer change in dementia, using optical coherence tomography. Alzheimers Dement (Amst). 2015;1(2):136–43.
66. Trebbastoni A, D'Antonio F, Bruscolini A, Marcelli M, Cecere M, Campanelli A, et al. Retinal nerve fibre layer thickness changes in Alzheimer's disease: results from a 12-month prospective case series. Neurosci Lett. 2016;629:165–70.
67. Valenti DA. Alzheimer's disease and glaucoma: imaging the biomarkers of neurodegenerative disease. Int J Alzheimers Dis. 2011;2010:793931.
68. Doustar J, Torbati T, Black KL, Koronyo Y, Koronyo-Hamaoui M. Optical coherence tomography in Alzheimer's disease and other neurodegenerative diseases. Front Neurol. 2017;8:701.
69. Koronyo-Hamaoui M, Koronyo Y, Ljubimov AV, Miller CA, Ko MK, Black KL, et al. Identification of amyloid plaques in retinas from Alzheimer's patients and noninvasive in vivo optical imaging of retinal plaques in a mouse model. NeuroImage. 2011;54(Suppl 1):S204–17.
70. Tsai Y, Lu B, Ljubimov AV, Girman S, Ross-Cisneros FN, Sadun AA, et al. Ocular changes in TgF344-AD rat model of Alzheimer's disease. Invest Ophthalmol Vis Sci. 2014;55(1):523–34.
71. Schon C, Hoffmann NA, Ochs SM, Burgold S, Filser S, Steinbach S, et al. Long-term in vivo imaging of fibrillar tau in the retina of P301S transgenic mice. PLoS One. 2012;7(12):e53547.

72. Koronyo Y, Biggs D, Barron E, Boyer DS, Pearlman JA, Au WJ, et al. Retinal amyloid pathology and proof-of-concept imaging trial in Alzheimer's disease. JCI Insight. 2017;2(16):e93621.
73. La Morgia C, Ross-Cisneros FN, Koronyo Y, Hannibal J, Gallassi R, Cantalupo G, et al. Melanopsin retinal ganglion cell loss in Alzheimer disease. Ann Neurol. 2016;79(1):90–109.
74. Koronyo Y, Salumbides BC, Black KL, Koronyo-Hamaoui M. Alzheimer's disease in the retina: imaging retinal Abeta plaques for early diagnosis and therapy assessment. Neurodegener Dis. 2012;10(1–4):285–93.
75. Hampel H, Toschi N, Babiloni C, Baldacci F, Black KL, Bokde ALW, et al. Revolution of Alzheimer precision neurology. Passageway of systems biology and neurophysiology. J Alzheimers Dis. 2018;64(s1):S47–S105.
76. Purves D, Fitzpatrick D. The retina. In: Purves DGJA, Fitzpatrick D, Katz LC, LaMantia A-S, McNamara JO, Williams SM, editor. 2nd ed. Sunderland: Sinauer Associates; 2001.
77. Byerly MS, Blackshaw S. Vertebrate retina and hypothalamus development. Wiley Interdiscip Rev Syst Biol Med. 2009;1(3):380–9.
78. Trost A, Lange S, Schroedl F, Bruckner D, Motloch KA, Bogner B, et al. Brain and retinal pericytes: origin, function and role. Front Cellular Neurosci. 2016;10:20.
79. Maude RJ, Dondorp AM, Abu Sayeed A, Day NP, White NJ, Beare NA. The eye in cerebral malaria: what can it teach us? Trans R Soc Trop Med Hyg. 2009;103(7):661–4.
80. Morin PJ, Abraham CR, Amaratunga A, Johnson RJ, Huber G, Sandell JH, et al. Amyloid precursor protein is synthesized by retinal ganglion cells, rapidly transported to the optic nerve plasma membrane and nerve terminals, and metabolized. J Neurochem. 1993;61(2):464–73.
81. Li L, Luo J, Chen D, Tong JB, Zeng LP, Cao YQ, et al. BACE1 in the retina: a sensitive biomarker for monitoring early pathological changes in Alzheimer's disease. Neural Regen Res. 2016;11(3):447–53.
82. Cai J, Qi X, Kociok N, Skosyrski S, Emilio A, Ruan Q, et al. beta-Secretase (BACE1) inhibition causes retinal pathology by vascular dysregulation and accumulation of age pigment. EMBO Mol Med. 2012;4(9):980–91.
83. Vecino E, Rodriguez FD, Ruzafa N, Pereiro X, Sharma SC. Glia-neuron interactions in the mammalian retina. Prog Retin Eye Res. 2016;51:1–40.
84. Johnson LV, Leitner WP, Rivest AJ, Staples MK, Radeke MJ, Anderson DH. The Alzheimer's Abeta-peptide is deposited at sites of complement activation in pathologic deposits associated with aging and age-related macular degeneration. Proc Natl Acad Sci U S A. 2002;99(18):11830–5.
85. Bambo MP, Garcia-Martin E, Gutierrez-Ruiz F, Pinilla J, Perez-Olivan S, Larrosa JM, et al. Analysis of optic disk color changes in Alzheimer's disease: a potential new biomarker. Clin Neurol Neurosurg. 2015;132:68–73.
86. Berisha F, Feke GT, Trempe CL, McMeel JW, Schepens CL. Retinal abnormalities in early Alzheimer's disease. Invest Ophthalmol Vis Sci. 2007;48(5):2285–9.
87. Iseri PK, Altinas O, Tokay T, Yuksel N. Relationship between cognitive impairment and retinal morphological and visual functional abnormalities in Alzheimer disease. J Neuroophthalmol. 2006;26(1):18–24.
88. Kirbas S, Turkyilmaz K, Anlar O, Tufekci A, Durmus M. Retinal nerve fiber layer thickness in patients with Alzheimer disease. J Neuroophthalmol. 2013;33(1):58–61.
89. Kromer R, Serbecic N, Hausner L, Froelich L, Aboul-Enein F, Beutelspacher SC. Detection of retinal nerve fiber layer defects in Alzheimer's disease using SD-OCT. Front Psychiatry. 2014;5:22.
90. Larrosa JM, Garcia-Martin E, Bambo MP, Pinilla J, Polo V, Otin S, et al. Potential new diagnostic tool for Alzheimer's disease using a linear discriminant function for Fourier domain optical coherence tomography. Invest Ophthalmol Vis Sci. 2014;55(5):3043–51.
91. Moncaster JA, Pineda R, Moir RD, Lu S, Burton MA, Ghosh JG, et al. Alzheimer's disease amyloid-beta links lens and brain pathology in Down syndrome. PLoS One. 2010;5(5):e10659.
92. Marziani E, Pomati S, Ramolfo P, Cigada M, Giani A, Mariani C, et al. Evaluation of retinal nerve fiber layer and ganglion cell layer thickness in Alzheimer's disease using spectral-domain optical coherence tomography. Invest Ophthalmol Vis Sci. 2013;54(9):5953–8.

93. Moreno-Ramos T, Benito-Leon J, Villarejo A, Bermejo-Pareja F. Retinal nerve fiber layer thinning in dementia associated with Parkinson's disease, dementia with Lewy bodies, and Alzheimer's disease. J Alzheimers Dis. 2013;34(3):659–64.
94. Moschos MM, Markopoulos I, Chatziralli I, Rouvas A, Papageorgiou SG, Ladas I, et al. Structural and functional impairment of the retina and optic nerve in Alzheimer's disease. Curr Alzheimer Res. 2012;9(7):782–8.
95. Parisi V. Correlation between morphological and functional retinal impairment in patients affected by ocular hypertension, glaucoma, demyelinating optic neuritis and Alzheimer's disease. Semin Ophthalmol. 2003;18(2):50–7.
96. Parisi V, Restuccia R, Fattapposta F, Mina C, Bucci MG, Pierelli F. Morphological and functional retinal impairment in Alzheimer's disease patients. Clin Neurophysiol. 2001;112(10):1860–7.
97. Sadun AA, Bassi CJ. Optic nerve damage in Alzheimer's disease. Ophthalmology. 1990;97(1):9–17.
98. Surguchov A, McMahan B, Masliah E, Surgucheva I. Synucleins in ocular tissues. J Neurosci Res. 2001;65(1):68–77.
99. Blanks JC, Hinton DR, Sadun AA, Miller CA. Retinal ganglion cell degeneration in Alzheimer's disease. Brain Res. 1989;501(2):364–72.
100. Blanks JC, Schmidt SY, Torigoe Y, Porrello KV, Hinton DR, Blanks RH. Retinal pathology in Alzheimer's disease. II. Regional neuron loss and glial changes in GCL. Neurobiol Aging. 1996;17(3):385–95.
101. Blanks JC, Torigoe Y, Hinton DR, Blanks RH. Retinal pathology in Alzheimer's disease. I. Ganglion cell loss in foveal/parafoveal retina. Neurobiol Aging. 1996;17(3):377–84.
102. Curcio CA, Drucker DN. Retinal ganglion cells in Alzheimer's disease and aging. Ann Neurol. 1993;33(3):248–57.
103. Hinton DR, Sadun AA, Blanks JC, Miller CA. Optic-nerve degeneration in Alzheimer's disease. N Engl J Med. 1986;315(8):485–7.
104. Patton N, Aslam T, Macgillivray T, Pattie A, Deary IJ, Dhillon B. Retinal vascular image analysis as a potential screening tool for cerebrovascular disease: a rationale based on homology between cerebral and retinal microvasculatures. J Anat. 2005;206(4):319–48.
105. Besser LM, Alosco ML, Ramirez Gomez L, Zhou XH, McKee AC, Stern RA, et al. Late-life vascular risk factors and Alzheimer disease neuropathology in individuals with normal cognition. J Neuropathol Exp Neurol. 2016;75(10):955–62.
106. Armstrong R, Kergoat H. Oculo-visual changes and clinical considerations affecting older patients with dementia. Ophthalmic Physiol Opt. 2015;35(4):352–76.
107. Chang LY, Lowe J, Ardiles A, Lim J, Grey AC, Robertson K, et al. Alzheimer's disease in the human eye. Clinical tests that identify ocular and visual information processing deficit as biomarkers. Alzheimers Dement. 2014;10(2):251–61.
108. Katz B, Rimmer S. Ophthalmologic manifestations of Alzheimer's disease. Surv Ophthalmol. 1989;34(1):31–43.
109. Nolan JM, Loskutova E, Howard AN, Moran R, Mulcahy R, Stack J, et al. Macular pigment, visual function, and macular disease among subjects with Alzheimer's disease: an exploratory study. J Alzheimers Dis. 2014;42(4):1191–202.
110. Sadun AA, Borchert M, DeVita E, Hinton DR, Bassi CJ. Assessment of visual impairment in patients with Alzheimer's disease. Am J Ophthalmol. 1987;104(2):113–20.
111. Salobrar-Garcia E, de Hoz R, Rojas B, Ramirez AI, Salazar JJ, Yubero R, et al. Ophthalmologic psychophysical tests support OCT findings in mild. Alzheimers Dis. 2015;2015:736949.
112. Trick GL, Barris MC, Bickler-Bluth M. Abnormal pattern electroretinograms in patients with senile dementia of the Alzheimer type. Ann Neurol. 1989;26(2):226–31.
113. Valenti DA. Alzheimer's disease: visual system review. Optometry (St Louis, Mo). 2010;81(1):12–21.
114. Alexandrov PN, Pogue A, Bhattacharjee S, Lukiw WJ. Retinal amyloid peptides and complement factor H in transgenic models of Alzheimer's disease. Neuroreport. 2011;22(12):623–7.

115. den Haan J, Morrema THJ, Verbraak FD, de Boer JF, Scheltens P, Rozemuller AJ, et al. Amyloid-beta and phosphorylated tau in post-mortem Alzheimer's disease retinas. Acta Neuropathol Commun. 2018;6(1):147.
116. Loffler KU, Edward DP, Tso MO. Immunoreactivity against tau, amyloid precursor protein, and beta-amyloid in the human retina. Invest Ophthalmol Vis Sci. 1995;36(1):24–31.
117. Luibl V, Isas JM, Kayed R, Glabe CG, Langen R, Chen J. Drusen deposits associated with aging and age-related macular degeneration contain nonfibrillar amyloid oligomers. J Clin Invest. 2006;116(2):378–85.
118. Anderson DH, Talaga KC, Rivest AJ, Barron E, Hageman GS, Johnson LV. Characterization of beta amyloid assemblies in drusen: the deposits associated with aging and age-related macular degeneration. Exp Eye Res. 2004;78(2):243–56.
119. Lu Y, Li Z, Zhang X, Ming B, Jia J, Wang R, et al. Retinal nerve fiber layer structure abnormalities in early Alzheimer's disease: evidence in optical coherence tomography. Neurosci Lett. 2010;480(1):69–72.
120. La Morgia C, Ross-Cisneros FN, Sadun AA, Carelli V. Retinal ganglion cells and circadian rhythms in Alzheimer's disease, Parkinson's disease, and beyond. Front Neurol. 2017;8:162.
121. Cheung CY, Ong YT, Ikram MK, Ong SY, Li X, Hilal S, et al. Microvascular network alterations in the retina of patients with Alzheimer's disease. Alzheimers Dement. 2014;10(2):135–42.
122. Frost S, Kanagasingam Y, Sohrabi H, Vignarajan J, Bourgeat P, Salvado O, et al. Retinal vascular biomarkers for early detection and monitoring of Alzheimer's disease. Transl Psychiatry. 2013;3:e233.
123. Frost S, Martins RN, Kanagasingam Y. Ocular biomarkers for early detection of Alzheimer's disease. J Alzheimers Dis. 2010;22(1):1–16.
124. Williams MA, McGowan AJ, Cardwell CR, Cheung CY, Craig D, Passmore P, et al. Retinal microvascular network attenuation in Alzheimer's disease. Alzheimers Dement (Amst). 2015;1(2):229–35.
125. Smith MZ, Nagy Z, Esiri MM. Cell cycle-related protein expression in vascular dementia and Alzheimer's disease. Neurosci Lett. 1999;271(1):45–8.
126. Bookheimer SY, Strojwas MH, Cohen MS, Saunders AM, Pericak-Vance MA, Mazziotta JC, et al. Patterns of brain activation in people at risk for Alzheimer's disease. N Engl J Med. 2000;343(7):450–6.
127. Kimbrough IF, Robel S, Roberson ED, Sontheimer H. Vascular amyloidosis impairs the gliovascular unit in a mouse model of Alzheimer's disease. Brain. 2015;138(Pt 12):3716–33.
128. Zlokovic BV, Ghiso J, Mackic JB, McComb JG, Weiss MH, Frangione B. Blood-brain barrier transport of circulating Alzheimer's amyloid beta. Biochem Biophys Res Commun. 1993;197(3):1034–40.
129. Do TM, Dodacki A, Alata W, Calon F, Nicolic S, Scherrmann JM, et al. Age-dependent regulation of the blood-brain barrier influx/efflux equilibrium of amyloid-beta peptide in a mouse model of Alzheimer's disease (3xTg-AD). J Alzheimers Dis. 2015;49(2):287–300.
130. Banks WA, Robinson SM, Verma S, Morley JE. Efflux of human and mouse amyloid beta proteins 1-40 and 1-42 from brain: impairment in a mouse model of Alzheimer's disease. Neuroscience. 2003;121(2):487–92.
131. DeMattos RB, Bales KR, Cummins DJ, Paul SM, Holtzman DM. Brain to plasma amyloid-beta efflux: a measure of brain amyloid burden in a mouse model of Alzheimer's disease. Science (New York, NY). 2002;295(5563):2264–7.
132. Sweeney MD, Sagare AP, Zlokovic BV. Blood-brain barrier breakdown in Alzheimer disease and other neurodegenerative disorders. Nat Rev Neurol. 2018;14(3):133–50.
133. Zhao Z, Sagare AP, Ma Q, Halliday MR, Kong P, Kisler K, et al. Central role for PICALM in amyloid-beta blood-brain barrier transcytosis and clearance. Nat Neurosci. 2015;18(7):978–87.
134. Michaud JP, Bellavance MA, Prefontaine P, Rivest S. Real-time in vivo imaging reveals the ability of monocytes to clear vascular amyloid beta. Cell Rep. 2013;5(3):646–53.
135. Iadanza MG, Jackson MP, Radford SE, Ranson NA. MpUL-multi: software for calculation of amyloid fibril mass per unit length from TB-TEM images. Sci Rep. 2016;6:21078.

136. Goldstein LE, Muffat JA, Cherny RA, Moir RD, Ericsson MH, Huang X, et al. Cytosolic beta-amyloid deposition and supranuclear cataracts in lenses from people with Alzheimer's disease. Lancet. 2003;361(9365):1258–65.
137. Kayabasi U, Sergott R, Rispoli M. Retinal examination for the diagnosis of Alzheimer's disease. Int J Ophthalmic Pathol. 2014;3:4.
138. Jentsch S, Schweitzer D, Schmidtke KU, Peters S, Dawczynski J, Bar KJ, et al. Retinal fluorescence lifetime imaging ophthalmoscopy measures depend on the severity of Alzheimer's disease. Acta Ophthalmol. 2015;93(4):e241–7.
139. Hedges TR 3rd, Perez Galves R, Speigelman D, Barbas NR, Peli E, Yardley CJ. Retinal nerve fiber layer abnormalities in Alzheimer's disease. Acta Ophthalmol Scand. 1996;74(3):271–5.
140. Tsai CS, Ritch R, Schwartz B, Lee SS, Miller NR, Chi T, et al. Optic nerve head and nerve fiber layer in Alzheimer's disease. Arch Ophthalmol. 1991;109(2):199–204.
141. Bambo MP, Garcia-Martin E, Otin S, Pinilla J, Larrosa JM, Polo V, et al. Visual function and retinal nerve fibre layer degeneration in patients with Alzheimer disease: correlations with severity of dementia. Acta Ophthalmol. 2015;93(6):e507–8.
142. Poroy C, Yücel A. Optical coherence tomography: is really a new biomarker for Alzheimer's disease? Ann Indian Acad Neurol. 2018;21(2):119–25.
143. O'Bryhim B, Apte RS, Kung N, Coble D, Van Stavern GP. Association of preclinical Alzheimer disease with optical coherence tomographic angiography findings. JAMA Ophthalmol. 2018;136(11):1242–8.
144. Cunha JP, Proenca R, Dias-Santos A, Almeida R, Aguas H, Alves M, et al. OCT in Alzheimer's disease: thinning of the RNFL and superior hemiretina. Graefes Arch Clin Exp Ophthalmol. 2017;255(9):1827–35.
145. Mutlu U, Colijn JM, Ikram MA, Bonnemaijer PWM, Licher S, Wolters FJ, et al. Association of retinal neurodegeneration on optical coherence tomography with dementia: a population-based study. JAMA Neurol. 2018;75(10):1256–63.
146. Einarsdottir AB, Hardarson SH, Kristjansdottir JV, Bragason DT, Snaedal J, Stefansson E. Retinal oximetry imaging in Alzheimer's disease. J Alzheimers Dis. 2015;49(1):79–83.
147. Ukalovic K, Cao S, Lee S, Tang Q, Beg MF, Sarunic MV, et al. Drusen in the peripheral retina of the Alzheimer's eye. Curr Alzheimer Res. 2018;15(8):743–50.
148. Danesh-Meyer HV, Birch H, Ku JY, Carroll S, Gamble G. Reduction of optic nerve fibers in patients with Alzheimer disease identified by laser imaging. Neurology. 2006;67(10):1852–4.
149. Bayer AU, Ferrari F, Erb C. High occurrence rate of glaucoma among patients with Alzheimer's disease. Eur Neurol. 2002;47(3):165–8.
150. Tamura H, Kawakami H, Kanamoto T, Kato T, Yokoyama T, Sasaki K, et al. High frequency of open-angle glaucoma in Japanese patients with Alzheimer's disease. J Neurol Sci. 2006;246(1–2):79–83.
151. Kerbage C, Sadowsky CH, Jennings D, Cagle GD, Hartung PD. Alzheimer's disease diagnosis by detecting exogenous fluorescent signal of ligand bound to beta amyloid in the lens of human eye: an exploratory study. Front Neurol. 2013;4:62.
152. Bei L, Shui YB, Bai F, Nelson SK, Van Stavern GP, Beebe DC. A test of lens opacity as an indicator of preclinical Alzheimer disease. Exp Eye Res. 2015;140:117–23.
153. Frederikse PH, Zigler JS Jr. Presenilin expression in the ocular lens. Curr Eye Res. 1998;17(9):947–52.
154. Gharbiya M, Trebbastoni A, Parisi F, Manganiello S, Cruciani F, D'Antonio F, et al. Choroidal thinning as a new finding in Alzheimer's disease: evidence from enhanced depth imaging spectral domain optical coherence tomography. J Alzheimers Dis. 2014;40(4):907–17.
155. Ning A, Cui J, To E, Ashe KH, Matsubara J. Amyloid-beta deposits lead to retinal degeneration in a mouse model of Alzheimer disease. Invest Ophthalmol Vis Sci. 2008;49(11):5136–43.
156. Liu B, Rasool S, Yang Z, Glabe CG, Schreiber SS, Ge J, et al. Amyloid-peptide vaccinations reduce {beta}-amyloid plaques but exacerbate vascular deposition and inflammation in the retina of Alzheimer's transgenic mice. Am J Pathol. 2009;175(5):2099–110.

157. Perez SE, Lumayag S, Kovacs B, Mufson EJ, Xu S. Beta-amyloid deposition and functional impairment in the retina of the APPswe/PS1DeltaE9 transgenic mouse model of Alzheimer's disease. Invest Ophthalmol Vis Sci. 2009;50(2):793–800.
158. Du LY, Chang LY, Ardiles AO, Tapia-Rojas C, Araya J, Inestrosa NC, et al. Alzheimer's disease-related protein expression in the retina of Octodon degus. PLoS One. 2015;10(8):e0135499.
159. Yang Y, Shiao C, Hemingway JF, Jorstad NL, Shalloway BR, Chang R, et al. Suppressed retinal degeneration in aged wild type and APPswe/PS1DeltaE9 mice by bone marrow transplantation. PLoS One. 2013;8(6):e64246.
160. He Y, Zhao H, Su G. Ginsenoside Rg1 decreases neurofibrillary tangles accumulation in retina by regulating activities of neprilysin and PKA in retinal cells of AD mice model. J Mol Neurosci. 2014;52(1):101–6.
161. Parthasarathy R, Chow KM, Derafshi Z, Fautsch MP, Hetling JR, Rodgers DW, et al. Reduction of amyloid-beta levels in mouse eye tissues by intra-vitreally delivered neprilysin. Exp Eye Res. 2015;138:134–44.
162. Gao L, Chen X, Tang Y, Zhao J, Li Q, Fan X, et al. Neuroprotective effect of memantine on the retinal ganglion cells of APPswe/PS1DeltaE9 mice and its immunomodulatory mechanisms. Exp Eye Res. 2015;135:47–58.
163. Ardiles AO, Tapia-Rojas CC, Mandal M, Alexandre F, Kirkwood A, Inestrosa NC, et al. Postsynaptic dysfunction is associated with spatial and object recognition memory loss in a natural model of Alzheimer's disease. Proc Natl Acad Sci U S A. 2012;109(34):13835–40.
164. Dutescu RM, Li QX, Crowston J, Masters CL, Baird PN, Culvenor JG. Amyloid precursor protein processing and retinal pathology in mouse models of Alzheimer's disease. Graefes Arch Clin Exp Ophthalmol. 2009;247(9):1213–21.
165. Edwards MM, Rodriguez JJ, Gutierrez-Lanza R, Yates J, Verkhratsky A, Lutty GA. Retinal macroglia changes in a triple transgenic mouse model of Alzheimer's disease. Exp Eye Res. 2014;127:252–60.
166. More SS, Vince R. Hyperspectral imaging signatures detect amyloidopathy in Alzheimer's mouse retina well before onset of cognitive decline. ACS Chem Neurosci. 2015;6(2):306–15.
167. Park SW, Kim JH, Mook-Jung I, Kim KW, Park WJ, Park KH. Intracellular amyloid beta alters the tight junction of retinal pigment epithelium in 5XFAD mice. Neurobiol Aging. 2014;35(9):2013–20.
168. Pogue AI, Dua P, Hill JM, Lukiw WJ. Progressive inflammatory pathology in the retina of aluminum-fed 5xFAD transgenic mice. J Inorg Biochem. 2015;152:206–9.
169. Williams PA, Thirgood RA, Oliphant H, Frizzati A, Littlewood E, Votruba M, et al. Retinal ganglion cell dendritic degeneration in a mouse model of Alzheimer's disease. Neurobiol Aging. 2013;34(7):1799–806.
170. Carmine-Simmen K, Proctor T, Tschape J, Poeck B, Triphan T, Strauss R, et al. Neurotoxic effects induced by the Drosophila amyloid-beta peptide suggest a conserved toxic function. Neurobiol Dis. 2009;33(2):274–81.
171. Greeve I, Kretzschmar D, Tschape JA, Beyn A, Brellinger C, Schweizer M, et al. Age-dependent neurodegeneration and Alzheimer-amyloid plaque formation in transgenic Drosophila. J Neurosci. 2004;24(16):3899–906.
172. Zhao H, Chang R, Che H, Wang J, Yang L, Fang W, et al. Hyperphosphorylation of tau protein by calpain regulation in retina of Alzheimer's disease transgenic mouse. Neurosci Lett. 2013;551:12–6.
173. Inestrosa NC, Reyes AE, Chacon MA, Cerpa W, Villalon A, Montiel J, et al. Human-like rodent amyloid-beta-peptide determines Alzheimer pathology in aged wild-type Octodon degu. Neurobiol Aging. 2005;26(7):1023–8.
174. Grimaldi A, Brighi C, Peruzzi G, Ragozzino D, Bonanni V, Limatola C, et al. Inflammation, neurodegeneration and protein aggregation in the retina as ocular biomarkers for Alzheimer's disease in the 3xTg-AD mouse model. Cell Death Dis. 2018;9(6):685.
175. Frederikse PH, Ren XO. Lens defects and age-related fiber cell degeneration in a mouse model of increased AbetaPP gene dosage in Down syndrome. Am J Pathol. 2002;161(6):1985–90.

176. Cutler T, Sarkar A, Moran M, Steffensmeier A, Puli OR, Mancini G, et al. Drosophila eye model to study neuroprotective role of CREB Binding Protein (CBP) in Alzheimer's disease. PLoS One. 2015;10(9):e0137691.
177. Finelli A, Kelkar A, Song HJ, Yang H, Konsolaki M. A model for studying Alzheimer's Abeta42-induced toxicity in Drosophila melanogaster. Mol Cell Neurosci. 2004;26(3):365–75.
178. Gupta VK, Chitranshi N, Gupta VB, Golzan M, Dheer Y, Wall RV, et al. Amyloid beta accumulation and inner retinal degenerative changes in Alzheimer's disease transgenic mouse. Neurosci Lett. 2016;623:52–6.
179. Chiasseu M, Alarcon-Martinez L, Belforte N, Quintero H, Dotigny F, Destroismaisons L, et al. Tau accumulation in the retina promotes early neuronal dysfunction and precedes brain pathology in a mouse model of Alzheimer's disease. Mol Neurodegener. 2017;12(1):58.
180. Rodriguez L, Mdzomba JB, Joly S, Boudreau-Laprise M, Planel E, Pernet V. Human tau expression does not induce mouse retina neurodegeneration, suggesting differential toxicity of tau in brain vs retinal neurons. Front Mol Neurosci. 2018;11:293.
181. Grammenoudi S, Kosmidis S, Skoulakis EM. Cell type-specific processing of human tau proteins in Drosophila. FEBS Lett. 2006;580(19):4602–6.
182. Bayhan HA, Aslan Bayhan S, Celikbilek A, Tanik N, Gurdal C. Evaluation of the chorioretinal thickness changes in Alzheimer's disease using spectral-domain optical coherence tomography. Clin Exp Ophthalmol. 2015;43(2):145–51.
183. Guo L, Duggan J, Cordeiro MF. Alzheimer's disease and retinal neurodegeneration. Curr Alzheimer Res. 2010;7(1):3–14.
184. Stefansson E, Olafsdottir OB, Einarsdottir AB, Eliasdottir TS, Eysteinsson T, Vehmeijer W, et al. Retinal oximetry discovers novel biomarkers in retinal and brain diseases. Invest Ophthalmol Vis Sci. 2017;58(6):BIO227–BIO33.
185. Kurna SA, Akar G, Altun A, Agirman Y, Gozke E, Sengor T. Confocal scanning laser tomography of the optic nerve head on the patients with Alzheimer's disease compared to glaucoma and control. Int Ophthalmol. 2014;34(6):1203–11.
186. Kerbage C, Sadowsky CH, Tariot PN, Agronin M, Alva G, Turner FD, et al. Detection of amyloid beta signature in the lens and its correlation in the brain to aid in the diagnosis of Alzheimer's disease. Am J Alzheimers Dis Other Dement. 2015;30(8):738–45.
187. Antes R, Ezra-Elia R, Weinberger D, Solomon A, Ofri R, Michaelson DM. ApoE4 induces synaptic and ERG impairments in the retina of young targeted replacement apoE4 mice. PLoS One. 2013;8(5):e64949.
188. Antes R, Salomon-Zimri S, Beck SC, Garcia Garrido M, Livnat T, Maharshak I, et al. VEGF mediates ApoE4-induced neovascularization and synaptic pathology in the choroid and retina. Curr Alzheimer Res. 2015;12(4):323–34.
189. Maharshak I, Salomon-Zimri S, Antes R, Liraz O, Nisgav Y, Livnat T, et al. The effects of the apoE4 genotype on the developing mouse retina. Exp Eye Res. 2015;145:17–25.
190. Perez de Lara MJ, Pintor J. Presence and release of ATP from the retina in an Alzheimer's disease model. J Alzheimers Dis. 2015;43(1):177–81.
191. Polans J, Keller B, Carrasco-Zevallos OM, LaRocca F, Cole E, Whitson HE, et al. Wide-field retinal optical coherence tomography with wavefront sensorless adaptive optics for enhanced imaging of targeted regions. Biomed Opt Express. 2017;8(1):16–37.
192. Polo V, Rodrigo MJ, Garcia-Martin E, Otin S, Larrosa JM, Fuertes MI, et al. Visual dysfunction and its correlation with retinal changes in patients with Alzheimer's disease. Eye (Lond). 2017;31(7):1034–41.
193. Gota VS, Maru GB, Soni TG, Gandhi TR, Kochar N, Agarwal MG. Safety and pharmacokinetics of a solid lipid curcumin particle formulation in osteosarcoma patients and healthy volunteers. J Agric Food Chem. 2010;58(4):2095–9.
194. Garcia-Alloza M, Borrelli LA, Rozkalne A, Hyman BT, Bacskai BJ. Curcumin labels amyloid pathology in vivo, disrupts existing plaques, and partially restores distorted neurites in an Alzheimer mouse model. J Neurochem. 2007;102(4):1095–104.
195. Airoldi C, Zona C, Sironi E, Colombo L, Messa M, Aurilia D, et al. Curcumin derivatives as new ligands of Abeta peptides. J Biotechnol. 2011;156(4):317–24.

196. Kumaraswamy P, Sethuraman S, Krishnan UM. Mechanistic insights of curcumin interactions with the core-recognition motif of beta-amyloid peptide. J Agric Food Chem. 2013;61(13):3278–85.
197. Masuda Y, Fukuchi M, Yatagawa T, Tada M, Takeda K, Irie K, et al. Solid-state NMR analysis of interaction sites of curcumin and 42-residue amyloid beta-protein fibrils. Bioorg Med Chem. 2011;19(20):5967–74.
198. Mutsuga M, Chambers JK, Uchida K, Tei M, Makibuchi T, Mizorogi T, et al. Binding of curcumin to senile plaques and cerebral amyloid angiopathy in the aged brain of various animals and to neurofibrillary tangles in Alzheimer's brain. J Vet Med Sci. 2012;74(1):51–7.
199. Yanagisawa D, Shirai N, Amatsubo T, Taguchi H, Hirao K, Urushitani M, et al. Relationship between the tautomeric structures of curcumin derivatives and their Abeta-binding activities in the context of therapies for Alzheimer's disease. Biomaterials. 2010;31(14):4179–85.
200. Yanagisawa D, Taguchi H, Yamamoto A, Shirai N, Hirao K, Tooyama I. Curcuminoid binds to amyloid-beta1-42 oligomer and fibril. J Alzheimers Dis. 2011;24(Suppl 2):33–42.
201. Cabrera DeBuc D, Somfai GM, Arthur E, Kostic M, Oropesa S, Mendoza Santiesteban C. Investigating multimodal diagnostic eye biomarkers of cognitive impairment by measuring vascular and neurogenic changes in the retina. Front Physiol. 2018;9:1721.
202. Rafii M, Wishnek H, Brewer J, Donohue M, Ness S, Mobley W, et al. The Down Syndrome Biomarker Initiative (DSBI) pilot: proof of concept for deep phenotyping of Alzheimer's disease biomarkers in down syndrome. Front Behav Neurosci. 2015;9:239.
203. Head E, Helman AM, Powell D, Schmitt FA. Down syndrome, beta-amyloid and neuroimaging. Free Radic Biol Med. 2018;114:102–9.
204. More SS, Beach JM, Vince R. Early detection of amyloidopathy in Alzheimer's mice by hyperspectral endoscopy. Invest Ophthalmol Vis Sci. 2016;57(7):3231–8.
205. Yang J, Yang J, Li Y, Xu Y, Ran C. Near-infrared Fluorescence Ocular Imaging (NIRFOI) of Alzheimer's disease. Mol Imaging Biol. 2019;21:35–43.
206. Hickman RA, Faustin A, Wisniewski T. Alzheimer disease and its growing epidemic: risk factors, biomarkers, and the urgent need for therapeutics. Neurol Clin. 2016;34(4):941–53.

Advances in Retinal Imaging: Real-Time Imaging of Single Neuronal Cell Apoptosis (DARC)

7

Timothy E. Yap, Maja Szymanska, and M. Francesca Cordeiro

7.1 Mechanisms of Cell Death and Apoptosis

Amongst the distinct pathways through which cells are pathways believed to die, increased rates of apoptosis are thought to play a key role in glaucoma and other neurodegenerative conditions such as Alzheimer's disease, Parkinson's disease and motor neurone disease [1]. 'Apoptosis' from the Greek for 'falling off' represents the pathway of programmed cell death by which cells are able to die in order to make way for new cells, without triggering inflammation that may threaten the health and function of neighbouring cells. The rate of this stereotyped behaviour occurs is important when considering the likely necessity of some neuronal cells to last the lifetime of an organisms in order to maintain learnt neurological functions, memories or motor units [1]. It follows the minimising the triggers of this process may prolong visual, neurological or neuromuscular function in certain neurodegenerative conditions. As far as we can conclude currently, trigger events of apoptosis

T. E. Yap
The Western Eye Hospital, Imperial College Healthcare NHS Trust (ICHNT), London, UK

The Imperial College Ophthalmic Research Group (ICORG), Imperial College London, London, UK
e-mail: timothyedward.yap@nhs.net

M. Szymanska
The Imperial College Ophthalmic Research Group (ICORG), Imperial College London, London, UK
e-mail: maja.szymanska15@imperial.ac.uk

M. F. Cordeiro (✉)
The Western Eye Hospital, Imperial College Healthcare NHS Trust (ICHNT), London, UK

The Imperial College Ophthalmic Research Group (ICORG), Imperial College London, London, UK

Glaucoma and Retinal Neurodegeneration Group, Department of Visual Neuroscience, UCL Institute of Ophthalmology, London, UK
e-mail: m.cordeiro@imperial.ac.uk

A. Grzybowski, P. Barboni (eds.), *OCT and Imaging in Central Nervous System Diseases*, https://doi.org/10.1007/978-3-030-26269-3_7

are likely to combine genetic susceptibility and environmental factors, progressing downstream to a highly conserved intracellular apoptotic pathway. Well-studied examples of chemical activation signals include lack of neurotrophic factor support, glutamate excitotoxicity, and oxidative, metabolic, and environmental stresses [1]. It is becoming increasingly apparent that mitochondrial events are crucial in this critical moment of apoptosis initiation [2]. Early cellular signals associated with an activated apoptosis pathway include the pro- and anti-apoptotic members of the B-cell lymphoma-2 (Bcl-2) family, upstream and downstream apoptosis-activating caspases, and telomerase activity [3]. The ensuing morphological changes involve shrinkage, membrane blebbing, chromatin condensation and the development of pyknotic neuclei [4]. This apoptotic pathway is distinct from primary necrosis whereby immediate, unregulated cell death occurs in response to extreme stress causing mass release of intracellular molecules, damage-associated molecular patterns (DAMPs) [5] and recruitment of cells mediating an acute inflammatory response. Less acute events sufficient to cause necrosis with delayed rupture of the cell membrane allows modification of intracellular components prior to release, presumably in an attempt to prune to inflammatory response [6].

Phosphatidylserine (PS) is a marker of early apoptosis of particular interest in diagnostics. This anionic phospholipid is usually maintained in an asymmetric distribution across the cell membrane by ATP-dependent flippases located on the inner leaflet of the cell membrane, in physiologic conditions [7]. In apoptotic conditions, flippases are downregulated which causes the increased externalisation of PS on the outer leaflet of the cell membrane. Scramblase proteins are another type of cell membrane protein thought to induce this change, enlisting their ability to facilitate bi-directional, non-specific movement of phospholipids across bilayers in a calcium-dependent manner [8], as in this instance.

In glaucoma in particular, apoptosis is believed to be the predominant mechanism of ganglion cell layer (GCL) loss in glaucoma. Ganglion cells reside in the inner retina, with their dendrites forming the inner plexiform layer and axons projecting over the inner surface of the retina, forming the retinal nerve fibre layer. Far from being an exclusively ophthalmic condition, a considerable body of evidence suggests neurodegeneration extending further into the central nervous system, specifically the lateral geniculate nucleus and visual cortex [9, 10]. Typically difficult to image due to their low-contrast edges, retinal ganglion cells (RGCs) vary in density across the retina, peaking at around 32,000–38,000 cells/mm^2 in the perifoveal region [11], whilst also varying throughout development and lifespans, and between healthy individuals. Unsatisfactorily, the evidence for RGC apoptosis mainly lies with the absence of features of necrosis such as ATP depletion, cell lysis and acute inflammation. However, in addition to this observation, primate studies have attempted to use DNA assays showing DNA fragmentation typical of apoptosis, examining primate ocular hypertension models of glaucoma. However, these are hampered by the low number of cells thought to be undergoing apoptosis at any one time [12]. Detection of the typical 180–200 base pair fragments created in apoptosis has proven a slightly more successful way forward, utilising the TUNEL (Terminal transferase dUTP Nick End Labelling) method of biotin-labelled deoxyuridine tagging of DNA fragments, showing significantly increased levels in experimental glaucoma eyes in comparison to their healthy, contralateral counterparts [13]. Such results have also since been replicated in human patients [14–16]. The trigger for apoptosis in the setting of glaucoma has been widely debated and may indeed be multiple, with several prominent theories. Deprivation of neurotrophic factor (e.g. brain derived neurotrophic factor, BDNF) support due to intraocular pressure (IOP) related congestion and restricted axoplasmic transport at the lamina cribrosa where the optic nerve exits the globe. In a similar manner, a vascular hypothesis behind glaucoma offering the concept of optic nerve head vaso-dysregulation [17] might also be involved in deficiencies in neurotrophic factor support. Glutamate excitotoxicity via NMDA receptor over-activation is another theory behind glaucoma and lends itself to the possibility of neuroprotective therapies. Conflicting findings exist with regards to whether glutamate is present in raised levels in the vitreous of glaucoma patients [18–22] and indeed the significance of this measure in the context of the overall theory [23]. Oxidative stress [24] and immunological factors [25, 26] are other factors that are suggested to have important and likely overlapping roles in instigating downstream apoptotic cascades.

7.2 DARC Technology

The molecular basis of DARC uses the affinity annexin A5 has for PS, therefore lending itself well to the application of labelling cells in the early phases of apoptosis. Annexin A5 is a 36 kDa protein that is ubiquitously expressed in humans. Its unique function is unclear, however it has been proposed to play a role in membrane repair and permeability [27, 28], autophagy [29], and anti-endotoxin activities [30], as well as working in combination with C1q complement protein as a ligand in the induction of apoptosis [31]. Annexin A5 electrostatically binds PS in strong but reversible, calcium-dependent fashion, taking advantage of the local high calcium (Ca^{2+}) concentrations found near the negatively charged cell surface [32, 33]. In-vitro use of fluorescently-labelled or biotinylated annexin A5 has therefore been used to detect apoptosing cells with both imaging and flow cytometry [34]. When used in combination with propidium iodide (PI), cells undergoing necrosis (annexin A5+/PI+) or apoptosis (annexin A5+/PI−) can be successfully identified. The high affinity with PS also brings about high levels of sensitivity for early apoptosis which favours annexin A5 as a detector of apoptosis, such that it has been translated into human studies as a radiolabelled marker investigating diseases where rates of apoptosis are altered such as malignancy [35–38], stroke, myocardial infarction [39, 40], organ transplantation [41] and inflammatory bowel disease [42]. However, in many of these applications, resolution and localisation is limited by tissue opacity. In contrast, the transparent media of the eye including the cornea, aqueous humour, lens and vitreous body allow direct visualisation of fluorescent markers in the retina, permitting cellular-resolution imaging using DARC, amongst other techniques [43, 44].

DARC technology uses Annexin A5 conjugated with either a 488 nm (ANX488) or 776 nm (ANX776) fluorophore in order to visualise apoptosing retinal cells. These probes have so far been administered intravitreally in animals [45] and intravenously in humans [46] as a novel type of contrast agent for retinal cell apoptosis. ANX488 has excitation/emission wavelengths of 495/519 nm, and ANX776, excitation/emission wavelengths in the near-infrared spectrum of 771/793 nm. ANX776 was developed using a human variant annexin molecule (RhAnnexin V128) permitting a single covalent bond between the maleimide form of Dy776 fluorescent marker (Dy-776-mal) and RhAnnexin V128. This provided a similar excitation/emission profile to indocyanine green (ICG), a fluorescent dye commonly used in the investigation of retinal vascular pathology such as idiopathic polypoidal choroidal vasculopathy (IPCV).

Confocal scanning laser ophthalmoscopy is an imaging technique that is able to provide high resolution imaging with depth selectivity in order to form optical cross-sections. The axial volume required is selected by passing the reflected light through an adjustable pinhole aperture, therefore improving axial resolution by minimising optical cross-talk [47]. For acquiring DARC images, two settings have been used in conjunction with cSLO according to the fluorescent marker in question. For earlier studies and the majority of the animal work completed, using ANX488 required illumination with argon laser of 488 nm, with a wide band-pass filter with short wavelength cut-off at 521 nm to select out the fluorescent signal. Using ANX776 however, meant the ICG set-up already in clinical use could be used to image 'DARC spots' with diode laser illumination of 786 nm and an 800 nm barrier filter. The resultant images show 'DARC spots' 12–16 μm in diameter that can be counted using an automated system based on a template-matching approach [48] after transformations to take into account large non-enhancing structures such as blood vessels and non-linear optical distortions. To maximise signal-to-noise ratio, the manufacturer's eye tracking technology was used in combination with 100-frame averaging.

7.3 DARC Investigating Disease Pathogenesis

DARC has been incorporated into a range of experimental studies using animal models of several neurodegenerative diseases including glaucoma, Alzheimer's disease, Parkinson's disease and diabetes (Table 7.1). The first study published in 2004 used rodent and primate glaucoma models to demonstrate proof of concept. The rat models included the Morrison's chronic ocular hypertension model involving episcleral vein injections of hypertonic saline resulting in chronic ocular hypertension (OHT) [9093024], another model using intravitreal injections of staurosporine, a non-selective protein kinase inhibitor causing neuronal cell death [60], and a further optic nerve transection (ONT) model of secondary neurodegeneration [49, 61]. DARC imaging was combined with histological analysis in order to determine the identity of DARC spots. Rats received intravitreal injections of ANX488 and retrograde labelling of RGCs was carried out using an injection of DiAsp

Table 7.1 Summary of DARC studies showing proof-of-concept and investigating pathogenesis

Factor of interest	Findings	Citation
Proof of concept	DARC demonstrating in-vivo apoptosing retinal cells using ANX488	[49]
Intraocular pressure	Correlation of DARC with intraocular pressure and changes in the extracellular matrix	[50]
DMSO	DMSO toxicity demonstrated with in-vivo DARC imaging and in-vitro studies	[51]
Staurosporine model	Staurosporine (SSP) induced RGC apoptosis confirmed with histological analysis	[52]
Partial optic nerve transection	Retinal apoptosis detected following pONT	[53]
Alzheimer's model	Triple transgenic model of Alzheimer's disease	[54]
Amyloid-β	Amyloid-β induction of RGC apoptosis and co-localization with DARC	[55]
Diabetic retinopathy	Raised DARC count in transgenic diabetic mice	[56]
Laser damage	Inner nuclear layer damage from lasers demonstrated with DARC	[57]
Blue light exposure	Photoreceptor death in response to blue light exposure investigated with DARC	[58]
Parkinson's model	DARC imaging used in a rotenone-induced model of Parkinson's disease.	[59]
Proof-of-concept	Longitudinal DARC using spectrally distinct fluorophores to image multiple phases of cell death in rats	[54]
Phase I clinical trial	Demonstration of DARC spot visualisation in humans, including demonstration of the safety and efficacy of intravenous ANX776	[46]

(4-(4-(didecylamino)styryl)-N-methylpyridinium iodide) to the superior colliculi of rats. After sacrifice, subsequent histological staining using Cy5-labeled anti-caspase-3 antibodies confirmed apoptosing cells, with 4,6-diamidino-2-phenylindole (DAPI) staining used to assess the nuclei. Anatomical reconstructions of in-vivo imaging and histological studies showed good correlation between staining patterns and DARC counts, supporting the identity of DARC spots as apoptosing RGCs [49]. DARC count was highest at 7 days in ONT and between 3–4 weeks in the OHT model. A correlation between the number of apoptosing cells and the magnitude of ocular hypertensive or staurosporine dose-related insult was also seen. Furthermore, using spectrally distinct fluorescent markers of early and late apoptosis DARC was shown to longitudinally image the same cells through time [54]. Thus, the ability of DARC to both identify and quantify retinal cell apoptosis suggested its capability as an outcome measure in future studies.

DARC has also been used to investigate the neurodegenerative mechanisms in glaucoma. A rat ocular hypertension model was used to investigate the effect of raised IOP on apoptosis of RGCs and expression of specific ECM components. Results showed a strong correlation between DARC count and the magnitude of IOP elevation. This study also demonstrated IOP-related alterations in extra-cellular matrix components including a positive correlation with matrix metalloproteinase-9 activity (MMP-9), tissue inhibitor of matrix metalloproteinase (TIMP-1) and collagen I, and negative correlations with laminin and TGF-beta2 deposition in the RGC layer [50] supporting the theory of glaucomatous RGC apoptosis relating to ECM remodelling, and the retina being the primary site of glaucomatous injury [15623771].

Another study of glaucoma pathogenesis examined the role of amyloid beta (Aβ) peptide in glaucoma, the production and deposition of which drives the pathogenesis of Alzheimer's disease [55, 62]. This study found that in a rat ocular hypertension model, amyloid beta not only co-localized with RGCs undergoing apoptosis, but also significantly contributed to their apoptosis in time and dose-dependent manner. These findings suggested that the amyloid beta pathway could be a therapeutic target in glaucoma, together with in vivo DARC imaging allowing to assess the efficacy of treatment [55].

In addition to glaucoma, DARC has been used to study the pathogenesis of other diseases in which neurodegeneration is implicated. DARC was able to provide the first in-vivo visualisation of apoptosing RGCs in a transgenic mouse model of diabetic retinopathy. This study suggested that the rate of apoptosis was highest early in the lifecycle of this model (8 weeks), suggesting DARC may have a future role as a detector of early diabetic retinopathy [56].

Retinal damage using light has also been examined with DARC, using Nd:YAG laser. This study found that the damage to the inner nuclear layer of rats was correlated with the power and duration of the laser insult, with DARC spot density showing a dose-dependent correlation with laser exposure [57]. Blue light damage has also been studied, with DARC demonstrating damage to the outer retinal layers, as confirmed by histological studies finding photoreceptor death [58].

7.4 DARC Investigating Novel Therapeutics

DARC has been used in pre-clinical studies to assess the neuroprotective efficacy of several novel therapeutic agents and new formulations of drugs already in clinical use (Table 7.2). In relation to glaucoma, the alpha agonist, brimonidine, has been suggested to have neuroprotective actions in addition to its anti-ocular hypertensive actions [67]. However, the human studies supporting this theory are plagued with difficulties surrounding high attrition rates due to drop intolerance [68]. Using DARC, systemic brimonidine and clonidine were shown to reduce apoptosis in a glaucoma-induced rodent model by 92.8% and 92.3% respectively via the non-amyloidogenic Aβ and secreted amyloid precursor protein α (sAPPα) pathways suggesting these drugs may have a role to play in other pathologies involving Aβ toxicity such as Alzheimer's disease [65]. In contrast to clonidine, no significant IOP lowering effect was seen with systemic brimonidine supporting the hypothesis of an IOP-independent neuroprotective mechanism.

Glutamate-induced excitotoxicity implicated in Alzheimer's disease [69] is also likely to play a role in glaucoma, causing RGC death. Furthermore, blocking

Table 7.2 Summary of DARC studies as an outcome measure

Factor of interest	Findings	Citation
NMDA receptor antagonists	DARC used to investigate NMDA receptor antagonism to target glutamate excitotoxicity as a neuroprotective strategy in rat models of glaucoma	[52]
Amyloid-β	Investigation of MRZ-99030, an amyloid-β aggregator	[63]
Schwann cell delivery	DARC used to help evaluate the efficacy of a novel direct Schwann cell delivery method in a partial optic nerve transection (ONT) model	[53]
Adenosine A3 agonism	Selective adenosine A3 agonism by 2-Cl-IB-MECA investigated with DARC as a neuroprotective treatment strategy in partial ONT	[64]
Rosiglitazone	The neuroprotective potential of liposome-encapsulated rosiglitazone investigated with DARC in a Parkinson's model	[59]
Alpha-agonists	DARC used to demonstrate IOP-independent neuroprotection in ocular hypertension model	[65]
Coenzyme Q10	Topical coenzyme Q10 investigated in an ocular hypertension model	[66]

N-Methyl-D-aspartate (NMDA) receptors has been reported to reduce RGC apoptosis [70–72]. Targeting the role glutamate excitotoxicity may play in glaucoma, non-selective (MK801) and selective (ifenprodil) NMDA receptor antagonists and a metabotropic glutamate receptor agonist (mGluR Group II, LY354740) were used in a study on rat models of glaucoma. All the glutamate modulation strategies employed were shown to have efficacy in neuroprotection in the staurosporine model seen with both in vivo imaging and histological analysis, in a dose-dependent manner. MK801 was shown to have greater efficacy than ifenprodil, however due to MK801's neurotoxic side effects, best results were achieved with low-dose MK801 combined with LY354740 [52]. Treatments were administered to an OHT model using DARC as an outcome measure, demonstrating maximal neuroprotective efficacy at the start of IOP elevation (day 0).

There is some evidence suggesting that targeting adenosine A1 receptors (A1Rs) may be a potentially useful neuroprotective therapeutic strategy [73], in at least part due to its inhibitory effect on glutaminergic activity. 2-Cl-IB-MECA, a selective (A3R) agonist was trialled with DARC in models of partial optic nerve transection (pONT). DARC showed significantly increased apoptosis after pONT, an effect reduced by intravitreal 2-Cl-IB-MECA [64].

The commonality in the excitotoxic pathogenesis of both glaucoma and Alzheimer's disease has led to the same drugs being used or trialled in both diseases [74]. Similarly, amyloid-beta (Aβ) central to the amyloid hypothesis of Alzheimer's disease [75], has been proposed as a potential therapeutic target in glaucoma. In a rat model of ocular hypertension, DARC imaging was used as an outcome measure in combination with histological studies to demonstrate the Aβ aggregation modulator MRZ-99030 could achieve dose-dependent neuroprotection, with MRZ-99030 achieving a 33% reduction of apoptosis without exhibiting any effect on the IOP [63].

DARC has also been used to study drugs more commonly used in another neurodegenerative condition, Parkinson's disease (PD). Using a rotenone-induced rat model, animals were treated with liposome-encapsulated rosiglitazone, a peroxisome proliferator-activated receptor gamma (PPAR-gamma) agonist [76]. The results of the treatment versus vehicle-only controls demonstrated a neuroprotective effect of intraperitoneal rosiglitazone in this formulation. More importantly for DARC, in-vivo apoptosis imaging detected a peak in counts at 20 days after rotenone administration in comparison to pathological studies at day 60. The earlier appearance of a significant rise in DARC count compared to the pathological finding of dopaminergic loss from the substantia nigra further supports the role of DARC as a useful tool for early diagnosis [59].

The role of impaired mitochondrial function and oxidative stress in triggering RGC apoptosis has been examined with DARC. Coenzyme Q10 (CoQ10) is a mitochondrial antioxidant, key to the normal function of the electron transport chain. CoQ10 has been shown to play a neuroprotective role in neurological conditions such as PD, AD, Huntington's disease [77] and experimental glaucoma [78]. In a rat OHT model, the effect of topically applied CoQ10 was examined, in a micellular α–tocopherol polyethylene glycol succinate (TPGS) formulation. DARC imaging revealed a significantly lower number of apoptosing retinal cells in those animal treated with CoQ10 compared to the TPGS-only controls at 3 weeks [66], suggesting translational therapeutic promise for this formulation of CoQ10.

A novel cell-based therapy using Schwann cells has also been investigated with DARC technology, comparing direct optic nerve sheath application (DONS) versus intravitreal injections, in a model of partial optic nerve transection. Although both methods reduced showed a significantly increased proportion of RGCs remaining at certain time points, the DONS method demonstrated delayed but had longer-lasting effects at 56 days. These histological results using Brn-3a-labelling were mirrored by using DARC, demonstrating significantly reduced rates of apoptosis in the DONS group compared to those untreated at days 7 and 21. Using DARC to provide *in vivo* observation of retinal cell apoptosis in this manner facilitated the comparison of effect on secondary degeneration through multiple time intervals in the same subject, instead of requiring sacrifice in order to complete histological analysis at each timepoint [53].

7.5 DARC in Humans

DARC has now been translated into investigating human disease, with a phase I trial published in 2017 [46]. This study set out to examine the safety and tolerability of DARC using intravenous ANX776. The study population included eight glaucoma patients proven to demonstrate disease progression, and eight healthy volunteers. Inclusion of glaucoma patients was based on having at least one progressing index from visual field testing or OCT/HRT (optical coherence imaging/Heidelberg retinal tomography) imaging. A storer design was used to allocate 4 groups of patients to each dose of ANX776. Each group consisted of 2 glaucoma and 2 healthy subjects. The doses given were 0.1, 0.2, 0.4 and 0.5 mg. The results showed that no serious adverse event occurred, with the six reported adverse events deemed not related to the ANX776 itself. Pharmacokinetic experiments showed a dose-dependent relationship with ANX776 administration. Clearance of the drug was also found to be high, with no drug accumulation.

With regards to efficacy of the investigation, DARC spots were successfully seen appearing in humans as they had previously had been in animals (Fig. 7.1). At the 0.4 mg dose, significantly more spots were seen in the glaucomatous group compared to healthy controls ($n = 4$, $p < 0.005$). DARC count was also seen to be significantly correlated with reduced central corneal thickness (Spearman's correlation $R = -0.68$, $p = 0.006$) and increased cup-to-disc ratio (Spearman's correlation $R = 0.47$, $p = 0.038$). Further post-hoc analysis was carried out using clinical follow up data for these patients, demonstrating that the DARC count was significantly higher in those patients who underwent increased rates of disease progression following ANX776 administration, compared to healthy controls. Phase II of the DARC project is currently underway and included a spectrum of neurodegenerative conditions compared to healthy controls. Five patient groups have been included in this study, including healthy volunteers, progressive glaucoma patients, optic neuritis patients, age-related macular degeneration patients, and subjects with Down's syndrome who are believed to demonstrate similar CNS pathology to Alzheimer's disease [79].

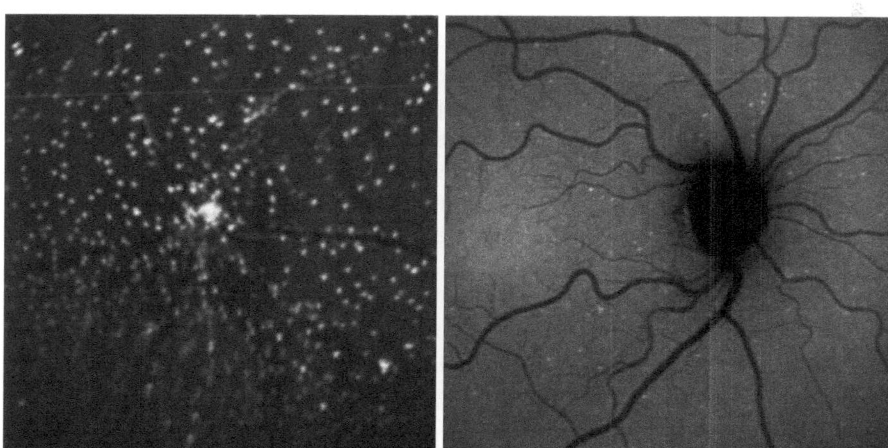

Fig. 7.1 DARC images from a rat model (left) and human (right)

7.6 Potential Implications for Clinical Practice in Glaucoma and Beyond

Neurodegenerative diseases have inherent challenges in their diagnosis, monitoring and treatment that may be overcome if DARC technology is able to be successfully translated to clinic and human research. In the case of glaucoma, subtle early visual field defects not affecting central vision are rarely detected by patients, with incidental findings of raised IOP, family history or fundus examination detecting more advanced disease all more common methods of presentation. The biomarker most commonly considered is intraocular pressure (IOP). IOP is carefully monitored, and the sole target of current glaucoma therapies. However its reliability is under constant scrutiny as measurements can vary by technique, corneal thickness and time of day, amongst other variables [80]. Also, deciding how low an individual's IOP should be is often a clinical decision that can influence whether or not a patient undergoes procedures that may involve lasers or intraocular surgery. Further complexity lies in the fact that intraocular pressure is not a universal surrogate marker for disease progression. From the ocular hypertension treatment study [81], we know that lowering IOP reduces the rate of conversion to glaucoma in patients with ocular hypertension to glaucoma (number needed to treat, NNT = 20). However, the fact remains that the majority of those with high IOP will not develop glaucomatous damage, and a small proportion of those with sufficiently treated IOP will still progress to disease. As a further complexity, the Collaborative Normal-Tension Glaucoma Study (CNTGS) has also shown that reducing IOP still reduces disease progression in 'normal-tension' glaucoma (NTG), where IOP is thought to be within 'normal' range. Therefore, knowing how low an individual patient's IOP should can be a complex and subjective decision.

Visual field tests are currently the gold standard investigation in glaucoma that demonstrate the extent and location of functional loss the patient is experiencing. As is the case with IOP, many variables affect the test reliability, with a stationary posture, good concentration and steady fixation required for up to 4–5 min at a time. This can be challenging for patients, especially those with musculoskeletal or cognition-related health problems that are common in the glaucoma population. Such is the difficulty many patients experience carrying out these tests, a significant 'learning effect' takes place whereby the first few visual fields may paradoxically improve with increasing reliability parameters [82]. There is also believed to be a significant lag-time between the onset of glaucoma and the appearance of visual field defects, with an estimated 20–30% RGC loss prior to the development of 'perimetric' glaucoma. This is also dependent on the test sensitivity, with recent studies suggesting that the standard 24-2 visual field testing algorithms may not detect early visual field defects [83]. A further limiting factor in visual field testing is the slow rate at which many patients progress [84], thus making the use of visual fields as a primary outcome in clinical trials an expensive option. Concomitant ophthalmic pathology may also affect visual field outcomes which may mask glaucomatous change in a subset of patients. These factors have led to the majority of glaucoma treatments proven on efficacy of IOP-lowering alone. The first large placebo-controlled study claiming to have shown visual field-sparing efficacy of a topical glaucoma therapy was published in 2015 [85].

OCT imaging in glaucoma has shown great promise in detecting 'pre-perimetric glaucoma' in patients who are yet to develop visual field defects. This period is reported to last between 2 and 8 years in the cohorts studied [86, 87]. Due to individual variation in optic disc and posterior pole morphologies, rate of progression indicated by longitudinal change is thought to be a good predictor of future visual field progression [87] but requires multiple timepoints for reliable trends to be detected, during which RGC loss may be continuing. OCT imaging in other neurodegenerative conditions where apoptosis has been implicated is also starting to be recognised, especially in the field of dementia. Alzheimer's disease similarly often has a lag-time between disease onset and diagnosis due to a non-specific early prodrome of symptoms. Both retinal nerve fibre layer (RNFL) and ganglion cell layers have been demonstrated to display thinning, especially in the superior and inferior peripapillary quadrants and may be used as part of a diagnostic or monitoring tool to provide easily accessible information on disease severity and progression [88]. However, in a similar manner to glaucoma, rate of progression in likely to be slow and require multiple visits over time.

The placing of DARC in human research or clinical practice is still yet to be fully clarified. What is very promising for the future is the first demonstration of in-vivo visualisation of apoptosing retinal cells in humans using a method that is easily achievable in the majority of clinical environments. Additionally, the ANX776 has been shown to be safe for use in humans with no adverse events thought to be related to the agent itself. The concepts of primary and secondary neurodegeneration suggest that early treatment in a range of diseases is crucial in order to have a hope of reducing increasingly convergent secondary pathways [89–92]. Given our current lack of ability to confidently diagnose early neurodegeneration, DARC is attempting to meet a crucial unmet clinical need both in terms of patient management and surrogate markers. The future for DARC will involve clearly demonstrating what DARC spots mean in humans, and whether these can be used in a meaningful way to reduce morbidity from visual or cognitive decline from the instigation of early treatment, or facilitate the study of novel therapeutics in order to abate neurodegenerative processes.

References

1. Mattson MP. Apoptosis in neurodegenerative disorders. Nat Rev Mol Cell Biol. 2000;1:120–9. https://doi.org/10.1038/35040009.
2. Kroemer G, Dallaporta B, Resche-Rigon M. The mitochondrial death/life regulator in apoptosis and necrosis. Annu Rev Physiol. 1998;60:619–42. https://doi.org/10.1146/annurev.physiol.60.1.619.
3. Liu JP. Studies of the molecular mechanisms in the regulation of telomerase activity. FASEB J. 1999;13:2091–104.
4. Zhang Y, Chen X, Gueydan C, et al. Plasma membrane changes during programmed cell deaths. Cell Res. 2018;28:9–21. https://doi.org/10.1038/cr.2017.133.

5. Schaefer L. Complexity of danger: the diverse nature of damage-associated molecular patterns. J Biol Chem. 2014;289:35237–45. https://doi.org/10.1074/jbc.R114.619304.
6. Sachet M, Liang YY, Oehler R. The immune response to secondary necrotic cells. Apoptosis. 2017;22:1189–204. https://doi.org/10.1007/s10495-017-1413-z.
7. Daleke DL. Phospholipid flippases. J Biol Chem. 2007;282:821–5. https://doi.org/10.1074/jbc.R600035200.
8. Hankins HM, Baldridge RD, Xu P, et al. Role of flippases, scramblases and transfer proteins in phosphatidylserine subcellular distribution. Traffic. 2015;16:35–47. https://doi.org/10.1111/tra.12233.
9. Danesh-Meyer HV, Levin LA. Glaucoma as a neurodegenerative disease. J Neuroophthalmol. 2015;35(Suppl 1):S22–8. https://doi.org/10.1097/WNO.0000000000000293.
10. Gupta N, Ang LC, Noel de Tilly L, et al. Human glaucoma and neural degeneration in intracranial optic nerve, lateral geniculate nucleus, and visual cortex. Br J Ophthalmol. 2006;90:674–8. https://doi.org/10.1136/bjo.2005.086769.
11. Curcio CA, Allen KA. Topography of ganglion cells in human retina. J Comp Neurol. 1990;300:5–25. https://doi.org/10.1002/cne.903000103.
12. Nickells RW. Retinal ganglion cell death in glaucoma: the how, the why, and the maybe. J Glaucoma. 1996;5:345–56.
13. Quigley HA, Nickells RW, Kerrigan LA, et al. Retinal ganglion cell death in experimental glaucoma and after axotomy occurs by apoptosis. Invest Ophthalmol Vis Sci. 1995;36:774–86.
14. Kyrylkova K, Kyryachenko S, Leid M, et al. Detection of apoptosis by TUNEL assay. Methods Mol Biol. 2012;887:41–7. https://doi.org/10.1007/978-1-61779-860-3_5.
15. Okisaka S, Murakami A, Mizukawa A, et al. Apoptosis in retinal ganglion cell decrease in human glaucomatous eyes. Jpn J Ophthalmol. 1997;41:84–8.
16. Kerrigan LA, Zack DJ, Quigley HA, et al. TUNEL-positive ganglion cells in human primary open-angle glaucoma. Arch Ophthalmol. 1997;115:1031–5.
17. Flammer J, Konieczka K, Flammer AJ. The primary vascular dysregulation syndrome: implications for eye diseases. EPMA J. 2013;4:14. https://doi.org/10.1186/1878-5085-4-14.
18. Dreyer EB, Zurakowski D, Schumer RA, et al. Elevated glutamate levels in the vitreous body of humans and monkeys with glaucoma. Arch Ophthalmol. 1996;114:299–305.
19. Brooks DE, Garcia GA, Dreyer EB, et al. Vitreous body glutamate concentration in dogs with glaucoma. Am J Vet Res. 1997;58:864–7.
20. Honkanen RA, Baruah S, Zimmerman MB, et al. Vitreous amino acid concentrations in patients with glaucoma undergoing vitrectomy. Arch Ophthalmol. 2003;121:183–8.
21. Levkovitch-Verbin H, Martin KR, Quigley HA, et al. Measurement of amino acid levels in the vitreous humor of rats after chronic intraocular pressure elevation or optic nerve transection. J Glaucoma. 2002;11:396–405.
22. Wamsley S, Gabelt BT, Dahl DB, et al. Vitreous glutamate concentration and axon loss in monkeys with experimental glaucoma. Arch Ophthalmol. 2005;123:64–70. https://doi.org/10.1001/archopht.123.1.64.
23. Salt TE, Cordeiro MF. Glutamate excitotoxicity in glaucoma: throwing the baby out with the bathwater? Eye (Lond). 2006;20:730–1. https://doi.org/10.1038/sj.eye.6701967. Author reply 731–732.
24. Izzotti A, Bagnis A, Sacca SC. The role of oxidative stress in glaucoma. Mutat Res. 2006;612:105–14. https://doi.org/10.1016/j.mrrev.2005.11.001.
25. Rieck J. The pathogenesis of glaucoma in the interplay with the immune system. Invest Ophthalmol Vis Sci. 2013;54:2393–409. https://doi.org/10.1167/iovs.12-9781.
26. Tezel G. The immune response in glaucoma: a perspective on the roles of oxidative stress. Exp Eye Res. 2011;93:178–86. https://doi.org/10.1016/j.exer.2010.07.009.
27. Bouter A, Gounou C, Berat R, et al. Annexin-A5 assembled into two-dimensional arrays promotes cell membrane repair. Nat Commun. 2011;2:270. https://doi.org/10.1038/ncomms1270.
28. Creutz CE, Hira JK, Gee VE, et al. Protection of the membrane permeability barrier by annexins. Biochemistry. 2012;51:9966–83. https://doi.org/10.1021/bi3013559.

29. Ghislat G, Aguado C, Knecht E. Annexin A5 stimulates autophagy and inhibits endocytosis. J Cell Sci. 2012;125:92–107. https://doi.org/10.1242/jcs.086728.
30. Park JH, Jang JH, Choi EJ, et al. Annexin A5 increases survival in murine sepsis model by inhibiting HMGB1-mediated pro-inflammation and coagulation. Mol Med. 2016;22:424–36. https://doi.org/10.2119/molmed.2016.00026.
31. Martin M, Leffler J, Blom AM. Annexin A2 and A5 serve as new ligands for C1q on apoptotic cells. J Biol Chem. 2012;287:33733–44. https://doi.org/10.1074/jbc.M112.341339.
32. Meers P, Mealy T. Calcium-dependent annexin V binding to phospholipids: stoichiometry, specificity, and the role of negative charge. Biochemistry. 1993;32:11711–21.
33. Andree HA, Reutelingsperger CP, Hauptmann R, et al. Binding of vascular anticoagulant alpha (VAC alpha) to planar phospholipid bilayers. J Biol Chem. 1990;265:4923–8.
34. Schutte B, Nuydens R, Geerts H, et al. Annexin V binding assay as a tool to measure apoptosis in differentiated neuronal cells. J Neurosci Methods. 1998;86:63–9.
35. Hofstra L, Dumont EA, Thimister PW, et al. In vivo detection of apoptosis in an intracardiac tumor. JAMA. 2001;285:1841–2.
36. Belhocine T, Steinmetz N, Hustinx R, et al. Increased uptake of the apoptosis-imaging agent (99m)Tc recombinant human annexin V in human tumors after one course of chemotherapy as a predictor of tumor response and patient prognosis. Clin Cancer Res. 2002;8:2766–74.
37. Kartachova M, Haas RL, Olmos RA, et al. In vivo imaging of apoptosis by 99mTc-annexin V scintigraphy: visual analysis in relation to treatment response. Radiother Oncol. 2004;72:333–9. https://doi.org/10.1016/j.radonc.2004.07.008.
38. Vermeersch H, Ham H, Rottey S, et al. Intraobserver, interobserver, and day-to-day reproducibility of quantitative 99mTc-HYNIC annexin-V imaging in head and neck carcinoma. Cancer Biother Radiopharm. 2004;19:205–10. https://doi.org/10.1089/108497804323071986.
39. Thimister PW, Hofstra L, Liem IH, et al. In vivo detection of cell death in the area at risk in acute myocardial infarction. J Nucl Med. 2003;44:391–6.
40. Hofstra L, Liem IH, Dumont EA, et al. Visualisation of cell death in vivo in patients with acute myocardial infarction. Lancet. 2000;356:209–12.
41. Narula J, Acio ER, Narula N, et al. Annexin-V imaging for noninvasive detection of cardiac allograft rejection. Nat Med. 2001;7:1347–52. https://doi.org/10.1038/nm1201-1347.
42. Van den Brande JM, Koehler TC, Zelinkova Z, et al. Prediction of antitumour necrosis factor clinical efficacy by real-time visualisation of apoptosis in patients with Crohn's disease. Gut. 2007;56:509–17. https://doi.org/10.1136/gut.2006.105379.
43. Yap TE, Donna P, Almonte MT, et al. Real-time imaging of retinal ganglion cell apoptosis. Cell. 2018;7 https://doi.org/10.3390/cells7060060.
44. Dong ZM, Wollstein G, Wang B, et al. Adaptive optics optical coherence tomography in glaucoma. Prog Retin Eye Res. 2017;57:76–88. https://doi.org/10.1016/j.preteyeres.2016.11.001.
45. Yap TE, Davis BM, Guo L, et al. Annexins in glaucoma. Int J Mol Sci. 2018;19 https://doi.org/10.3390/ijms19041218.
46. Cordeiro MF, Normando EM, Cardoso MJ, et al. Real-time imaging of single neuronal cell apoptosis in patients with glaucoma. Brain. 2017;140:1757–67. https://doi.org/10.1093/brain/awx088.
47. Webb RH, Hughes GW, Delori FC. Confocal scanning laser ophthalmoscope. Appl Opt. 1987;26:1492–9. https://doi.org/10.1364/AO.26.001492.
48. Brunelli R. Template matching techniques in computer vision: theory and practice. Chichester: Wiley; 2009.
49. Cordeiro MF, Guo L, Luong V, et al. Real-time imaging of single nerve cell apoptosis in retinal neurodegeneration. Proc Natl Acad Sci U S A. 2004;101:13352–6. https://doi.org/10.1073/pnas.0405479101.
50. Guo L, Moss SE, Alexander RA, et al. Retinal ganglion cell apoptosis in glaucoma is related to intraocular pressure and IOP-induced effects on extracellular matrix. Invest Ophthalmol Vis Sci. 2005;46:175–82. https://doi.org/10.1167/iovs.04-0832.
51. Galvao J, Davis B, Tilley M, et al. Unexpected low-dose toxicity of the universal solvent DMSO. FASEB J. 2014;28:1317–30. https://doi.org/10.1096/fj.13-235440.

52. Guo L, Salt TE, Maass A, et al. Assessment of neuroprotective effects of glutamate modulation on glaucoma-related retinal ganglion cell apoptosis in vivo. Invest Ophthalmol Vis Sci. 2006;47:626–33. https://doi.org/10.1167/iovs.05-0754.
53. Guo L, Davis B, Nizari S, et al. Direct optic nerve sheath (DONS) application of Schwann cells prolongs retinal ganglion cell survival in vivo. Cell Death Dis. 2014;5:e1460. https://doi.org/10.1038/cddis.2014.399.
54. Cordeiro MF, Guo L, Coxon KM, et al. Imaging multiple phases of neurodegeneration: a novel approach to assessing cell death in vivo. Cell Death Dis. 2010;1:e3. https://doi.org/10.1038/cddis.2009.3.
55. Guo L, Salt TE, Luong V, et al. Targeting amyloid-beta in glaucoma treatment. Proc Natl Acad Sci U S A. 2007;104:13444–9. https://doi.org/10.1073/pnas.0703707104.
56. Borrie SC, Cheung W, Guo L, et al. Diabetic retinal neurodegeneration: in vivo imaging of retinal ganglion cell apoptosis in the Ins2Akita/J mouse. Invest Ophthalmol Vis Sci. 2008;49:4924.
57. Schmitz-Valckenberg S, Guo L, Maass A, et al. Real-time in vivo imaging of retinal cell apoptosis after laser exposure. Invest Ophthalmol Vis Sci. 2008;49:2773–80. https://doi.org/10.1167/iovs.07-1335.
58. Schmitz-Valckenberg S, Guo L, Cheung W, et al. In vivo imaging of retinal cell apoptosis following acute light exposure. Ophthalmologe. 2010;107:22–9. https://doi.org/10.1007/s00347-009-1952-y.
59. Normando EM, Davis BM, De Groef L, et al. The retina as an early biomarker of neurodegeneration in a rotenone-induced model of Parkinson's disease: evidence for a neuroprotective effect of rosiglitazone in the eye and brain. Acta Neuropathol Commun. 2016;4:86. https://doi.org/10.1186/s40478-016-0346-z.
60. Koh JY, Wie MB, Gwag BJ, et al. Staurosporine-induced neuronal apoptosis. Exp Neurol. 1995;135:153–9. https://doi.org/10.1006/exnr.1995.1074.
61. Levkovitch-Verbin H, Quigley HA, Martin KR, et al. A model to study differences between primary and secondary degeneration of retinal ganglion cells in rats by partial optic nerve transection. Invest Ophthalmol Vis Sci. 2003;44:3388–93.
62. Murphy MP, LeVine H 3rd. Alzheimer's disease and the amyloid-beta peptide. J Alzheimers Dis. 2010;19:311–23. https://doi.org/10.3233/JAD-2010-1221.
63. Salt TE, Nizari S, Cordeiro MF, et al. Effect of the Abeta aggregation modulator MRZ-99030 on retinal damage in an animal model of glaucoma. Neurotox Res. 2014;26:440–6. https://doi.org/10.1007/s12640-014-9488-6.
64. Galvao J, Elvas F, Martins T, et al. Adenosine A3 receptor activation is neuroprotective against retinal neurodegeneration. Exp Eye Res. 2015;140:65–74. https://doi.org/10.1016/j.exer.2015.08.009.
65. Nizari S, Guo L, Davis BM, et al. Non-amyloidogenic effects of alpha2 adrenergic agonists: implications for brimonidine-mediated neuroprotection. Cell Death Dis. 2016;7:e2514. https://doi.org/10.1038/cddis.2016.397.
66. Davis BM, Tian K, Pahlitzsch M, et al. Topical coenzyme Q10 demonstrates mitochondrial-mediated neuroprotection in a rodent model of ocular hypertension. Mitochondrion. 2017;36:114–23. https://doi.org/10.1016/j.mito.2017.05.010.
67. Saylor M, McLoon LK, Harrison AR, et al. Experimental and clinical evidence for brimonidine as an optic nerve and retinal neuroprotective agent: an evidence-based review. Arch Ophthalmol. 2009;127:402–6. https://doi.org/10.1001/archophthalmol.2009.9.
68. Krupin T, Liebmann JM, Greenfield DS, et al. A randomized trial of brimonidine versus timolol in preserving visual function: results from the Low-Pressure Glaucoma Treatment Study. Am J Ophthalmol. 2011;151:671–81. https://doi.org/10.1016/j.ajo.2010.09.026.
69. Hynd MR, Scott HL, Dodd PR. Glutamate-mediated excitotoxicity and neurodegeneration in Alzheimer's disease. Neurochem Int. 2004;45:583–95. https://doi.org/10.1016/j.neuint.2004.03.007.
70. WoldeMussie E, Yoles E, Schwartz M, et al. Neuroprotective effect of memantine in different retinal injury models in rats. J Glaucoma. 2002;11:474–80.

71. Hare WA, WoldeMussie E, Lai RK, et al. Efficacy and safety of memantine treatment for reduction of changes associated with experimental glaucoma in monkey, I: functional measures. Invest Ophthalmol Vis Sci. 2004;45:2625–39. https://doi.org/10.1167/iovs.03-0566.
72. Hare WA, WoldeMussie E, Weinreb RN, et al. Efficacy and safety of memantine treatment for reduction of changes associated with experimental glaucoma in monkey, II: structural measures. Invest Ophthalmol Vis Sci. 2004;45:2640–51. https://doi.org/10.1167/iovs.03-0567.
73. Cunha RA. Neuroprotection by adenosine in the brain: from A(1) receptor activation to A (2A) receptor blockade. Purinergic Signal. 2005;1:111–34. https://doi.org/10.1007/s11302-005-0649-1.
74. Weinreb RN, Liebmann JM, Cioffi GA, et al. Oral memantine for the treatment of glaucoma: design and results of 2 randomized, placebo-controlled, phase 3 studies. Ophthalmology. 2018;125:1874–85. https://doi.org/10.1016/j.ophtha.2018.06.017.
75. Selkoe DJ. Toward a comprehensive theory for Alzheimer's disease. Hypothesis: Alzheimer's disease is caused by the cerebral accumulation and cytotoxicity of amyloid beta-protein. Ann N Y Acad Sci. 2000;924:17–25.
76. Bove J, Perier C. Neurotoxin-based models of Parkinson's disease. Neuroscience. 2012;211:51–76. https://doi.org/10.1016/j.neuroscience.2011.10.057.
77. McMonnies C. Reactive oxygen species, oxidative stress, glaucoma and hyperbaric oxygen therapy. J Optom. 2018;11:3–9. https://doi.org/10.1016/j.optom.2017.06.002.
78. Nucci C, Tartaglione R, Cerulli A, et al. Retinal damage caused by high intraocular pressure-induced transient ischemia is prevented by coenzyme Q10 in rat. Int Rev Neurobiol. 2007;82:397–406. https://doi.org/10.1016/S0074-7742(07)82022-8.
79. Cork LC. Neuropathology of Down syndrome and Alzheimer disease. Am J Med Genet Suppl. 1990;7:282–6.
80. Yap TE, Normando EM, Cordeiro MF. Redefining clinical outcomes and endpoints in glaucoma. Expert Rev Ophthalmol. 2018;13:113–27. https://doi.org/10.1080/17469899.2018.1465820.
81. Kass MA, Heuer DK, Higginbotham EJ, et al. The Ocular Hypertension Treatment Study: a randomized trial determines that topical ocular hypotensive medication delays or prevents the onset of primary open-angle glaucoma. Arch Ophthalmol. 2002;120:701–13. Discussion 829–730.
82. Castro DP, Kawase J, Melo LA Jr. Learning effect of standard automated perimetry in healthy individuals. Arq Bras Oftalmol. 2008;71:523–8.
83. De Moraes CG, Hood DC, Thenappan A, et al. 24-2 visual fields miss central defects shown on 10-2 tests in glaucoma suspects, ocular hypertensives, and early glaucoma. Ophthalmology. 2017;124:1449–56. https://doi.org/10.1016/j.ophtha.2017.04.021.
84. Heijl A, Buchholz P, Norrgren G, et al. Rates of visual field progression in clinical glaucoma care. Acta Ophthalmol. 2013;91:406–12. https://doi.org/10.1111/j.1755-3768.2012.02492.x.
85. Garway-Heath DF, Crabb DP, Bunce C, et al. Latanoprost for open-angle glaucoma (UKGTS): a randomised, multicentre, placebo-controlled trial. Lancet. 2015;385:1295–304. https://doi.org/10.1016/S0140-6736(14)62111-5.
86. Kuang TM, Zhang C, Zangwill LM, et al. Estimating lead time gained by optical coherence tomography in detecting Glaucoma before development of visual field defects. Ophthalmology. 2015;122:2002–9. https://doi.org/10.1016/j.ophtha.2015.06.015.
87. Yu M, Lin C, Weinreb RN, et al. Risk of visual field progression in glaucoma patients with progressive retinal nerve fiber layer thinning: a 5-year prospective study. Ophthalmology. 2016;123:1201–10. https://doi.org/10.1016/j.ophtha.2016.02.017.
88. Chan VTT, Sun Z, Tang S, et al. Spectral-domain OCT measurements in Alzheimer's disease: a systematic review and meta-analysis. Ophthalmology. 2018; https://doi.org/10.1016/j.ophtha.2018.08.009.
89. Glass CK, Saijo K, Winner B, et al. Mechanisms underlying inflammation in neurodegeneration. Cell. 2010;140:918–34. https://doi.org/10.1016/j.cell.2010.02.016.
90. Gauthier SG. Alzheimer's disease: the benefits of early treatment. Eur J Neurol. 2005;12(Suppl 3):11–6. https://doi.org/10.1111/j.1468-1331.2005.01322.x.

91. Heijl A, Leske MC, Bengtsson B, et al. Reduction of intraocular pressure and glaucoma progression: results from the Early Manifest Glaucoma Trial. Arch Ophthalmol. 2002;120:1268–79.
92. Davis BM, Guo L, Brenton J, et al. Automatic quantitative analysis of experimental primary and secondary retinal neurodegeneration: implications for optic neuropathies. Cell Death Discov. 2016;2:16031. https://doi.org/10.1038/cddiscovery.2016.31.

Retinal Oximetry in Central Nervous System Diseases

8

Anna Bryndis Einarsdottir, Olof Birna Olafsdottir, and Sveinn Hakon Hardarson

8.1 Introduction

Retinal imaging is gaining interest for diagnostics of central nervous system (CNS) diseases and to evaluate progression of CNS diseases. The retina is part of the central nervous system and is the only part of the CNS that can be visualized non-invasively with visible light. It is easy to image structural and metabolic changes in the retina, which reflect abnormalities in the CNS.

The fundus of the eye provides the only opportunity for visible light imaging of central nervous system tissue and circulation. The notion of using the eye to learn about the brain dates back to ancient Rome and the proverb "the eyes are the mirror of the soul" exists in many languages. It is however only recently that modern imaging technologies have realized this potential. Optical coherence tomography images the structure of the retina and retinal oximetry documents the oxygen metabolism and both reflect changes in the wider CNS.

Optical coherence tomography of the retina has demonstrated changes in the retinal structure in CNS diseases. Thinning of the retinal nerve fiber layer and other structural anomalies in the retina have been found in Alzheimer's disease [1, 2], mild cognitive impairment [3, 4], multiple sclerosis (MS) [5, 6] and Parkinson's disease [7] and suggest that OCT imaging may help to diagnose and evaluate progression of CNS disease.

A. B. Einarsdottir (✉)
Department of Neurology, Odense University Hospital, Odense, Denmark
e-mail: abe1@hi.is

O. B. Olafsdottir
Faculty of Medicine, University of Iceland, Reykjavik, Iceland
e-mail: olofbo@hi.is

S. H. Hardarson
Institute of Physiology, Faculty of Medicine, University of Iceland, Reykjavik, Iceland
e-mail: sveinnha@hi.is

A. Grzybowski, P. Barboni (eds.), *OCT and Imaging in Central Nervous System Diseases*, https://doi.org/10.1007/978-3-030-26269-3_8

The fundus of the eye provides direct view of retinal blood vessels, which are part of CNS vasculature. Imaging them provides information on oxygen saturation in CNS vessels. Metabolic imaging with retinal oximetry involves noninvasive spectrophotometric imaging of retinal blood vessels. This fairly new clinical technology has led to discovery of new biomarkers in several retinal diseases, such as diabetic retinopathy [8, 9], glaucoma [10–12], central retinal vein occlusion [13], age-related macular degeneration [14], retinitis pigmentosa [15, 16], and CNS diseases, such as Alzheimer's disease [17], mild cognitive impairment [18] and MS [19, 20].

8.2 Retinal Oximetry: The Technology

Retinal oximetry is an imaging technique that allows the visualization and measurement of oxygen saturation of hemoglobin in retinal arterioles and venules. The most common form of retinal oximetry uses conventional fundus cameras to image retinal vessels. The only inconvenience for the patient is pupil dilation and the light flash, which can be less intense than in conventional fundus photography [21, 22].

The technology has been described in detail [23]. Retinal oximetry typically involves specialized optics and camera(s) that are coupled to a fundus camera to capture images at two different wavelengths simultaneously. Optical density (light absorbance) of retinal vessels is calculated at both wavelengths and the ratio of the optical densities at these wavelengths is calculated (optical density ratio, ODR). If one of the wavelengths is relatively insensitive to oxygen and the other is sensitive, there is a nearly linear relationship between hemoglobin oxygen saturation and the optical density ratio. Analysis software displays the results as a pseudocolor fundus image as shown in Fig. 8.1. This approach to oximetry has been commercialized by two companies, Oxymap in Reykjavik, Iceland, and Imedos in Jena, Germany.

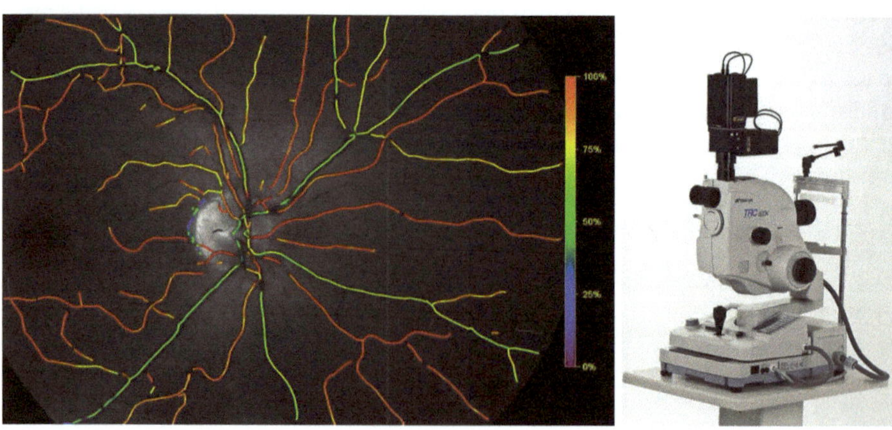

Fig. 8.1 Left: Retinal oximetry image of a normal fundus. Color indicates oxygen saturation in retinal vessels (pseudocolor scale to the right of the image; red is fully saturated, blue and purple is low oxygen saturation). Right: Dual wavelength non-invasive retinal oximeter Oxymap T1 (Oxymap ehf., Reykjavik, Iceland) coupled to a fundus camera (Topcon TRC-50DX) [24]

Retinal oximetry is as easy and safe to perform as regular fundus photography and provides robust and reproducible data on retinal oxygen metabolism [25].

8.3 Retinal Oximetry Is Affected in Alzheimer's Disease

Einarsdottir et al. were first to report oximetry abnormalities in retinas of individuals with moderate stage Alzheimer's disease compared with a healthy cohort [17]. Alzheimer's patients showed increased oxygen saturation in retinal arterioles and venules compared to healthy individuals (Fig. 8.2) [17]. While the oximetry findings in Alzheimer's disease are similar to diabetic retinopathy [8, 9] and neovascular age-related macular degeneration [14], the biological basis behind these findings has not been fully elucidated and need not be the same for all diseases.

Thal et al. found that 82–98% of individuals with Alzheimer's disease have cerebral amyloid angiopathy [26]. This leads to thickening of vessel walls and to decreased diffusion of glucose and oxygen from the vessels, which could increase venular oxygen saturation. This could also explain the increase in arteriolar oxygen saturation, as arterioles lose oxygen by diffusion and this loss would decrease with thicker walls. Similar results have been demonstrated in diabetic retinopathy (increased arteriolar and venular oxygen saturation), and it has been suggested that thickening of the vessel wall could partly explain those results [27]. Another possible explanation for increased arteriolar oxygen saturation could be an effect of atrophy and a thinner retinal nerve fiber layer and a resultant decreased oxygen consumption and uptake by tissue adjacent to an arteriole. Decreased difference in oxygen concentration between the arterioles (arteries) and adjacent venules (veins) could also decrease counter current diffusion of oxygen directly between these arterioles and venules. This would result in increased arterial levels.

Retinal oximetry studies on Alzheimer's patients indicate that retinal oxygen metabolism is affected in patients with Alzheimer's disease. Retinal oximetry may be a useful objective biomarker for patients with Alzheimer's disease. Further and larger studies are needed to confirm these findings.

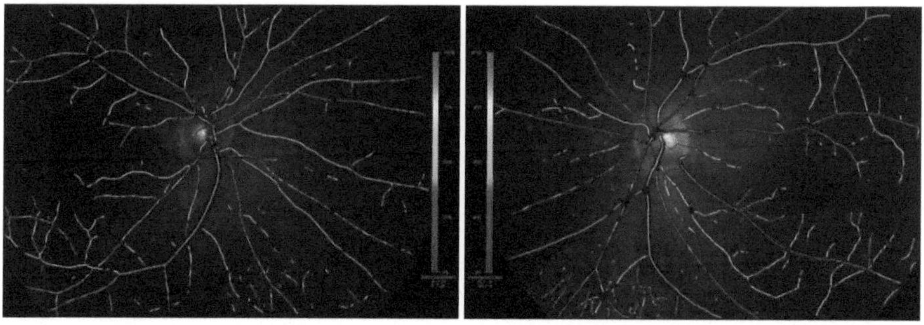

Fig. 8.2 Oximetry fundus images from healthy subject (left image) and patient with Alzheimer's disease (right image). Color indicates oxygen saturation in retinal vessels (pseudocolor scale to the right of the image; red is fully saturated, blue and purple is low oxygen saturation) [17]

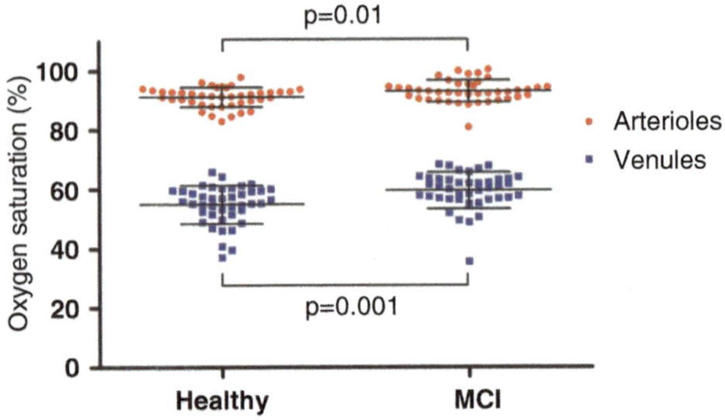

Fig. 8.3 Oxygen saturation in retinal arterioles and venules in patients with mild cognitive impairment (MCI) and healthy controls [18]

8.4 Retinal Oxygen Metabolism Changes in Mild Cognitive Impairment

The findings from retinal oximetry in Alzheimer's disease have recently been confirmed and extended to individuals with mild cognitive impairment. Olafsdottir et al. showed increased retinal arteriolar and venular oxygen saturation and decreased arteriovenous difference in individuals with mild cognitive impairment compared to healthy subjects (Fig. 8.3) [18]. These changes could reflect decreased oxygen extraction by retinal tissue in individuals with mild cognitive impairment, compared with healthy subjects. Fluorodeoxyglucose positron emission tomography studies have showed that metabolism could be decreased in the brain of individuals with mild cognitive impairment [28, 29]. The findings by Olafsdottir et al. could indicate less metabolic activity in the retinal tissue due to atrophy and thinner retinal nerve fiber layer and less metabolically active retina in mild cognitive impairment [18].

Retinal oxygen metabolism is affected in patients with Alzheimer's disease and mild cognitive impairment. The value of these biomarkers in clinical practice remains to be elucidated as well as what insights this provides into the pathophysiology of these disorders.

8.5 Retinal Oxygen Metabolism Is Affected in Multiple Sclerosis and Optic Neuritis

Recent studies have suggested that retinal oxygen metabolism is abnormal in individuals with MS compared to a healthy cohort [19, 20]. Lucero et al. reported oximetry abnormalities in retinas of individuals with MS compared to healthy subjects [20]. Einarsdottir et al. showed increased venular oxygen saturation and decreased arteriovenous difference in patients with MS compared to healthy individuals [19]. These results may indicate reduced oxygen uptake, which may be due to less oxygen demand following retinal atrophy.

Optic neuritis is a common presenting symptom of MS [30]. In 1989 Sebag et al. studied retinal oxygen saturation in individuals with optic neuritis with an early prototype retinal oximeter [31]. They compared eyes with optic neuritis with the healthy fellow eye and found optic neuritis eyes to have increased arteriovenous difference and reduced blood flow. The net result of these changes was decreased oxygen delivery. On the other hand, Einarsdottir et al., in a small study, did not find difference in retinal vessel oxygen saturation between MS patients eyes with optic neuritis compared to fellow eyes without optic neuritis [19]. A recent study by Svrčinová et al. assessed acute optic neuritis in individuals with MS [32]. They found increased arteriovenous difference in eyes affected by optic neuritis in MS compared to patients unaffected eye. This is in accordance with report by Sebag et al. [31]. This could suggest that in the early stage of optic neuritis, arteriovenous difference could reflect inflammatory and metabolic changes in the optic neuritis eye. They suggest that retinal oximetry could be used as a diagnostic tool in MS patients with suspicion of optic neuritis [32].

It remains to be seen whether the retinal oximetry findings in Alzheimer's disease, mild cognitive impairment and multiple sclerosis are a consequence of tissue atrophy and reduced oxygen consumption and thereby a simple consequence of the disease processes; or whether they reflect metabolic changes earlier in the pathophysiological process.

8.6 Correlation Between Retinal and Transcranial Oximetry

Cerebral ischemia and hypoxia may exist in the absence of systemic hypoxia and there is a need for selective assessment of central nervous system oxygenation [33, 34]. Non-invasive techniques to measure cerebral vessel saturation exist, but they have some drawbacks. Transcranial near-infrared spectroscopy (NIRS) can be used to measure cerebral vessel saturation, but the oxygen saturation is affected by superficial peripheral circulation. Also, oxygen saturation measured by NIRS is a combination of arterial, capillary and venous blood.

The retina offers an opportunity to evaluate central nervous system vasculature and oxygen metabolism. Embryologically, the retina is an extension of the diencephalon and the retina and cerebral circulation share a common anatomical and physiological background. Retinal oximetry is able to measure arterial and venous oxygen saturation separately without being affected by superficial peripheral circulation. Van Keer et al. reported a positive correlation between transcranial oxygen blood vessel saturation and retinal arteriolar and venular saturation [35]. Retinal oximetry may be useful to estimate cerebral oxygen saturation in clinical settings such as intensive care and with major surgery and injuries.

8.7 Conclusion

Retinal oximetry and metabolic imaging of the retina show abnormalities in central nervous system diseases, such as Alzheimer's disease, mild cognitive impairment and multiple sclerosis.

The pathophysiological mechanism behind these changes is not fully elucidated. The oximetry findings may be a simple consequence of tissue atrophy and reduced oxygen consumption. Alternatively, they may be involved in the pathophysiological process and reflect features such as vessel wall thickening and changes in energy metabolism.

There is a correlation between oxygen metabolism in the brain and retina. This may be useful to monitor brain oxygenation in intensive care, surgery and major injuries.

Retinal oximetry may offer insights into the pathophysiology of central nervous system diseases and also has the potential to be provide biomarkers to diagnose central nervous system diseases and evaluate their progression. More extensive studies are indicated to realize this potential.

References

1. Bambo MP, Garcia-Martin E, Pinilla J, Herrero R, Statue M, Otin S, et al. Detection of retinal nerve fiber layer degeneration in patients with Alzheimer's disease using optical coherence tomography: searching new biomarkers. Acta Ophthalmol. 2014;92(7):e581–2.
2. Marziani E, Pomati S, Ramolfo P, Cigada M, Giani A, Mariani C, et al. Evaluation of retinal nerve fiber layer and ganglion cell layer thickness in Alzheimer's disease using spectral-domain optical coherence tomography. Invest Ophthalmol Vis Sci. 2013;54(9):5953–8.
3. Lad EM, Mukherjee D, Stinnett SS, Cousins SW, Potter GG, Burke JR, et al. Evaluation of inner retinal layers as biomarkers in mild cognitive impairment to moderate Alzheimer's disease. PLoS One. 2018;13(2):e0192646.
4. Paquet C, Boissonnot M, Roger F, Dighiero P, Gil R, Hugon J. Abnormal retinal thickness in patients with mild cognitive impairment and Alzheimer's disease. Neurosci Lett. 2007;420(2):97–9.
5. Garcia-Martin E, Pablo LE, Herrero R, Ara JR, Martin J, Larrosa JM, et al. Neural networks to identify multiple sclerosis with optical coherence tomography. Acta Ophthalmol. 2013;91(8):e628–34.
6. Park KA, Kim J, Oh SY. Analysis of spectral domain optical coherence tomography measurements in optic neuritis: differences in neuromyelitis optica, multiple sclerosis, isolated optic neuritis and normal healthy controls. Acta Ophthalmol. 2014;92(1):e57–65.
7. Lee JY, Ahn J, Kim TW, Jeon BS. Optical coherence tomography in Parkinson's disease: is the retina a biomarker? J Park Dis. 2014;4(2):197–204.
8. Hammer M, Vilser W, Riemer T, Mandecka A, Schweitzer D, Kühn U, et al. Diabetic patients with retinopathy show increased retinal venous oxygen saturation. Graefes Arch Clin Exp Ophthalmol. 2009;247(8):1025–30.
9. Hardarson SH, Stefánsson E. Retinal oxygen saturation is altered in diabetic retinopathy. Br J Ophthalmol. 2012;96(4):560–3.
10. Olafsdottir OB, Hardarson SH, Gottfredsdottir MS, Harris A, Stefánsson E. Retinal oximetry in primary open-angle glaucoma. Invest Ophthalmol Vis Sci. 2011;52(9):6409–13.
11. Olafsdottir OB, Vandewalle E, Abegão Pinto L, Geirsdottir A, De Clerck E, Stalmans P, et al. Retinal oxygen metabolism in healthy subjects and glaucoma patients. Br J Ophthalmol. 2014;98(3):329–33.
12. Vandewalle E, Abegão Pinto L, Olafsdottir OB, De Clerck E, Stalmans P, Van Calster J, et al. Oximetry in glaucoma: correlation of metabolic change with structural and functional damage. Acta Ophthalmol. 2014;92(2):105–10.
13. Hardarson SH, Stefánsson E. Oxygen saturation in central retinal vein occlusion. Am J Ophthalmol. 2010;150(6):871–5.
14. Geirsdottir A, Hardarson SH, Olafsdottir OB, Stefánsson E. Retinal oxygen metabolism in exudative age-related macular degeneration. Acta Ophthalmol. 2014;92(1):27–33.

15. Eysteinsson T, Hardarson SH, Bragason D, Stefánsson E. Retinal vessel oxygen saturation and vessel diameter in retinitis pigmentosa. Acta Ophthalmol. 2014;92(5):449–53.
16. Türksever C, Valmaggia C, Orgül S, Schorderet DF, Flammer J, Todorova MG. Retinal vessel oxygen saturation and its correlation with structural changes in retinitis pigmentosa. Acta Ophthalmol. 2014;92(5):454–60.
17. Einarsdottir AB, Hardarson SH, Kristjansdottir JV, Bragason DT, Snaedal J, Stefánsson E. Retinal oximetry imaging in Alzheimer's disease. J Alzheimers Dis. 2016;49(1):79–83.
18. Olafsdottir OB, Saevarsdottir HS, Hardarson SH, Hannesdottir KH, Traustadottir VD, Karlsson RA, et al. Oxygen metabolism in patients with mild cognitive impairment. Alzheimers Dement (Amst). 2018;10:340–5.
19. Einarsdottir AB, Olafsdottir OB, Hjaltason H, Hardarson SH. Retinal oximetry is affected in multiple sclerosis. Acta Ophthalmol. 2018;96(5):528–30.
20. Lucero M, Conger A, Conger D, Sobhanian M, Stokes V, Frohman T, et al. Retinal oximetry-derived biomarkers of metabolic dysfunction in MS. Neurology. 2015;84(14 Supplement):P5.307.
21. Geirsdottir A, Palsson O, Hardarson SH, Olafsdottir OB, Kristjansdottir JV, Stefánsson E. Retinal vessel oxygen saturation in healthy individuals. Invest Ophthalmol Vis Sci. 2012;53(9):5433–42.
22. Hardarson SH, Harris A, Karlsson RA, Halldorsson GH, Kagemann L, Rechtman E, et al. Automatic retinal oximetry. Invest Ophthalmol Vis Sci. 2006;47(11):5011–6.
23. Beach J. Pathway to retinal oximetry. Transl Vis Sci Technol. 2014;3(5):2.
24. Stefánsson E, Olafsdottir OB, Einarsdottir AB, Eliasdottir TS, Eysteinsson T, Vehmeijer W, et al. Retinal oximetry discovers novel biomarkers in retinal and brain diseases. Invest Ophthalmol Vis Sci. 2017;58(6):BIO227–33.
25. Palsson O, Geirsdottir A, Hardarson SH, Olafsdottir OB, Kristjansdottir JV, Stefánsson E. Retinal oximetry images must be standardized: a methodological analysis. Invest Ophthalmol Vis Sci. 2012;53(4):1729–33.
26. Thal DR, Griffin WS, de Vos RA, Ghebremedhin E. Cerebral amyloid angiopathy and its relationship to Alzheimer's disease. Acta Neuropathol. 2008;115(6):599–609.
27. Hardarson SH, Olafsdottir OB, Karlsson RA, Beach JM, Eysteinsson T, Benediktsson JA, et al. Retinal vessel oxygen saturation in patients with diabetic retinopathy. Invest Ophthalmol Vis Sci. 2009;50:1328.
28. Mosconi L, Tsui WH, Herholz K, Pupi A, Drzezga A, Lucignani G, et al. Multicenter standardized 18F-FDG PET diagnosis of mild cognitive impairment, Alzheimer's disease, and other dementias. J Nucl Med. 2008;49(3):390–8.
29. Perani D, Della Rosa PA, Cerami C, Gallivanone F, Fallanca F, Vanoli EG, et al. Validation of an optimized SPM procedure for FDG-PET in dementia diagnosis in a clinical setting. Neuroimage Clin. 2014;6:445–54.
30. Sørensen TL, Frederiksen JL, Brønnum-Hansen H, Petersen HC. Optic neuritis as onset manifestation of multiple sclerosis: a nationwide, long-term survey. Neurology. 1999;53(3):473–8.
31. Sebag J, Delori FC, Feke GT, Weiter JJ. Effects of optic atrophy on retinal blood flow and oxygen saturation in humans. Arch Ophthalmol. 1989;107(2):222–6.
32. Svrčinová T, Mareš J, Chrapek O, Šínová I, Rybariková M, Otruba P, et al. Changes in oxygen saturation and the retinal nerve fibre layer in patients with optic neuritis – a pilot study. Acta Ophthalmol. 2018;96(3):e309–14.
33. Hadolt I, Litscher G. Noninvasive assessment of cerebral oxygenation during high altitude trekking in the Nepal Himalayas. Neurol Res. 2003;25:183–8.
34. Yeh T Jr, Gouldman J, Auden SM, Seremet V, Edmonds HL Jr, Cerrito PB, et al. Mixed venous oxygen saturation does not adequately predict cerebral perfusion during pediatric cardiopulmonary bypass. J Thorac Cardiovasc Surg. 2001;122(1):192–3.
35. Van Keer K, Van Keer J, Barbosa Bred J, Nassiri V, De Deyne C, Genbrugge C, et al. Noninvasive assessment of cerebral oxygenation: a comparison of retinal and transcranial oximetry. PLoS One. 2018;13(1):e0190612.

Optical Coherence Tomography and Optic Nerve Edema

9

Laurel N. Vuong and Thomas R. Hedges III

9.1 Papilledema

Information given to us by optical coherence tomography (OCT) has advanced our understanding of the pathophysiology of papilledema and pseudopapilledema. In 1860, von Graefe described engorgement and distention of the retinal veins as an early manifestation of papilledema, suggesting that increased intracranial pressure led to increased intracranial venous pressure and eventual venous stasis [1]. Subsequent investigators described dilatation of the optic nerve sheath in cases of papilledema, suggesting that increased pressure within the sheath could obstruct the central retinal vein [2, 3].

In 1963, in a study of rhesus monkeys, Hedges showed that, with acute and subacute increases in intracranial pressure, there was always an associated rise in ophthalmic vein pressure. He proposed that impairment of orbital venous outflow at the level of the cavernous sinus, arterial pressure elevation, and a local hemodynamic effects within the orbit all contribute to the elevation if orbital venous pressure [4]. In 1977, in an experimental model of rhesus monkeys, Tso and Hayreh demonstrated that, unlike swelling in the central nervous system which is characterized by fluid accumulation in glial cells and extracellular space, the primary pathologic change in papilledema is severe swelling of axons with disruption of mitochondria and neurotubules [5]. The Tso and Hayreh study also demonstrated that the edematous axons displaced the peripapillary retinal laterally, with extension of tracer into the subretinal space surrounding the optic nerve head. This idea of a direct communication between the swollen optic disc and the submacular space was first put forth by Samuel's histopathologic study in 1938, suggesting that the intermediary tissue of Kuhnt can be disrupted from optic nerve swelling with subsequent escape of peripapillary fluid [6]. Visual acuity loss, when it is seen in papilledema, is typically in conjunction with these macular changes [7].

L. N. Vuong (✉) · T. R. Hedges III
Tufts University School of Medicine, New England Eye Center, Neuro-Ophthalmology Service, Boston, MA, USA

A. Grzybowski, P. Barboni (eds.), *OCT and Imaging in Central Nervous System Diseases*, https://doi.org/10.1007/978-3-030-26269-3_9

Visual acuity loss is infrequent in papilledema. More commonly, chronic papilledema leads to degeneration of optic nerve fibers with resultant peripheral visual field loss [7]. In 1980, Morris and Sanders described visual acuity loss from papilledema due to macular changes, including retinal hemorrhages, macular exudates and choroidal folds. They suggested that cerebrospinal fluid pressure in the optic nerve sheath produces hemodynamic and mechanical effects causing compensatory dilatation of the retinal papillary and peripapillary plexus and distention of the optic nerve sheath, indenting the posterior globe causing choroidal and pigment epithelial wrinkling in the macula [8].

Shortly after, Corbett et al. showed that peripapillary fluid in the context of papilledema could lead to enlargement of the blind spot, hyperopia, and refractive scotoma [9]. In some patients with papilledema, macular retinal pigment epithelial changes, as seen in cases of chronic macular edema, have also been observed [10]. Even choroidal neovascular membranes have been described in patients with papilledema [11–19].

In 2001, Hoye et al. evaluated 55 patients with papilledema from increased intracranial pressure using time-domain OCT to measure the retinal nerve fiber layer (RNFL) thickness. Nineteen of the patients also had OCT of the macula during times of acute, subacute, or recurrent papilledema. OCT showed subretinal fluid in association with decreased visual acuity in a subset of patients. In some cases, this fluid was localized to the subfoveal region, and in others the fluid appeared to be continuous from the optic disc to the subfoveal region, suggesting fluid leakage from the optic nerve head. In these cases, fluorescein angiography, however, failed to demonstrate leakage from the retinal or choroidal vasculature. In cases in which the visual acuity was not substantially affected, there was thickening of the maculopapillary retina on OCT, suggesting intraretinal edema, without clear separation of the retina and underlying choroid. The authors further noted improvement in visual acuity after resolution of subretinal fluid [7].

A common clinical problem is the inability to clinically differentiate mild papilledema from pseudopapilledema. Although following these patients with repeated clinical examinations will eventually yield an answer, such action is subjective and could delay diagnosis.

In a study of patients under 20 years of age, time-domain OCT measurements of peripapillary RNFL thickness was found to be a reliable tool in assisting in the differentiation between frank papilledema and pseudopapilledema. The mean RNFL thickness in eyes with papilledema was 218% (340 μm versus 156 μm) thicker than the eyes with pseudopapilledema [20]. However, patients with moderate to severe papilledema can be readily distinguished from pseudopapilledema on clinical examination. Differentiating cases of *mild* papilledema from congenital crowding without optic disc drusen, however, is much more challenging. In 2005, Karam and Hedges showed that mean RNFL thicknesses, measured with a time-domain OCT, were significantly increased in patients with congenital crowding and mild papilledema in comparison to normal control patients. Although the patients with mild papilledema had higher RNFL values than those with congenital crowding, the difference was not statistically significant, and it was concluded that distinction between these similar appearing entities could not be made by OCT RNFL analysis alone. However, this finding suggests pseudopapilledema and papilledema share a similar pathogenesis, in which axonal swelling is the result of delayed axoplasmic transport [21].

Fard et al. studied 42 eyes with mild papilledema, 37 eyes with pseudopapilledema from congenitally crowded discs, and 34 normal eyes with spectral-domain OCT (SD-OCT). Patients with optic disc drusen, moderate to severe papilledema, atrophic papilledema, and previous retinal disease were excluded. As previously found, eyes with both papilledema and pseudopapilledema had statistically significant increased RNFL thickness in comparison to normal subjects. In addition, the authors measured the peripapillary total retinal volume, which they defined as a volumetric region between the inner limiting membrane and the outer aspect of the retinal pigment epithelial complex in a defined space circumferential to the optic disc. Two peripapillary total retinal volumes were calculated as volumes (inner versus outer), from ring-shape areas concentric to the optic nerve. They found that the difference between the average outer peripapillary total retinal volume in the papilledema and pseudopapilledema groups was statistically significant. However, the difference between the outer ring peripapillary total retinal volume in pseudopapilledema and normal eyes was not. They concluded that outer peripapillary total retinal ring volumes might be useful in helping to differentiate between papilledema and pseudopapilledema [22].

Kupersmith, Sibony, and et al. have used OCT in a different manner to try to distinguish papilledema from other types of optic disc edema. In 2011, the authors published two articles studying the biomechanical changes of the optic nerve head in patients with papilledema secondary to elevated intracranial pressure, optic neuritis and non-arteritic anterior ischemic optic neuropathy (NAION). Specifically, the authors measured the angle of the peripapillary retinal pigment epithelium and Bruch's membrane (pRPE/BM) at the temporal and nasal borders of the neural canal opening. The angle was measured as positive with inward (toward the vitreous) angulation and as negative with outward angulation (away the vitreous) amongst the patients in the three categories. Only OCTs from patients with papilledema showed a positive angulation. Since, the same angulation was not seen in NAION or optic neuritis, the angulation was concluded to be secondary to elevated intracranial pressure [23, 24]. A follow-up study by Sibony et al. [25] and data from the idiopathic intracranial hypertension treatment trial [26], showed that the pRPE/BM positive angulation in patients with papilledema became more negative as the intracranial pressure decreased through any means, thus confirming their previous conclusion. Interestingly, Sibony et al. also found the same positive angulation in patients with presumed optic nerve sheath meningioma. While the authors were uncertain of the mechanism, they postulated it might involve a change in the compliance of the nerve or localized sequestration of cerebrospinal fluid in the distal optic nerve sheath or a combination of both [27].

OCT has also been valuable in demonstrating the natural history of optic disc edema from a variety of causes by measuring the RNFL thickness. OCT can objectively quantify the amount of RNFL swelling, and thus axonal swelling, which is the main pathological event in optic nerve edema; conversely, confocal scanning laser ophthalmoscope cannot due to disruption of mitochondria and neurotubules in the swelling axons [5, 28]. OCT can thus be an objective tool in following the clinical course of optic disc edema. After the period of acute edema, during which the RNFL is diffusely thickened, OCT can be used to monitor resolution of axonal swelling and thinning of the RNFL. Long term, RNFL thinning on OCT can be used to monitor for evolution towards optic atrophy [28].

Monteiro and Afonso analyzed SD-OCT findings in patients with pseudotumor cerebri with clinically resolved papilledema and stable visual fields for at least 6 months. They found that macular and RNFL thickness measurements were significantly reduced when compared with normal eyes, and that the degree of RNFL and retinal axonal loss correlated with visual field loss. This study highlights that OCT can be used as an objective tool in guiding management and may estimate axonal loss following chronic papilledema [29].

The retinal nerve fiber layer is composed of the unmyelinated axons that originate from ganglion cell bodies in the macula [30]. Therefore, degeneration of the RNFL may lead to decreased average macular thickness reductions, at least in part secondary to ganglion cell death from retrograde axonal degeneration [31].

Papchenko et al. demonstrated a robust association between visual field sensitivity using automated perimetry and structural changes in OCT macular thickness in patients with NAION, suggesting macular thickness could be a surrogate for determining the extent of neuronal damage in non-glaucomatous optic neuropathy. Further, there was a topographical correlation between regions of macular thinning with corresponding visual field loss [32].

Average macular thickness measurements are the summation of multiple layers of the macula, including diverse cell types with diverse functions. However, recent advancements in segmentation algorithms have made it possible to measure some discrete retinal layers. Quantification of the retinal ganglion cell layer in the macula, therefore, may provide a more specific assessment of a discrete retinal neuronal population. Analysis of the ganglion cell layer complex (GCC), which is a combination of the ganglion cell and inner plexiform layers, in the macula has become an important tool in assessing various optic neuropathies [33–35].

Marzoli et al. showed that measurements of GCC thickness correlated better with decreases in visual field mean deviation than RNFL measurements in papilledema. They concluded that mean GCC thickness measurements give a more reliable estimate and an objective estimate of early retrograde optic nerve damage even in cases without papilledema or visual loss [36]. The NORDIC trial, which included patients with idiopathic intracranial hypertension (IIH) with mild visual fields loss, showed a correlation between the GCC measurements below the control fifth percentile and higher mean deviations on visual fields. Correlations were not seen with mean deviations and increased RNFL thickness [37]. Chen et al. reviewed the OCTs of 31 IIH patients in a retrospective study to determine the prognosis of visual acuity loss at initial presentation. Using a custom programmed analysis software, they found GCC thickness was a reliable objective measurement in predicting visual outcome [38]. Athappilly et al. [39] studied IIH patients with significant papilledema and vision loss (RNFL thicknesses greater than 200 μm and an average mean deviation on initial visual fields of −9.0). GCC analysis generated from commercially available software showed evidence of optic nerve injury as early as the first follow-up visit. Despite the presence of papilledema, GCC, in contrast to RNFL, was found to be a more reliable indicator of optic nerve injury and predictor of symptomatic vision loss. It was suggested that close follow-up and, if necessary, more aggressive management when GCC thinning is present could halt, or even reverse visual field loss.

The authors found that in cases where the RNFL thickness was greater than 200 μm, GCC analysis was not always reliable, presumably because of axon swelling as well as subretinal and intraretinal fluid obscuring the GCC (Fig. 9.1).

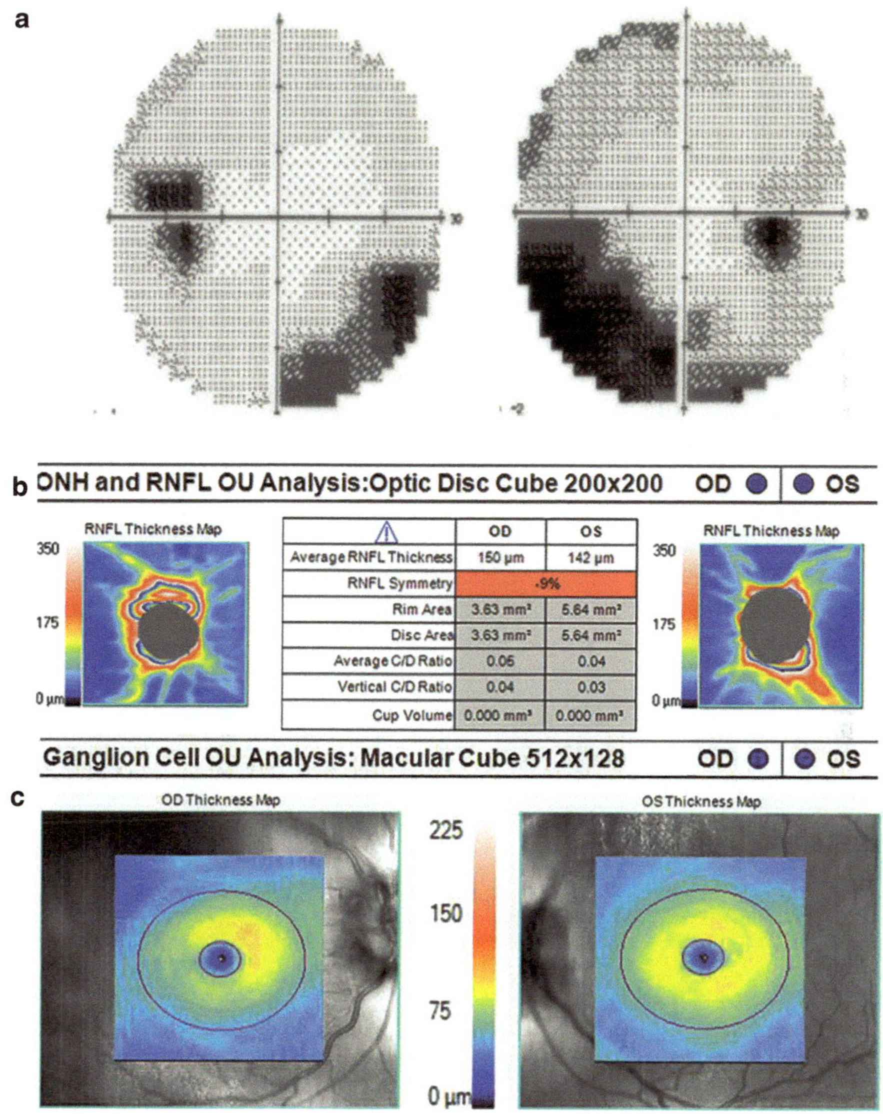

Fig. 9.1 A 33-year-old man with idiopathic intracranial hypertension treated with daily acetazolamide and optic nerve sheath fenestration in both eyes 5 years prior presented with blurred vision in both eyes and headache. There was moderate papilledema on fundoscopy and visual field examination revealed inferior arcuate scotomata in the right and left eyes (**a**). OCT demonstrated diffuse thickening on the RNFL bilaterally (**b**). Ganglion cell layer complex (GCC) analysis revealed segmental thinning, despite the papilledema (**c**). The opening pressure was elevated on lumbar puncture, and he underwent left transverse sinus stenting. Post stenting, his visual field examination remained largely unchanged in the right and left eyes (**d**). Although the optic disc swelling significantly improved (**e**), segmental GCC loss remained apparent in (**f**)

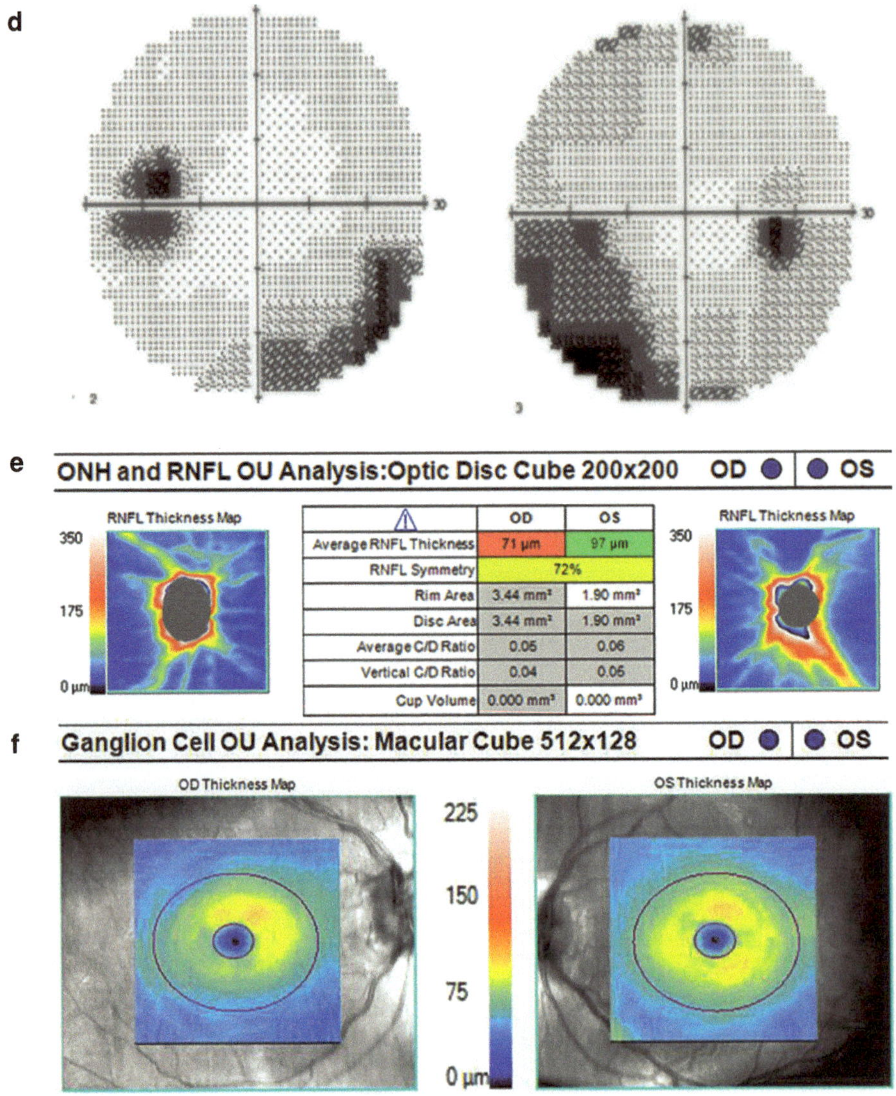

Fig. 9.1 (continued)

9.2 Optic Disc Edema Secondary to Ischemia

Non-arteritic anterior ischemic optic neuropathy (NAION) is characterized by abrupt visual loss with associated optic disc edema [40]. It is believed to be secondary to disrupted blood flow in a disc with retinal nerve fiber crowding and minimal to no physiologic cup. Although typically occurring unilaterally, optic disc edema secondary to NAION can be confused with papilledema resulting from increased intracranial pressure. Both conditions have been associated with axonal swelling and axoplasmic flow stasis in the optic nerve head and can appear similar on ophthalmoscopy with disc swelling, obscured disc margins, and peripapillary hemorrhages [41].

NAION occurs acutely, and is followed by a period of axonal swelling and subsequent thinning. After atrophy of the retinal ganglion cells has occurred, the optic neuropathy remains relatively stable [28].

OCT can detect RNFL edema in NAION. In the acute phase, the RNFL of the involved eye is significantly thicker than the fellow eye, and can be nearly doubled [42–44]. The mean RNFL from superior, inferior, temporal, and nasal quadrants have been shown to all be significantly higher than the corresponding normal values [6]. This corresponds to histopathologic studies [45–48].

Over time, the optic disc edema decreases, and the RNFL undergoes thinning, corresponding to progressive optic atrophy and pallor. OCT can follow this evolution of initial thickening and progressive thinning of the RNFL as a proxy for estimating optic disc damage. By 2 months after the NAION event, the RNFL thickness is similar to the fellow eye, marking resolution of optic disc edema. By 3–4 months, RNFL thickness is decreased nearly 40% in comparison to the fellow eye. By 12 months, the retinal nerve fiber loss is typically stabilized, with only a 6% further reduction in RNFL thickness [42, 43]. Resolution of optic disc edema from the onset of visual acuity loss may be longer in patients with diabetes and maybe shorter in patients with worse initial visual field and visual acuity loss. Resolution of edema may be quicker in patients with more severe vision loss because the greater destruction of axons results in fewer axons to swell and cause edema [44].

Bellusci et al. used OCT to detect different patterns of RNFL damage in 16 eyes with NAION, classified by visual field (VF) loss. They found that eyes with NAION and VF loss limited to the inferior hemifield had RNFL atrophy limited to the superior half of the optic nerve head. Patients with diffuse VF loss had diffuse RNFL atrophy involving all quadrants around the disc. Patients with central or centrocecal scotomas had RNFL atrophy limited to the superior and temporal sectors [44]. Alasil et al. found a similar correlation between the peripapillary nerve fiber layer thinning on OCT and the severity and location of visual field defects. They also showed that the division between affected and nonaffected hemispheres is more complicated than the altitudinal defects seen on visual field testing, illustrated by the greatest relative loss of RNFL to be in the superior quadrant and superotemporal octant, correlating with visual field loss greatest inferonasally [49].

OCT demonstrates that some patients with optic disc edema secondary to NAION develop subretinal fluid, similar to that which occurs in papilledema [7, 50]. Hedges et al. found 8 out of 76 patients with NAION had subfoveal fluid when examined within 4 weeks of developing acute vision loss. Additional patients had peripapillary subretinal fluid and peripapillary subretinal fluid extending toward, but not involving, the fovea. OCT findings in the patients with subfoveal fluid included peripapillary subretinal hyporeflectivity adjacent to the elevated optic nerve head with retinal nerve fiber thickening and hyporeflectivity under the fovea. Decreased visual acuity corresponded to degree of macular thickening. Similar to the subretinal fluid reported in some patients with papilledema, in half of the NAION patients with subretinal fluid, the fluid appeared to extend from the optic disc to the fovea.

The other half of the patients had subretinal fluid in the peripapillary region and a separate area of subfoveal fluid. Reduction in OCT RNFL thickness and resolution of subretinal fluid corresponded to improvement in visual acuity [50].

Optic disc edema as demonstrated by increased RNFL thickness on OCT has limited prognostic value in patients with NAION; it is not correlated with final RNFL thickness, visual acuity, or visual field mean deviation. In non-glaucomatous optic neuropathies, like NAION, greater damage occurs in the papillomacular fibers, with resultant loss of central acuity. Therefore, although the site of damage occurs at the optic nerve head, axons have cell bodies in the macula and contribute to macular thickness [51]. Papchenko et al. studied the macular thickness in addition to the retinal nerve fiber layer thickness in patients with NAION, and found a stronger correlation between macular thickness and Humphrey visual field sensitivity than RNFL parameters, suggesting that macular thickness may be a surrogate marker for determining the extent of nerve injury in NAION. They found that in patients with inferior visual field defects, the total macula thickness and temporal thickness were thinner when compared to control eyes [32]. Similarly, Fernandez-Beunaga et al. found that nasal macular thickness correlated with visual acuity in ischemic optic neuropathy [51].

When it became possible to measure the GCC directly, Aggarwal et al. showed a high correlation of GCC thickness with visual field losses in both magnitude and location in patients with NAION, with hemispheric GCC loss correlating with altitudinal visual field loss [33]. Larrea et al. showed a significant correlation between GCC averages at the onset of NAION and visual field losses in both acute and chronic stages, suggesting that GCC thickness in the acute stage may be a determining factor to predict final visual field defects, with good correlation between location of damage in the GCC in the macular region and location of the scotoma [34].

Erlich et al. compared the pattern of GCC loss between NAION and patients with optic neuritis at time points less than 2 weeks from onset of symptom, 5–8 weeks, 9–16 weeks, and greater than 16 weeks and found there was a significantly greater hemispheric difference in GCC thickness in NAION patients than optic neuritis at every time-point measured [52]. However, the GCC hemispheric difference in NAION lessened at time points greater than 16 weeks. This may be explained by the observation that ganglion cell atrophy extends to a greater area, beyond one hemisphere, with time. The initial segmental ischemia of the optic nerve is associated with edema, which may lead to subsequent damage in other areas of the optic nerve [53, 54] (Fig. 9.2).

In early studies using OCT angiography (OCTA) to analyze the microvasculature of the retina and choroid nerve in NAION patients, flow impairment of the retinal peripapillary capillaries and peripapillary choriocapillaris was found to correspond with changes seen in the OCT measurements of the retinal nerve fiber layer and ganglion cell layer complex and to visual fields defects [55]. Comparison of acute and chronic NAION showed vessel density was significantly less in chronic NAION. No difference was seen in the microvasculature of the unaffected fellow eye of patients with NAION when compared to normal eyes. These findings suggest that OCTA may be a usual tool in diagnosing NAION and monitoring the course [56].

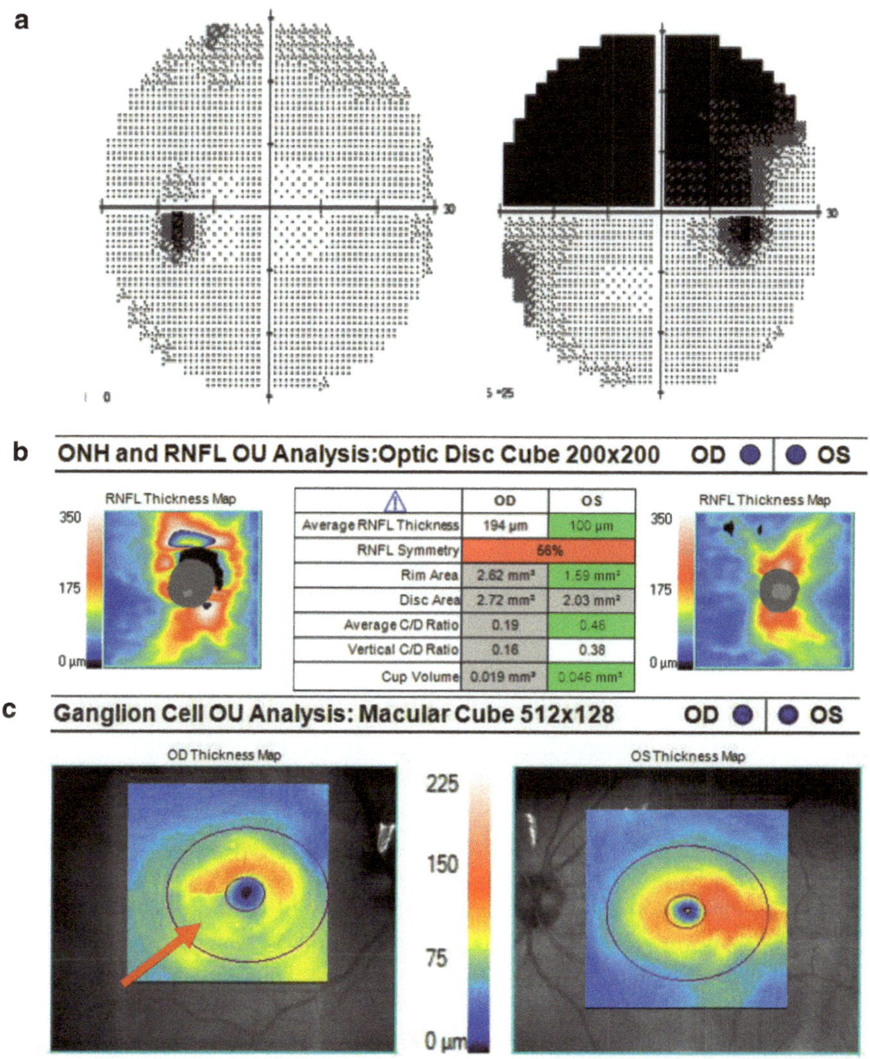

Fig. 9.2 A 78-year-old man with hypertension awoke with a dark shadow in his right eye upon awakening. Humphrey visual fields showed a superior altitudinal visual field defect OD and the visual field was full OS (**a**). Fundoscopy and OCT RNFL analysis showed diffuse swelling of the optic nerve in the right eye (**b**). Despite the edema on RNFL analysis, there was thinning inferiorly in the right eye on ganglion cell layer complex (GCC) analysis, suggesting neuronal loss (**c**). Two months later, the RNFL measurement normalized (**d**) in the right eye and GCC showed thinning, inferior greater than superior (**e**)

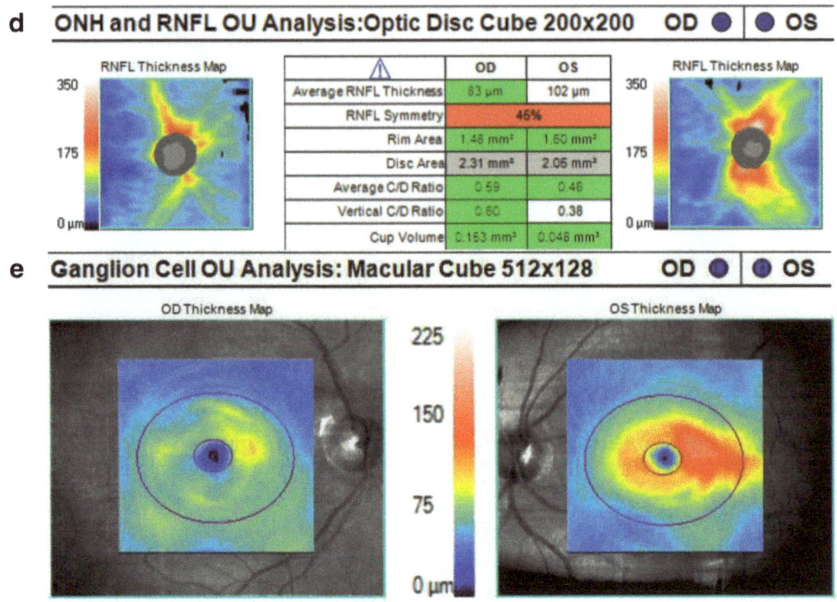

Fig. 9.2 (continued)

9.3 Optic Disc Edema Secondary to Toxic/Hereditary/Nutritional Optic Neuropathies

SD-OCT has shed some light on the events occurring at the optic nerve head in Leber Hereditary Optic Neuropathy (LHON), including a clearer depiction of axonal swelling, which precedes and is present at the time of visual loss. Furthermore, OCT clearly shows, and can be used to measure, atrophy of the nerve fiber layer (RNFL) following the acute event, which in most cases, is confined to the papillomacular bundle [57–59]. Hedges et al. found that in the early phases of LHON, when visual acuity begins to decline, the GCC remains relatively normal, while the RNFL becomes swollen and is frequently associated with peripapillary telangiectasias. Within days, as the vision further declines, the GCC starts to thin. The RNFL thickening resolves or becomes thin only until the chronic phase in most patients. In some cases, average RNFL thickness remains relatively normal despite GCC loss, creating a mismatch between RNFL and GCC thickness measurements. In cases where RNFL loss is mild, the papillomacular bundle is affected. The degree of GCC thinning or RNFL loss does not correlate with final visual acuity or visual fields even if there is visual recovery [60] (Fig. 9.3).

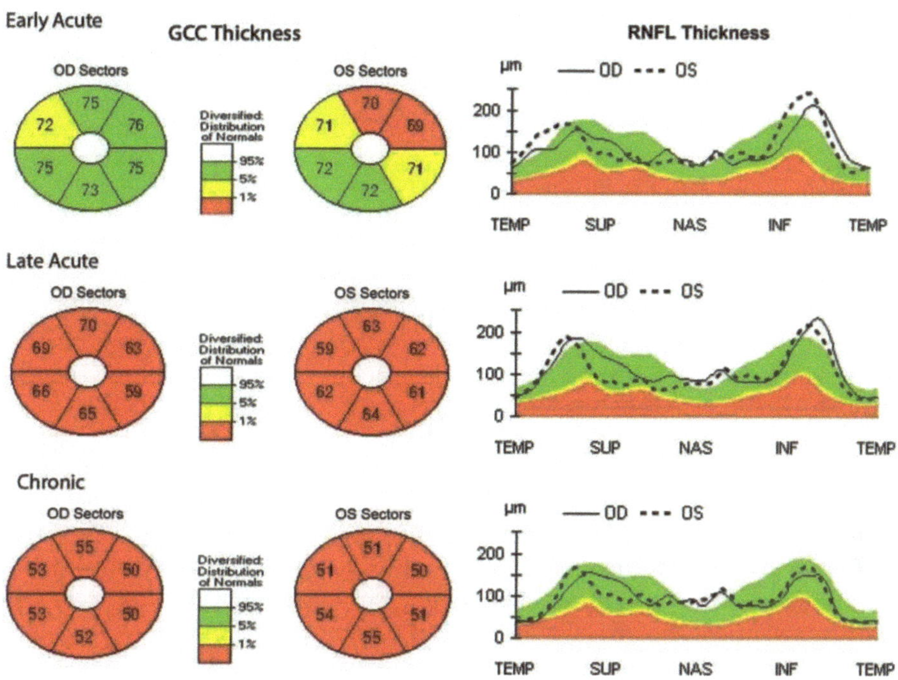

Fig. 9.3 OCT findings throughout the early acute, late acute, and chronic phases in a 44-year-old woman LHON with 11,778 mutation. She had decreased vision bilaterally (20/30 and 20/50) 3 weeks after symptom onset. In the early acute phase, ganglion cell layer complex (GCC) defects are noted bilaterally with RNFL swelling. In the late acute phase, severe GCC thinning is present with persistent RNFL swelling. In the chronic phase, severe GCC thinning is present with RNFL thinning noted temporally

In a handful of case reports using OCTA to evaluate LHON, results have shown that there is temporal radial peripapillary capillaries (RPC) thinning, in the papillomacular bundle, associated with LHON [61, 62]. Matszuki et al., were able to follow a patient with acute symptoms in one eye and pre-symptomatic in the other. They found that the RPC thinning and its spread did not precede the symptomatic vision loss. The authors suggest that based on this finding that it is reasonable to assume the spreading of the RPC less was a secondary association of RNFL thinning [62].

Barboni et al. analyzed the OCT RNFL and GCC thicknesses of patients with dominant optic atrophy (DOA) diagnosed with a mutation in the OPA1 gene and found that, overall, DOA patients have thinner RNFL and GCC measurements compared to age matched healthy subjects. The temporal RNFL was particularly thin regardless of patients' visual acuities. Inferior and superior quadrants of the RNFL were thinner in the DOA patients with the worse visual acuities compared to those with milder vision loss. While, the GCC thinning was mostly similar despite different visual acuities, further analysis did show significant thinning in the superotemporal and superior sectors in the patients with visual acuities between 0.6–1.0 and 0.4–0.5 [63].

In a small case series of three patients, Moura and Monteiro found that 2 of their patients with a chronic history of vision loss related to excessive alcohol intake and cigarette smoking showed temporal RNFL thinning using time-domain OCT. The third patient, whose vision loss had only been present for half of year, very mild temporal RNFL loss in one eye, but overall the RNFL was thick [64]. Kee and Hwang, published a case report of one patient with progressive vision loss over the course of 4 years who had a similar RNFL pattern of thinning and thickening. Increased RNFL thickness was found to be consistent with OCT findings in a case of methanol poisoning with severe peripapillary nerve fiber swelling and intraretinal fluid accumulation [65], and may be explained with pathologic findings of mitochondrial swelling and vacuolation in the retinal pigment epithelium, photoreceptor inner segments, and optic nerve verified in a rodent model [66, 67]. Klein et al. showed nasal GCC thinning in one patient who presented 1 month after bilateral decreased vision from methanol and then in follow-up 8 months later. The selective involvement of the papillomacular bundle fibers is common in toxic optic neuropathies and represents damage to the small caliber axons rich in mitochondria. Despite severe systemic toxicity, the relative sparing of the optic nerve in this case enabled characterization of the evolution of methanol toxicity with segmental GCL involvement and preservation of the RNFL, corresponding to the papillomacular bundle [68] (Fig. 9.4).

9.4 Pseudopapilledema

9.4.1 Pseudopapilledema: Vitreopapillary Traction

OCT has been useful in distinguishing other causes of pseudopapilledema, such as vitreopapillary traction, optic nerve head drusen, myelinated nerve fiber layer, and Bergmeister papillae.

Posterior vitreous detachment is a dynamic process characterized by the liquefaction and separation of the posterior vitreous cortex from the inner limiting membrane of the retina. Proliferative disorders, such as the development of premacular membranes, and tractional disorders, such as macular hole formation can result from faulty separation at this interface. If the vitreous partially or anomalously separates from the internal limiting membrane, it can lead to persistent adhesion and even traction on posterior pole structures [69].

Vitreomacular traction syndrome, a result of a partially or anomalously separated vitreous face, is a well-known clinical entity that has been well described in the literature. In 1954, Schepens used the term pseudopapilledema when he demonstrated

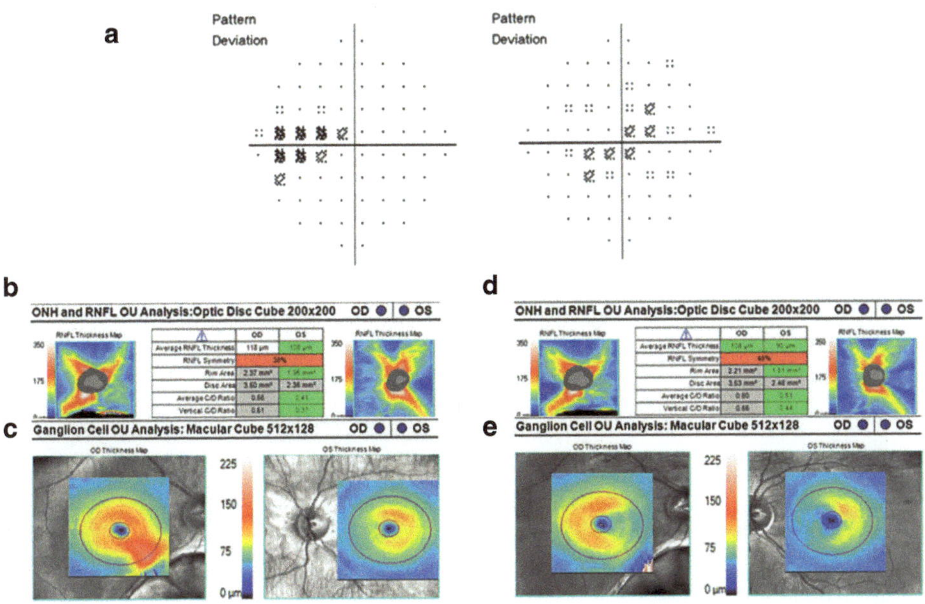

Fig. 9.4 A 19-year-old woman presented with 1 month of bilateral blurred vision, photophobia and a central scotoma after traveling abroad and ingesting methanol in local made liquor and requiring hospitalization for methanol toxicity. Visual fields showed bilateral ceocentral defects (**a**). OCTs of the RNFL and ganglion cell layer complex (GCC) were unremarkable (**b, c**). At her 8 month follow-up, there was some mild temporal RNFL thinning OU (**d**) and binasal GCC thinning (**e**). The selective involvement of the papillomacular bundle fibers is common in toxic optic neuropathies and represents damage to the small caliber axons rich in mitochondria

the histopathology of partially detached vitreous at the optic nerve head, usually in the context of co-existing retinal disease [70], such as proliferative diabetic retinopathy [71], central retinal vein occlusion [72], and non-arteritic ischemic optic neuropathy [73]. Using slit lamp biomicroscopy and ultrasonography, Katz and Hoyt observed peripapillary and intrapapillary hemorrhage in 8 young patients with mildly dysplastic discs and persistent vitreopapillary traction, postulating that transmitted forces traumatized disc vessels [74]. In addition, Wisotsky et al. demonstrated in two patients that vitreopapillary traction could cause highly elevated optic discs with blurring of the margins [75].

In 2006, Hedges et al. demonstrated by OCT that persistent vitreopapillary traction could occur as an isolated phenomenon, in the absence of proliferative fibrocellular membranes or vascular insult [76]. Tractional forces from vitreous adhesion on the optic nerve alone were sufficient in causing optic disc elevation, obscured disc margins, and peripapillary hemorrhage in these patients [76]. Vitreopapillary traction has even been shown to cause focal disc leakage on fluorescein angiography [77]. When occurring bilaterally, vitreopapillary traction can be confused with papilledema, potentially leading to costly and invasive diagnostic procedures and even unnecessary treatment [77] (Fig. 9.5).

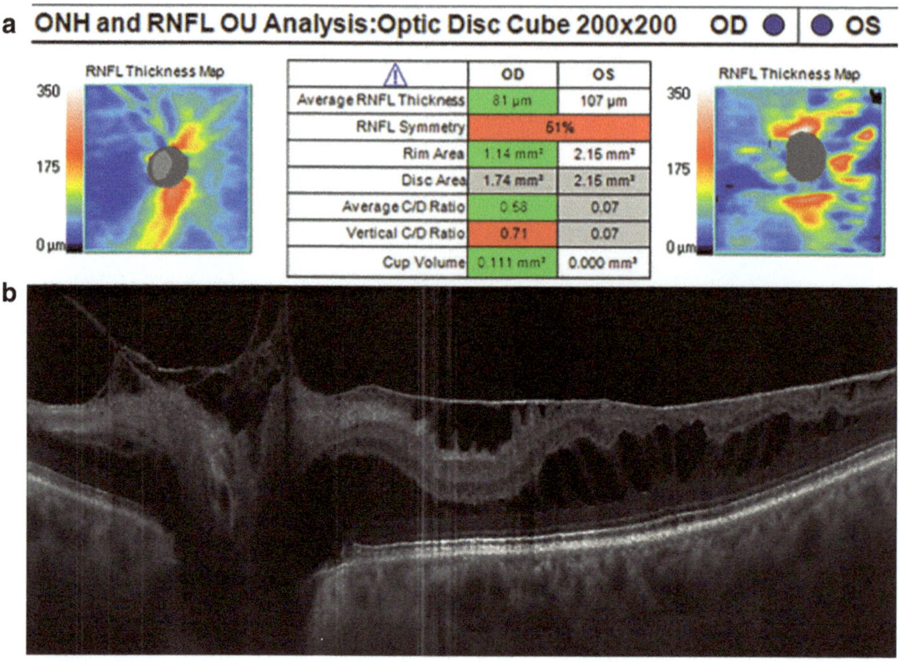

Fig. 9.5 A 74-year-old man was referred for transient flashes of color in the left eye. Automated perimetry testing showed minimal temporal enlargement of the bilind spot with no other visual field loss. Dilated funduscopic examination showed optic disc edema. OCT of the RNFL showed mild disc edema in the left eye (**a**). OCT through the macular and optic nerve of the left eye showed vitreopapilllary and vitreomacular traction (**b**)

9.4.2 Pseudopapilledema: Optic Nerve Head Drusen

Optic nerve head drusen (ONHD) are calcified hyaline deposits and have been associated with small, crowded optic discs [78]. Histopathologically, they are associated with elevation of the optic nerve head, compression of optic nerve fibers, disc hemorrhages, and juxtapapillary retinal scarring [79]. Several predisposing factors for the development of ONHD have been proposed, including a small scleral canal, altered axoplasmic transport, and abnormal vasculature [80].

When ONHD are superficially located on the nerve, they can be recognized as refractile deposits. When they are buried within the optic nerve head, however, they can be much more difficult to identify by ophthalmoscopy alone. Further, they can elevate the optic nerve head and obscure the margins of the optic disc. It is estimated that in approximately 2/3 to 4/5 of cases, ONHD occurs bilaterally [80]. In these cases, ONHD can simulate papilledema. This pseudopapilledema secondary to ONHD is typically benign, whereas true papilledema requires emergent work-up for a potentially life-threatening condition. Thus, differentiating true optic disc edema caused by papilledema or other optic neuropathies is crucial for the ophthalmologist.

Various methods have been used to study buried ONHD, including B-scan ultrasonography, fluorescein angiography, computerized tomography, and fundus autofluoresence [81]. Currently, B-scan ultrasonography is the gold standard in the clinical evaluation of ONHD. Although useful, B-scan ultrasonography necessitates a skilled ultrasonographer and interpreter, and is not always available. Fluorescein angiography is also not readily available and may not be compatible for patients with allergies to shellfish and iodine, which cross react with fluorescein dye. While fundus autofluorescence is a non-invasive way to diagnose ONHD, buried drusen may be missed using this modality. Ophthalmologist are unlikely to subject their patients to radiation to diagnose ONHD with a computerized tomography. OCT, however, is a widely available and has been shown to give information regarding the size, structure, and location of ONHD within the optic disc.

Thinning of the RNFL OCT is often associated with optic atrophy, and thickening of the RNFL OCT is often associated with optic disc edema [82]. However, both ONHD and optic disc edema can present with either RNFL thinning or RNFL thickening on OCT [83]. Therefore, the presence or absence of RNFL thinning or thickening alone does not help the clinician distinguish between ONHD and optic disc edema [84].

Savini et al. examined 9 patients with optic disc edema due to various causes. In addition to noting a significant increase in the mean RNFL thickness in all optic nerve quadrants in patients with optic disc edema, they described a triangular-shaped hyporeflective subretinal space above the retinal pigment epithelium, possibly representing subretinal fluid, with the widest part of the triangle abutting the optic nerve head and the tapered apex pointing away. They hypothesized that swelling induced by the optic disc edema could produce an upward traction producing a subretinal space with the hydrostatic forces overcoming osmotic forces [28].

Expanding on this idea of subretinal hyporeflective space, Johnson et al., used OCT images to examine the qualitative and quantitative differences between ONHD and optic disc edema. They found that patients with ONHD tended to have an elevated optic nerve head with a "lumpy bumpy" internal optic nerve contour, a rapid and abrupt decline in subretinal hyporeflective space with a normal thickness at the 2.0 mm radius, and normal or mildly increased RNFL thickness with the nasal RNFL being less than 86 μm. Patients with optic disc edema, on the other hand, had an elevated optic nerve head with a smooth internal contour, a recumbent "lazy V" pattern of the subretinal hyporeflective space with an increased thickness at the 2.0 mm radius, and an increased RNFL thickness with a nasal RNFL greater than 86 μm. They found a nasal RNFL thickness greater than 86 μm has 80% specificity and a subretinal hyporeflective space thickness greater than 169 μm at 2.0 mm radius has 90% specificity in differentiating between optic disc edema and ONHD [81].

Using SD-OCT, Lee et al. found ONHD to be focal, hyperreflective subretinal masses with distinct margins. They found the RNFL to be deformed with high reflectance and the ONHD to be beneath the outer nuclear layer and on the retinal pigment epithelium. They proposed that the increased thickness and deposition of axonal transport materials in the RNFL in optic disc edema could increase peripapillary RNFL reflectance and induce shadowing of the underlying retinal layers, mimicking subretinal fluid space rather than representing it. Like Johnson et al., they found RNFL thickness in the nasal section to be a good differential marker for optic disc edema from ONHD, with a thinner cut-off value of 78 μm [84].

Enhanced depth imaging OCT (EDI-OCT), a technique developed to give superior imaging quality of the deeper structures of the retina and optic nerve head, has also shown useful in detecting ONHD. Merchant et al., in an analysis of 34 patients with clinically visible or suspected ONHD based on ophthalmoscopy or optic disc stereophotography, EDI OCT had a significantly higher ONHD detection rate than B-scan ultrasound [85] (Fig. 9.6).

9.4.3 Pseudopapilledema: Bergmeister's Papilla and Myelinated Nerve Fiber Layer

OCT can help characterize other conditions causing pseudopapilledema. In cases of myelinated retinal nerve fiber layer, OCT can show significant hyper-reflectivity and increased thickness of the RNFL in the area of the myelinated fibers [86, 87]. The recent use of wide field three-dimensional swept source OCT (SS-OCT), which utilizes better sensitivity with imaging depth and longer imaging range, has enabled enhanced imaging of vitreous and vitreo-retinal interface. SS-OCT can offer superior resolution of vitreo-retinal entities, such as Bergmeister's papillae that may simulate papilledema [88] (Fig. 9.7).

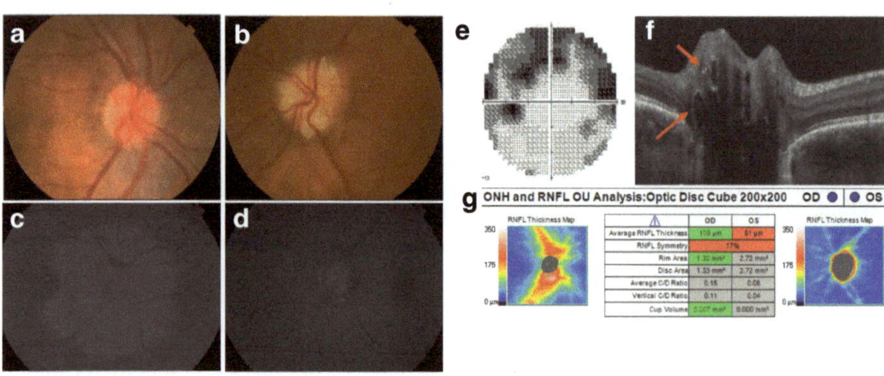

Fig. 9.6 A 16-year-old woman was referred for left visual field loss. On examination, visual acuities were 20/20 in both eyes, there was no afferent papillary defect, and color vision was preserved. The optic discs were crowded in both eyes (**a**, **b**) with multiple optic nerve head drusen (ONHD) in the left eye (**b**). Fundus auto-fluorescence was unremarkable in the right eye (**c**) and revealed numerous round lesions with hyper auto-fluorescence on the optic nerve head in the left eye corresponding with ONHD (**d**). Visual fields showed superior arcuate defect in the left eye (**e**). OCT through the optic nerve showed multiple rings of hyper-reflectivity with internal hypo-reflectivity corresponding with the ONHD (**f**). OCT of the RNFL showed thinning superiorly and inferiorly in the left eye (**g**)

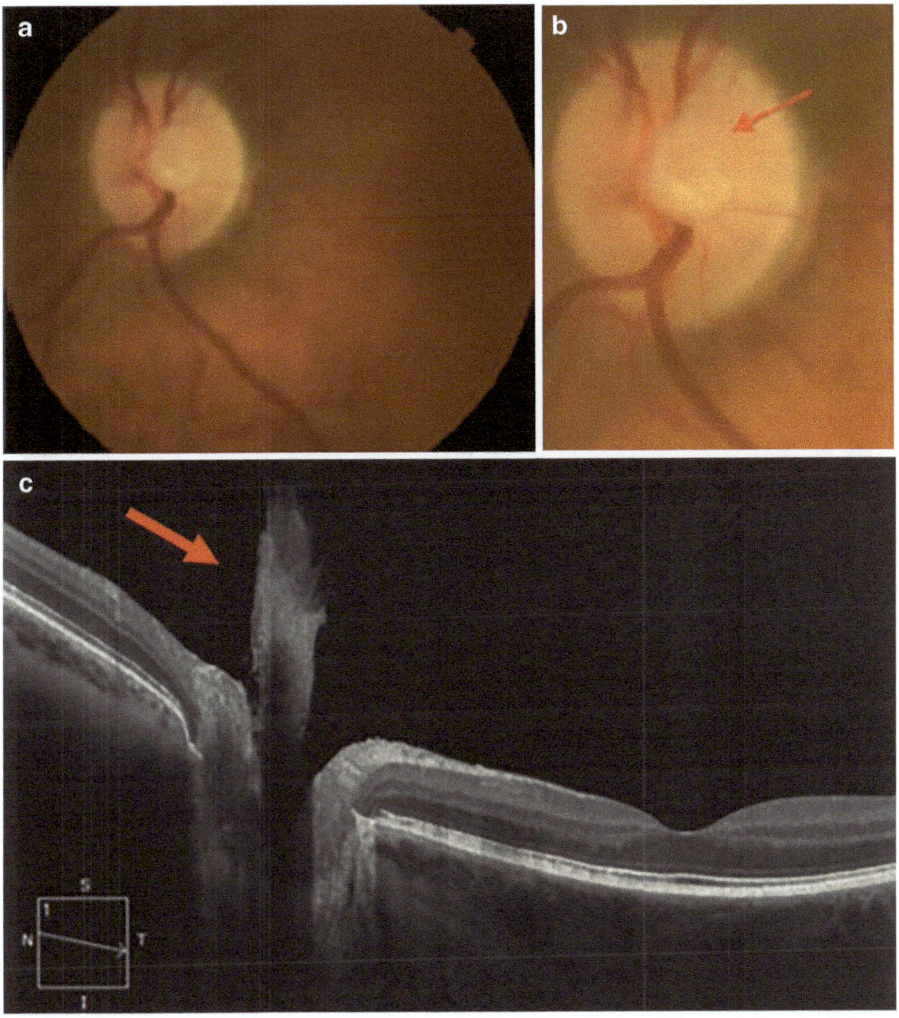

Fig. 9.7 A 43-year-old woman was referred for pain in her left eye. Incidentally, a small tuft of tissue was visualized at the optic disc (**a**, **b**) and appeared to be continuous with the optic disc on OCT (**c**), consistent with Bergmeister papillae

References

1. Von Graefe A. Ueber Komplikation von Sehnervenentzundung mit Gehirnkrankheiten. Arch F Ophth. 1860;7:58–71.
2. Paton L, Holmes G. The pathology of papilledema. Brain. 1911;33:289–432.
3. Fry WE. The pathology of papilledema. Am J Ophthalmol. 1931;14:874–83.
4. Hedges TR. A correlative study of orbital vascular and intracranial pressure in the rhesus monkey. Trans Am Ophthalmol Soc. 1963;61:589–637.
5. Tso MO, Hayreh SS. Optic disc edema in raised intracranial pressure III: a pathologic study of experimental papilledema. Arch Ophthalmol. 1977;95:1448–57.

6. Samuels B. Histopathology of papilledema. Am J Ophthalmol. 1938;21:1242–8.
7. Hoye VJ III, Berrocal AM, Hedges TR III, Amaro-Quireza ML. Optic coherence tomography demonstrates subretinal macular edema from papilledema. Arch Ophthalmol. 2001;119:1287–9.
8. Morris AT, Sanders MD. Macular changes resulting from papilloedema. Br J Ophthalmol. 1980;64:211–6.
9. Corbett JJ, Jacobson DM, Mauer RC, Thompson HS. Enlargement of the blind spot caused by papilledema. Am J Ophthalmol. 1988;105:261–5.
10. Gittinger JW Jr, Asdourian GK. Macular abnormalities in papilledema from pseudotumor cerebri. Ophthalmology. 1989;96:192–4.
11. Jamerson SC, Arunagiri G, Ellis BD, Leys MJ. Intravitreal bevacizumab for the treatment of choroidal neovascularization secondary to pseudotumor cerebri. Int Ophthalmol. 2009;29:183–5.
12. Jamison RR. Subretinal neovascularization and papilledema associated with pseudotumor cerebri. Am J Ophthalmol. 1978;85:78–81.
13. Mas AM, Villegas VM, Garcia JM, Acevedo S, Serrrano L. Intravitreal bevacizumab for peripapillary subretinal neovascular membrane associated to papilledema: a case report. P R Health Sci J. 2012;31:148–50.
14. Lee IJ, Maccheron LJ, Kwan AS. Intravitreal bevacizumab in the treatment of peripapillary choroidal neovascular membrane secondary to idiopathic intracranial hypertension. J Neuroophthalmol. 2013;33:155–7.
15. Morse PH, Leveille AS, Antel JP, Burch JV. Bilateral juxtapapillary subretinal neovascularization associated with pseudotumor cerebri. Am J Ophthalmol. 1981;91:312–7.
16. Caballero-Presencia A, Diaz-Guia E, Martinex-Perez M, Lopez-Lopez J. Neo-vascularisation sous-retinienne jiuxtapapillaire bilaterale dans un cas de pseudotumor cerebri. J Fr Ophtalmol. 1986;9:105–10.
17. Sathornsumetee B, Webb A, Hill DL, Newman NJ, Biousse V. Subretinal hemorrhage from a peripapillary choroidal neovascular membrane in papilledema caused by idiopathic intracranial hypertension. J Neuroophthalmol. 2006;26:197–9.
18. Kaeser PF, Borruat FX. Peripapillary neovascular membrane: a rare cause of acute vision loss in pediatric idiopathic intracranial hypertension. J AAPOS. 2011;15:83–6.
19. Troost BT, Sufit RL, Grand MG. Sudden monocular visual loss in pseudotumor cerebri. Arch Neurol. 1979;36:440–2.
20. Martinez MR, Ophir A. Optical coherence tomography as an adjunctive tool for diagnosing papilledema in young patients. J Pediatr Ophthalmol Strabismus. 2011;48:174–81.
21. Karam EZ, Hedges TR. Optical coherence tomography of the retinal nerve fibre layer in mild papilloedema and pseudopapilloedema. Br J Ophthalmol. 2005;89:294–8.
22. Fard MA, Fakhree S, Abdi P, Hassanpoor N, Subramanian PS. Quantification of peripapillary total retinal volume in pseudopapilledema and mild papilledema using spectral-domain optical coherence tomography. Am J Ophthalmol. 2014;158:136–43.
23. Kupersmith MJ, Sibony P, Mandel G, Durbin M, Kardon RH. Optical coherence tomography of the swollen optic nerve head: deformation of the peripapillary retinal pigment epithelium layer in papilledema. Invest Ophthalmol Vis Sci. 2011;52(9):6558–64.
24. Sibony P, Kupersmith MJ, Rohlf FJ. Shape analysis of the peripapillary RPE layer in papilledema and ischemic optic neuropathy. Invest Ophthalmol Vis Sci. 2011;52(11):7987–95.
25. Sibony P, Kupersmith MJ, Honkanen R, Rohlf FJ, Torab-Parhiz A. Effects of lowering cerebrospinal fluid pressure on the shape of the peripapillary retina in intracranial hypertension. Invest Ophthalmol Vis Sci. 2014;55(12):8223–31.
26. Wang JK, Kardon RH, Ledolter J, Sibony PA, Kupersmith MJ, Garvin MK, OCT Sub-Study Committee and the NORDIC Idiopathic. Peripapillary retinal pigment epithelium layer shape changes from acetazolamide treatment in the idiopathic intracranial hypertension treatment trial. Intracranial Hypertension Study Group. Invest Ophthalmol Vis Sci. 2017;58(5):2554–65.
27. Sibony P, Straachovsky M, Honkanen R, Kupersmith MJ. Optical coherence tomography shape analysis of the peripapillary retinal pigment epithelium layer in presumed optic nerve sheath meningiomas. J Neuroophthalmol. 2014;34:130–6.

28. Savini G, Bellusci C, Carbonelli M, Zanini M, Carelli V, Sadun AA, Barboni P. Detection and quantification of retinal nerve fiber layer thickness in optic disc edema using stratus OCT. Arch Ophthalmol. 2006;124:1111–7.
29. Monteiro ML, Afonso CL. Macular thickness measurements with frequency domain-OCT for quantification of axonal loss in chronic papilledema from pseudotumor cerebri syndrome. Eye (Lond). 2014;28:390–8.
30. Perry VH, Lund RD. Evidence that the lamina cribrosa prevents intraretinal myelination of retinal ganglion cell axons. J Neurocytol. 1990;19:265–72.
31. Burkholder BM, Osborne B, Loguidice MJ, Bisker E, Frohman TC, Conger A, Ratchford JN, Warner C, Markowitz CE, Jacobs DA, Galetta SL, Cutter GR, Maguire MG, Calabresi PA, Balcer LJ, Frohman EM. Macular volume determined by optical coherence tomography as a measure of neuronal loss in multiple sclerosis. Arch Neurol. 2009;66:1366–72.
32. Papchenko T, Grainger BT, Savino PJ, Gamble GD, Danesh-Meyer HV. Macular thickness predictive of visual field sensitivity in ischaemic optic neuropathy. Acta Ophthalmol. 2012;90:e463–9.
33. Aggarwal D, Tan O, Huang D, Sadun AA. Patterns of ganglion cell complex and nerve fiber layer loss in nonarteritic ischemic optic neuropathy by Fourier-domain optical coherence tomography. Invest Ophthalmol Vis Sci. 2012;53:4539–45.
34. Larrea BA, Iztueta MG, Indart LM, Alday NM. Early axonal damage detection by ganglion cell complex analysis with optical coherence tomography in nonarteritic anterior ischaemic optic neuropathy. Graefes Arch Clin Exp Ophthalmol. 2014;252:1839–46.
35. Syc SB, Saidha S, Newsome SD, Ratchford JN, Levy M, Ford E, Crainiceanu CM, Durbin MK, Oakley JD, Meyer SA, Frohman EM, Calabresi PA. Optical coherence tomography segmentation reveals ganglion cell layer pathology after optic neuritis. Brain. 2012;135:521–33.
36. Marzoli SB, Ciasca P, Curone M, Cammarata G, Melzi L, Criscuoli A, Bussone G, D'Amico D. Quantitative analysis of optic nerve damage in idiopathic intracranial hypertension (IIH) at diagnosis. Neurol Sci. 2013;34(Suppl 1):S143–5.
37. Optical Coherence Tomography Substudy Committee, NORDIC Idiopathic Intracranial Hypertension Study Group. Papilledema outcomes from the optical coherence tomography substudy of the idiopathic intracranial hypertension treatment trial. Ophthalmology. 2015;122(9):1939–45.
38. Chen JJ, Thurtell MJ, Longmuir RA, Garvin MK, Wang JK, Wall M, Kardon RH. Causes and prognosis of visual acuity at the time of initial presentation in idiopathic intracranial hypertension. Invest Ophthalmol Vis Sci. 2015;56(6):3850–9.
39. Athappilly G, Garcia-Basterra I, Machado-Miller F, Hedges TR, Mendoza-Santiesteban C, Vuong L. Ganglion cell complex analysis as a potential indicator of early neuronal loss in idiopathic intracranial hypertension. Neuroophthalmology. 2018;43(1):10–7.
40. Hayreh SS. Anterior ischemic optic neuropathy. Arch Neurol. 1981;38:675–8.
41. Hayreh SS. Fluids in the anterior part of the optic nerve in health and disease. Surv Ophthalmol. 1978;23:1–25.
42. Contreras I, Noval S, Rebolleda G, Munoz-Negrete FJ. Follow-up of nonarteritic anterior ischemic optic neuropathy with optical coherence tomography. Ophthalmology. 2007;114:2338–44.
43. Contreras I, Rebolleda G, Noval S, Munoz-Negrete FJ. Optic disc evaluation by optical coherence tomography in nonarteritic anterior ischemic optic neuropathy. IOVS. 2007;48:4087–92.
44. Bellusci C, Savini G, Carbonelli M, Carelli V, Sadun AA, Barboni P. Retinal nerve fiber layer thickness in nonarteritic ischemic optic neuropathy: OCT characterization of the acute and resolving phases. Graefes Arch Clin Exp Ophthalmol. 2008;246:641–7.
45. Quigley HA, Miller NR, Green WR. The pattern of optic nerve fiber loss in anterior ischemic optic neuropathy. Am J Ophthalmol. 1985;100:769–76.
46. Traustason OI, Feldon SE, Leemaster JE, Weiner JM. Anterior ischemic optic neuropathy: classification of field defects by Octopus automated static perimetry. Graefes Arch Clin Exp Ophthalmol. 1988;226:206–12.

47. Hayreh SS, Zimmerman MB. Visual field abnormalities in nonarteritic anterior ischemic optic neuropathy: their pattern and prevalence at initial examination. Arch Ophthalmol. 2005;23:1554–62.
48. Hayreh SS, Zimmerman MB. Optic disc edema in non-arteritic anterior ischemic optic neuropathy. Graefes Arch Clin Exp Ophthalmol. 2007;245:1107–21.
49. Alasil T, Tan O, Lu ATH, Huang D, Sadun AA. Correlation of Fourier domain optical coherence tomography retinal nerve fiber layer maps with visual fields in nonarteritic ischemic optic neuropathy. Ophthalmic Surg Lasers Imaging. 2008;39:S71–9.
50. Hedges TR III, Vuong LN, Gonzalez-Garcia AO, Mendoza-Santiesteban CE, Amaro-Quierza ML. Subretinal fluid from anterior ischemic optic neuropathy demonstrated by optical coherence tomography. Arch Ophthalmol. 2008;126:812–5.
51. Fernandez-Buenaga R, Rebolleda G, Munoz-Negrete FJ, Contreras I, Casas-Llera P. Macular thickness. Ophthalmology. 2009;116:1587–1587.e3.
52. Erlich-Malona N, Mendoza-Santiesteban CE, Hedges TR 3rd, Patel N, Monaco C, Cole E. Distinguishing ischaemic optic neuropathy from optic neuritis by ganglion cell analysis. Acta Ophthalmol. 2016;94(8):721–6.
53. Miller NR, Arnold AC. Current concepts in the diagnosis, pathogenesis and management of nonarteritic anterior ischaemic optic neuropathy. Eye. 2015;29:65–79.
54. Ho JK, Stanford MP, Shariati MA, Dalal R, Liao YJ. Optical coherence tomography study of experimental anterior ischemic optic neuropathy and histologic confirmation. Invest Ophthalmol Vis Sci. 2013;54:5981–8.
55. Wright-Mayes E, Cole ED, Dang S, Novais EA, Vuong L, Mendoza-Santiesteban C, Duker JS, Hedges TR 3rd. Optical coherence tomography angiography in non-arteritic anterior ischemic optic neuropathy. J Neuroophthalmol. 2017;37(4):358–64.
56. Song Y, Min JY, Mao L, Gong YY. Microvasculature dropout detected by the optical coherence tomography angiography in nonarteritic anterior ischemic optic neuropathy. Lasers Surg Med. 2018;50(3):194–201.
57. Barboni P, Savini G, Valentino ML, et al. Retinal nerve fiber layer evaluation by optical coherence tomography in Leber's hereditary optic neuropathy. Ophthalmology. 2005;112:120–6.
58. Zhang Y, Huang H, Wei S, et al. Characterization of macular thickness changes in Leber's hereditary optic neuropathy by optical coherence tomography. BMC Ophthalmol. 2014;14:105.
59. Savini G, Barboni P, Valentino ML, et al. Retinal nerve fiber layer evaluation by optical coherence tomography in unaffected carriers with Leber's hereditary optic neuropathy mutations. Ophthalmology. 2005;112:127–31.
60. Hedges TR, Gobuty M, Manfreddy RA, Erlich-Malona N, Monaco C, Mendoza-Santiesteban CE. The optic coherence tomography profile of Leber hereditary optic neuropathy. Neuroophthalmology. 2016;40(3):107–12.
61. De Rojas JO, Rasool N, Chen RW, Horowitz J, Odel JG. Optical coherence tomography angiography in Leber hereditary optic neuropathy. Neurology. 2016;87(19):2065–6.
62. Matsuzaki M, Hirami Y, Uyama H, Kurimoto Y. Optic coherence tomography angiography changes in radial peripapillary capillaries in Leber hereditary optic neuropathy. Am J Ophthalmol Case Rep. 2018;9:51–5.
63. Barboni P, Savini G, Cascavilla ML. Early macula retinal ganglion cell loss in dominant optic atrophy: genotype-phenotype correlation. Am J Ophthalmol. 2014;158(3):62–636.
64. Moura F, Monteiro M. Evaluation of retinal nerve fiber layer thickness measurements using optical coherence tomography in patient with tobacco-alcohol-induced toxic optic neuropathy. Indian J Ophthalmol. 2010;58(2):143–6.
65. Kee C, Hwang JM. Optical coherence tomography in a patient with tobacco-alcohol amblyopia. Eye (Lond). 2008;22(3):469–70.
66. Fujihara M, Kikuchi M, Kurimoto Y. Methanol-induced retinal toxicity patient examined by optic coherence tomography. Jpn J Ophthalmol. 2006;50:239–41.
67. Eells JT, Henry MM, Lewandowski MF, Seme MT, Murray TG. Development and characterization of a rodent model of methanol induced retinal and optic nerve. Neurotoxicology. 2000;21:321–30.

68. Klein KA, Warren AK, Baumal CR, Hedges TR III. Optical coherence tomography findings in methanol toxicity. Int J Retina Vitreous. 2017;3:36.
69. Sebag J. Anatomy and pathology of the vitreo-retinal interface. Eye. 1992;6(6):541–52.
70. Schepens CL. Clinical aspects of pathologic changes in the vitreous body. Am J Ophthalmol. 1954;38:8–21.
71. Kroll P, Weigrand W, Schmidt J. Vitreopapillary traction in proliferative diabetic vitreoretinopathy. Br J Ophthalmol. 1999;83:261–4.
72. Rumelt S, Karatas M, Pikkel J, Majlin M, Ophir A. Optic disc traction syndrome associated with central retinal vein occlusion. Arch Ophthalmol. 2003;121:1093–7.
73. Modarres M, Sanjari MS, Falavarjani KG. Vitrectomy and release of presumed epipapillary vitreous traction for treatment of nonarteritic anterior ischemic optic neuropathy associated with partial posterior vitreous detachment. Ophthalmology. 2007;114(2):340–4.
74. Katz B, Hoyt WF. Intrapapillary and peripapillary hemorrhage in young patients with incomplete posterior vitreous detachment: signs of vitreopapillary traction. Ophthalmology. 1995;102:349–54.
75. Wisotsky BJ, Magat-Gordon CB, Puklin JE. Vitreopapillary traction as a cause of elevated optic nerve head. Am J Ophthalmol. 1998;126:137–9.
76. Hedges TR, Flattem NL, Bagga A. Vitreopapillary traction confirmed by optical coherence tomography. Arch Ophthalmol. 2006;124(2):349–54.
77. Houle E, Miller NR. Bilateral vitreopapillary traction demonstrated by optical coherence tomography mistaken for papilledema. Case Rep Ophthalmol Med. 2012;2012:682659.
78. Lam BL, Morais CG Jr, Pasol J. Drusen of the optic disc. Curr Neurol Neurosci Rep. 2008;8:404–8.
79. Friedman AH, Gartner S, Modi SS. Drusen of the optic disc: a retrospective study in cadaver eyes. Br J Ophthalmol. 1975;59:413–21.
80. Auw-Haedrich C, Staubach F, Witschel H. Major review: optic disk drusen. Surv Ophthalmol. 2002;47:515–32.
81. Johnson LN, Diehl ML, Hamm CW, Sommerville DN, Petroski GF. Differentiating optic disc edema from optic nerve head drusen on optical coherence tomography. Arch Ophthalmol. 2009;127:45–9.
82. Katz BJ, Pomeranz HD. Visual field defects and retinal nerve fiber layer defects in eyes with buried optic nerve drusen. Am J Ophthalmol. 2006;141:248–53.
83. Roh S, Noecker RJ, Schuman JS, Hedges TR III, Weiter JJ, Mattox C. Effect of optic nerve head drusen on nerve fiber layer thickness. Ophthalmology. 1998;105:878–85.
84. Lee KM, Woo SJ, Hwang JM. Differentiation of optic nerve head drusen and optic disc edema with spectral domain optical coherence tomography. Ophthalmology. 2011;118:971–7.
85. Merchant KY, Su D, Park SC, Qayum S, Banik R, Liebmann JM, Ritch R. Enhanced depth imaging optical coherence tomography of optic nerve head drusen. Ophthalmology. 2013;120:1409–14.
86. Salvatore S, Iannetti L, Fragiotta S, Vingolo EM. Optical coherence tomography and myelinated retinal nerve fibers: anatomical description and comparison between time-domain and spectral domain OCT. Minerva Oftalmol. 2011;53:31–8.
87. Nourinia R, Behdad B, Montahaei T. Optical coherence tomography findings in a patient with myelinated retinal nerve fiber layer. J Ophthalmic Vis Res. 2013;8:280–1.
88. Liu JJ, Witkin AJ, Adhi M, Grulkowski I, Kraus MF, Dhalla AH, Lu CD, Hornegger J, Duker JS, Fukimoto JG. Enhanced vitreous imaging in healthy eyes using swept source optical coherence tomography. PLoS One. 2014;9(7):e102950.

OCT and Compressive Optic Neuropathy 10

Mário Luiz Ribeiro Monteiro

10.1 Introduction

Compressive optic neuropathies are among the most important diseases of the anterior visual pathway and can lead to severe visual handicap particularly when an early diagnosis is not obtained. It encompass a wide array of conditions including optic nerve glioma and meningioma, extrinsic optic nerve compression by orbital tumor, enlarged muscles in Graves' orbitopathy, sinus expansive disease or intracranial tumors affecting the optic nerve and chiasm such as occurs in pituitary adenomas, craniopharyngiomas, aneurysms, meningioma, glioma, germ cell tumors and metastases [1].

The diagnosis of compressive optic neuropathy usually relies on the history of progressive visual loss and on imaging studies, particularly modern magnetic resonance imaging (MRI) and computed tomography (CT) scanning devices. On ophthalmic examination patients with tumors compressing the anterior visual pathway usually present with visual acuity (VA) and visual field (VF) loss in one or both eyes. Visual loss may occur rapidly in fast growing or hemorrhagic tumors but most of the times visual loss (either central or in the peripheral field) is slow. Optic disc pallor is also commonly found in longstanding diseases while proptosis may be present when optic nerve compression occurs at the orbit.

Traditionally evaluation of the visual pathway in such cases is restricted to VA, color vision and VF assessment as well as fundus observation of structural abnormalities in the optic nerve head such as optic disc pallor or edema and peripapillary retinal nerve fiber layer (RNFL) loss. However, the development of technology that enables to objective measure retinal and optic nerve neuronal integrity has greatly modified our ability to evaluate fundoscopic abnormalities in anterior visual pathway diseases with the introduction of imaging equipments such as scanning laser

M. L. R. Monteiro (✉)
Division of Ophthalmology, Department of Ophthalmology and Otolaryngology, University of São Paulo Medical School, São Paulo, Brazil

A. Grzybowski, P. Barboni (eds.), *OCT and Imaging in Central Nervous System Diseases*, https://doi.org/10.1007/978-3-030-26269-3_10

polarimetry, confocal laser scanning and particularly optical coherence tomography (OCT) [2–5]. Among those technologies, OCT is the most useful instrument for structural evaluation of the fundus. The instrument was introduced as a means of detecting retinal abnormalities but quickly progressed to include measurements that estimate axonal loss in diseases such as glaucoma and hereditary, demyelinating, degenerative diseases of the central nervous system or compressive lesions affecting the optic pathways [6–10].

OCT became particularly useful in neuro-ophthalmology after the introduction of spectral-domain OCT (SD-OCT) and swept-source OCT (SS-OCT) technology that replaced earlier generation time-domain (TD) technology and achieved a resolution of 5–7 μm [11, 12]. The current technologies allow for OCT to be of help in the diagnosis and follow-up of compressive optic neuropathies both by quantifying peripapillary RNFL and also by measuring retinal thickness in the macular area for estimating particularly macular RNFL and ganglion cell layer (GCL) loss [9, 13–15]. Furthermore, other retinal layers in the macular area, such as the inner nuclear layer (INL) and even outer retinal layers that may also be evaluated and may be affected in optic pathway diseases [16–19]. OCT may also be of help in optic neuropathies associated with optic disc edema by estimating the severity of disc edema and helping analyzing the shape of the peripapillary retinal pigment epithelium layer on linear high-resolution scans passing through the optic disc [20, 21].

Compressive lesions of the anterior visual pathways may go unnoticed by examiners until a significant amount of retinal axonal loss has occurred and clinically detected optic atrophy is present [6]. In such conditions, OCT-measured RNFL and macular thickness measurements may be reduced, indicating retinal neuronal loss. By quantifying RNFL and retinal ganglion cells, the technology can therefore be very useful both in the early diagnosis as well as in the follow-up of compressive diseases of the optic pathway.

Reduced OCT-measured perpipapillary RNFL and macular thickness measurements may help detecting optic neuropathies occurring from intrinsic or extrinsic optic nerve tumors. When visual loss is subtle, with mild decrease in VA, VF and color vision, the finding of RNFL thinning provides more objective evidence that there is an optic neuropathy. Since compressive optic neuropathies usually have an insidious presentation such finding can be extremely important to raise suspicion and pursue with further investigation [22].

In patients with compressive optic neuropathies OCT may not only be of help in the diagnosis but also be useful for estimating the chances of visual improvement after treatment. Ideally such conditions should be detected before retinal axonal loss is present based on history, ophthalmic examination and neuroimaging studies. In such cases, the finding of normal or only mildly reduced OCT measurements in a patient with significant visual loss from compressive optic neuropathy indicates that visual recovery is possible at least to a large extent. Finally, detailed analysis with high-resolution OCT examinations can be of help when judging treatment efficacy, particularly when complete removal of lesions is not possible. Efficacy of treatment can be estimated with OCT by repeating retinal and optic nerve measurements over time [23].

While not all conditions have been studied using OCT, the technology should probably provide important data in all compressive optic neuropathies. Irrespective of the etiology the most frequent utility of OCT is to assess optic neuropathy through quantification of peripapillary RNFL thickness measurements. More recently macular thickness measurements, particularly segmented measurements of macular RNFL and GCL (usually measured together with the inner plexiform layer, and labeled GCL+), as well as the combined measurement of both macular RNFL and GCL+, have been introduced in practice and are available in most modern OCT equipments [9, 14, 15]. In the following paragraphs, we discuss briefly the most important compressive lesions of the anterior visual pathway, particularly those that have been evaluated in previous studies with regard to the use of OCT.

10.2 Optic Nerve Tumors

Tumors of the optic nerve represent approximately 4–10% of all orbital tumors [24–26]. Although uncommon lesions such as hemangiopericytomas and medulloepitheliomas are occasionally reported, the great majority are either optic nerve gliomas or optic nerve meningiomas. Gliomas usually occur in children while most optic nerve meningiomas are tumors affecting middle-aged persons with progressive visual loss, proptosis, disc edema and optociliary veins on fundus examination [24, 26].

Meningiomas of the anterior visual pathway are important compressive lesions of the optic nerve that usually occur in middle aged patients leading to progressive VA and VF loss, optic atrophy or optic disc edema and abnormalities on imaging studies such as MRI and CT scan. The tumors can originate from the sheaths of the optic nerve or from the meninges near the nerves [1].

Optic nerve sheath meningiomas (ONSM) are tumors that originate from the meninges of the optic nerve and account for one-third of primary optic nerve tumors [24, 27]. The tumor shows a female predominance, with a mean age at diagnosis of around 40 years [28]. The lesions generally have a slow rate of growing but usually lead to gradual visual deterioration. Some tumors are localized to a small segment of the optic nerve while others surround the entire length of the nerve in the orbit and the optic canal [27]. Patients with ONSM and progressive but recent visual loss or those with long-standing loss but still visual function can be treated with conformational fractioned radiation therapy [29, 30]. By contrast, surgical resection of ONSM leads to significant or complete visual loss and should be restricted to patients with severe irreversible visual loss for correction of disfiguring proptosis or preventing intracranial extension.

ONSM classically present with slowly progressive visual loss, optic atrophy and optociliary shunt vessels [28, 31]. In many patients there is optic disc edema preceding the development of optic atrophy [31]. However, although optic disc edema or atrophy is very often, in some patients the fundus may appear normal causing diagnostic confusion, particularly because when the tumor is small neuroimaging studies are frequently inconclusive. In such cases, OCT may be of help in the diagnosis by confirming the existence of peripapillary RNFL and/or macular GCL+ loss (Fig. 10.1).

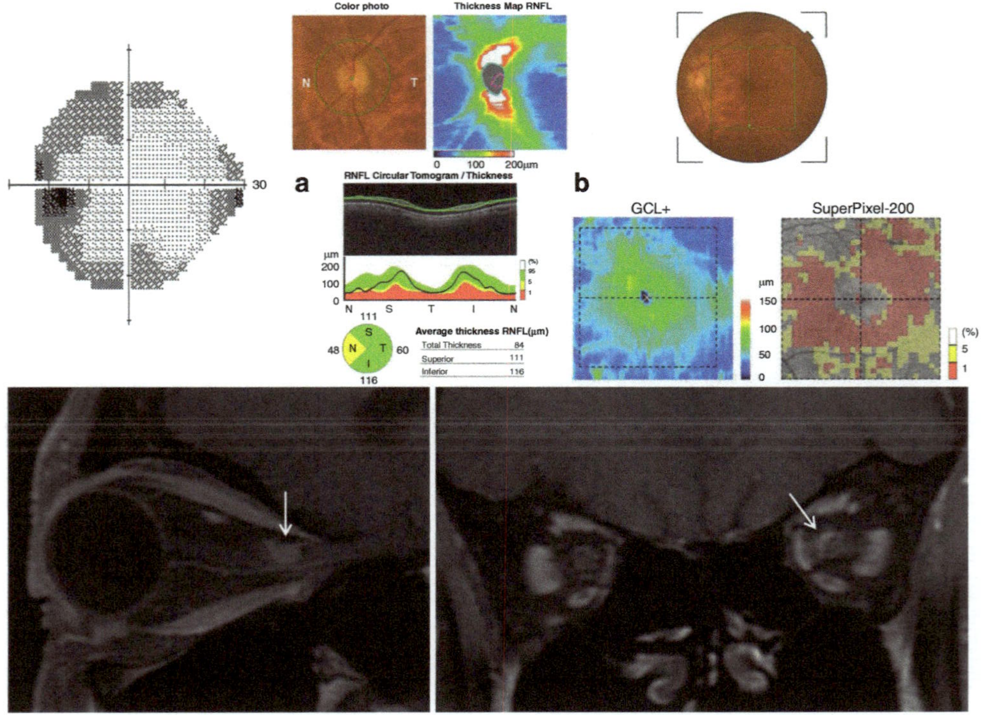

Fig. 10.1 A 72-year-old woman complained of progressive visual loss in the left eye for 1 year. Visual field showed reduced peripheral sensitivity (upper left) but neuroimaging studies were unrevealing and a diagnosis was not established. Optical coherence tomography (DRI OCT Triton Plus®, Topcon) revealed borderline reduction of the peripapillary retinal nerve fiber layer in the nasal quadrant of the disc (upper middle, **a**). Segmented macular thickness measurements indicated reduced macular ganglion cell layer (GCL+) volume, significantly reduced compared to normative data (upper right, **b**). Because of OCT findings a repeat magnetic resonance imaging of the orbit disclosed a small meningioma affecting a segment of the optic nerve on sagittal (lower left, arrow) and coronal cuts (lower right, arrow)

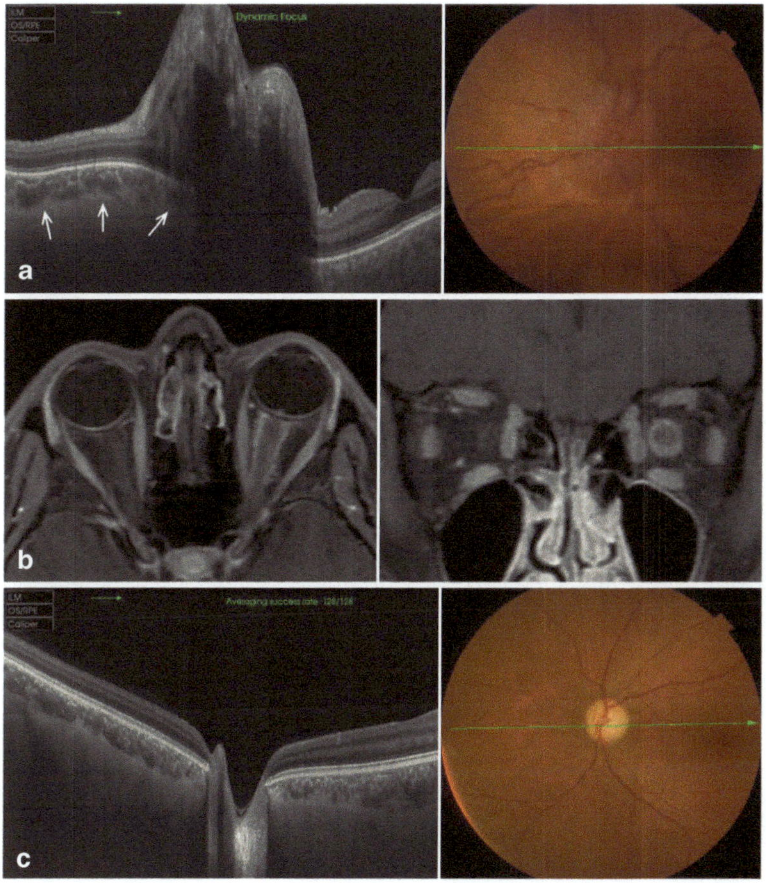

Fig. 10.2 A 26-year-old man presented with blurred vision and optic disc edema in the left eye. Above: swept source optical coherence tomography (DRI OCT Triton Plus®, Topcon) 12-mm linear horizontal scan passing through the optic disc revealing deformation of the peripapillary retinal pigment epithelium layer, with the appearance previously described as an inverted-U shape image (arrows) [20]. Middle: magnetic resonance imaging revealed enhancing lesion around the optic nerve, later confirmed to be an optic nerve sheath meningioma. Below: linear scanning showing the normal V-shape of the peripapillary retinal pigment epithelium layer

When optic disc edema is present in patients with ONSM the diagnosis is frequently confused with other causes of optic disc edema such as optic neuritis and papilledema. In such cases, OCT may be of help in the diagnosis by showing indentation of the retinal pigment epithelium (on high-resolution linear scans passing through the nerve) presumably because of lack of compliance of the nerve that exerts pressure on the posterior pole (Fig. 10.2) [20]. However, it is important that while such deformation is not encountered in ischemic or inflammatory optic neuropathies it may also occur in papilledema and is not specific for ONSM [21].

OCT can be important not only in the diagnosis of ONSM but also in estimating the chances of visual recovery. When visual loss occurs in a patient with little or no retinal neuronal loss visual improvement may be expected (Fig. 10.3). On the other

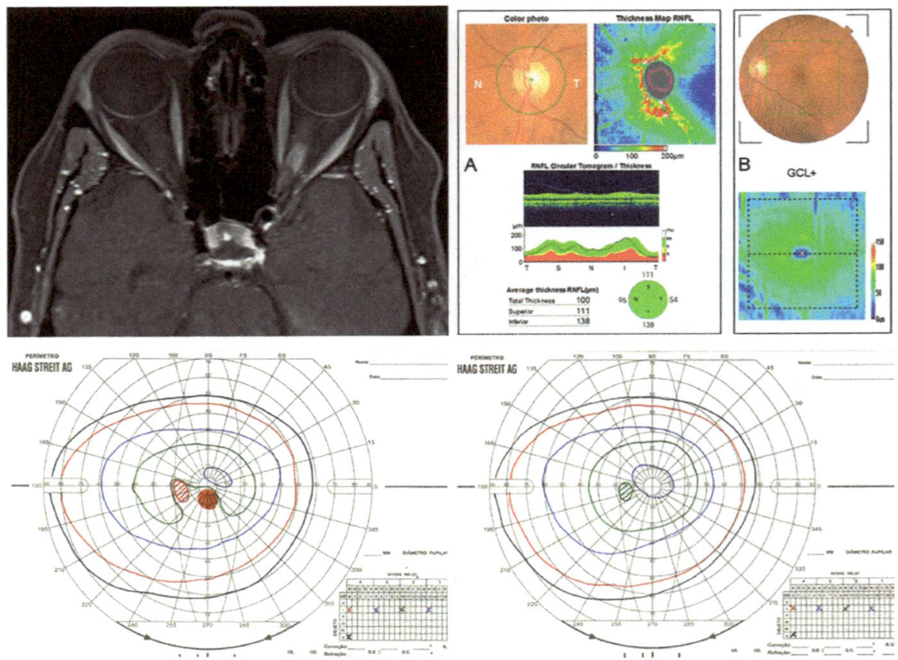

Fig. 10.3 A 51-year-old woman with progressive visual loss in the left eye for 1 year was found to have an optic nerve sheath meningioma (upper left). Optical coherence tomography (Topcon 3D-OCT 2000™) revealed normal peripapillary retinal nerve fiber layer (upper right, **a**). Segmented macular thickness measurements indicated normal macular ganglion cell layer (upper right, **b**). The patient presented with an inferior paracentral scotoma and constricted field (lower left) and showed significant improvement after conformational radiation therapy (lower right)

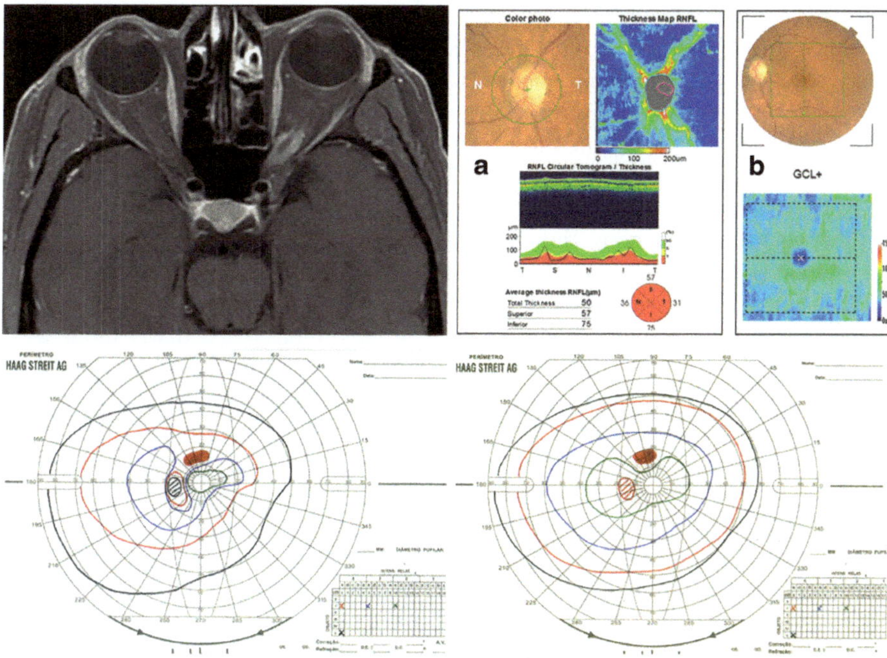

Fig. 10.4 A 49-year-old woman with a 7-year history of visual loss in the left eye from an optic nerve sheath meningioma (upper left). Optical coherence tomography (Topcon 3D-OCT 2000™) revealed severely reduced peripapillary retinal nerve fiber layer (upper right, **a**). Segmented macular thickness measurements indicated markedly reduced macular ganglion cell layer (upper right, **b**). The patient presented with a severe constriction, enlarged blind spot and superior paracentral scotoma (lower left). There was only mild visual improvement after conformational radiation therapy (lower right)

hand, when significant RNFL and macular GCL is present indicating established axonal loss, successful treatment should be aimed at preventing further visual loss and absence of visual improvement is not an indication of treatment failure (Fig. 10.4).

While ONSM are usually treated with radiotherapy, patients with tumors from the skull base meninges but compressing the optic pathway are usually treated with surgery. Visual outcome after decompressive surgery however is variable; while a significant number of patients experience improvement or stability of vision, 20–30% deteriorate [32]. Although several risk factors for poor visual outcomes are known including prolonged duration of symptoms, the presence of disc pallor and incomplete tumor resection, estimating the potential for visual recovery may be difficult based on the clinical exam and imaging finding alone. Loo et al. [19] performed a study to determine the prognostic value of pretreatment OCT measurement of the peripapillary RNFL in final visual outcomes of patients with anterior visual pathway meningioma and optic neuropathy. The authors evaluated the outcome of 14 eyes of 12 patients treated in which pretreatment and post-treatment OCT along with clinical examination were performed. After treatment, the group with normal RNFL experienced significant improvement in the VA, color vision, and VF compared with the group with reduced peripapillary RNFL. The findings in this study is a further indication that patients with compressive optic neuropathy due to anterior pathway meningioma are more likely to improve post-treatment if they have a normal pretreatment RNFL.

Optic nerve gliomas are the most common tumors of the optic nerve but represent only 1% of all intracranial tumors [33]. While malignant gliomas may occur in the adult, the large majority of gliomas are benign juvenile pilocytic astrocytomas that present primarily among children in the first decade of life. The natural history of childhood optic nerve gliomas is almost always benign and most patients retain stable visual function without treatment. A conservative management is usually recommended to patients with unilateral optic nerve gliomas, particularly those with neurofibromatosis type 1 (NF-1) [34]. On the other hand in uncommon cases of more aggressive tumors, particularly those near of affecting the optic chiasm chemotherapy can be used to help stabilize the lesion [35].

Both in patients with optic pathway gliomas (OPG) followed with conservatively without treatment and in those submitted to chemotheraphy, assessment of visual function along with imaging studies is the main parameters used to evaluate disease progression on follow-up examinations. However, monitoring young children with OPGs for visual deterioration can be difficult owing to age-related noncompliance. OCT measures of peripapillary RNFL and macular thickness can be of significant help in monitoring the integrity of the visual pathway and has been proposed as a surrogate marker of vision in previous studies evaluating OCT findings in patients with OPG.

Chang et al. [36] evaluated, using TD-OCT, both macular and RNFL thickness measurements in patients with NF-1 with or without optic gliomas and controls. The authors found that NF-1 subjects with OPG had average RNFL thickness and macular volume significantly reduced compared to those without gliomas. The study suggests that OCT can be used to detect RNFL thinning secondary to NF-1 related OPGs and that it may be a useful adjunct to routine clinical ophthalmologic evaluation in children with NF-1.

Avery et al. [37] prospectively evaluated 62 patients with NF-1 and optic nerve gliomas submitted to neuro-ophthalmic examination including TD-OCT of the optic nerve head. Eighty-nine eyes of patients with OPG were included and 41 classified as having abnormal VA or VF loss. Reduced RNFL thickness was associated significantly reduced VA and contrast sensitivity. The study indicated that reduced OCT-measured RNFL is a sensitive technology to detect visual loss in OPG.

Parrozzoni et al. [38] compared visual function and SD-OCT measured RNFL thickness for the screening of OPG in 57 pediatric patients affected by NF-1. Visual function assessment, RNFL analysis, and optic disc evaluation results correlated with the presence of OPGs, but only RNFL analysis reached statistically significant sensitivity and positive predictive value. The authors concluded that RNFL analysis assessment using SD-OCT is superior to visual function assessment and optic disc evaluation as a clinical screening tool for OPGs. Macular thickness measurements were not investigated.

Fard et al. [39] studied 38 eyes of 23 children with OPG and evaluated the relationship between SD-OCT findings and clinical/radiological changes at diagnosis and on a 24-month follow-up evaluation. Mean changes in average RNFL and macular thickness measurements were significantly higher in patients that had clinical/radiological progression of the gliomas compared to those that did not progressed. OCT measurements were significantly different in patients with tumor progression compared to those that did not progress indicating that OCT measurements may be helpful in monitoring OPG. Gu et al. [40] evaluated the macular GC-inner plexiform layer (GC-IPL) thickness in children with or without visual loss from OPG using SD-OCT. Decreased GC-IPL thickness was able to discriminate between children with and without vision loss from their OPG. The authors concluded that GC-IPL thickness could be used as a surrogate marker of vision in children with OPGs. Two other reports have also indicated the value of OCT-measured peripapillary RNFL and macular thickness parameters in the diagnosis and follow-up of patients with OPG [41, 42].

While the above-mentioned studies have indicated the value of OCT in monitoring visual function in OPG, an important limitation for obtaining OCT measurements in this condition is that gliomas usually occur in young patients, when the technique is also limited by patient cooperation. However, Avery et al. [43] used a hand-held OCT to obtain optic nerve and retinal thickness measurements during sedation in 33 young children with OPGs. The authors concluded that for young children who do not cooperate with vision testing, hand-held OCT measures may be a surrogate marker of vision. More recently, the same authors [44] reported the results of an investigation in 55 eyes of patients with OPG that were followed longitudinally and completed 250 OCT examinations. They concluded that children experiencing visual loss frequently demonstrate a decline $\geq 10\%$ of peripapillary RNFL thickness measurements in one or more sectors of the disc further emphasizing that peripapillary RNFL thickness measurements may be helpful in the follow up of OPG.

10.3 Dysthyroid Optic Neuropathy

Graves' orbitopathy (GO) is an autoimmune inflammatory process affecting the orbital and periorbital tissues, mainly the extraocular muscles but also the retrobulbar fat. GO occurs before, during or after the onset of hyperthyroidism and, less frequently, in euthyroid or hypothyroid patients [45]. The enlargement of the extraocular muscles is responsible for most of the debilitating manifestations of the disease, including proptosis, diplopia, congestive signs and dysthyroid optic neuropathy (DON) [45, 46].

DON is a serious complication of GO occurring in 3.4% of patients [47], almost always as a result of optic nerve compression at the orbital apex by enlarged extraocular muscles. The diagnosis of DON rests mainly on clinical findings, such as decreased VA, abnormal VF, altered color and brightness perception, delayed visual evoked potentials, afferent pupillary defects and edema or atrophy of the optic nerve head [48]. Nevertheless, DON is often subclinical and in many cases difficult to diagnose due to confounding signs and symptoms, especially significant orbital congestion or decreased corneal transparency due to exposure keratopathy. Establishing a diagnosis may also be difficult because many tests of optic nerve dysfunction, such as VA, color and brightness perception and VF, especially when performed with standard automated perimetry, require full cooperation of an alert and motivated patient and will not infrequently render false positive results, particularly in patients with congestive GO.

Because the prognosis of DON improves significantly with early diagnosis and treatment, much effort has been put into designing objective tests capable of identifying patients at high risk for developing DON. Therefore imaging studies, particularly CT scanning of the orbit are often used to investigate the possibility of DON [49]. Several studies have tested the ability of CT parameters (linear, area and volume measurements of the orbital muscles) to raise suspicion and facilitate the diagnosis of DON [49, 50]. More recently, OCT measurements have been introduced in the management of GO.

In patients with GO, OCT can be of help in the diagnosis and in follow-up of DON. Because DON can present with optic disc edema, OCT can help its detection and measurement to monitor treatment efficacy. While no previous studies have specifically evaluated the use of OCT for monitoring optic disc edema in GO, many studies have documented the ability of the equipment for that purpose in patients with papilledema [51, 52]. Presumably the same rationale applies for measuring optic disc edema in patients with DON. On the other hand, many patients with DON present without optic disc edema, either with atrophy or with normal optic disc appearance. As in any other compressive optic neuropathy, OCT thickness measurements can help quantifying axonal loss in patients with DON both help establishing the diagnosis as well as to estimate the chances of reversing visual loss (Fig. 10.5).

Very few studies, however, have critically evaluated OCT in GO and in special those with DON. Forte et al. [53] evaluated the RNFL in patients with GO and ocular hypertension using OCT. The authors found that RNFL loss on OCT was found in 9 of the 30 patients evaluated. However, apparently the patients did not have well-defined DON and the authors concluded that RNFL loss was important to detect the presence of optic neuropathy but could not differentiate whether the causative effect was DON or the elevated intraocular pressures.

One study evaluated patients with DON using OCT but as a secondary measurements when investigating the value of multifocal visual evoked potentials (mfVEP). Perez-Rico et al. [54] evaluated 65 eyes of 34 consecutive patients with GO using mfVEP, SAP and OCT (Stratus TD-OCT). The authors found mfVEP abnormalities in 27% of eyes and diffuse VF defects in 20% indicating that a significant number of eyes had DON. OCT-measured RNFL did not differ from normal and no correlation was found between mfVEP, VF and OCT data. While the study might indicate a poor sensitivity to detect abnormalities on OCT it may also be interpreted as indicating reversibility of visual function abnormalities in the patients.

It is widely known that visual loss in DON can be reversible when properly treated, provided there is no significant permanent optic nerve damage. The finding of normal RNFL in a patient with significant visual loss would therefore be a strong indicator for further treatment to obtain visual recovery (Fig. 10.5).

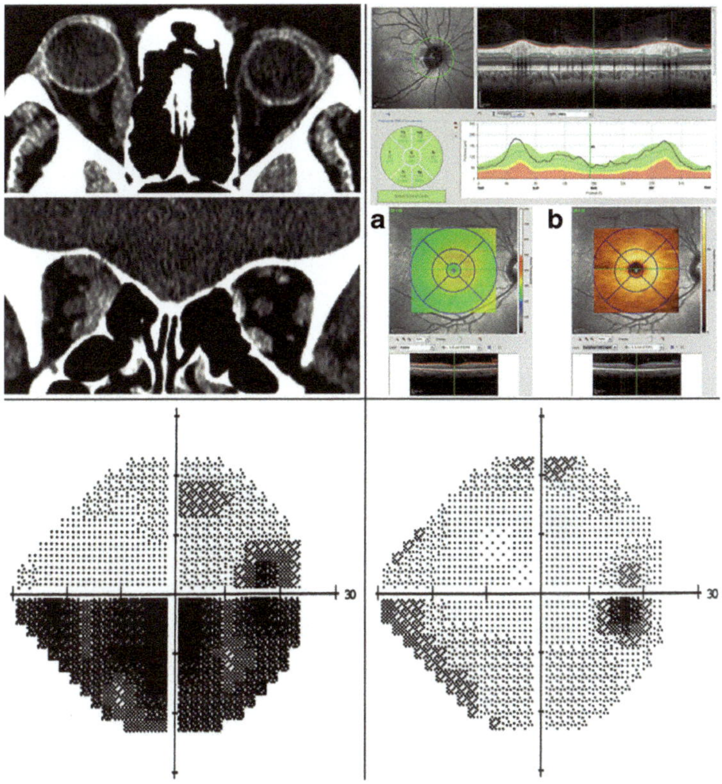

Fig. 10.5 A 50-year-old woman with Graves' orbitopathy presented with double vision, proptosis for 3 months and a 2-week history of visual loss in the right eye (OD). Computerized tomography scan showed enlarged medial and inferior rectus muscles and crowding at the orbital apex (upper left). Visual acuity was 20/200 and there was inferior altitudinal field loss (lower left). Optical coherence tomography (OCT) scan (HRA Spectralis™, Heidelberg Engineering) showed normal peripapillary retinal nerve fiber layer (upper right). Macular thickness measurements showed normal full-thickness (**a**) and normal macular ganglion cell layer (**b**). There was marked improvement of both visual acuity and visual field after orbital decompressive surgery (lower right) in accordance with the normal retinal neural integrity as assessed by OCT

10.4 Other Compressive Optic Nerve Diseases

Optic nerve compression can also be due to a number of orbital and adnexal conditions including extrinsic tumors of the orbit, osseous diseases leading to optic nerve compression at the canal, sinusal processes invading the orbit, metastases and lymphoproliferative diseases that can lead to optic nerve dysfunction. Very few of these conditions have been evaluated systematically using OCT but the instrument can certainly be an important additional data in the diagnosis by characterizing the presence of an optic neuropathy as well as estimating the chances of visual recovery after treatment (Fig. 10.6).

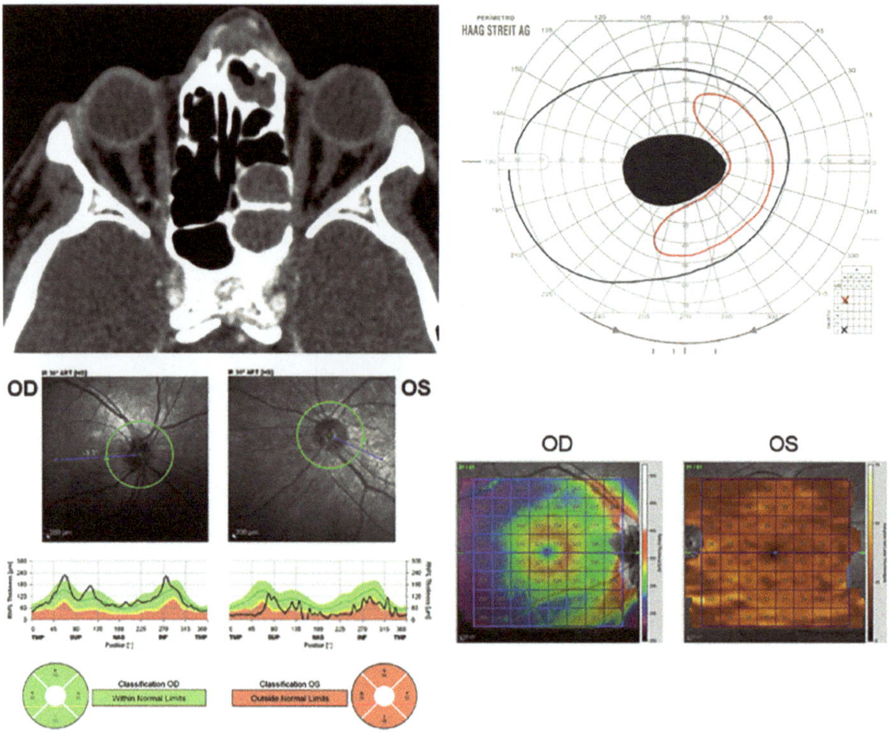

Fig. 10.6 A 52-year-old man had severe visual loss in the left eye (OS) due to a spheno-ethmoidal mucocele compressing the optic nerve at the optic canal and the orbital apex (upper left). Visual field showed a dense central scotoma (upper right) and visual acuity was reduced to finger counting. Optical coherence tomography (OCT) scan (HRA Spectralis™, Heidelberg Engineering) showed severely reduced peripapillary retinal nerve fiber layer in OS and was normal in the right eye (OD) (lower left). Segmented macular scans showed normal macular ganglion cell layer in OD and severely reduced in OS (lower right). There was no significant improvement of vision after surgery in accordance with the severe retinal neural loss observed on OCT

10.5 Compressive Chiasmal Diseases

Compressive lesions at the optic chiasmal region are among the most important lesions of the anterior visual pathway and can be caused by a number of lesions including pituitary adenoma, craniopharyngioma, meningioma, Rathke cleft cysts, aneurism and metastatic lesions. Pituitary tumors are the most common cause of chiasmal compression, representing 10–15% of intracranial tumors [55]. Visual loss is a frequent finding and occurs in 32–70% of patients [55]. Functioning tumors can present with clinical symptoms related to hormonal abnormalities, such as impotence, amenorrhea, galactorrhea, acromegaly and Cushing's syndrome, but in many cases visual complaints are the most relevant symptoms at presentation. On the other hand, in nonfunctioning pituitary adenomas visual complaints are generally the only symptoms. The lesions produce reduced VA, loss of color vision and particularly VF defects. However, because visual symptoms are usually vague early on the course of the disease, the diagnosis may be delayed until later stages when permanent damage of the visual pathway has already occurred.

Chiasmal lesions can lead to a wide variety of visual and axonal damage to the visual pathway fibers, ranging from mild VF defect and focal peripapillary RNFL and macular GCL loss to severe and diffuse visual loss and optic nerve atrophy and retinal GCL loss. In most cases, however, typical bitemporal VF defect occur and a specific pattern of axonal loss develops. In patients with mid-chiasmal lesions, temporal hemianopia and preserved nasal field, the crossed nerve fibers are lost with preservation of the uncrossed nerve fibers, which originate in the temporal hemiretina and penetrate the optic nerve through the superior and inferior arcuate fiber bundles. Thus, RNFL loss occurs predominantly on the nasal and temporal side of the optic disc, a pattern identified on ophthalmoscopy as band atrophy (BA) of the optic nerve [56], and the retina may show a clear distinction in the pattern of axonal loss when the temporal hemiretina is compared with the affected nasal hemiretina (Fig. 10.7).

Chiasmal lesions were the first compressive anterior visual pathway diseases to be evaluated using OCT when we and other authors have demonstrated that retinal thickness measurements could detect neural loss in patients with temporal hemianopia caused by suprasellar tumors and that such measurements were able to identify the BA pattern of axonal loss found in this condition, based peripapillary RNFL thickness measurements using early generation TD-OCT devices (Fig. 10.8) [4, 57–59]. Later studies with SD and SS-OCT equipments [14, 16, 60–62] largely confirmed the ability of the technology to detect peripapillary RNFL loss in pituitary tumors, including the characteristic pattern of BA of the optic nerve (Fig. 10.9).

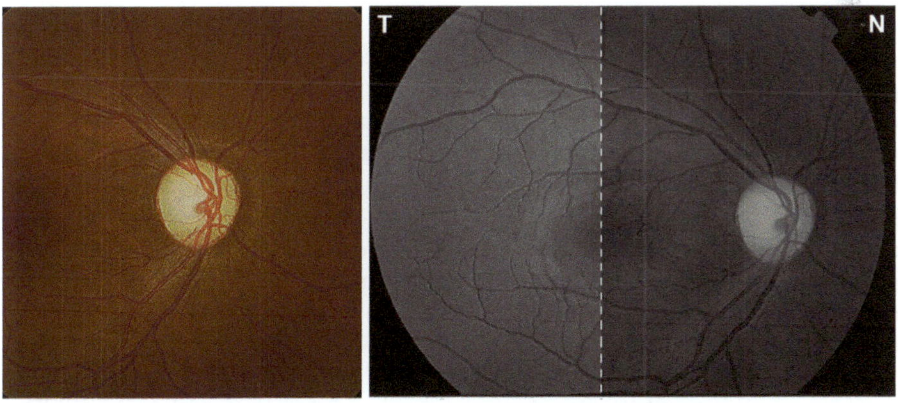

Fig. 10.7 Optic nerve (left) and fundus photograph (right) of a patient complete temporal hemianopia with normal nasal hemifield, band atrophy of the optic nerve and a pattern of retinal nerve fiber layer loss in the temporal and nasal portions of the optic nerve with relative preservation of the superior and inferior arcuate fibers (left) and the demarcation between the retinal area with preserved ganglions cells (temporal) and the areas with atrophic ganglion cells (nasal). T = temporal; N = nasal (modified from Cunha LP, et al., Doc Ophthalmol 2008; 117:223–32)

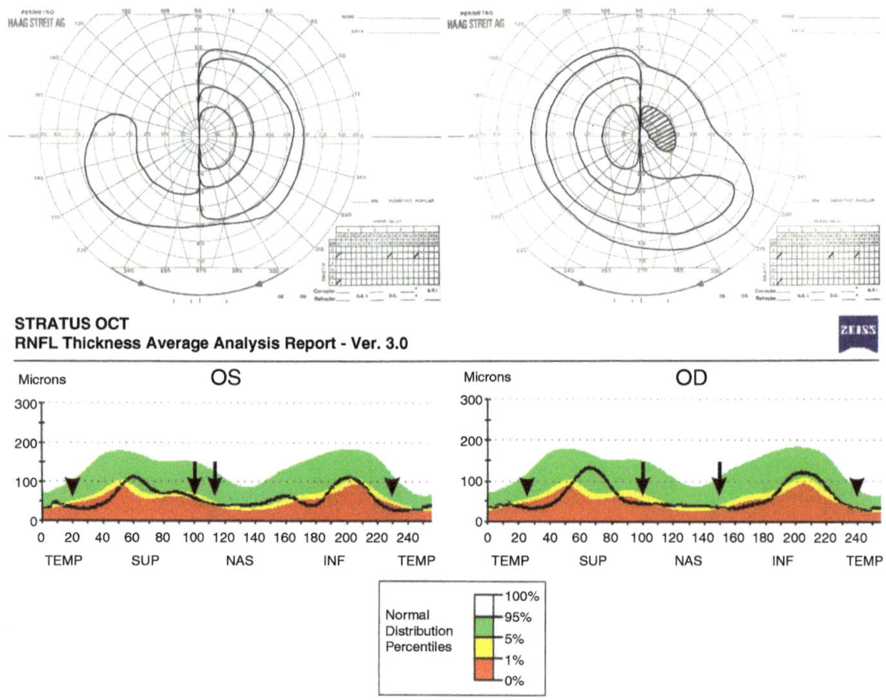

Fig. 10.8 Above, Goldmann visual fields showing bitemporal severe loss in a patient with pituitary adenoma. Below, Stratus™ (Carl Zeiss, Meditec), time-domain Optical coherence tomography showing diffuse retinal nerve fiber layer loss in both eyes mostly in the nasal (arrows) and temporal (arrowheads) aspects of the optic nerve (from Leal BC, et al., Arq Bras Oftalmol 2006; 69:251–4)

A few years after the initial studies evaluating only peripapillary RFNL thickness parameters, we have demonstrated that full-thickness macular thickness measurements were also able to detect axonal loss in chiasmal compression and correlated well both with peripapillary RNFL and with VF defects [13, 60, 63]. Discrimination ability and the relationship between OCT thickness measurements and VF loss were similar with both sets of measurements although macular thickness measurements allowed a better correlation when quadrantic measurements of the macula were obtained [13]. Because the RNFL of different quadrants and different hemifields enter the optic disc in a way that the fibers from different quadrants superimpose one with the other, specific correlation of RNFL with VF is somewhat cumbersome at the optic disc. With the exception of the nasal area of the disc all other sectors receive retinal nerve fibers from both the nasal and the temporal hemiretina. The result is a lack of specificity between VF loss and optic disc sectors in patients with lesions of the optic chiasm [13, 14]. For example, when a VF defect affecting the superotemporal quadrant is present, it results in RNFL loss in the nasal, temporal and inferior regions of the optic disc. Since the inferior region of the optic disc also receives nerve fibers from the unaffected nasal VF, there is presumably a lack of specificity in the structure-function relationship.

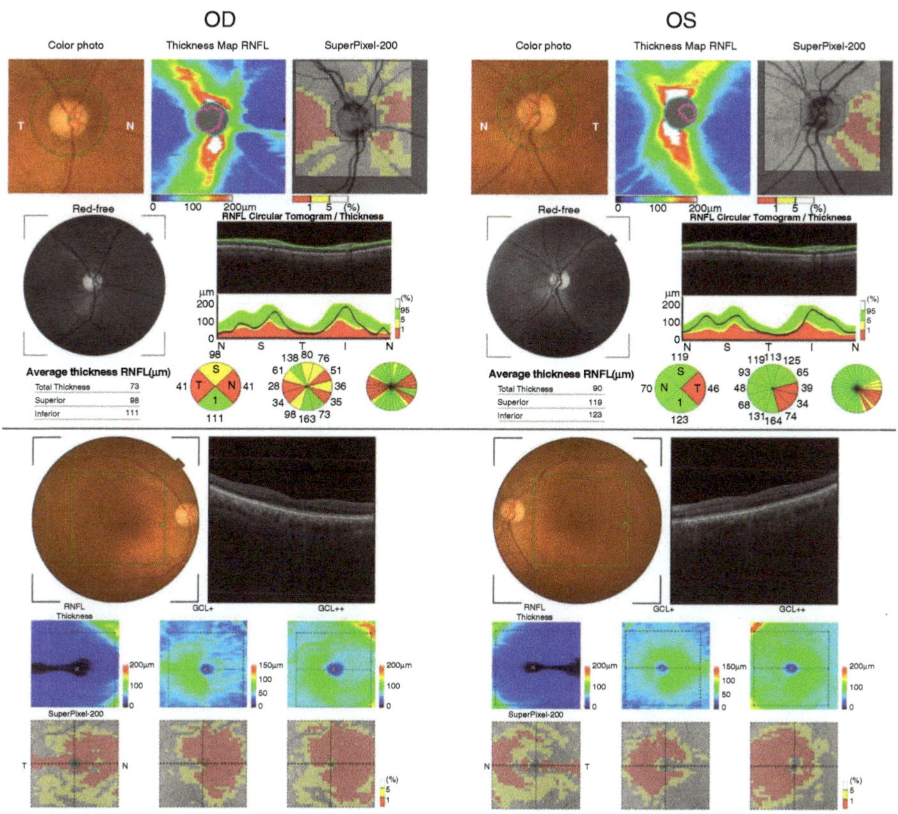

Fig. 10.9 Optical coherence tomography (DRI OCT Triton Plus®, Topcon, Japan) of a 56-year-old woman with a large pituitary adenoma compressing the optic chiasm and bitemporal hemianopia. Above, note significantly reduced peripapillary retinal nerve fiber layer in the nasal and temporal quadrants of the right eye (OD) and in the temporal quadrant in the left eye (OS). Below, scanning of the macular areas showing marked thinning of the ganglion cell layer in the nasal hemiretina of both eyes

On the other hand, with macular thickness measurements a superotemporal VF defect may be related to reduced macular thickness below and nasally to the fovea, with a direct correspondence to the quadrantic VF defect. The advantage of macular thickness measurements is even greater in patients with temporal hemianopia, affecting both the superior and the inferior temporal quadrants. Based on the distribution of the RNFL on the optic disc [64], such patients may be expected to have RNFL loss in every quadrant of the optic disc, with a resultant lack of specificity in the structure-function relationship, while macular thickness reduction would be observed almost exclusively nasally to the fovea, probably with a much higher specificity. In previous studies we have demonstrated a closest structure-function relationships observed between macular thickness measurements and VF abnormalities compared to the relationship between peripapillary RNFL thickness measurements and VF defects [13]. The relationship between OCT-measured macular thickness parameters and VF defects were even greater when segmented macular thickness measurements were used and separate analysis of the retina GCL is possible (Figs. 10.9 and 10.10), and a number of studies have confirmed the greater sensitivity of inner macular thickness parameters to detect neural loss in chiasmal compression [9, 14, 62, 65–71].

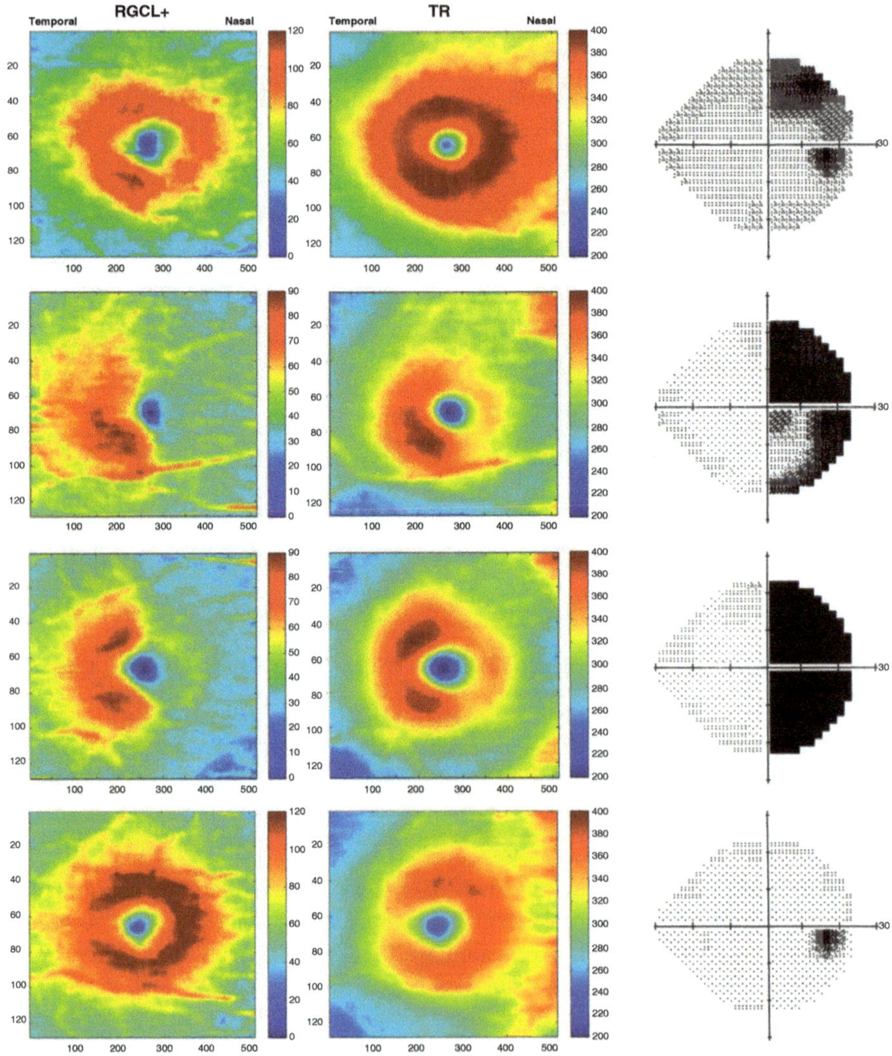

Fig. 10.10 Pseudo-color thickness map generated from cube scan based on the thickness of the macular layers obtained using spectral-domain optical coherence tomography (Topcon 3D-OCT 1000™). First, second and third lines = eyes with band atrophy of the optic nerve and different degrees of visual field loss. Fourth line = a normal control. RGCL+ = retinal ganglion cell layer associated with the inner plexiform layer. TR = total retinal thickness. Notice that thickness reduction in the nasal hemiretinas is more evident in the RGCL+ when compared to TR (modified from Monteiro MLR, et al. Invest Ophthalmol Vis Sci 2014; 55:3328–36)

Several studies have evaluated the relationship between OCT findings and VF or electrophysiological testing. In one study, we have also shown that OCT measurements correlated well both with VF and the finding on pattern electroretinogram in patients with chiasmal compression [72]. In another study we have even demonstrated a significant correlation between OCT and multifocal pattern electroretinogram measurements in such patients [73]. Moon et al. [74] showed an important correlation between reduced peripapillary RNFL thickness and decreased b wave on the photopic negative response, both associated with worse VF outcome. More recently we have documented significant correlation between OCT and multifocal visual evoked potential measurements [61]. Therefore, OCT can also be associated with other electrophysiological methods as prognostic indicator in the preoperative assessment of chiasmal compression.

While in most patients with chiasmal compression treatment is usually necessary, estimating the prognosis for visual recovery is particularly important in patients with recurrent tumors where the need for further surgery is in question. Although it is expected that visual improvement may occur after optic pathway decompression, in many cases such recovery is variable and many times difficult to predict [75–78]. Although other predictive values such as duration of symptoms, age, size of tumor, the severity of VA and VF loss as the presence or absence of optic disc pallor have been used to estimate visual recovery, the results are far from ideal [76–80]. The grading of optic disc pallor is difficult and subjective [79]. Therefore the use of OCT to quantify axonal loss through peripapillary RNFL and macular thickness measurements seems to be one of the most important predictor of visual recovery (Figs. 10.11 and 10.12).

While both peripapillary RNFL and macular thickness measurements are important for estimating retinal axonal loss in chiasmal compression, studies using

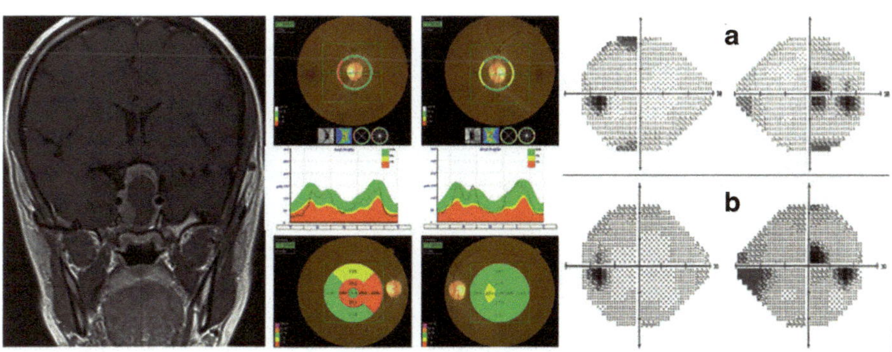

Fig. 10.11 32-year-old woman with a large pituitary adenoma with chiasmal compression (left). Middle: optical coherence tomography (OCT) scan (Topcon 3D-OCT 1000™) revealed reduced peripapillary retinal nerve fiber layer in the temporal portion of the right eye (in red) and in the nasal and temporal portions of the left eye (in yellow). Full-thickness macular measurements showed thinning mostly of the nasal macula (in red or yellow) indicating retinal axonal loss. Right: visual fields showing bilateral defect pre-operatively (**a**) and no significant improvement after surgery (**b**) in accordance with the finding of permanent retinal axonal loss on OCT

high-resolution OCT with segmented analysis of macular thickness measurements demonstrates that GCL+ measurements show abnormality before peripapillary RNFL loss is detectable (Figs. 10.13 and 10.14) [14, 65–68, 71].

Several studies have evaluated prospectively the ability of OCT in predicting visual improvement in chiasmal compression. Such studies have shown a significant correlation between the depth and thickness of the RNFL measured by OCT and the possibility of improvement in patients that undergo surgery for tumors involving the chiamal region [22, 81]. Danesh-Meyer et al. [22] evaluated 40 patients with chiasmal compression with TD-OCT and VF both pre- and post-surgical decompression. Patients with preoperative RNFL below 97.5% of normal values did not demonstrate significant improvement in VA and VF mean deviation in the post-operative period while those with normal RNFL thickness had significant improvement in VA. The authors found that there was an increased likelihood of postoperative improvement with thicker preoperative RNFL until approximately 85 um. In a subsequent study, Danesh-Meyer et al. [82] evaluated the data of 107 patients with pituitary tumor that underwent surgical treatment evaluating pre-operatively peripapillary RNFL and the VF mean deviation (MD). Patients with thin pre-operative RNFL (defined as the fifth percentile of normative values) had more severe VF defects than the group with normal RNFL thickness. Long-term follow up showed that 81% of eyes with normal RNFL, compared to 37.1% with thin RNFL, achieved an MD of 2.00 dB at the final visit. The results showed that long-term visual recovery after surgical decompression of pituitary lesions can be predicted by pre-operative OCT-measured peripapillary RNFL.

Jacob et al. [81] showed that the odds of complete VF recovery in patients with pituitary adenomas compressing the visual pathways that underwent trans-sphenoidal surgery was multiplied by 1.29 for each increase in 1 micron of mean RNFL. The

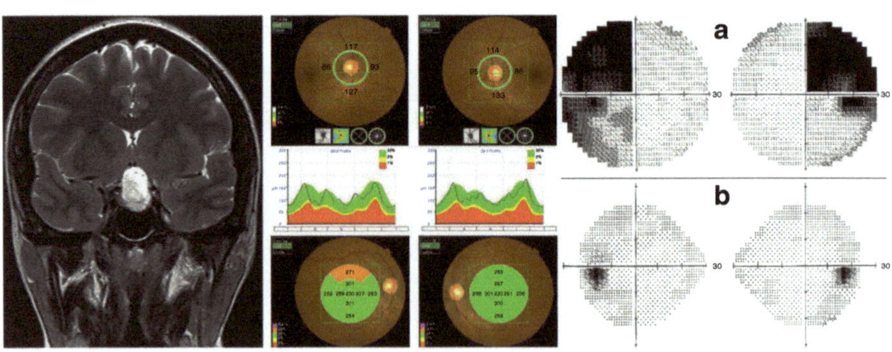

Fig. 10.12 A 24-year-old pregnant woman developed a large pituitary adenoma with chiasmal compression (left). Middle: optical coherence tomography (Topcon 3D-OCT 1000™) revealed normal peripapillary retinal nerve fiber layer in both eyes. Full-thickness macular measurements showed normal measurements indicating retinal axonal normality. Right: visual fields showing bitemporal quadrantic defect pre-operatively (**a**) and normal visual field after surgery (**b**) in accordance with normal OCT findings

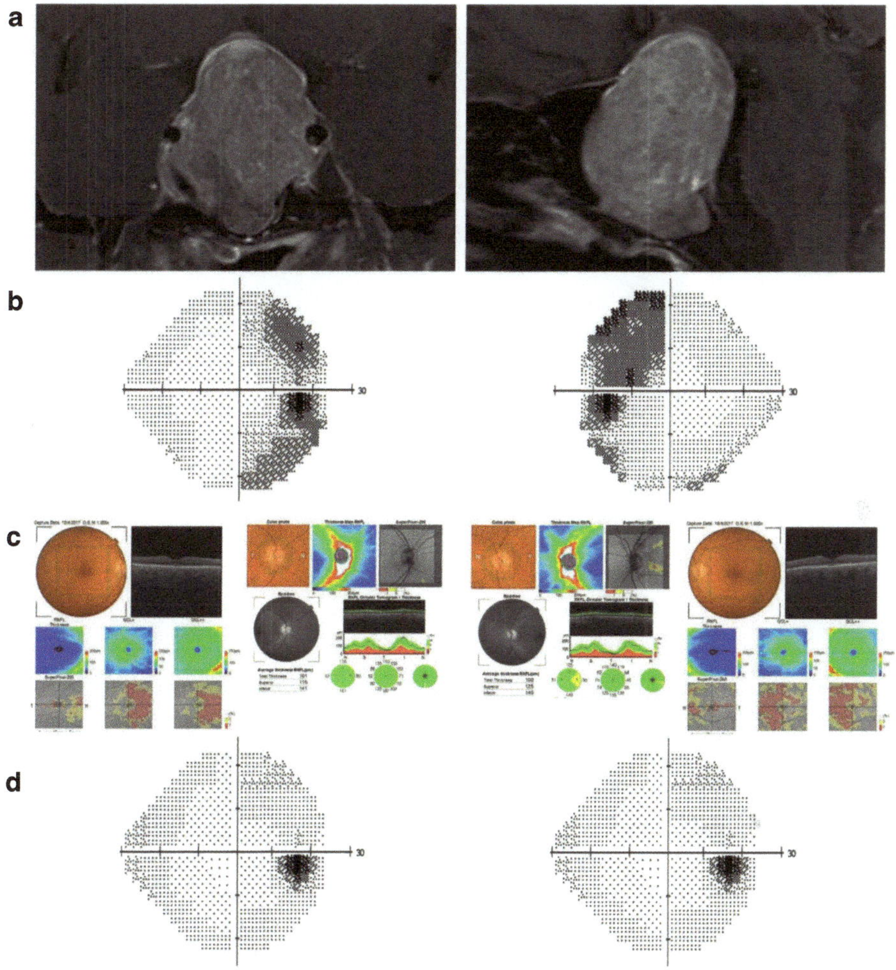

Fig. 10.13 A 45-year-old man underwent neuroimaging studies because of headache. Magnetic resonance imaging on coronal (left) and sagittal (right) cuts showed a large non-secreting pituitary adenoma (**a**). Standard automated perimetry (24-2 threshold test) revealed bitemporal visual field defects (**b**). Optical coherence tomography (DRI OCT Triton Plus®, Topcon, Japan) revealed peripapillary retinal nerve fiber layer within normal limits in the right eye and borderline reduction in the temporal quadrant in the left eye (**c**). Macular thickness measurements revealed significant macular ganglion cell layer loss in the nasal hemiretina of both eyes (**c**). After surgery, there was significant improvement of visual fields (**d**) on both eyes. Note that there was significant reduction in macular ganglion cell layer despite only minor abnormalities in the peripapillary retinal nerve fiber (**c**). Also, note that there was significant improvement in the visual field defect despite the presence of macular ganglion cell layer thinning in both eyes

authors concluded that RNFL thinning measured by OCT leads to a decreased chance of recovery of an initial VF defect 3 months after treatment.

Ohkubo et al. [83] evaluated the relationship between macular GCL and VF parameters in chiasmal compression and the potential for GCL parameters in order to predict the short-term post-surgical VF. Examining the macular GCL

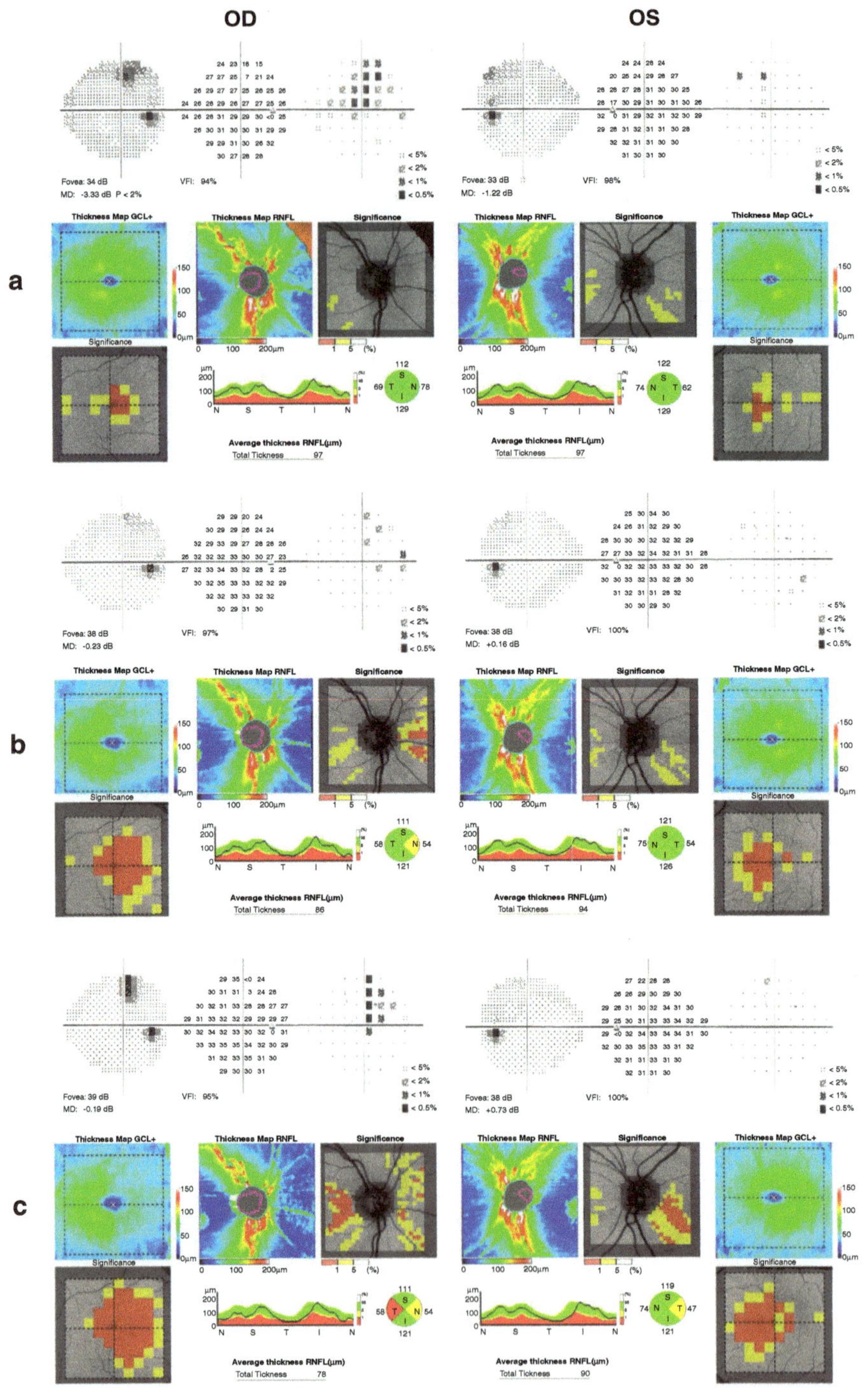
OD
OS
a
b
c
Fovea: 34 dB
MD: -3.33 dB P < 2%
VFI: 94%
Fovea: 33 dB
MD: -1.22 dB
VFI: 98%
Fovea: 38 dB
MD: -0.23 dB
VFI: 97%
Fovea: 38 dB
MD: +0.16 dB
VFI: 100%
Fovea: 39 dB
MD: -0.19 dB
VFI: 95%
Fovea: 38 dB
MD: +0.73 dB
VFI: 100%
< 5%
< 2%
< 1%
< 0.5%
Thickness Map GCL+
Thickness Map RNFL
Significance
Average thickness RNFL(μm)
Total Tickness 97
Total Tickness 97
Total Tickness 86
Total Tickness 94
Total Tickness 78
Total Tickness 90

Fig. 10.14 Data for the right (OD, left row) and left eye (OS, right row) of a patient with a large pituitary tumor compressing the optic chiasm, obtained at three sequential examinations (**a**: November 2015, **b**: August 2016, and **c**: August 2017). The upper row of each point in time shows the visual field (VF) gray scale (left), sensitivity data in decibels (center) and pattern deviation plot (right). The mid and lower rows are optical coherence tomography findings (OCT-2000, Topcon corporation, Tokyo, Japan): pseudo-colored thickness maps of the macular ganglion cell layer + the inner plexiform layer (Thickness Map GCL+) and, immediately below, significance patterns with color-coded grids (no color = within normal limits; yellow = outside the 95% normal limit; red = outside the 99% normal limit); pseudo-colored map of the peripapillary retinal nerve fiber layer (Thickness Map RNFL) and corresponding significance patterns with color-coded grids. Peripapillary global average and quadrantic and RFNL thickness measurements as well as a graphic demonstration of the thickness profile are also presented. Note that retinal GCL+ was abnormal on the first examination although peripapillary RNFL were still within normal limits (**a**). Also, note definite worsening of peripapillary RNFL thickness profile as well as nasal hemiretina RGC+ layer in both eyes, on the follow-up examinations (**b** and **c**) despite only mild worsening of VF defect in the right and none in the left eye (modified from Monteiro MLR. J Neuroophthalmol. 2018; 38:124–127)

was useful for evaluating structural damage in patients with chiasmal compression. Preoperative GCL parameters, especially focal loss of GCL, seemed useful in predicting visual function following surgical decompression of chiasmal compression.

However, while GCL loss certainly indicates that permanent damage exists, it is important to know that presence of GCL+ thinning does not exclude the possibility of significant recovery of VF defect. Tieger et al. [66] reported a series of 23 patients with chiasmal compression evaluated with OCT and standard automated perimetry (SAP) before and after surgical treatment. Because some of their patients showed complete VF recovery despite persistent macular GCL layer thinning on OCT, the authors suggested that RGC loss may precede VF defect, at least when assessed with standard 24-2 or 30-2 threshold strategies with size III target on SAP. Recently, I was able to confirm such suggestion in a patient with a pituitary tumor compressing the chiasm that was followed for 21 months with OCT, SAP (using the 24-2 threshold strategy) and manual Goldmann perimetry [84]. Although surgery was indicated, the patient declined it and opted for conservative management. Sequential examinations clearly showed that GCL+ loss preceded the development of peripapillary RNFL reduction (Fig. 10.14). Also, while there was only mild deterioration of the VF over the follow-up period, OCT data (especially GCL+ thickness) displayed significant worsening in both eyes, indicating that in chronic compressive lesions, retinal structures may be impaired prior to clinically detectable VF loss, at least with most commonly used strategies [84].

On the other hand, it is important to consider that axonal loss may appear later in the course of the disease, even after optic pathway decompression has occurred. Moon et al. [70] evaluated 19 patients undergoing chiasmal decompression before and 1 and 3 months after surgery. Visual recovery was significantly correlated with the changes in retinal GCL and RNFL thickness measurements. However, prolonged retrograde degeneration progressed for some period, even after surgical decompression and visual recovery occurred.

10.6 Conclusions

With progressive improvement in technology OCT has become an extremely useful instrument in a number of neuro-ophthalmic diseases. While continued research on the subject is necessary to better understand the precise relationship between OCT and VA, VF and other modalities of visual function evaluation, a large number of previous studies as well as clinical observation clearly indicate the importance of using OCT in diagnosis, treatment as well as follow-up of compressive optic neuropathies. As both technology and interpretation of data advances we expect the use of OCT in the management of this important group of optic nerve diseases will certainly continue to increase.

References

1. Chan JW. Compressive and infiltrative optic neuropathies. In: Chan JW, editor. Optic nerve disorders diagnosis and management. New York: Springer; 2007. p. 88–129.
2. Monteiro ML, Medeiros FA, Ostroscki MR. Quantitative analysis of axonal loss in band atrophy of the optic nerve using scanning laser polarimetry. Br J Ophthalmol. 2003;87(1):32–7.
3. Sergott RC, Balcer LJ. The latest on optical coherence tomography. J Neuroophthalmol. 2014;34(Suppl):S1–2.
4. Monteiro ML, Leal BC, Rosa AA, Bronstein MD. Optical coherence tomography analysis of axonal loss in band atrophy of the optic nerve. Br J Ophthalmol. 2004;88(7):896–9.
5. Mendoza-Santiesteban CE, Lopez-Felipe D, Fernandez-Cherkasova L, Hernandez-Echavarria O, Hernandez-Silva Y, Gonzalez-Garcia A. Microperimetry in the study of neuro-ophthalmic diseases. Semin Ophthalmol. 2010;25(4):136–43.
6. Pasol J. Neuro-ophthalmic disease and optical coherence tomography: glaucoma look-alikes. Curr Opin Ophthalmol. 2011;22(2):124–32.
7. Chen JJ. Optical coherence tomography and neuro-ophthalmology. J Neuroophthalmol. 2018;38(1):e5–8.
8. Monteiro ML. Optical coherence tomography in neuro-ophthalmology: do we really need it? J Neuroophthalmol. 2016;36(4):353–5.
9. Kardon RH. Role of the macular optical coherence tomography scan in neuro-ophthalmology. J Neuroophthalmol. 2011;31(4):353–61.
10. Costello F. Optical coherence tomography in neuro-ophthalmology. Neurol Clin. 2017;35(1):153–63.
11. Adhi M, Duker JS. Optical coherence tomography--current and future applications. Curr Opin Ophthalmol. 2013;24(3):213–21.
12. Mrejen S, Spaide RF. Optical coherence tomography: imaging of the choroid and beyond. Surv Ophthalmol. 2013;58(5):387–429.
13. Monteiro ML, Costa-Cunha LV, Cunha LP, Malta RF. Correlation between macular and retinal nerve fibre layer Fourier-domain OCT measurements and visual field loss in chiasmal compression. Eye (Lond). 2010;24(8):1382–90.

14. Monteiro ML, Hokazono K, Fernandes DB, Costa-Cunha LV, Sousa RM, Raza AS, et al. Evaluation of inner retinal layers in eyes with temporal hemianopic visual loss from chiasmal compression using optical coherence tomography. Invest Ophthalmol Vis Sci. 2014;55(5):3328–36.
15. Lam BL. Retinal ganglion cell thickness to assess the optic nerve. J Neuroophthalmol. 2015;35(2):107–8.
16. de Araujo RB, Oyamada MK, Zacharias LC, Cunha LP, Preti RC, Monteiro MLR. Morphological and functional inner and outer retinal layer abnormalities in eyes with permanent temporal hemianopia from chiasmal compression. Front Neurol. 2017;8:619.
17. Abegg M, Dysli M, Wolf S, Kowal J, Dufour P, Zinkernagel M. Microcystic macular edema: retrograde maculopathy caused by optic neuropathy. Ophthalmology. 2014;121(1):142–9.
18. Fernandes DB, Raza AS, Nogueira RG, Wang D, Callegaro D, Hood DC, et al. Evaluation of inner retinal layers in patients with multiple sclerosis or neuromyelitis optica using optical coherence tomography. Ophthalmology. 2013;120(2):387–94.
19. Loo JL, Tian J, Miller NR, Subramanian PS. Use of optical coherence tomography in predicting post-treatment visual outcome in anterior visual pathway meningiomas. Br J Ophthalmol. 2013;97(11):1455–8.
20. Sibony P, Strachovsky M, Honkanen R, Kupersmith MJ. Optical coherence tomography shape analysis of the peripapillary retinal pigment epithelium layer in presumed optic nerve sheath meningiomas. J Neuroophthalmol. 2014;34(2):130–6.
21. Sibony P, Kupersmith MJ, Rohlf FJ. Shape analysis of the peripapillary RPE layer in papilledema and ischemic optic neuropathy. Invest Ophthalmol Vis Sci. 2011;52(11):7987–95.
22. Danesh-Meyer HV, Papchenko T, Savino PJ, Law A, Evans J, Gamble GD. In vivo retinal nerve fiber layer thickness measured by optical coherence tomography predicts visual recovery after surgery for parachiasmal tumors. Invest Ophthalmol Vis Sci. 2008;49(5):1879–85.
23. Subei AM, Eggenberger ER. Optical coherence tomography: another useful tool in a neuro-ophthalmologist's armamentarium. Curr Opin Ophthalmol. 2009;20(6):462–6.
24. Dutton JJ. Optic nerve sheath meningiomas. Surv Ophthalmol. 1992;37(3):167–83.
25. Spencer WH. Primary neoplasms of the optic nerve and its sheaths: clinical features and current concepts of pathogenetic mechanisms. Trans Am Ophthalmol Soc. 1972;70:490–528.
26. Dutton JJ. Optic nerve gliomas and meningiomas. Neurol Clin. 1991;9(1):163–77.
27. Miller NR. New concepts in the diagnosis and management of optic nerve sheath meningioma. J Neuroophthalmol. 2006;26(3):200–8.
28. Parker RT, Ovens CA, Fraser CL, Samarawickrama C. Optic nerve sheath meningiomas: prevalence, impact, and management strategies. Eye Brain. 2018;10:85–99.
29. Saeed P, Blank L, Selva D, Wolbers JG, Nowak PJ, Geskus RB, et al. Primary radiotherapy in progressive optic nerve sheath meningiomas: a long-term follow-up study. Br J Ophthalmol. 2010;94(5):564–8.
30. Solda F, Wharram B, De Ieso PB, Bonner J, Ashley S, Brada M. Long-term efficacy of fractionated radiotherapy for benign meningiomas. Radiother Oncol. 2013;109(2):330–4.
31. Imes RK, Schatz H, Hoyt WF, Monteiro ML, Narahara M. Evolution of optociliary veins in optic nerve sheath meningioma. Evol Arch Ophthalmol. 1985;103(1):59–60.
32. Rosenberg LF, Miller NR. Visual results after microsurgical removal of meningiomas involving the anterior visual system. Arch Ophthalmol. 1984;102(7):1019–23.
33. Dutton JJ. Gliomas of the anterior visual pathway. Surv Ophthalmol. 1994;38(5):427–52.
34. Miller NR. Primary tumours of the optic nerve and its sheath. Eye (Lond). 2004; 18(11):1026–37.
35. Kelly JP, Leary S, Khanna P, Weiss AH. Longitudinal measures of visual function, tumor volume, and prediction of visual outcomes after treatment of optic pathway gliomas. Ophthalmology. 2012;119(6):1231–7.
36. Chang L, El-Dairi MA, Frempong TA, Burner EL, Bhatti MT, Young TL, et al. Optical coherence tomography in the evaluation of neurofibromatosis type-1 subjects with optic pathway gliomas. J AAPOS. 2010;14(6):511–7.

37. Avery RA, Liu GT, Fisher MJ, Quinn GE, Belasco JB, Phillips PC, et al. Retinal nerve fiber layer thickness in children with optic pathway gliomas. Am J Ophthalmol. 2011;151(3):542–9 e2.
38. Parrozzani R, Clementi M, Kotsafti O, Miglionico G, Trevisson E, Orlando G, et al. Optical coherence tomography in the diagnosis of optic pathway gliomas. Invest Ophthalmol Vis Sci. 2013;54(13):8112–8.
39. Fard MA, Fakhree S, Eshraghi B. Correlation of optical coherence tomography parameters with clinical and radiological progression in patients with symptomatic optic pathway gliomas. Graefes Arch Clin Exp Ophthalmol. 2013;251(10):2429–36.
40. Gu S, Glaug N, Cnaan A, Packer RJ, Avery RA. Ganglion cell layer-inner plexiform layer thickness and vision loss in young children with optic pathway gliomas. Invest Ophthalmol Vis Sci. 2014;55(3):1402–8.
41. Hepokur M, Sarici AM. Investigation of retinal nerve fiber layer thickness and ganglion cell layer-inner plexiform layer thickness in patients with optic pathway gliomas. Graefes Arch Clin Exp Ophthalmol. 2018;256(9):1757–65.
42. Sahinoglu-Keskek N, Altan-Yaycioglu R, Canan H, Coban-Karatas M, Erbay A, Yazici N, et al. Measurements of retinal nerve fiber thickness and ganglion cell complex in neurofibromatosis type 1, with and without optic pathway gliomas: a case series. Curr Eye Res. 2018;43(3):424–7.
43. Avery RA, Hwang EI, Ishikawa H, Acosta MT, Hutcheson KA, Santos D, et al. Handheld optical coherence tomography during sedation in young children with optic pathway gliomas. JAMA Ophthalmol. 2014;132(3):265–71.
44. Avery RA, Cnaan A, Schuman JS, Trimboli-Heidler C, Chen CL, Packer RJ, et al. Longitudinal change of circumpapillary retinal nerve fiber layer thickness in children with optic pathway gliomas. Am J Ophthalmol. 2015;160(5):944–52 e1.
45. McKeag D, Lane C, Lazarus JH, Baldeschi L, Boboridis K, Dickinson AJ, et al. Clinical features of dysthyroid optic neuropathy: a European Group on Graves' Orbitopathy (EUGOGO) survey. Br J Ophthalmol. 2007;91(4):455–8.
46. Hallin ES, Feldon SE, Luttrell J. Graves' ophthalmopathy: III. Effect of transantral orbital decompression on optic neuropathy. Br J Ophthalmol. 1988;72(9):683–7.
47. Ben Simon GJ, Syed HM, Douglas R, Schwartz R, Goldberg RA, McCann JD. Clinical manifestations and treatment outcome of optic neuropathy in thyroid-related orbitopathy. Ophthalmic Surg Lasers Imaging. 2006;37(4):284–90.
48. Neigel JM, Rootman J, Belkin RI, Nugent RA, Drance SM, Beattie CW, et al. Dysthyroid optic neuropathy. The crowded orbital apex syndrome. Ophthalmology. 1988;95(11):1515–21.
49. Goncalves AC, Gebrim EM, Monteiro ML. Imaging studies for diagnosing Graves' orbitopathy and dysthyroid optic neuropathy. Clinics (Sao Paulo). 2012;67(11):1327–34.
50. Goncalves AC, Silva LN, Gebrim EM, Monteiro ML. Quantification of orbital apex crowding for screening of dysthyroid optic neuropathy using multidetector CT. AJNR Am J Neuroradiol. 2012;33(8):1602–7.
51. Wang JK, Kardon RH, Kupersmith MJ, Garvin MK. Automated quantification of volumetric optic disc swelling in papilledema using spectral-domain optical coherence tomography. Invest Ophthalmol Vis Sci. 2012;53(7):4069–75.
52. Kupersmith MJ, Sibony P, Mandel G, Durbin M, Kardon RH. Optical coherence tomography of the swollen optic nerve head: deformation of the peripapillary retinal pigment epithelium layer in papilledema. Invest Ophthalmol Vis Sci. 2011;52(9):6558–64.
53. Forte R, Bonavolonta P, Vassallo P. Evaluation of retinal nerve fiber layer with optic nerve tracking optical coherence tomography in thyroid-associated orbitopathy. Ophthalmologica. 2010;224(2):116–21.
54. Perez-Rico C, Rodriguez-Gonzalez N, Arevalo-Serrano J, Blanco R. Evaluation of multifocal visual evoked potentials in patients with Graves' orbitopathy and subclinical optic nerve involvement. Doc Ophthalmol. 2012;125(1):11–9.

55. Anderson D, Faber P, Marcovitz S, Hardy J, Lorenzetti D. Pituitary tumors and the ophthalmologist. Ophthalmology. 1983;90(11):1265–70.
56. Unsold R, Hoyt WF. Band atrophy of the optic nerve. The histology of temporal hemianopsia. Arch Ophthalmol. 1980;98(9):1637–8.
57. Kanamori A, Nakamura M, Matsui N, Nagai A, Nakanishi Y, Kusuhara S, et al. Optical coherence tomography detects characteristic retinal nerve fiber layer thickness corresponding to band atrophy of the optic discs. Ophthalmology. 2004;111(12):2278–83.
58. Danesh-Meyer HV, Carroll SC, Foroozan R, Savino PJ, Fan J, Jiang Y, et al. Relationship between retinal nerve fiber layer and visual field sensitivity as measured by optical coherence tomography in chiasmal compression. Invest Ophthalmol Vis Sci. 2006;47(11):4827–35.
59. Monteiro ML, Leal BC, Moura FC, Vessani RM, Medeiros FA. Comparison of retinal nerve fibre layer measurements using optical coherence tomography versions 1 and 3 in eyes with band atrophy of the optic nerve and normal controls. Eye (Lond). 2007;21(1):16–22.
60. Costa-Cunha LV, Cunha LP, Malta RF, Monteiro ML. Comparison of Fourier-domain and time-domain optical coherence tomography in the detection of band atrophy of the optic nerve. Am J Ophthalmol. 2009;147(1):56–63 e2.
61. Sousa RM, Oyamada MK, Cunha LP, Monteiro MLR. Multifocal visual evoked potential in eyes with temporal hemianopia from chiasmal compression: correlation with standard automated perimetry and OCT findings. Invest Ophthalmol Vis Sci. 2017;58(11):4436–49.
62. Al-Louzi O, Prasad S, Mallery RM. Utility of optical coherence tomography in the evaluation of sellar and parasellar mass lesions. Curr Opin Endocrinol Diabetes Obes. 2018;25(4):274–84.
63. Moura FC, Medeiros FA, Monteiro ML. Evaluation of macular thickness measurements for detection of band atrophy of the optic nerve using optical coherence tomography. Ophthalmology. 2007;114(1):175–81.
64. Garway-Heath DF, Poinoosawmy D, Fitzke FW, Hitchings RA. Mapping the visual field to the optic disc in normal tension glaucoma eyes. Ophthalmology. 2000;107(10):1809–15.
65. Shin HY, Park HY, Choi JA, Park CK. Macular ganglion cell-inner plexiform layer thinning in patients with visual field defect that respects the vertical meridian. Graefes Arch Clin Exp Ophthalmol. 2014;252(9):1501–7.
66. Tieger MG, Hedges TR 3rd, Ho J, Erlich-Malona NK, Vuong LN, Athappilly GK, et al. Ganglion cell complex loss in chiasmal compression by brain tumors. J Neuroophthalmol. 2017;37(1):7–12.
67. Sun M, Zhang Z, Ma C, Chen S, Chen X. Quantitative analysis of retinal layers on three-dimensional spectral-domain optical coherence tomography for pituitary adenoma. PLoS One. 2017;12(6):e0179532.
68. Yum HR, Park SH, Park HY, Shin SY. Macular ganglion cell analysis determined by cirrus HD optical coherence tomography for early detecting chiasmal compression. PLoS One. 2016;11(4):e0153064.
69. Moon CH, Lee SH, Kim BT, Hwang SC, Ohn YH, Park TK. Diagnostic ability of retinal nerve fiber layer thickness measurements and neurologic hemifield test to detect chiasmal compression. Invest Ophthalmol Vis Sci. 2012;53(9):5410–5.
70. Moon CH, Hwang SC, Ohn YH, Park TK. The time course of visual field recovery and changes of retinal ganglion cells after optic chiasmal decompression. Invest Ophthalmol Vis Sci. 2011;52(11):7966–73.
71. Akashi A, Kanamori A, Ueda K, Matsumoto Y, Yamada Y, Nakamura M. The detection of macular analysis by SD-OCT for optic chiasmal compression neuropathy and nasotemporal overlap. Invest Ophthalmol Vis Sci. 2014;55(7):4667–72.
72. Monteiro ML, Cunha LP, Costa-Cunha LV, Maia OO Jr, Oyamada MK. Relationship between optical coherence tomography, pattern electroretinogram and automated perimetry in eyes with temporal hemianopia from chiasmal compression. Invest Ophthalmol Vis Sci. 2009;50(8):3535–41.

73. Monteiro ML, Hokazono K, Cunha LP, Oyamada MK. Correlation between multifocal pattern electroretinography and Fourier-domain OCT in eyes with temporal hemianopia from chiasmal compression. Graefes Arch Clin Exp Ophthalmol. 2012;251(3):903–15.
74. Moon CH, Hwang SC, Kim BT, Ohn YH, Park TK. Visual prognostic value of optical coherence tomography and photopic negative response in chiasmal compression. Invest Ophthalmol Vis Sci. 2011;52(11):8527–33.
75. Kerrison JB, Lynn MJ, Baer CA, Newman SA, Biousse V, Newman NJ. Stages of improvement in visual fields after pituitary tumor resection. Am J Ophthalmol. 2000;130(6):813–20.
76. Findlay G, McFadzean RM, Teasdale G. Recovery of vision following treatment of pituitary tumours; application of a new system of assessment to patients treated by transsphenoidal operation. Acta Neurochir. 1983;68(3–4):175–86.
77. Gnanalingham KK, Bhattacharjee S, Pennington R, Ng J, Mendoza N. The time course of visual field recovery following transphenoidal surgery for pituitary adenomas: predictive factors for a good outcome. J Neurol Neurosurg Psychiatry. 2005;76(3):415–9.
78. Monteiro ML, Zambon BK, Cunha LP. Predictive factors for the development of visual loss in patients with pituitary macroadenomas and for visual recovery after optic pathway decompression. Can J Ophthalmol. 2010;45(4):404–8.
79. Cohen AR, Cooper PR, Kupersmith MJ, Flamm ES, Ransohoff J. Visual recovery after transsphenoidal removal of pituitary adenomas. Neurosurgery. 1985;17(3):446–52.
80. Barzaghi LR, Medone M, Losa M, Bianchi S, Giovanelli M, Mortini P. Prognostic factors of visual field improvement after trans-sphenoidal approach for pituitary macroadenomas: review of the literature and analysis by quantitative method. Neurosurg Rev. 2012;35(3):369–78. Discussion 78–9.
81. Jacob M, Raverot G, Jouanneau E, Borson-Chazot F, Perrin G, Rabilloud M, et al. Predicting visual outcome after treatment of pituitary adenomas with optical coherence tomography. Am J Ophthalmol. 2009;147(1):64–70 e2.
82. Danesh-Meyer HV, Wong A, Papchenko T, Matheos K, Stylli S, Nichols A, et al. Optical coherence tomography predicts visual outcome for pituitary tumors. J Clin Neurosci. 2015;22(7):1098–104.
83. Ohkubo S, Higashide T, Takeda H, Murotani E, Hayashi Y, Sugiyama K. Relationship between macular ganglion cell complex parameters and visual field parameters after tumor resection in chiasmal compression. Jpn J Ophthalmol. 2012;56(1):68–75.
84. Monteiro MLR. Macular ganglion cell complex reduction preceding visual field loss in a patient with chiasmal compression with a 21-month follow-up. J Neuroophthalmol. 2018;38(1):124–7.

OCT and Multiple Sclerosis

11

James V. M. Hanson, Carla A. Wicki, Praveena Manogaran, Axel Petzold, and Sven Schippling

J. V. M. Hanson
Department of Ophthalmology, University Hospital Zurich and University of Zurich, Zurich, Switzerland

Neuroimmunology and Multiple Sclerosis Research, Department of Neurology, University Hospital Zurich and University of Zurich, Zurich, Switzerland
e-mail: James.Hanson@usz.ch

C. A. Wicki
Neuroimmunology and Multiple Sclerosis Research, Department of Neurology, University Hospital Zurich and University of Zurich, Zurich, Switzerland

Department of Health Sciences and Technology, Swiss Federal Institute of Technology, Zurich, Switzerland
e-mail: Carla.Wicki@usz.ch

P. Manogaran
Neuroimmunology and Multiple Sclerosis Research, Department of Neurology, University Hospital Zurich and University of Zurich, Zurich, Switzerland

Department of Information Technology and Electrical Engineering, Swiss Federal Institute of Technology, Zurich, Switzerland
e-mail: Praveena.Manogaran@usz.ch

A. Petzold
Moorfields Eye Hospital, London, UK

National Hospital for Neurology and Neurosurgery, London, UK

Department of Neurology, Amsterdam Neuroscience, VUmc MS Center Amsterdam and Dutch Expertise Centre for Neuro-Ophthalmology, VU University Medical Center, Amsterdam, The Netherlands

Institute of Neurology, University College London, London, UK
e-mail: A.Petzold@nhs.net

S. Schippling (✉)
Neuroimmunology and Multiple Sclerosis Research, Department of Neurology, University Hospital Zurich and University of Zurich, Zurich, Switzerland

Neuroscience Center Zurich, University of Zurich and Federal Institute of Technology (ETH) Zurich, Zurich, Switzerland
e-mail: Sven.Schippling@usz.ch

A. Grzybowski, P. Barboni (eds.), *OCT and Imaging in Central Nervous System Diseases*, https://doi.org/10.1007/978-3-030-26269-3_11

11.1 Background

Multiple sclerosis (MS) is a highly heterogeneous autoimmune neurological disorder characterized by inflammation, demyelination, and neuroaxonal degeneration within the central nervous system (CNS), and the leading cause of neurological disability among young adults worldwide [1]. The precise aetiology remains unknown and may be multifactorial, with a range of environmental factors appearing to act against the background of a complex polygenetic trait [2]. It is believed that, initially, the disease is predominantly driven by aberrant peripheral immune cells, including T- and B-cells, that, upon (re)activation, target CNS myelin antigens [2]. MS frequently manifests with an initial inflammatory and demyelinating event affecting the CNS, termed clinically isolated syndrome (CIS) [3]. Current diagnostic criteria require evidence of clinical or radiological disease activity dissemination in both time and space, and allow a diagnosis of MS to be made based on a single clinical event when confirmed by radiological evidence of previous disease activity [4]. Relapsing-remitting MS (RRMS) is the most common form of the disease and is characterised by clinical episodes of inflammatory demyelination ('relapses') followed by periods of variable recovery and relatively stable neurological status ('remissions') [3, 4]. Patients initially diagnosed with RRMS may develop a gradual, progressive accumulation of disability independently of relapses, defined as secondary progressive MS (SPMS); alternatively, a minority of patients may exhibit progressive disease activity in the absence of relapses from disease onset, defined as primary progressive MS (PPMS) [3, 4]. In addition to these phenotypical classifications, MS may also be described as clinically or radiologically active, with or without evidence of disease progression [3].

Despite a highly heterogeneous clinical presentation and disease course, involvement of the visual system is a near-ubiquitous hallmark of the disease [5, 6]. In the afferent visual pathway, optic neuritis (ON; an acute or subacute inflammation of the optic nerve) is the most common manifestation of MS [7]. ON may occur within the context of previously-diagnosed MS, or as an initial clinical event strongly suggestive of MS but not immediately fulfilling diagnostic criteria for the disease [4] (CIS). It should be noted that ON may also occur idiopathically, in systemic disease, and in immunological conditions other than MS [8]; however, for the purpose of this overview, the nomenclature ON should be understood to refer only to that associated with MS and CIS. This prevalence of anterior visual pathway involvement, the accessibility of the retina for viewing retinal neurons and their axons *in vivo*, and the unmyelinated nature of ganglion cell axons within the retina (unique within the CNS), have ensured that the anterior visual pathway has generated considerable interest as a model for research in MS [9]. Much of this interest has been facilitated by the development of optical coherence tomography (OCT) and its increasing use in neurological clinics.

Since the first retinal OCT scans were acquired in 1991 [10], the introduction of spectral-domain OCT (SD-OCT), offering higher resolution and acquisition speed than previous time-domain OCT (TD-OCT) technology, has permitted the development of automated or semi-automated software algorithms enabling the definition and delineation of the boundaries separating the retinal layers (Fig. 11.1), in addition to coarse measures of retinal thickness such as total macular volume (TMV). These layers and complexes include the retinal nerve fibre layer (RNFL), which is most commonly measured around the optic nerve head (pRNFL) but may also be measured at the central macular region (mRNFL); the ganglion cell layer (GCL); inner plexiform layer (IPL); the inner nuclear layer (INL); the outer plexiform layer (OPL); the outer nuclear layer (ONL); and the photoreceptor layer (PRL). As the boundary between GCL and IPL may be difficult to visualise and accurately define, these layers are typically combined and described as the ganglion cell and inner plexiform layer (GCIP or GCIPL are equally acceptable abbreviations [11];

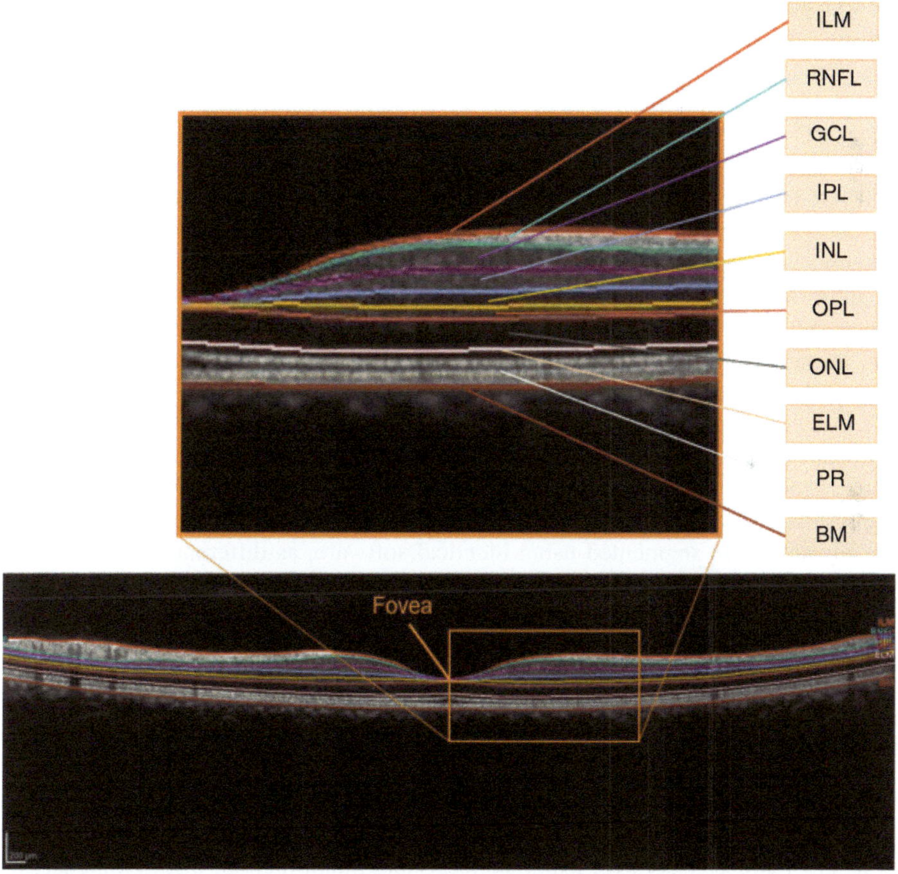

Fig. 11.1 Segmented macular OCT B-scan of a healthy individual, showing the delineation of the retinal layers. *ILM* inner limiting membrane, *RNFL* retinal nerve fibre layer, *GCL* ganglion cell layer, *IPL* inner plexiform layer, *INL* inner nuclear layer, *OPL* outer plexiform layer, *ONL* outer nuclear layer, *ELM* external limiting membrane, *PRL* photoreceptor layers, *BM* Bruch's membrane. Note that GCL and IPL are typically aggregated to form the ganglion cell and inner plexiform layer (GCIP), and other layers may also be aggregated, depending on the segmentation software used and/or aims of individual studies

throughout this work, GCIP will be used for consistency). However, different proprietary software algorithms and studies may choose to additionally aggregate or otherwise classify layers of the retina (e.g., INL-OPL; outer retinal layers, ORL; ganglion cell complex, GCC). Whichever approach individual laboratories or researchers choose when conducting OCT research in MS patients, transparent and precise definition of the relevant retinal structures is vital [11]. This process of retinal layer delineation, referred to as segmentation, has led to a large and growing body of literature examining the structure of the full range of retinal layers and complexes in the eyes of patients with MS.

Image quality is paramount for accurate and reliable definition and verification of the intra-retinal boundaries, and early recognition of this fact by MS researchers led to the development of the first OCT quality guidelines validated for use in MS research, the OSCAR-IB consensus criteria [12]. These guidelines emphasise the importance of signal strength, scan centration, algorithm performance (i.e., errors of automated segmentation), absence of co-existing retinal pathology (which may affect OCT interpretation), fundus illumination, beam placement, and exclusion of any other obvious acquisition errors when assessing OCT data. Application of the OSCAR-IB criteria has been shown to result in high inter-rater agreement regarding the acceptance or rejection of scans in multi-centre studies [12, 13], and may thus maximise the reproducibility of OCT studies. Recent work analysing the reliability of inter-rater, multi-centre manual correction of automatically segmented OCT scans, utilising the OSCAR-IB criteria, recorded excellent agreement between raters, in particular for the inner retinal layers [14]. The agreement between raters appeared to be greater than in previous work predating the OSCAR-IB criteria [15]. We therefore recommend adherence to the OSCAR-IB criteria at all times when evaluating OCT scans, and to the APOSTEL recommendations for describing OCT scan protocols and analyses [11] (described in detail in Chap. 3), whenever publishing results of OCT studies in MS patients. We also recommend that all OCT scans for any study are segmented using identical software, as different versions of the same proprietary software have been shown to produce small but significant differences in axonal thickness in patients with MS and in control subjects [16].

11.2 OCT Findings in Patients with MS

Findings to date consistently show that pRNFL thickness is reduced in the eyes of MS patients without previous ON relative to healthy control subjects [17–25] (Fig. 11.2), although this may not necessarily be the case in patients with CIS [26] or newly diagnosed MS [27]. Meta-analyses have quantified this loss of thickness in MS patients as being on average just over 7 μm whether measured with SD-OCT or TD-OCT technology [28, 29]. Thickness of the temporal quadrant of pRNFL has been suggested to be preferentially affected by MS [23], although other studies failed to observe this pattern in eyes without previous ON [21]. Likewise, sparing of the nasal quadrant has been proposed [23] but not confirmed [21]. Some of these differences may be attributable to subtly different RNFL quantifications obtained by

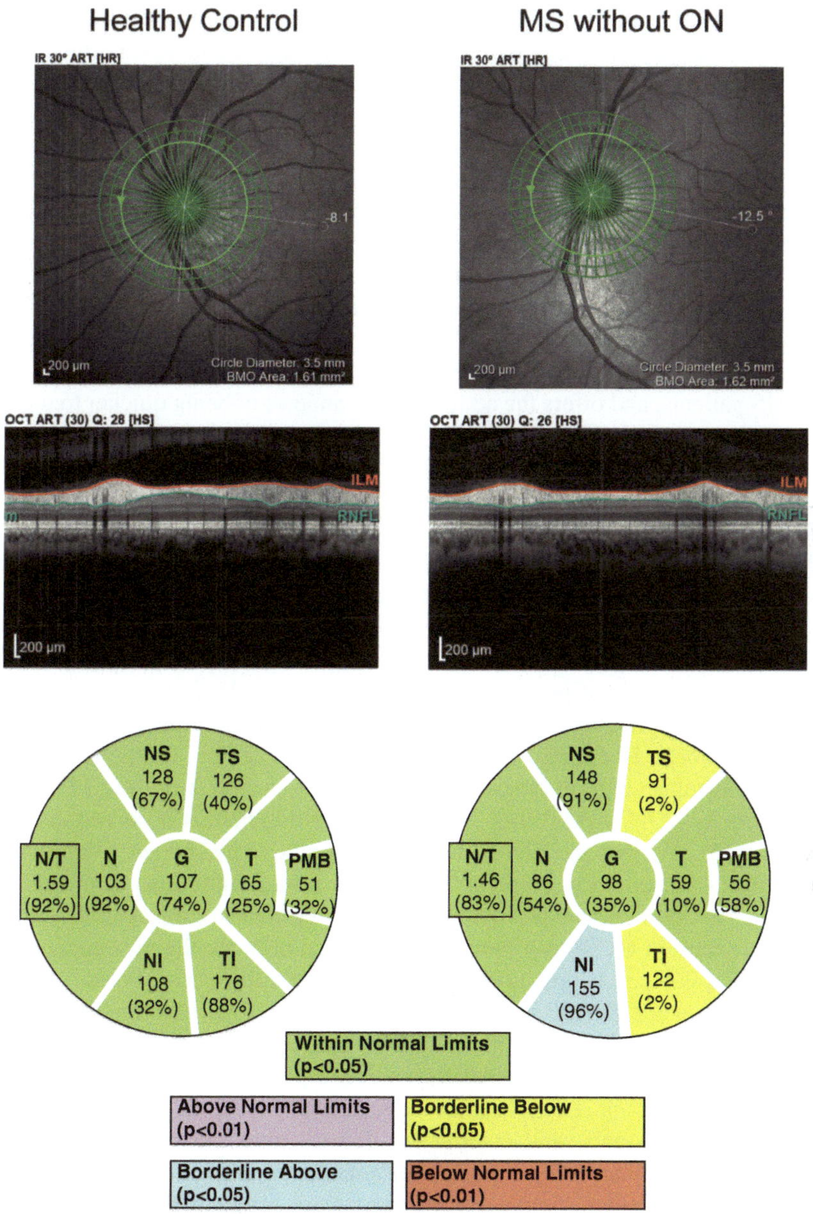

Fig. 11.2 pRNFL analysis from the left eyes of a healthy individual and a multiple sclerosis (MS) patient without previous optic neuritis (ON), obtained from a Spectralis OCT device (Heidelberg Engineering, Heidelberg, Germany). The global averaged (G) thickness is reduced in the patient with MS, as are the thicknesses of the majority of the individual sectors; in the case of the temporal superior (TS) and temporal inferior (TI) sectors, thickness is below the 95th percentile of age-matched normal values and so is classified as borderline below average (and colour-coded yellow) by the proprietary software. The borderline above average thickness in the nasal inferior (NI) sector in the MS patient is an artefact caused by a retinal blood vessel

different OCT devices [30]. Longitudinal studies of RNFL atrophy show that MS eyes without a history of ON undergo an average decline in RNFL thickness of between 0.5–1.5 μm per year [31–33], approximately 3–10 times faster than healthy control subjects. This rate of decline is highest in the early stages of the disease (up to approximately 10 years of disease duration) and thereafter declines, consistent with a plateau effect [31]. The inverse relationship between RNFL atrophy rate and disease duration (Fig. 11.3) may explain the different annual RNFL loss rates obtained in different studies in cohorts with varying average disease duration, and should thus be considered when planning and evaluating future research.

MRNFL has also been shown to be thinned in MS patients [18, 19, 26], but by an average of just over 2 μm relative to normal individuals [28]; therefore it appears that pRNFL may offer more power than mRNFL when investigating axonal integrity in MS patients, and offers the additional advantages of being quicker to measure and requiring less post-hoc correction (typically one B-scan rather than, e.g., 19). Additionally, as an outcome measure mRNFL has been suggested to be less reliable than pRNFL due to the density of vascular perfusion between the fovea and optic nerve head potentially causing artefact-based segmentation errors [34]. These factors, combined with the relatively recent development of macular segmentation algorithms compared to software able to reliably quantify pRNFL, have ensured that pRNFL remains the more widely studied outcome measure in MS research.

In addition to the RNFL, thickness of the GCIP is also reduced in the eyes of MS and CIS patients without previous ON [17–19, 24–27, 35–37], by an average of 6.3 μm relative to control subjects [28]. Using the 1, 2.22, and 3.45 mm Early Treatment Diabetic Retinopathy Study (ETDRS) grid centred on the fovea, it was shown that average GCIP thickness declined by 0.9 μm over 2 years in MS patients without previous ON, a rate of loss approximately double that observed in healthy individuals [31]. As with the RNFL, annual rates of GCIP loss appear to be inversely related to disease duration (Fig. 11.3) [31]. A similar study also found that MS patients lost GCIP thickness just over twice as fast as control subjects [32], although quantitative rates of GCIP loss cannot be compared between the two studies due to different OCT devices, acquisition protocols, and retinal areas analysed.

In contrast to the RNFL and GCIP of the inner retina, INL thickness in MS patients seems to not differ significantly from that of control subjects [17, 18, 37, 38] and appears to remain stable in the eyes of MS patients without ON irrespective of disease duration (Fig. 11.3), at least over a 2 year period [31]. However, disease activity, treatment status, and (indirectly) disease duration may influence these results [24]. Rather than being a marker for neurodegeneration like the inner retina, the INL currently holds promise as a biomarker for inflammatory disease activity and response to disease-modifying therapy in MS. OCT thus has the potential to objectively capture and quantify the two main hallmarks of MS disease activity, neuronal degeneration and inflammation. A detailed discussion of the potential role of the INL in MS research can be found in Sect. 11.5.

Studies of the structure of the retina distal to INL are relatively sparse at the time of writing, and interpretation is made more challenging by the fact that some studies aggregate two or more of the retinal layers for analyses (e.g., INL and OPL [19];

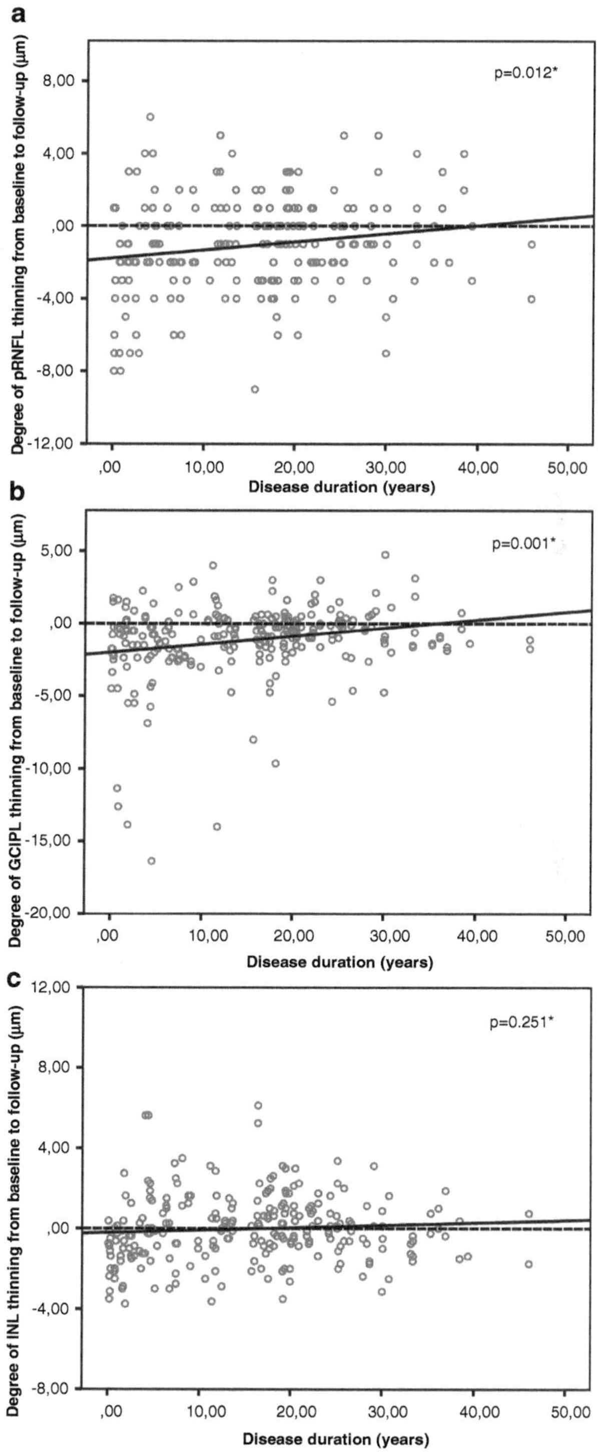

Fig. 11.3 Scatter plots showing the degree of thinning of the peripapillary retinal nerve fibre layer (pRNFL, **a**), ganglion cell and inner plexiform layer (GCIP; here GCIPL, **b**), and inner nuclear layer (INL, **c**) over a 2 year period in patients with multiple sclerosis (MS). RNFL and GCIP loss was greater in patients with a lower disease duration, whilst INL remained approximately constant over the study period irrespective of disease duration. Reproduced from Balk et al. Journal of Neurology 263, 1323–1331 (2016) under the terms of the Creative Commons CC BY license

ONL and PRL [36]). However, published studies to date have consistently found no effects of MS on the thickness of the retinal layers distal to INL [18, 19, 24, 25, 39].

Although the majority of patients with MS exhibit a relapsing-remitting disease course (RRMS), and thus the majority of the studies above relate mainly to RRMS and CIS patients, researchers have also measured differences in OCT parameters between the different MS phenotypes. Patients with progressive forms of MS (PPMS; SPMS) show reduced RNFL thickness compared to patients with RRMS [20, 40] and healthy control subjects [25, 40, 41]. As would be expected, GCIP is similarly reduced [25, 40, 41]. INL, but not ONL, is also thinned in patients with progressive forms of MS relative to control subjects [25, 40]. Findings with regard to the OPL in progressive MS are not unanimous [25, 40], whilst PRL thickness has been reported to be thinner in patients with progressive MS relative to control subjects but comparable to that of patients with RRMS [40].

Due to the historical lack of medical therapy for patients with PPMS (thereby reducing the need for frequent clinic visits to monitor effectiveness and side-effects of treatment) and the relative rarity of this phenotype relative to RRMS and CIS, PPMS patients are arguably underrepresented in OCT studies and, when included, it may only be possible to recruit a relative small cohort in single centre studies (e.g., 12 PPMS patients [25]). Such difficulties are likely to have the effect of decreasing the potential statistical power in studies of PPMS. This situation may improve in the future, following the recent licensing of ocrelizumab (Ocrevus®), a monoclonal antibody targeting the CD20 antigen expressed on B-cells and (to a lesser extent) T-cells, as the first treatment for use in patients with PPMS. This may lead to an increase the numbers of PPMS patients regularly attending neurology clinics for reasons of efficacy and safety monitoring.

It has been proposed that OCT may be used to define novel MS phenotypes defined by primary retinal pathology (i.e., structural and/or functional changes unrelated to a history of ON) [42]. These authors documented a subset of their MS cohort who exhibited thinning of the macula in the presence of normal RNFL thickness relative to normative data, with segmentation revealing thinning of both the INL and ONL, a phenotype the authors named "macular thinning predominant" (MTP) [42]. No MTP eyes had a prior history of ON, and no significant differences in INL or ONL thickness were observed between non-MTP MS patients and healthy controls [42]. Clinically, MTP-MS patients were found to have reduced high- and low-contrast visual acuity (HCVA; LCVA) and higher Expanded Disability Status Scale (EDSS; the most widely accepted and most broadly applied measure of clinical disability in MS patients) scores when compared to non-MTP MS patients [42]. Subsequent works were unable to confirm the existence of a distinct subset of MS patients consistent with the proposed MTP phenotype [19, 43] and found INL thinning in the absence of ONL changes only in patients with PPMS [25]. Differences in OCT hardware, software, and manufacturer-specific normative databases, as well as in patient populations, doubtless contribute to this apparent dichotomy. However, functional evidence consistent with similarly ON-independent abnormalities of the retinal layers distal to GCIP in patients with MS has been credibly reported by a number of authors working independently [35, 39, 44–47], and INL atrophy in MS eyes has been histologically confirmed post-mortem [48].

In MS, patients of African-American ethnicity have been shown to accumulate disability more rapidly [49, 50], and exhibit more cerebellar dysfunction [49], compared to Americans of Caucasian ethnicity; they are also more likely to have PPMS and less likely to have RRMS [49]. Using OCT, it has also been found that African-American MS patients have thinner RNFL (in the temporal quadrant only) and GCIP, which decline in thickness more rapidly, than Caucasian Americans [51, 52]. Thus, OCT results appear to be consistent with a more neurodegenerative phenotype in African-Americans [51].

Fingolimod (Gilenya®) is a modulator of sphingosine 1-phosphate receptors prescribed as an immunomodulatory therapy in MS. Whilst its high efficacy [53, 54] and oral administration are attractive, a small number of patients (up to 1% of treated RRMS patients [55, 56]) develop cystoid macula oedema (CMO; an accumulation of fluid in the central retina most likely consequent to breakdown of the blood-retinal barrier [57]) as a side-effect of the treatment (Fig. 11.4). It is therefore recommended that patients undergo ophthalmological examination before commencing therapy, and again 3–4 months afterwards, a time interval in which the

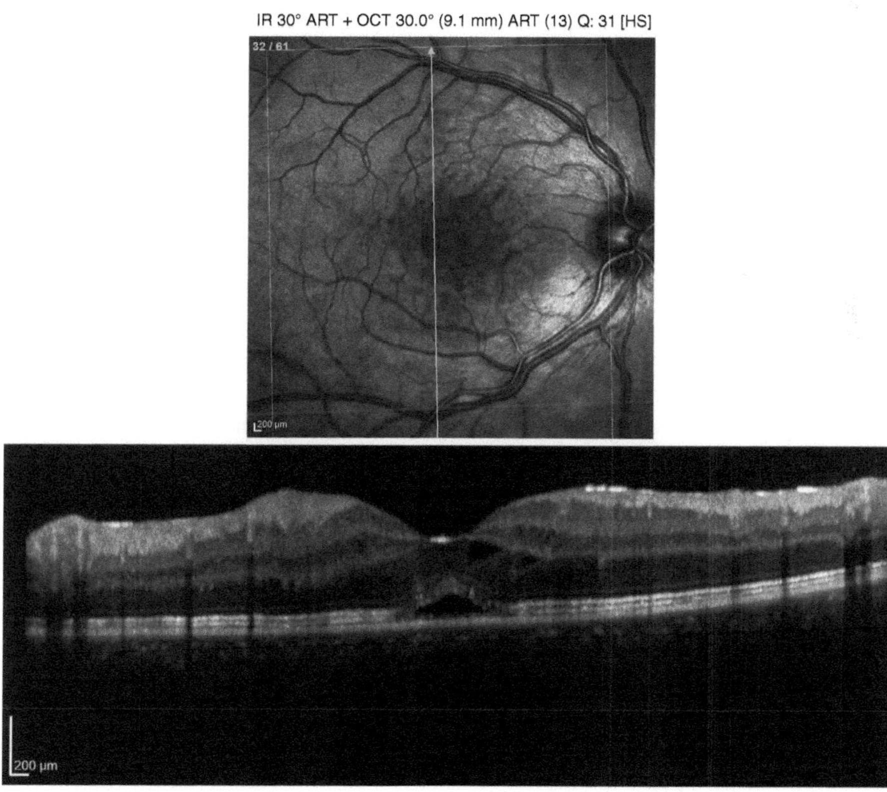

Fig. 11.4 OCT scan of the right eye of a patient with multiple sclerosis (MS) who has developed cystoid macula oedema (CMO) consequent to medical treatment with fingolimod (Gilenya®). Cystoid spaces are visible in the outer and (to a lesser extent) inner nuclear layers, as well as a small subfoveal accumulation of subretinal fluid

majority of CMO cases manifest [58]. OCT has been demonstrated to be significantly more sensitive than fundoscopy in detecting CMO [59], and therefore is of utility when assessing and monitoring MS patients undergoing treatment with fingolimod.

Recent developments in OCT technology have led to the development of OCT angiography (OCT-A), which is able to evaluate both arterial and venous density at the retina and optic nerve head down to the capillary level (OCT-A is described in detail in Chap. 4). Retinal vascular abnormalities such as periphlebitis have long been known to exist in some patients with MS [23, 60], but precise examination and quantification of the vessels with OCT was not possible until the introduction of OCT-A. Perfusion of the optic nerve head (as quantified by the density of visible vessels) has been shown to be reduced in MS eyes without previous ON compared to control subjects [61]. Results regarding macular perfusion are mixed at the time of writing, with a single study showing reduced vessel density in MS patients without ON [62] but other studies recording no differences with healthy control subjects [63, 64]. Increased vessel density in the choriocapillaris may be associated with prospective disease activity in MS [64], via an as-yet unknown mechanism. Future OCT-A studies are vital in order to elucidate the precise role of the retinal and choroidal vessels in MS.

11.3 OCT Findings in Patients with Optic Neuritis (ON)

ON is the most frequent manifestation of anterior visual pathway involvement in MS [7], being the first clinical sign of CIS in over a fifth of patients [8], and postmortem evidence of pathological changes to the optic nerve has been documented in up to 86% of MS eyes [48, 65]. Clinically confirmed episodes of ON occur in approximately 70% of MS patients during their disease course, typically during the relapsing-remitting phase [8]. Although presentation is variable, symptoms of ON commonly include reduced vision, periocular or retrobulbar pain (which typically worsens upon eye movements), and altered colour perception [66, 67]. Visual phenomena such as scintillations and/or phosphenes may also be reported [67]. Clinical signs upon examination may include reduced high- and/or low-contrast visual acuity (HCVA; LCVA), a relative afferent pupillary defect (RAPD), perimetric abnormalities (central scotoma [68], centrocecal scotoma, paracentral scotoma, or diffusely reduced sensitivity [69]), and abnormalities on colour vision testing [66] (although note that MS patients without previous ON may display similar abnormalities of colour vision [70]). Swelling of the optic nerve head is visible on fundoscopy in approximately one third of patients [66], with the remainder presenting with a normal fundus appearance due to inflammation being confined to the retrobulbar portion of the optic nerve and not extending to the optic nerve head. Visual function typically recovers spontaneously over a period of weeks to months [71], however many patients experience persistent visual impairment such as reduced LCVA and residual impairment of colour vision perception, with corresponding measures of vision-related quality of life being reduced [72]. The Pulfrich phenomenon, caused by inter-ocular differences in afferent conduction velocity consequent to unilateral demyelination, may be noticed by patients during the recovery phase [67]. These visual findings may be recorded even when HCVA returns to normal or near-normal levels [22, 73, 74]. Treatment with corticosteroids may accelerate clinical recovery after ON [75] and reduce the risk of progression to MS over approximately 2 years [76], but has minimal effect on visual outcome [75, 76]. Given these factors, and the fact that MS patients have been shown to rate vision as their most important bodily function irrespective of disease duration and disability [77], it is clear that ON is of vital importance in the study of MS. Retinal injury is currently believed to occur following inflammatory demyelination and axonal damage of the optic nerve by a process of retrograde degeneration toward the retinal ganglion cells [78].

OCT examination of MS or CIS patients with a history of ON almost invariably reveals reduced pRNFL [18–20, 28, 29, 34, 36, 38, 39, 79–84]. Meta-analyses have quantified this loss of pRNFL as an average of just over 20 μm relative to healthy control subjects both with SD-OCT and TD-OCT [28, 29]. Considerable inter-individual variation has been documented [83], most likely reflecting the heterogeneity both of clinical outcomes after ON and in MS generally. However, this figure of 20 μm refers to the pRNFL averaged over 360° around the optic nerve head; when the superior, inferior, temporal and nasal quadrants are compared, the temporal quadrant may be the most sensitive in visualising and quantifying axonal loss after ON [21, 80, 85–88]. Thickness of the pRNFL in the papillomacular bundle (PMB), comprised of axons from the foveal region and the area between the fovea and optic nerve head which are anatomically distinct from the predominating arcuate organisation of RNFL axons, has been reported to be the most sensitive individual OCT parameter in blinded detection of previous ON despite its inclusion not increasing the overall sensitivity of such analyses [86]. Preferential involvement of the temporal and PMB RNFL would be consistent with the reported predominance of central and centrocecal visual field defects in ON [68, 69]. Thickness of the superior and inferior quadrants is also significantly reduced after ON in MS patients [23, 80, 85, 89], whilst the balance of evidence to date suggests that the nasal quadrant is relatively unaffected [23, 80, 85, 86, 89]. Loss of pRNFL appears to have plateaued by approximately 6–12 months after the first symptoms of ON [80, 82, 83]. An inter-ocular pRNFL thickness difference of more than 5–6 μm is strongly suggestive of a previous unilateral ON [90].

In addition to subacute axonal loss following ON, patients experience ongoing loss of RNFL as a consequence both of MS itself and the normal aging process (as discussed above in Sect. 11.2). The majority of evidence to date suggests that the underlying rate of RNFL loss does not differ between MS eyes with and without previous ON [31, 33]; in other words, the significant insult to RNFL after ON is independent of, and does not affect, the insidious neurodegenerative processes ongoing in the majority of MS patients. In both of these studies, the effect of subacute axonal loss was removed from the analyses by excluding patients with a history of ON within the previous 6 months [31, 33].

In addition to pRNFL, the thickness of mRNFL is also reduced after ON in MS and CIS patients [18, 19, 28, 34] by, on average, just over 6 μm [28]. As in MS without confounding ON (Sect. 11.2), mRNFL may be of lesser utility as an outcome measure in MS and ON than pRNFL.

As with RNFL, GCIP thickness has almost universally been found to be reduced following an episode of ON in MS (Fig. 11.5) and CIS patients [18, 19, 28, 34, 36, 39, 72, 82, 83, 87, 91], with meta-analysis suggesting an average thickness loss of just over 16 μm [28]. Also similarly to RNFL, despite subacute loss of GCIP following ON, the underlying rate of GCIP loss does not differ between MS eyes with and without ON [31, 33]. Despite this similarity, GCIP offers important advantages over pRNFL as an outcome measure following ON. One factor already alluded to is that while approximately two thirds of ON patients present with retrobulbar inflammation of the optic nerve, the remaining third present with peripapillary oedema visible on fundoscopy [66]. (In fact, subsequent work employing OCT has suggested that as many as 82% of patients may have increased pRNFL thickness during the acute phase of ON [92], suggesting superior sensitivity of OCT at enabling detection of peripapillary oedema compared to traditional fundoscopy). A consequence of this is that pRNFL thickness during the acute phase of ON, when baseline OCT measurements are ideally acquired, is frequently increased relative to the fellow eye and/or control subjects due to inflammatory oedema [72, 82, 83, 91, 92]. Therefore, reduction of pRNFL thickness after the acute phase of ON cannot be ascribed to either resolution of oedema or axonal loss in isolation, and it has been suggested by some authors that it may be prudent to wait at least 3 months following an episode of ON before attempting to quantify pRNFL loss (Fig. 11.6) [8, 93]. In contrast, the evidence to date shows that GCIP thickness is not increased relative to that of unaffected contralateral eyes of ON patients [36, 91] or healthy control subjects [91, 94] during the acute phase of ON, and thus assessment of GCIP may enable earlier detection of inner retinal atrophy after ON in MS patients [83]. Supporting this hypothesis, thinning of GCIP appears to have plateaued by approximately 3 to 6 months following the clinical onset of ON [82, 83], a considerably shorter period than for pRNFL. Recent evidence suggests that analysis of inter-ocular differences in GCIP thickness is more sensitive in detecting a previous unilateral ON episode than pRNFL thickness differences [95]. An additional consideration is that GCIP may be less likely to be affected by the presence of non-pathological anatomical variations such as optic disc drusen or ectopically myelinated retinal nerve fibres. Despite these undoubted advantages of GCIP, pRNFL remains a useful and robust measure of retinal atrophy following ON, with the practical advantage that its segmentation and quantification is quicker and easier than that of GCIP. An understanding of the potential confounding factors described above will assist the clinician when assessing patients with ON using OCT.

With regard to the effects of ON upon the INL, results are more mixed than for the inner retinal layers, with some authors recording some small degree of INL thickening (Fig. 11.7) [18, 39, 91, 96] and others finding INL thickness comparable to normal values [34, 36, 72, 83]. Results may differ even between separate

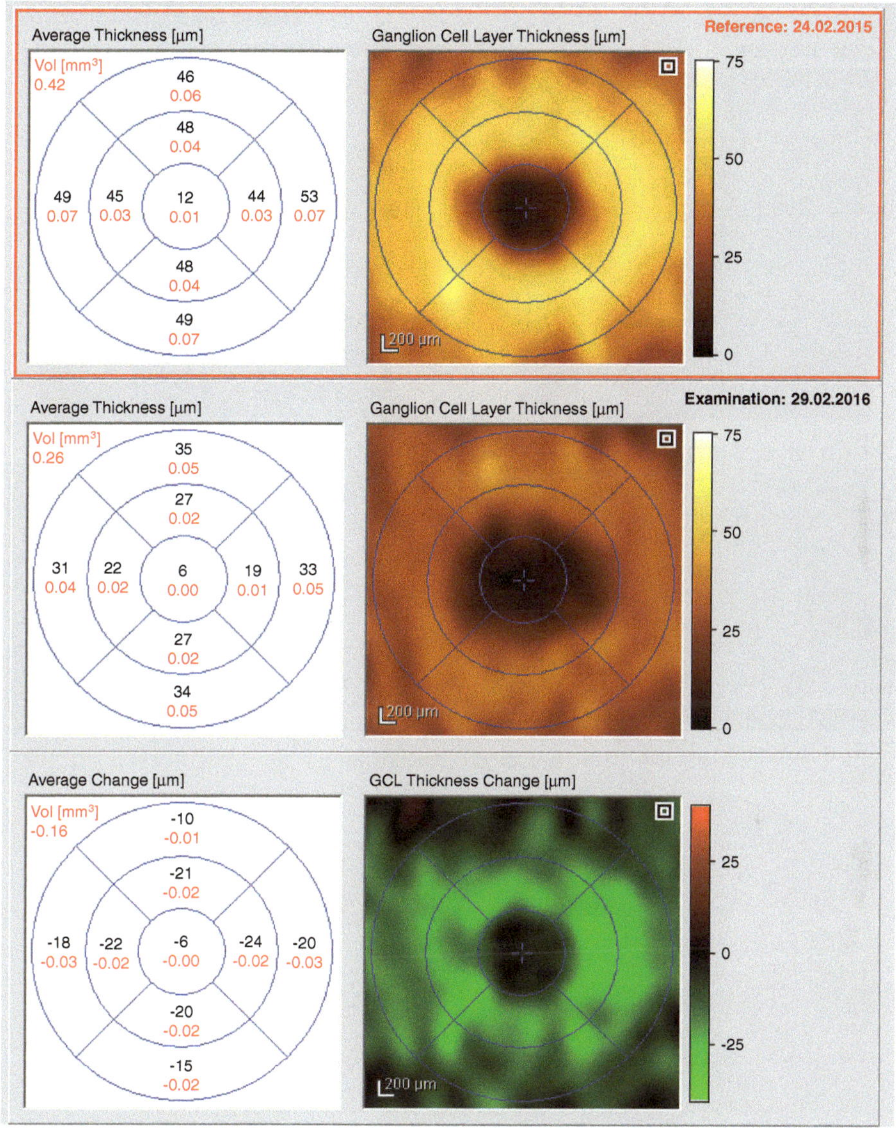

Fig. 11.5 OCT thickness maps of the ganglion cell layer (GCL) of a multiple sclerosis (MS) patient with optic neuritis (ON), showing OCT data acquired in the acute phase of ON (top) and 12 months later (middle). Atrophy of the GCL has followed ON, reflected in the thinner GCL at follow-up and in the negative thickness change values when the two examinations are compared (bottom). Although GCP is typically aggregated with the inner plexiform layer (IPL) as ganglion cell and inner plexiform layer (GCIP) for quantitative analysis, with this particular proprietary software it is not possible to generate thickness maps for GCIP and so only GCL is shown

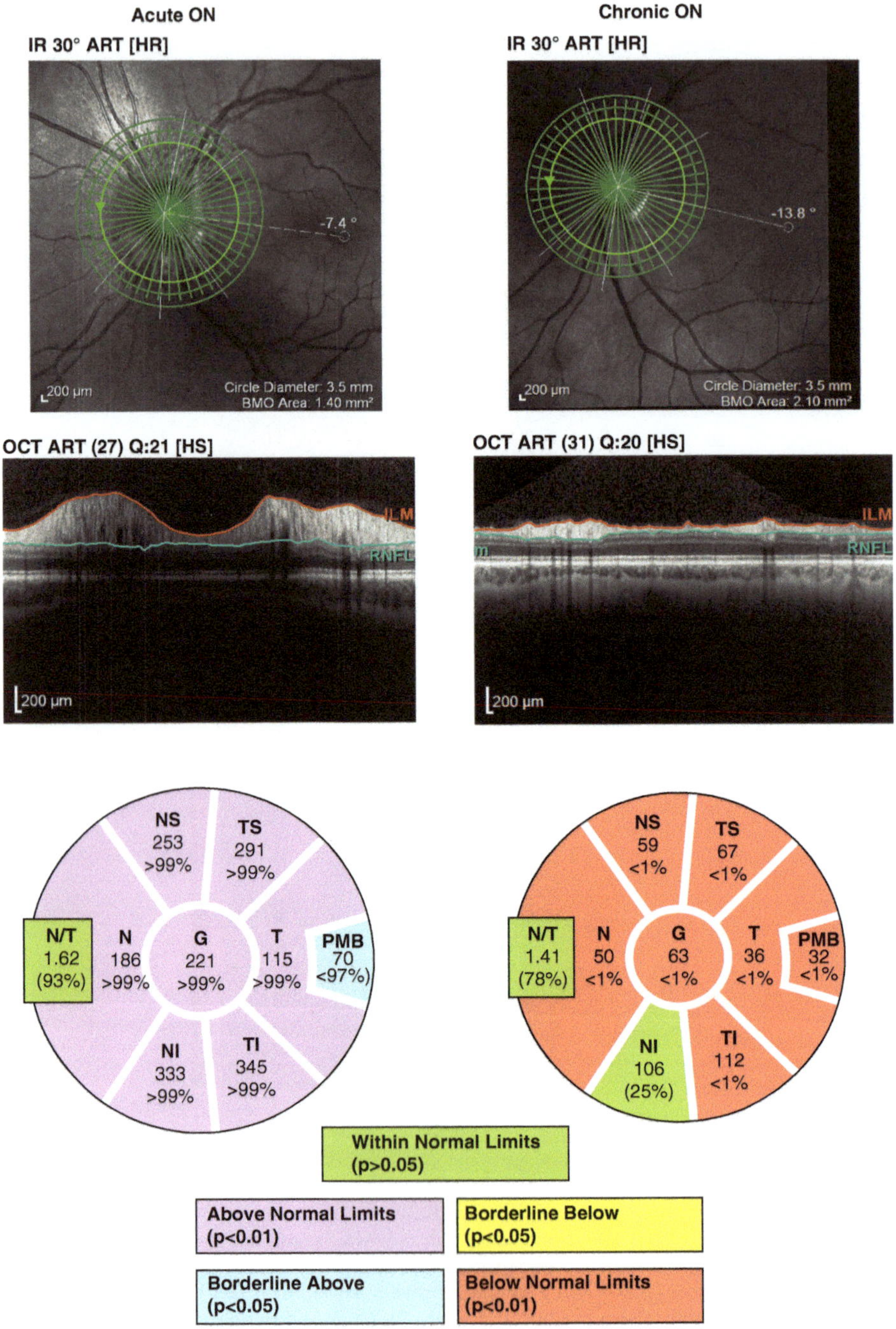

Fig. 11.6 OCT scans of the peripapillary retinal nerve fibre layer (pRNFL) in a patient with acute optic neuritis (ON) (left), and in a patient 12 months after ON (right). The patient with acute ON has inflammatory oedema around the optic nerve head, which is reflected in pRNFL thickness measurements significantly greater than normal values, whereas the patient with chronic ON shows significant atrophy of the pRNFL, with thickness values reduced compared to normal values

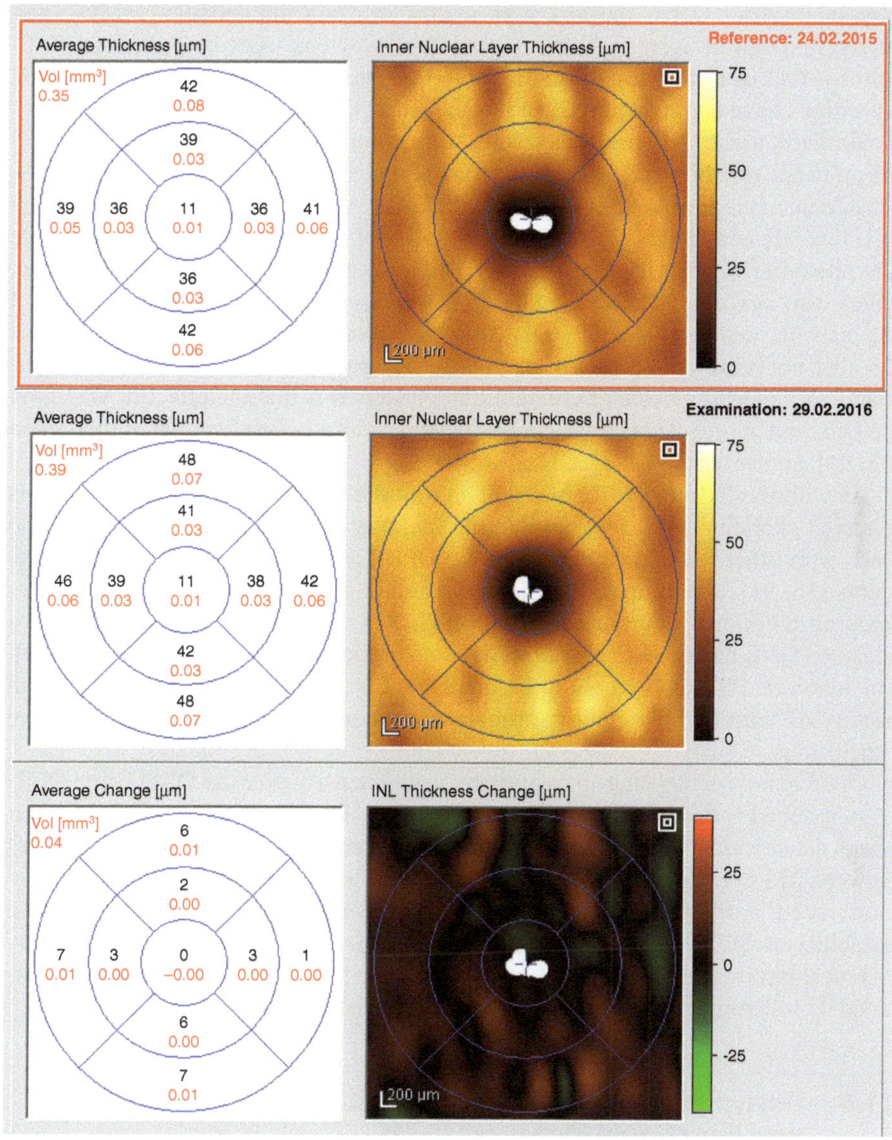

Fig. 11.7 OCT thickness maps of the inner nuclear layer (INL) of a multiple sclerosis (MS) patient with optic neuritis (ON), showing OCT data acquired in the acute phase of ON (top) and 12 months later (middle). INL is slightly thicker at follow-up, reflected in the small positive thickness change values when the two examinations are compared (bottom)

studies from the same laboratory [36, 91], which may reflect differences in sample size and thus statistical power. A meta-analysis including many hundreds of eyes detected an average macular INL thickening in MS eyes with previous ON of 0.77 µm relative to control subjects, and 0.61 µm relative to MS eyes without previous ON [28]. An important potential confounding factor associated with INL assessment after ON is the link with microcystic macula oedema (MMO), discussed in detail in Sect. 11.5. Interpretation of previous work is made more difficult by the fact that some studies and versions of proprietary segmentation algorithms have aggregated INL and OPL [36, 91].

Similarly to the INL, previous studies have reported conflicting results regarding the influence of ON upon the OPL, with some reporting no influence of ON [36, 39, 72] and others reporting mild thickening [83, 91]. Aggregation of the OPL with the INL [36, 91] and ONL [72, 83] in the majority of studies may mask any possible ON-related effect restricted to the OPL; the only meta-analysis available to date, which also aggregated OPL and ONL, showed minimal thickening in the eyes of MS patients with previous ON relative to those of MS patients without previous ON, but not relative to those of healthy control subjects [28]. An additional confounding factor as revealed by longitudinal analyses is that the effect of ON upon the OPL and aggregated layers appears dynamic, varying as a function of time since [83, 91], and severity of [83], ON.

As with the INL and OPL, interpretation of the effects of ON upon the ONL is rendered challenging by the fact that the majority of studies have aggregated the ONL with other retinal layers such as the OPL [28, 72, 83] or photoreceptor segments [36, 91]. Again, the likely dynamic nature of any thickness changes represents an additional confounding factor [83, 91]. The only study to date which analysed ONL thickness in isolation found no measurable effect related to ON [39]. Thickness of PRL also seems to be unaffected by ON [39], although the current paucity of corroborative data is problematic when attempting to draw definitive conclusions.

Optic nerve perfusion, as measured by vessel density over the ONH using OCT-A, is reduced following ON in MS patients [61]. Current data regarding macular vessel density after ON is not unanimous, with an early study finding no differences between MS eyes both with and without ON and healthy control subjects [63], but more recent work recording that vessel density is reduced after ON [62, 64]. The reliability of OCT-A examination in MS patients with acute ON may be limited by technical issues such as reduced signal strength and shadowing phenomena exacerbated by inflammatory oedema at the optic nerve head.

11.4 Association of OCT Outcomes with Clinical, Structural, and Functional Measures in MS

Despite the manifold benefits of OCT, it remains fundamentally an examination of retinal and optic nerve head structure only; it is currently not possible to perform concurrent measurements of retinal, optic nerve head, or visual function in a manner analogous to (e.g.) functional magnetic resonance imaging (MRI) of the brain. In MS clinics and research settings, OCT is frequently combined with quantification of global disability and other structural (e.g., MRI) and/or functional (e.g., visual acuity, retinal and/or cortical electrophysiology) measures. Here, we examine the relationships between OCT and these different outcome measures.

11.4.1 Disability

Global disability in MS can be assessed using clinical scales such as the EDSS or the Multiple Sclerosis Functional Composite (MSFC). EDSS scores have been reported as being negatively correlated with RNFL [97–104], although this effect has not consistently been shown in all studies [105, 106]. EDSS also negatively correlates with GCIP thickness [97, 101, 102, 107], although not with TMV [100]. Significant correlations have also been recorded between EDSS and macular thickness in RRMS and SPMS, although not PPMS, patients [97]. Multiple Sclerosis Severity Score (MSSS) appears to be unrelated to RNFL thickness [106]. As the majority of MS disability scales may not sufficiently capture all aspects of disability beyond that in the realms of motor function and mobility, and in particular may not adequately reflect visual disability [108], the heterogeneous nature of results regarding the relationships between such scales and OCT is perhaps unsurprising. Despite this, OCT-derived TMV has been found to correlate with ambulatory ability in MS patients [109]. Rating scales focussed on visual function, such as the National Eye Institute Visual Function Questionnaire-25 (NEI-VFQ-25) have been used successfully to capture subjective visual dysfunction in MS patients following ON [72, 110], and this approach may hold promise for future studies in the broader MS population.

In addition to cross-sectional associations with disability, OCT has also been shown to predict disability progression in MS patients. Patients with averaged pRNFL thickness of less than 87–88 μm at baseline were approximately twice as likely to show evidence of disability progression (measured by EDSS) over up to 3 years, and almost four times as likely over 5 years, as those with an RNFL thickness above this threshold at baseline [111]. The same study did not observe any prognostic power of TMV [111]. Another study also found that an averaged RNFL thickness of 88 μm was associated with a threefold increased risk of disability (EDSS) worsening over 3 years and a slightly lower, though comparable, risk of accumulating cognitive deficits over the same period [112]; a cross-sectional investigation has also shown a link between RNFL, as well as GCIP, with cognitive ability in MS patients [113]. Baseline atrophy of the temporal RNFL quadrant is associated with worsening of EDSS and increased risk of clinical relapses over 2 years [23], whilst averaged RNFL thickness has been shown to be of some utility in predicting a conversion to clinically definite MS over 12 months in CIS patients [114]. CIS patients with GCIP thinning are more likely to convert to MS within 3 years, and less likely to remain free of clinical disease activity, than those with thicker GCIP [115]. Finally, increased INL thickness at baseline is associated with a future increase in EDSS [116]. From these studies, it can be seen that OCT may enable clinicians to identify those MS and CIS patients at highest risk of relapses and disease progression, who may benefit from earlier and/or more efficacious treatment.

11.4.2 Magnetic Resonance Imaging (MRI)

MRI remains of vital importance in diagnosis and monitoring of MS patients, with improvements to conventional technology and the development of new imaging techniques increasing sensitivity and permitting measurement of more diffuse CNS pathology [117]. To date, evidence suggests that RNFL thickness in MS patients is related to measures of brain parenchymal fraction (BPF) [118–120] and bicaudate ratio [101], with thinner RNFL being associated with greater brain atrophy, and also positively correlated with volume of both white and grey matter [23, 121]. However, the correlation between RNFL and grey matter may only be significant in more advanced MS, rather than at early stages of the disease [122], and some authors have reported that the relationship with white and grey matter may be significant only in eyes without previous ON [107, 121, 123]. RNFL thickness is also associated with MRI lesions in the optic radiations [17, 124, 125] and visual cortex [124]. However, RNFL appears not to be associated with non-specific MRI measures of MS disease activity such as T1 hypo-intense or T2 hyper-intense lesion volumes [23, 122]. GCIP is correlated with brain volume and white matter volume [121], but (as with RNFL) some of these relationships may be significant only in those eyes without previous ON [107, 123]. Faster rates of GCIP loss are associated with correspondingly increased rates of cerebral volume fraction (CVF; a measure of brain volume analogous to BPF) reduction, as well as cortical grey matter and thalamic atrophy, over a 4-year period [126]. INL thickening is associated with prospective T2 hyper-intense and gadolinium-enhancing lesion volume [116].

A particularly interesting aspect of the relationships between OCT and MRI parameters is the finding that different OCT-derived retinal structural measures may be correlated with different MRI outcome measures. For example, in MS eyes RNFL and GCIP thickness were positively correlated with both grey matter and caudate volumes, whilst INL thickness was correlated positively with fluid-attenuated inversion recovery (FLAIR) lesion volume and negatively with normal-appearing white matter (NAWM) volume [107]. The authors reported that whilst these correlations were true of their MS cohort as a whole, they were driven primarily by MS eyes without previous ON [107]. It has been proposed that these differences in the pattern of results between the inner (RNFL; GCIP) and outer (INL) retina may reflect pathologically distinct disease processes in MS [107], a hypothesis supported by subsequent work investigating the relationships between OCT and immune cells and immunoglobulin indices in cerebrospinal fluid (CSF) [116]. This subsequent study found that both GCIP and INL thickness were inversely correlated with CSF $CD19^{+}$ B-cell count, immunoglobulin G (IgG) and immunoglobulin A (IgA) synthesis, but that INL thickness was additionally positively correlated with $CD56^{bright}$ natural killer cell count [116].

Whilst all of these results are of interest, it remains challenging to compare the correlation of OCT findings with MRI parameters in MS patients due to the considerable heterogeneity in devices used, acquisition techniques, and analyses and outcome measures employed, particularly in MRI. Additional challenges arise from the fact that it is not currently possible to correlate MRI data from the brain as a whole with OCT data from individual eyes [127], and previous ON appears to affect correlations with MRI parameters in individual eyes considerably [121]. Whether OCT can to some extent replace MRI, along with the relative utilities of each technique, has been the subject of some debate [128, 129]. We suggest that whilst neither OCT nor MRI are without disadvantages as tools for MS research, both will remain vital, complementary investigatory techniques in the future. Robust, long-term longitudinal data may enable better characterisation of the relative merits of both examinations [130].

11.4.3 Visual Function

Clinical tests of visual function have also been employed in the study of patients with MS. Perhaps the most fundamental and widely-used test of visual function is the measurement of visual acuity, in which the patient must correctly identify letters, numbers or symbols of diminishing size at a pre-defined test distance. In routine ophthalmological or optometric practice, the test is typically performed using black letters on a retro-illuminated white background, with contrast between target and background maximized; this measure is therefore described as high-contrast visual acuity (HCVA). By using grey letters instead of black, the contrast between letter and background is reduced (e.g., to 2.5% or 1.25% contrast rather than close to 100% in HCVA) and thus the measure becomes that of low-contrast visual acuity (LCVA). Examples of charts for measuring HCVA and LCVA can be seen in Fig. 11.8.

Patients with MS are frequently found to have reduced LCVA even when HCVA is normal [98, 131, 132], and thus LCVA is considered the more sensitive visual outcome measure in MS [132]. Reduced LCVA is correlated with RNFL thinning cross-sectionally [19, 22, 35, 97, 133–135] and longitudinally [133], although more strongly correlated with thinning of GCIP [19, 97]. LCVA correlates also with PMB thickness, TMV, and foveal volume [135]. Studies have also documented correlations between HCVA and RNFL [19, 22, 97, 133, 135], GCIP [19, 97, 133], and PMB [135] thickness, as well as TMV and foveal volume [135], although some of these relationships are likely to be weaker in comparison to 2.5% contrast LCVA [133] and have not been observed in all studies [35]. A clinically significant decrease in HCVA, 2.5% and 1.25% contrast LCVA is associated with a decrease in pRNFL thickness of 2.2, 3.3 and 3.3 μm as well as a decrease in GCIP thickness of 1.3, 1.9 and 2.4 μm, respectively [19].

In addition to impaired LCVA, patients with MS are commonly found to have impaired colour vision, in eyes both with and without a history of ON [70, 136], with up to two thirds of patients failing at least one screening test [136]. Studies using OCT have observed that performance in colour vision testing is strongly correlated with thickness of pRNFL [135, 137] and PMB [135, 137], as well as TMV [137], in MS patients. Given that the thicknesses of these retinal layers are reduced in MS eyes with previous ON relative to those without a history of ON [28, 29], it is intuitive that performance in colour vision testing appears worse in those eyes with previous ON [70, 135]. The correlations between OCT and colour vision outcome measures are stronger when using SD-OCT technology than with TD-OCT, likely reflecting the superior resolution and accuracy of the former [135].

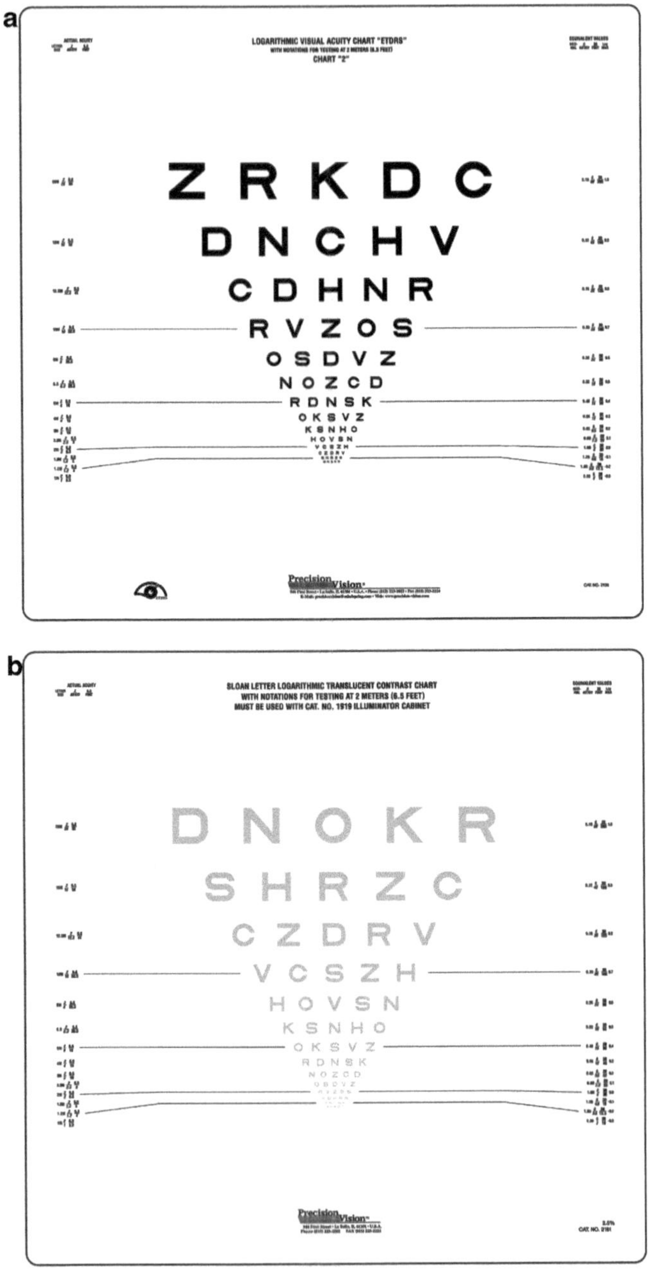

Fig. 11.8 Testing charts for measuring high- and low-contrast visual acuity (HCVA, LCVA). In order to measure HCVA, the contrast between target and background must be as close to 100% as possible, accomplished by using black targets on a white retro-illuminated background (**a**). Decreasing contrast can be accomplished by altering the colour of the targets from black to grey; the example chart shown here measures 2.5% contrast LCVA (**b**), but other contrast levels (e.g., 10%) are also possible. Images courtesy of Precision Vision, La Salle IL, U.S.A.

Perimetry, the subjective measurement of the visual field, may also be employed in order to ascertain the effects of disease on visual function. The technique is frequently utilized in patients with optic neuropathy (e.g. glaucoma), assessing the integrity of the entire visual pathway rather than specifically RGC or optic nerve function [138]. Visual field sensitivity (as measured by the mean deviation (MD) from age-matched normal values in decibels) is reduced in MS patients relative to normal subjects, with the greatest reduction being observed in those eyes with a history of ON [37, 139]. MD is correlated with TD-OCT-derived pRNFL thickness in MS eyes with a history of ON [140, 141]; at the time of writing, the quantitative relationship with deeper retinal layers remains unstudied. Given the high prevalence of fatigue symptoms in patients with MS [142] and the adverse effects of fatigue on both visual sensitivity and reliability when performing perimetry [138], it is likely that more objective measures of visual function, less dependent on alertness and cognitive performance, may be of more utility when studying patients with MS.

11.4.4 Electrophysiological Assessment of the Visual Pathway

Electrophysiological tests such as the visual evoked potential (VEP) and electroretinogram (ERG) quantify the electrical response of the visual cortex and retina, respectively, in response to precisely-defined visual stimuli. Using the ERG, the function of the photoreceptors and bipolar cells over the entire retina can be measured [143]. The multifocal ERG (MF-ERG) also measures the function of the photoreceptors and bipolar cells [144], but from discrete regions of the macula only [145]. The function of the ganglion cells of the inner retina can be measured using the pattern electroretinogram (PERG) or the photopic negative response (PhNR) of the ERG [146, 147]. The multifocal VEP (MF-VEP), in a manner analogous to the MF-ERG, allows functional assessment of smaller, localized areas of cortex and smaller bundles of axons in the visual pathway [148]. The utility of MF-VEP in clinical routine remains debated by experts in the field for a number of technical reasons, however it remains frequently used within MS research [35, 114, 149–152].

A number of studies have recorded significant correlations between electrophysiological and OCT parameters in MS patients. The response latency of the VEP or MF-VEP is correlated with mean RNFL thickness [35, 99, 153, 154], TMV [153], and GCIP thickness [35]. Evidence suggests that this relationship with RNFL is significant in eyes both with and without a history of ON but stronger in ON eyes [99]. Combining OCT measures of RNFL thickness with VEP ensures greater sensitivity in detecting anterior visual pathway damage after ON in MS patients than using either test alone [99]. PERG amplitudes are correlated with pRNFL thickness [37, 153, 154], TMV [153], GCIP thickness [37], and total retinal thickness [37]. Normalized PERG amplitudes (the ratio of the amplitudes of the N95 and P50 components) are also correlated with TMV [153, 154]. PhNR is correlated with RNFL thickness in MS eyes without previous ON and with an ON event at least 6 months previously, but not those with a history of ON less than 6 months previously [155];

this finding likely reflects the temporal dynamics of RNFL loss after ON as discussed in Sect. 11.3. The cone-driven ERG b-wave response latency has also been found to inversely correlate with RNFL and GCIP thickness, although its predictive power for these OCT parameters was significantly weaker than was the MF-VEP latency [35], doubtless reflecting the fact that this ERG component is generated by the bipolar cells and not the ganglion cells or their axons [156]. More recent work has documented some degree of negative correlation between ERG a-wave amplitudes and ONL thickness, as well as ERG b-wave amplitudes and INL thickness, in MS patients [39]; however, this study (and others) also recorded that ERG amplitudes are mostly normal in MS patients [35, 39, 46, 157–159]. Conversely, the latency of the ERG, particularly those responses driven in whole or in part by the cone system, has been shown to be abnormal to varying degrees in MS patients [35, 39, 46, 47, 157] whilst being uncorrelated with OCT-derived measures of ONL or INL [39]. This lack of correlation is compatible with dysfunctional, but not atrophic, photoreceptors and bipolar cells in patients with MS. The same study also failed to observe any correlations between MF-ERG parameters and INL structure, despite recording evidence of abnormal MF-ERG P1 latency [39].

With modification of the standard MF-ERG test protocol it is possible to visualize an additional component of the MF-ERG, the optic nerve head component (ONHC), which is generated at the optic nerve head [160]. Abnormalities of the OHNC have been documented in the ipsilateral and (to a lesser extent) contralateral eyes of MS patients with a history of unilateral ON [161]. The number of abnormal ONHC responses correlates strongly with RNFL thickness, so that a 10 μm reduction in pRNFL thickness is associated with 6.8 additional abnormal ONHC responses (from a total of 103 responses) [161]. The relationship between the ONHC and other OCT parameters remains unclear at the time of writing.

11.5 The Inner Nuclear Layer (INL)

Recent years have seen the emergence of interest regarding the potential importance of OCT-derived measurements of the INL in patients with MS. The INL contains the nuclei of the second-order retinal neurons, bipolar cells, as well as horizontal cells, amacrine cells, and the cell bodies of Müller glia [162]. This recent interest was arguably initially driven by an influential post-mortem histological study which recorded atrophy of the INL in addition to the ganglion cells [48]. Other authors, using OCT, have suggested that INL (in addition to ONL) may be reduced in thickness in a subset of MS patients exhibiting a severe clinical phenotype [42], and that increased INL thickness is associated with higher levels of disease activity, as evidenced both clinically and through MRI [163]. In addition, it has been proposed that the INL responds dynamically to MS disease activity and treatment; untreated MS patients were found to have a greater INL volume than healthy control subjects, yet this volume appeared to normalise following successful disease-modifying therapy (as evidenced by no clinical relapses or new MRI lesions during the follow-up period) yet remain elevated in patients in whom therapy was unsuccessful (Fig. 11.9) [24]. A particularly noteworthy aspect of this work [24] is that eyes with previous ON were excluded

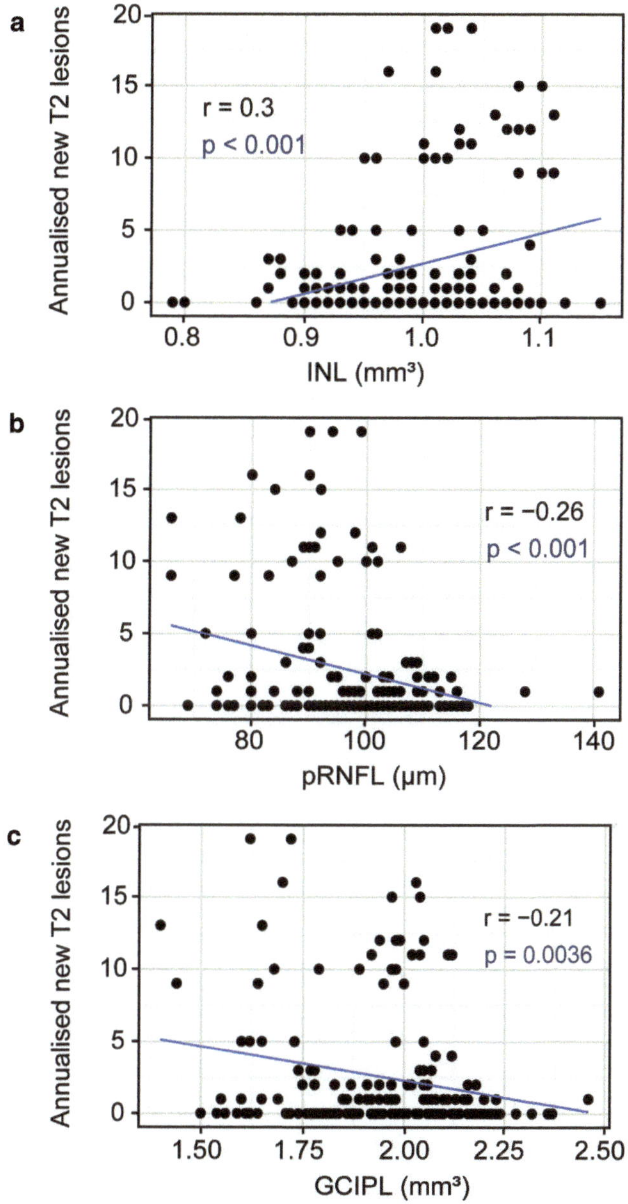

Fig. 11.9 Correlations between baseline inner nuclear layer (INL) volume (**a**), peripapillary retinal nerve fibre layer (pRNFL) thickness (**b**), and ganglion cell and inner plexiform layer (GCIP) volume (here named GCIPL; **c**) and prospective multiple sclerosis (MS) disease activity, as measured by annualised development of new T2 lesions visible using magnetic resonance imaging (MRI). INL volume is positively correlated with the number of new lesions, meaning that higher baseline INL volume is associated with an increased chance of developing new T2 lesions. Conversely, pRNFL thickness and GCIP volume are negatively correlated with the development of new T2 lesions, meaning that higher pRNFL thickness/GCIP volume is associated with a decreased chance of developing new lesions. Adapted from Knier et al. Brain 139, 2855–2863 (2016) with the permission of Oxford University Press and Prof. Thomas Korn

from analysis, ensuring that measures of INL thickness were uncontaminated by potential post-ON thickening [28]. Given that INL does not show atrophy after ON despite the well-documented thinning of the adjacent inner retina [18, 28], it may be that changes to INL thickness reflect inflammatory, rather than neurodegenerative, processes in MS [24].

Microcystic macular oedema (MMO) may also be observed in the INL of patients with MS. MMO was initially described as discrete, cyst-like spaces, visible on at least two adjacent OCT B-scans and predominantly confined to the INL, in 4.7% of MS patients (Fig. 11.10); these patients had, on average, higher EDSS and MSSS scores and reduced visual acuity, and were more likely to have previously suffered an episode of ON, in comparison to those without comparable changes to the INL [164]. These findings appear to be transient in the majority of patients (Fig. 11.11) [165]. The appropriate nomenclature of these findings has been a subject of debate; whilst originally described as microcystic macular oedema [164], the intraretinal

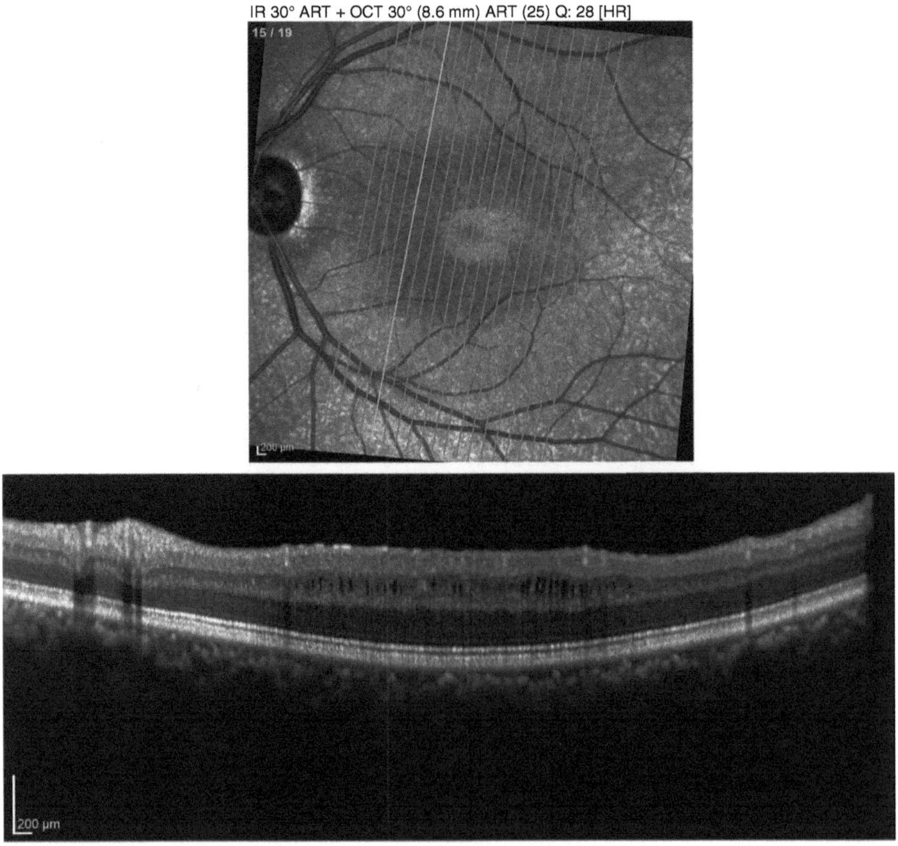

Fig. 11.10 OCT B-scan of the left eye of a patient with multiple sclerosis (MS) and microcystic macular oedema (MMO). The B-scan shows cystoid lesions confined to the inner nuclear layer (INL), pathognomonic for MMO

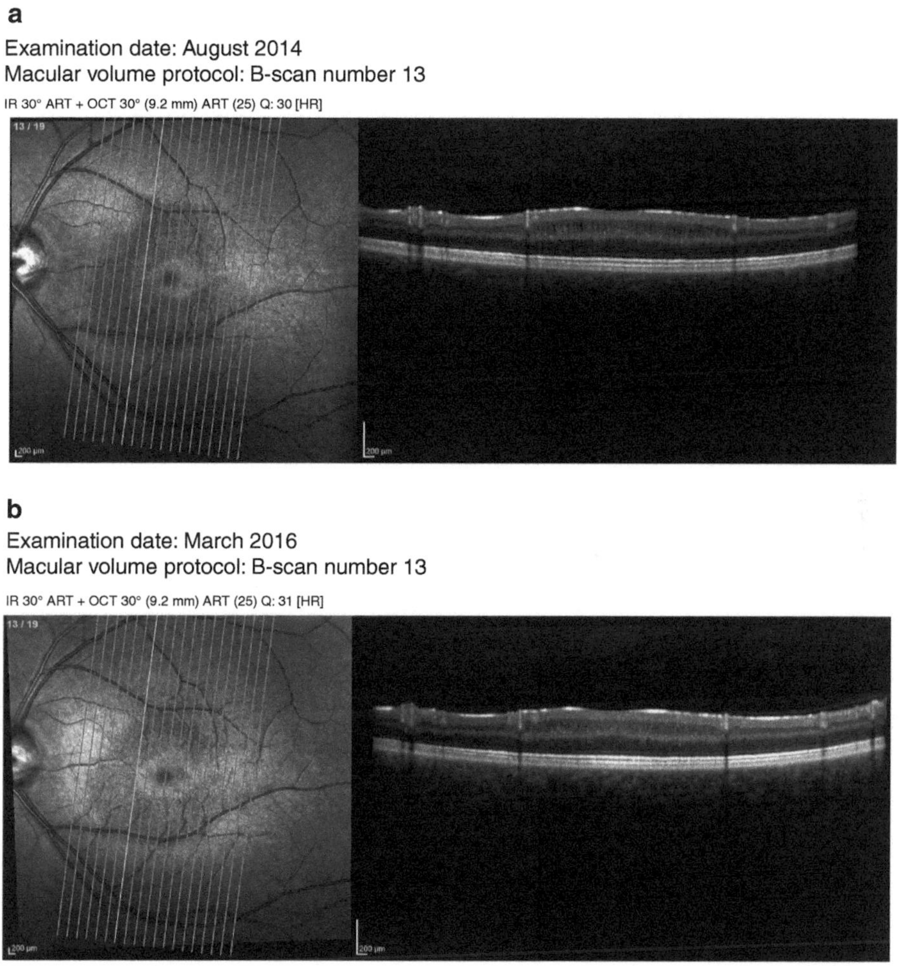

Fig. 11.11 Illustration of the transient nature of microcystic macular oedema (MMO) in a multiple sclerosis (MS) patient. The initial OCT scan revealed the presence of microcystoid lesions in the inner nuclear layer (INL), thereby confirming MMO in this patient (**a**). At follow-up 19 months later (at the same retinal location, as seen by the identical B-scan numbers), no more cystoid lesions were visible, indicating resolution of MMO (**b**)

spaces appear not to be lined with epithelium and are therefore not truly cystic, but rather cystoid, in nature [166]. When associated with optic atrophy, it has been suggested that INL thickening with or without cystoid lesions in the INL should be termed 'retrograde maculopathy' [167]. Nevertheless, the term MMO has persisted and will be used for familiarity here.

Although MMO was initially described in MS patients [163, 164], particularly in those with a history of ON [163, 164, 168], it rapidly became apparent from subsequent reports that MMO-like OCT findings can be observed in a range of non-MS disease states, including neuromyelitis optica spectrum disease (NMOSD)

[168–170], relapsing isolated optic neuritis (RION) [171], chronic relapsing inflammatory optic neuropathy (CRION) [168], glaucoma [172, 173], Leber's hereditary optic neuropathy (LHON) [174], dominant optic atrophy [174, 175], chronic compressive optic neuropathy secondary to glioma in a patient with neurofibromatosis type 1 [176], Tanzanian endemic optic neuropathy [177], traumatic optic neuropathy [172], hydrocephalus [172], tobacco-alcohol optic neuropathy [178], following phacoemulsification [179], and consequent to combined vitrectomy and inner limiting membrane removal [180]. The finding that cystoid changes in INL are observed post-vitrectomy (i.e., following surgical removal of the vitreous body) [180] is particularly relevant, as it provides clear evidence against previous hypotheses [174, 175] that vitreo-retinal traction is necessary for the formation of MMO, but is consistent with the proposal that MMO can occur independently of vitreo-retinal traction [170]. Changes in INL volume such as that seen in MMO have been hypothesised to be mediated by the Müller glial cells (the cell bodies of which are found in the INL) [171], and as potentially representing evidence of a glymphatic system (similar to that found in the brain) within the retina [181].

Despite a considerable lack of specificity, it is important to recognize that MMO in MS patients has to date, without exception, been found to be associated with increased disease severity [163, 164, 168]. This increased severity is observed in OCT scans as decreased RNFL [164] and GCIP [163] thickness, as well as increased INL thickness [163]; currently, there is no unanimity with regard to differences in TMV between MS eyes with and without MMO [164, 168]. Clinical indicators of increased disease severity in MS patients with MMO are reduced HCVA [163, 164, 168] and LCVA [163], higher MSSS values [163, 164, 168], higher EDSS values [164, 168], as well as an increased likelihood of developing Gadolinium-enhancing and T2-weighted MRI lesions [163]. African-American MS patients have a higher prevalence of MMO [51], consistent with the more aggressive disease course typically observed in this population [49–52]. Thus, a finding of MMO upon OCT examination may assist clinicians in their decision-making process when considering, for example, whether to recommend medical treatment (or a more efficacious treatment) to a MS patient. It may also lead the clinician to consider the possibility of an earlier insult to the optic nerve and initiate further diagnostic tests, for example VEP.

Although the evidence to date suggests that the INL is of great importance in MS, and may reflect inflammatory processes and response to treatment, at the time of writing the body of research is still nascent and thus the precise role of the INL arguably remains unclear. OCT-derived measures of INL structure may be confounded both by ON [28] and MMO, as discussed above, in patients with MS. An additional potential confound is that the INL contains nuclei of bipolar cells in addition to horizontal cells, amacrine cells, and the cell bodies of the Müller glia [162], meaning that structural changes to INL may be of multiple aetiologies and may not be ascribed to specific cell types (neuronal or glial) or specific types of neuron. Functional tests such as the ERG may measure bipolar integrity in isolation, however abnormal functional parameters appear not to correlate with OCT-derived INL structural measures [39]. More detailed characterisation of the role of the INL in MS, including longitudinal studies, is necessary.

11.6 OCT Findings in Experimental Models of MS

Although OCT has become a prominent tool in the clinical setting of MS diagnosis, it has only more recently begun to be explored in experimental animal, particularly rodent, models. Human and murine retinae share a similar laminar structure, with the primary difference between the two species being the lack of fovea in mice [182]. Therefore, the majority of studies utilizing OCT in murine models have obtained scans centred upon the optic nerve head, which provides a clear anatomical landmark for consistent longitudinal measurements (Fig. 11.12). OCT measures in mice are robust, with studies finding almost constant inner retinal layer (IRL)

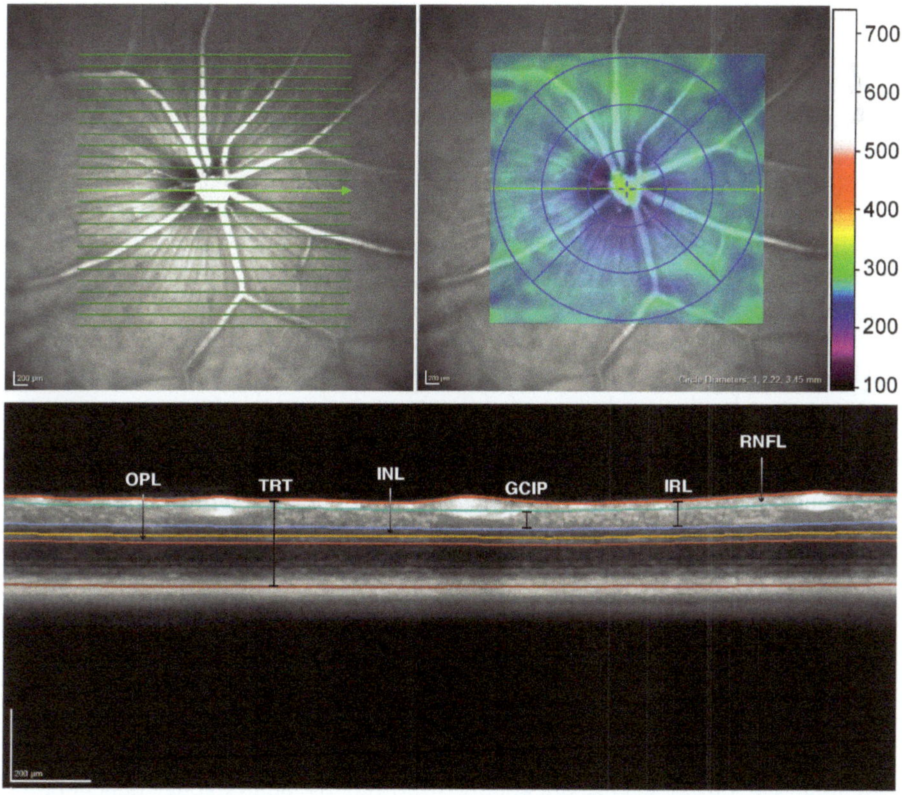

Fig. 11.12 Illustration of a typical scan in a healthy C57BL/6J (wild-type) mouse. The volume scan is centred upon the optic nerve head, rather than the fovea. After manual segmentation, the retinal layers can be defined as seen in the bottom panel: the retinal nerve fibre layer (RNFL) and ganglion cell and inner plexiform layer (GCIP) are aggregated together to give a thickness measure of the inner retinal layers (IRL), whilst the inner nuclear layer (INL) and outer plexiform layer (OPL) are analysed separately. A coarse but reliable measure of retinal structure is provided by the total retinal thickness (TRT), reflecting the thickness of all retinal layers combined

thickness over time in healthy controls [183–185] and excellent test-retest reliability [185, 186].

An early study utilizing a custom-built OCT device assessed the visual pathway in a transgenic mouse model of MS (using ND4 mice), in which animals spontaneously undergo demyelination after 3 months of age [187]. Qualitative OCT assessments of the retina and the optic nerve head areas were not significantly different between control mice or ND4 mice even though impaired ganglion cell function (as evidenced by reduced PERG amplitudes) was observed [187]. Furthermore, the authors observed no difference between groups when evaluating immunohistochemical retinal ganglion cell markers [187], suggesting that the ND4 murine model of MS may not be the most suitable for assessing structural damage to the visual pathway.

Experimental autoimmune encephalomyelitis (EAE) is an older and more widely employed model of MS, in which animals are injected with CNS proteins such as myelin oligodendrocyte glycoprotein (MOG) emulsified in an adjuvant, inducing an inflammatory response. Immunised animals develop demyelinating lesions in the CNS, including the optic nerve and retina [188–190]. Between 70–92% of eyes in these animals develop ON, making the model ideal for investigating therapies targeting visual impairment [78, 183, 185].

GCIP thinning around the optic nerve head has been observed in EAE mice 23–25 days post immunisation (dpi) compared to healthy control animals [191]. Similarly, significant RNFL thinning has been observed in EAE, specifically in the later stages of the disease course [186, 191, 192]. A previous study using EAE rats also recorded significant RNFL thinning prior to clinical manifestation of the disease [186], however another report in EAE mice did not observe differences in RNFL thickness relative to controls at similarly early timepoints [192]. These differences may be due to the use of different animal species (mouse vs. rat) and immunisation (MOG_{35-55} vs. MOG_{1-125}). An additional consideration is that the RNFL is a relatively thin layer in rodents compared to humans and it is difficult to distinguish between the RNFL and the ganglion cell layer, and therefore difficult to accurately and reproducibly quantify.

More recent studies have addressed this issue by aggregating the RNFL, GCL and IPL together; this complex is known as the IRL and provides a more robust measure of EAE-induced neuro-axonal degeneration [183–185]. IRL thickness significantly increases at clinical onset of the disease in EAE mice, followed by a steady decline as the disease progresses [185]. Another study following EAE mice up to 4 months post-immunisation found a continued and steady decline in IRL thickness throughout the later stages of the disease [183]. These findings resemble the initial RNFL thickening followed by neuroaxonal degeneration observed in many human studies of ON in MS, as summarised in Sect. 11.3. Interestingly, similar findings were also observed in a model of chronic MS, where IRL thickening was perceived after 2 weeks of EAE followed by significant thinning after 8 weeks of disease compared to healthy controls [184]. There is also evidence for early neurodegeneration in the retina, which may be initially masked by inflammatory oedema and become more visible only at later timepoints, after the inflammation has reduced [184–186]. Total retinal thickness (TRT) also increased during peak disease and decreased during recovery of clinical symptoms in EAE mice [191]. Since the TRT by definition includes the IRL, the increase in thickness at earlier time points is consistent. Conversely, INL thickness did not change during the disease course in both healthy and EAE mice [191]. However, this is a relatively thin structure and with currently available segmentation tools, involving primarily manual correction, it is challenging to obtain reliable measures of INL in mice.

As in humans [193], OCT findings of rodent retinal thickness correlate significantly with histological measurements of the retina at various time points in the disease course [184, 186, 194]. Discrepancies between retinal histology and OCT measurements can be attributable to tissue shrinkage following fixation [186]. Therefore, *in vivo* OCT measurements of the retina may provide a more accurate representation of retinal thickness changes compared to post-mortem histological analysis. OCT measures of IRL thinning are also inversely correlated with functional measures of visual impairment such as spatial frequency optokinetic response thresholds [183]. MRI measures of the visual pathway correlate strongly with OCT findings in EAE. Earlier in the disease course, IRL thickening correlates with T2 signal hyperintensities in the optic nerve, providing further support for inflammation in EAE mice [185]. Conversely, IRL thinning in later stages of the disease is associated with changes in the optic nerve [184, 185] and optic tracts [185] as detected with DTI, consistent with retrograde degeneration in the retina originating from lesions in more posterior parts of the visual pathway. However, the literature to date is not unanimous regarding the relationship between EAE scores and OCT measures, as one study recorded a significant negative correlation between EAE scores and IRL thickness [183], and others have reported no relationship [184, 185]. The EAE score does not incorporate visual outcomes but rather focuses on measurements of motor impairment, and therefore the lack of correlation observed in some studies may be due to atypical mice that present with ON and retinal damage but exhibit little or no clinical disability.

Overall, the retinal thinning observed longitudinally in EAE mice is representative of neuro-axonal degeneration independent of demyelination. This retinal degeneration in EAE parallels that observed in ON in humans (Sect. 11.3) but occurs in a much shorter time frame, making OCT an ideal tool for use in preclinical trials. The fact that structural damage to the visual pathway can precede clinical symptoms in EAE reinforces the need for early therapeutic interventions in ON.

Increasingly, pre-clinical trials in experimental models of MS are using OCT to assess structural damage to the anterior visual pathway and neuro-axonal degeneration following ON. For example, one such trial studied EAE-MOG_{35-55} mice which had been injected with antibodies against IL-17, a pro-inflammatory cytokine which is thought to play an important role in the development of ON and axonal atrophy in EAE. RNFL and GCIP were both significantly thicker in mice treated with anti-IL-17 compared to untreated EAE mice, and discontinuing anti-IL-17 treatment after the peak of clinical symptoms did not increase RNFL thinning [191]. This suggests that damage to the optic nerve and retina in EAE may occur, at least partly, due to an IL-17 mediated inflammatory response.

Another pre-clinical trial examined the effect of gypenosides, which are saponins with antioxidative and neuroprotective properties extracted from the *Gynostemma pentaphyllum* plant [192]. The authors administered either daily injections of gypenoside monotherapy with three different densities, methylprednisolone, or a combination of the two treatments to MOG_{35-55} immunized EAE mice. Attenuation of RNFL degeneration was observed in mice treated with gypenoside and combination therapy compared to untreated EAE mice 30 dpi [192]. Interestingly, at 40 dpi, RNFL thinning was observed in both untreated EAE mice and in mice treated with methylprednisolone compared to healthy controls, suggesting that gypenoside, rather than methylprednisolone, may have neuroprotective effects [192]. Results of previous human studies have suggested that corticosteroids may reduce the severity of symptoms at presentation but are not protective against neurodegeneration [75, 195], a finding reinforced by these more recent murine OCT findings [192]. Although gypenoside was not directly linked to decreased inflammation, it does appear to have some effect on reducing demyelination in the visual pathway, while a combination of both gypenoside and methylprednisolone appeared to have the best effect on reducing demyelination in the acute phase of ON [192].

Most recently, a pre-clinical OCT trial [183] was performed using alpha-lipoic acid (LA), a naturally occurring sulfhydryl compound with strong antioxidant and anti-inflammatory properties [196, 197]. In this study [183], LA was offered both as prophylactic and therapeutic treatment for mice immunised with EAE-MOG_{35-55}. Prophylactic LA treatment appeared to reduce IRL degeneration in EAE mice, while therapeutic treatment had no effect on IRL [183]. Therapeutic LA resulted in reduced clinical disability and preserved ganglion cells, yet IRL thinning and functional visual impairment was still observed [183], suggesting that early damage to IRL cannot be repaired or protected by LA administered after clinical disease onset. This suggests that early therapeutic intervention is essential to reducing degeneration following acute ON. Though these pre-clinical trials provide promising prophylactic treatment options in mice, there is still a need for viable therapeutic treatment options for ON in humans, as clinical trials usually involve treatment after the onset of clinical symptoms of ON, when the opportunity for prophylaxis has passed.

11.7 Summary

Patients with MS without previous ON exhibit thinning of the inner retina (pRNFL; GCIP), but not of the deeper layers such as INL, OPL, ONL, and PRL. Eyes with previous ON exhibit, on average, significantly more thinning of the inner retina. Although there is credible evidence of mild INL thickening in MS eyes with previous ON, this appears to be smaller in magnitude and more variable. Interpretation of OCT results pertaining to OPL, ONL, and PRL (and, to a lesser extent, the INL) is complicated by inconsistency of aggregation of these layers between different studies and software versions, although it appears that any documented changes to the thickness of these layers occur only after ON, are dynamic in nature, and also of considerably lesser magnitude than those observed in the inner retinal layers. With these factors in mind, we suggest that future studies examining outer, rather than inner, retinal structure in MS patients with or without ON may require much larger cohorts in order to achieve sufficient statistical power to detect potentially small differences between patient groups. OCT can be used to identify those patients at risk of a rapid or severely disabling disease course, and initiate timely intervention. In particular, analysis of the INL may in future assist in differentiating degenerative from inflammatory disease activity, and in monitoring treatment efficacy. Although it is unlikely to replace MRI, OCT provides valuable complementary information in patients with MS. OCT-A holds promise as a new outcome measure in MS, although at the time of writing the body of research is still nascent. Findings from studies using experimental models of MS may inform the clinical development of future prophylactic and/or therapeutic neuroprotective treatments for use in humans.

References

1. Kingwell E, Marriott JJ, Jette N, et al. Incidence and prevalence of multiple sclerosis in Europe: a systematic review. BMC Neurol. 2013;13:128.
2. Sospedra M, Martin R. Immunology of multiple sclerosis. Semin Neurol. 2016;36:115–27.
3. Lublin FD, Reingold SC, Cohen JA, et al. Defining the clinical course of multiple sclerosis: the 2013 revisions. Neurology. 2014;83:278–86.
4. Thompson AJ, Banwell BL, Barkhof F, et al. Diagnosis of multiple sclerosis: 2017 revisions of the McDonald criteria. Lancet Neurol. 2018;17:162–73.
5. McDonald WI, Barnes D. The ocular manifestations of multiple sclerosis. 1. Abnormalities of the afferent visual system. J Neurol Neurosurg Psychiatry. 1992;55:747–52.
6. Graham SL, Klistorner A. Afferent visual pathways in multiple sclerosis: a review. Clin Exp Ophthalmol. 2017;45:62–72.
7. Costello F. Vision disturbances in multiple sclerosis. Semin Neurol. 2016;36:185–95.
8. Toosy AT, Mason DF, Miller DH. Optic neuritis. Lancet Neurol. 2014;13:83–99.
9. Costello F. The afferent visual pathway: designing a structural-functional paradigm of multiple sclerosis. ISRN Neurol. 2013;2013:134858.
10. Huang D, Swanson EA, Lin CP, et al. Optical coherence tomography. Science (New York, NY). 1991;254:1178–81.
11. Cruz-Herranz A, Balk LJ, Oberwahrenbrock T, et al. The APOSTEL recommendations for reporting quantitative optical coherence tomography studies. Neurology. 2016;86:2303–9.
12. Tewarie P, Balk L, Costello F, et al. The OSCAR-IB consensus criteria for retinal OCT quality assessment. PLoS One. 2012;7:e34823.
13. Schippling S, Balk LJ, Costello F, et al. Quality control for retinal OCT in multiple sclerosis: validation of the OSCAR-IB criteria. Mult Scler. 2015;21:163–70.
14. Oberwahrenbrock T, Traber GL, Lukas S, et al. Multicenter reliability of semiautomatic retinal layer segmentation using OCT. Neurol Neuroimmunol Neuroinflamm. 2018;5:e449.
15. Seigo MA, Sotirchos ES, Newsome S, et al. In vivo assessment of retinal neuronal layers in multiple sclerosis with manual and automated optical coherence tomography segmentation techniques. J Neurol. 2012;259:2119–30.
16. Coric D, Petzold A, Uitdehaag BMJ, Balk LJ. Software updates of OCT segmentation algorithms influence longitudinal assessment of retinal atrophy. J Neurol Sci. 2018;387:16–20.

17. Klistorner A, Sriram P, Vootakuru N, et al. Axonal loss of retinal neurons in multiple sclerosis associated with optic radiation lesions. Neurology. 2014;82:2165–72.
18. Balk LJ, Twisk JW, Steenwijk MD, et al. A dam for retrograde axonal degeneration in multiple sclerosis? J Neurol Neurosurg Psychiatry. 2014;85:782–9.
19. Walter SD, Ishikawa H, Galetta KM, et al. Ganglion cell loss in relation to visual disability in multiple sclerosis. Ophthalmology. 2012;119:1250–7.
20. Oberwahrenbrock T, Schippling S, Ringelstein M, et al. Retinal damage in multiple sclerosis disease subtypes measured by high-resolution optical coherence tomography. Mult Scler Int. 2012;2012:530305.
21. Bock M, Brandt AU, Dorr J, et al. Patterns of retinal nerve fiber layer loss in multiple sclerosis patients with or without optic neuritis and glaucoma patients. Clin Neurol Neurosurg. 2010;112:647–52.
22. Fisher JB, Jacobs DA, Markowitz CE, et al. Relation of visual function to retinal nerve fiber layer thickness in multiple sclerosis. Ophthalmology. 2006;113:324–32.
23. Sepulcre J, Murie-Fernandez M, Salinas-Alaman A, Garcia-Layana A, Bejarano B, Villoslada P. Diagnostic accuracy of retinal abnormalities in predicting disease activity in MS. Neurology. 2007;68:1488–94.
24. Knier B, Schmidt P, Aly L, et al. Retinal inner nuclear layer volume reflects response to immunotherapy in multiple sclerosis. Brain. 2016;139:2855–63.
25. Albrecht P, Ringelstein M, Muller AK, et al. Degeneration of retinal layers in multiple sclerosis subtypes quantified by optical coherence tomography. Mult Scler. 2012;18:1422–9.
26. Knier B, Berthele A, Buck D, et al. Optical coherence tomography indicates disease activity prior to clinical onset of central nervous system demyelination. Mult Scler. 2016;22:893–900.
27. Pietroboni AM, Dell'Arti L, Caprioli M, et al. The loss of macular ganglion cells begins from the early stages of disease and correlates with brain atrophy in multiple sclerosis patients. Mult Scler. 2019;25:31–8.
28. Petzold A, Balcer LJ, Calabresi PA, et al. Retinal layer segmentation in multiple sclerosis: a systematic review and meta-analysis. Lancet Neurol. 2017;16:797–812.
29. Petzold A, de Boer JF, Schippling S, et al. Optical coherence tomography in multiple sclerosis: a systematic review and meta-analysis. Lancet Neurol. 2010;9:921–32.
30. Rebolleda G, Gonzalez-Lopez JJ, Munoz-Negrete FJ, Oblanca N, Costa-Frossard L, Alvarez-Cermeno JC. Color-code agreement among stratus, cirrus, and spectralis optical coherence tomography in relapsing-remitting multiple sclerosis with and without prior optic neuritis. Am J Ophthalmol. 2013;155:890–7.
31. Balk LJ, Cruz-Herranz A, Albrecht P, et al. Timing of retinal neuronal and axonal loss in MS: a longitudinal OCT study. J Neurol. 2016;263:1323–31.
32. Garcia-Martin E, Ara JR, Martin J, et al. Retinal and optic nerve degeneration in patients with multiple sclerosis followed up for 5 years. Ophthalmology. 2017;124(5):688–96.
33. Narayanan D, Cheng H, Bonem KN, Saenz R, Tang RA, Frishman LJ. Tracking changes over time in retinal nerve fiber layer and ganglion cell-inner plexiform layer thickness in multiple sclerosis. Mult Scler. 2014;20:1331–41.
34. Oberwahrenbrock T, Ringelstein M, Jentschke S, et al. Retinal ganglion cell and inner plexiform layer thinning in clinically isolated syndrome. Mult Scler. 2013;19:1887–95.
35. Sriram P, Wang C, Yiannikas C, et al. Relationship between optical coherence tomography and electrophysiology of the visual pathway in non-optic neuritis eyes of multiple sclerosis patients. PLoS One. 2014;9:e102546.
36. Syc SB, Saidha S, Newsome SD, et al. Optical coherence tomography segmentation reveals ganglion cell layer pathology after optic neuritis. Brain. 2012;135:521–33.
37. Hokazono K, Raza AS, Oyamada MK, Hood DC, Monteiro ML. Pattern electroretinogram in neuromyelitis optica and multiple sclerosis with or without optic neuritis and its correlation with FD-OCT and perimetry. Doc Ophthalmol. 2013;127:201–15.
38. Manogaran P, Vavasour IM, Lange AP, et al. Quantifying visual pathway axonal and myelin loss in multiple sclerosis and neuromyelitis optica. NeuroImage Clin. 2016;11:743–50.

39. Hanson JVM, Hediger M, Manogaran P, et al. Outer retinal dysfunction in the absence of structural abnormalities in multiple sclerosis. Invest Ophthalmol Vis Sci. 2018;59:549–60.
40. Behbehani R, Abu Al-Hassan A, Al-Salahat A, Sriraman D, Oakley JD, Alroughani R. Optical coherence tomography segmentation analysis in relapsing remitting versus progressive multiple sclerosis. PLoS One. 2017;12:e0172120.
41. Petracca M, Cordano C, Cellerino M, et al. Retinal degeneration in primary-progressive multiple sclerosis: a role for cortical lesions? Mult Scler. 2017;23:43–50.
42. Saidha S, Syc SB, Ibrahim MA, et al. Primary retinal pathology in multiple sclerosis as detected by optical coherence tomography. Brain. 2011;134:518–33.
43. Brandt AU, Oberwahrenbrock T, Ringelstein M, et al. Primary retinal pathology in multiple sclerosis as detected by optical coherence tomography. Brain. 2011;134:e193. Author reply e4.
44. Gills JP Jr. Electroretinographic abnormalities and advanced multiple sclerosis. Investig Ophthalmol. 1966;5:555–9.
45. Papakostopoulos D, Fotiou F, Hart JC, Banerji NK. The electroretinogram in multiple sclerosis and demyelinating optic neuritis. Electroencephalogr Clin Neurophysiol. 1989;74:1–10.
46. Forooghian F, Sproule M, Westall C, et al. Electroretinographic abnormalities in multiple sclerosis: possible role for retinal autoantibodies. Doc Ophthalmol. 2006;113:123–32.
47. You Y, Graham EC, Shen T, et al. Progressive inner nuclear layer dysfunction in non-optic neuritis eyes in MS. Neurol Neuroimmunol Neuroinflamm. 2018;5:e427.
48. Green AJ, McQuaid S, Hauser SL, Allen IV, Lyness R. Ocular pathology in multiple sclerosis: retinal atrophy and inflammation irrespective of disease duration. Brain. 2010;133:1591–601.
49. Naismith RT, Trinkaus K, Cross AH. Phenotype and prognosis in African-Americans with multiple sclerosis: a retrospective chart review. Mult Scler. 2006;12:775–81.
50. Kister I, Chamot E, Bacon JH, et al. Rapid disease course in African Americans with multiple sclerosis. Neurology. 2010;75:217–23.
51. Caldito NG, Saidha S, Sotirchos ES, et al. Brain and retinal atrophy in African-Americans versus Caucasian-Americans with multiple sclerosis: a longitudinal study. Brain. 2018;141:3115–29.
52. Kimbrough DJ, Sotirchos ES, Wilson JA, et al. Retinal damage and vision loss in African American multiple sclerosis patients. Ann Neurol. 2015;77:228–36.
53. Guarnera C, Bramanti P, Mazzon E. Comparison of efficacy and safety of oral agents for the treatment of relapsing-remitting multiple sclerosis. Drug Des Devel Ther. 2017;11:2193–207.
54. Derfuss T, Bergvall NK, Sfikas N, Tomic DL. Efficacy of fingolimod in patients with highly active relapsing-remitting multiple sclerosis. Curr Med Res Opin. 2015;31:1687–91.
55. Kappos L, Cohen J, Collins W, et al. Fingolimod in relapsing multiple sclerosis: an integrated analysis of safety findings. Mult Scler Relat Disord. 2014;3:494–504.
56. Calabresi PA, Radue EW, Goodin D, et al. Safety and efficacy of fingolimod in patients with relapsing-remitting multiple sclerosis (FREEDOMS II): a double-blind, randomised, placebo-controlled, phase 3 trial. Lancet Neurol. 2014;13:545–56.
57. Rotsos TG, Moschos MM. Cystoid macular edema. Clin Ophthalmol. 2008;2:919–30.
58. Novartis. Gilenya full prescribing information. Novartis; 2018.
59. Hajali M, Fishman GA. The prevalence of cystoid macular oedema on optical coherence tomography in retinitis pigmentosa patients without cystic changes on fundus examination. Eye (Lond). 2009;23:915–9.
60. Ortiz-Perez S, Martinez-Lapiscina EH, Gabilondo I, et al. Retinal periphlebitis is associated with multiple sclerosis severity. Neurology. 2013;81:877–81.
61. Spain RI, Liu L, Zhang X, et al. Optical coherence tomography angiography enhances the detection of optic nerve damage in multiple sclerosis. Br J Ophthalmol. 2018;102:520–4.
62. Lanzillo R, Cennamo G, Criscuolo C, et al. Optical coherence tomography angiography retinal vascular network assessment in multiple sclerosis. Mult Scler. 2018;24:1706–14.
63. Wang X, Jia Y, Spain R, et al. Optical coherence tomography angiography of optic nerve head and parafovea in multiple sclerosis. Br J Ophthalmol. 2014;98:1368–73.

64. Feucht N, Maier M, Lepennetier G, et al. Optical coherence tomography angiography indicates associations of the retinal vascular network and disease activity in multiple sclerosis. Mult Scler. 2019;25:224–34.
65. Ikuta F, Zimmerman HM. Distribution of plaques in seventy autopsy cases of multiple sclerosis in the United States. Neurology. 1976;26:26–8.
66. The clinical profile of optic neuritis. Experience of the Optic Neuritis Treatment Trial. Optic Neuritis Study Group. Arch Ophthalmol. 1991;109:1673–8.
67. Petzold A, Wattjes MP, Costello F, et al. The investigation of acute optic neuritis: a review and proposed protocol. Nat Rev Neurol. 2014;10:447–58.
68. Gerling J, Meyer JH, Kommerell G. Visual field defects in optic neuritis and anterior ischemic optic neuropathy: distinctive features. Graefes Arch Clin Exp Ophthalmol. 1998;236:188–92.
69. Halilovic EA, Alimanovic I, Suljic E, Hassan NA. Optic neuritis as first clinical manifestations the multiple sclerosis. Materia Socio Medica. 2014;26:246–8.
70. Moura AL, Teixeira RA, Oiwa NN, et al. Chromatic discrimination losses in multiple sclerosis patients with and without optic neuritis using the Cambridge Colour Test. Vis Neurosci. 2008;25:463–8.
71. Shams PN, Plant GT. Optic neuritis: a review. Int MS J. 2009;16:82–9.
72. Sanchez-Dalmau B, Martinez-Lapiscina EH, Torres-Torres R, et al. Early retinal atrophy predicts long-term visual impairment after acute optic neuritis. Mult Scler. 2018;24:1196–204.
73. Hickman SJ, Dalton CM, Miller DH, Plant GT. Management of acute optic neuritis. Lancet. 2002;360:1953–62.
74. Raz N, Dotan S, Chokron S, Ben-Hur T, Levin N. Demyelination affects temporal aspects of perception: an optic neuritis study. Ann Neurol. 2012;71:531–8.
75. Beck RW, Cleary PA, Anderson MM Jr, et al. A randomized, controlled trial of corticosteroids in the treatment of acute optic neuritis. The Optic Neuritis Study Group. N Engl J Med. 1992;326:581–8.
76. Beck RW, Cleary PA, Trobe JD, et al. The effect of corticosteroids for acute optic neuritis on the subsequent development of multiple sclerosis. The Optic Neuritis Study Group. N Engl J Med. 1993;329:1764–9.
77. Heesen C, Haase R, Melzig S, et al. Perceptions on the value of bodily functions in multiple sclerosis. Acta Neurol Scand. 2018;137:356–62.
78. Shindler KS, Ventura E, Dutt M, Rostami A. Inflammatory demyelination induces axonal injury and retinal ganglion cell apoptosis in experimental optic neuritis. Exp Eye Res. 2008;87:208–13.
79. Trip SA, Schlottmann PG, Jones SJ, et al. Retinal nerve fiber layer axonal loss and visual dysfunction in optic neuritis. Ann Neurol. 2005;58:383–91.
80. Costello F, Hodge W, Pan YI, Eggenberger E, Coupland S, Kardon RH. Tracking retinal nerve fiber layer loss after optic neuritis: a prospective study using optical coherence tomography. Mult Scler. 2008;14:893–905.
81. Henderson AP, Altmann DR, Trip AS, et al. A serial study of retinal changes following optic neuritis with sample size estimates for acute neuroprotection trials. Brain. 2010;133:2592–602.
82. Costello F, Pan YI, Yeh EA, Hodge W, Burton JM, Kardon R. The temporal evolution of structural and functional measures after acute optic neuritis. J Neurol Neurosurg Psychiatry. 2015;86:1369–73.
83. Gabilondo I, Martinez-Lapiscina EH, Fraga-Pumar E, et al. Dynamics of retinal injury after acute optic neuritis. Ann Neurol. 2015;77:517–28.
84. Parisi V, Manni G, Spadaro M, et al. Correlation between morphological and functional retinal impairment in multiple sclerosis patients. Invest Ophthalmol Vis Sci. 1999;40:2520–7.
85. Bertuzzi F, Suzani M, Tagliabue E, et al. Diagnostic validity of optic disc and retinal nerve fiber layer evaluations in detecting structural changes after optic neuritis. Ophthalmology. 2010;117:1256–64.e1.
86. Laible M, Jarius S, Mackensen F, et al. Adding papillomacular bundle measurements to standard optical coherence tomography does not increase sensitivity to detect prior optic neuritis in patients with multiple sclerosis. PLoS One. 2016;11:e0155322.

87. Schneider E, Zimmermann H, Oberwahrenbrock T, et al. Optical coherence tomography reveals distinct patterns of retinal damage in neuromyelitis optica and multiple sclerosis. PLoS One. 2013;8:e66151.
88. Neroev VV, Eliseeva EK, Zueva MV, et al. Demyelinating optic neuritis: optical coherence tomography and multifocal electroretinography data correlation. Hum Physiol. 2016;42:879–84.
89. Loughran-Fjeldstad AS, Carlson NG, Husebye CD, Cook LJ, Rose JW. Retinal nerve fiber layer sector-specific compromise in relapsing and remitting multiple sclerosis. eNeurologicalSci. 2015;1:30–7.
90. Nolan RC, Galetta SL, Frohman TC, et al. Optimal intereye difference thresholds in retinal nerve fiber layer thickness for predicting a unilateral optic nerve lesion in multiple sclerosis. J Neuroophthalmol. 2018;38:451–8.
91. Al-Louzi OA, Bhargava P, Newsome SD, et al. Outer retinal changes following acute optic neuritis. Mult Scler. 2016;22:362–72.
92. Kupersmith MJ, Mandel G, Anderson S, Meltzer DE, Kardon R. Baseline, one and three month changes in the peripapillary retinal nerve fiber layer in acute optic neuritis: relation to baseline vision and MRI. J Neurol Sci. 2011;308:117–23.
93. Costello F, Coupland S, Hodge W, et al. Quantifying axonal loss after optic neuritis with optical coherence tomography. Ann Neurol. 2006;59:963–9.
94. Garas A, Simo M, Hollo G. Nerve fiber layer and macular thinning measured with different imaging methods during the course of acute optic neuritis. Eur J Ophthalmol. 2011;21:473–83.
95. Xu SC, Kardon RH, Leavitt JA, Flanagan EP, Pittock SJ, Chen JJ. Optical coherence tomography is highly sensitive in detecting prior optic neuritis. Neurology. 2019;92.
96. Kaushik M, Wang CY, Barnett MH, et al. Inner nuclear layer thickening is inversley proportional to retinal ganglion cell loss in optic neuritis. PLoS One. 2013;8:e78341.
97. Saidha S, Syc SB, Durbin MK, et al. Visual dysfunction in multiple sclerosis correlates better with optical coherence tomography derived estimates of macular ganglion cell layer thickness than peripapillary retinal nerve fiber layer thickness. Mult Scler. 2011;17:1449–63.
98. Garcia-Martin E, Rodriguez-Mena D, Herrero R, et al. Neuro-ophthalmologic evaluation, quality of life, and functional disability in patients with MS. Neurology. 2013;81:76–83.
99. Di Maggio G, Santangelo R, Guerrieri S, et al. Optical coherence tomography and visual evoked potentials: which is more sensitive in multiple sclerosis? Mult Scler. 2014;20:1342–7.
100. Tugcu B, Soysal A, Kilic M, et al. Assessment of structural and functional visual outcomes in relapsing remitting multiple sclerosis with visual evoked potentials and optical coherence tomography. J Neurol Sci. 2013;335:182–5.
101. Abalo-Lojo JM, Limeres CC, Gomez MA, et al. Retinal nerve fiber layer thickness, brain atrophy, and disability in multiple sclerosis patients. J Neuroophthalmol. 2014;34:23–8.
102. Tatrai E, Simo M, Iljicsov A, Nemeth J, Debuc DC, Somfai GM. In vivo evaluation of retinal neurodegeneration in patients with multiple sclerosis. PLoS One. 2012;7:e30922.
103. Soufi G, AitBenhaddou E, Hajji Z, et al. Evaluation of retinal nerve fiber layer thickness measured by optical coherence tomography in Moroccan patients with multiple sclerosis. J Fr Ophtalmol. 2015;38:497–503.
104. Spain RI, Maltenfort M, Sergott RC, Leist TP. Thickness of retinal nerve fiber layer correlates with disease duration in parallel with corticospinal tract dysfunction in untreated multiple sclerosis. J Rehabil Res Dev. 2009;46:633–42.
105. Jeanjean L, Castelnovo G, Carlander B, et al. Retinal atrophy using optical coherence tomography (OCT) in 15 patients with multiple sclerosis and comparison with healthy subjects. Rev Neurol (Paris). 2008;164:927–34.
106. Naismith RT, Tutlam NT, Xu J, et al. Optical coherence tomography is less sensitive than visual evoked potentials in optic neuritis. Neurology. 2009;73:46–52.
107. Saidha S, Sotirchos ES, Oh J, et al. Relationships between retinal axonal and neuronal measures and global central nervous system pathology in multiple sclerosis. JAMA Neurol. 2013;70:34–43.

108. Ontaneda D, LaRocca N, Coetzee T, Rudick R. Revisiting the multiple sclerosis functional composite: proceedings from the National Multiple Sclerosis Society (NMSS) Task Force on clinical disability measures. Mult Scler. 2012;18:1074–80.
109. Balantrapu S, Sandroff BM, Pula JH, Motl RW. Integrity of the anterior visual pathway and its association with ambulatory performance in multiple sclerosis. Mult Scler Int. 2013;2013:481035.
110. Sabadia SB, Nolan RC, Galetta KM, et al. 20/40 or better visual acuity after optic neuritis: not as good as we once thought? J Neuroophthalmol. 2016;36:369–76.
111. Martinez-Lapiscina EH, Arnow S, Wilson JA, et al. Retinal thickness measured with optical coherence tomography and risk of disability worsening in multiple sclerosis: a cohort study. Lancet Neurol. 2016;15:574–84.
112. Bsteh G, Hegen H, Teuchner B, et al. Peripapillary retinal nerve fibre layer as measured by optical coherence tomography is a prognostic biomarker not only for physical but also for cognitive disability progression in multiple sclerosis. Mult Scler. 2019;25:196–203.
113. Coric D, Balk LJ, Verrijp M, et al. Cognitive impairment in patients with multiple sclerosis is associated with atrophy of the inner retinal layers. Mult Scler. 2018;24:158–66.
114. Perez-Rico C, Ayuso-Peralta L, Rubio-Perez L, et al. Evaluation of visual structural and functional factors that predict the development of multiple sclerosis in clinically isolated syndrome patients. Invest Ophthalmol Vis Sci. 2014;55:6127–31.
115. Zimmermann HG, Knier B, Oberwahrenbrock T, et al. Association of retinal ganglion cell layer thickness with future disease activity in patients with clinically isolated syndrome. JAMA Neurol. 2018;75:1071–9.
116. Knier B, Leppenetier G, Wetzlmair C, et al. Association of retinal architecture, intrathecal immunity, and clinical course in multiple sclerosis. JAMA Neurol. 2017;74:847–56.
117. Miller TR, Mohan S, Choudhri AF, Gandhi D, Jindal G. Advances in multiple sclerosis and its variants: conventional and newer imaging techniques. Radiol Clin N Am. 2014;52:321–36.
118. Dörr J, Wernecke KD, Bock M, et al. Association of retinal and macular damage with brain atrophy in multiple sclerosis. PLoS One. 2011;6:e18132.
119. Pfueller CF, Brandt AU, Schubert F, et al. Metabolic changes in the visual cortex are linked to retinal nerve fiber layer thinning in multiple sclerosis. PLoS One. 2011;6:e18019.
120. Gordon-Lipkin E, Chodkowski B, Reich DS, et al. Retinal nerve fiber layer is associated with brain atrophy in multiple sclerosis. Neurology. 2007;69:1603–9.
121. Zimmermann H, Freing A, Kaufhold F, et al. Optic neuritis interferes with optical coherence tomography and magnetic resonance imaging correlations. Mult Scler. 2013;19:443–50.
122. Young KL, Brandt AU, Petzold A, et al. Loss of retinal nerve fibre layer axons indicates white but not grey matter damage in early multiple sclerosis. Eur J Neurol. 2013;20:803–11.
123. Balk LJ, Steenwijk MD, Tewarie P, et al. Bidirectional trans-synaptic axonal degeneration in the visual pathway in multiple sclerosis. J Neurol Neurosurg Psychiatry. 2015;86:419–24.
124. Gabilondo I, Martinez-Lapiscina EH, Martinez-Heras E, et al. Trans-synaptic axonal degeneration in the visual pathway in multiple sclerosis. Ann Neurol. 2014;75:98–107.
125. Scheel M, Finke C, Oberwahrenbrock T, et al. Retinal nerve fibre layer thickness correlates with brain white matter damage in multiple sclerosis: a combined optical coherence tomography and diffusion tensor imaging study. Mult Scler. 2014;20:1904–7.
126. Saidha S, Al-Louzi O, Ratchford JN, et al. Optical coherence tomography reflects brain atrophy in multiple sclerosis: a four-year study. Ann Neurol. 2015;78:801–13.
127. Manogaran P, Hanson JV, Olbert ED, et al. Optical coherence tomography and magnetic resonance imaging in multiple sclerosis and neuromyelitis optica spectrum disorder. Int J Mol Sci. 2016;17:E1894.
128. Sotirchos ES, Saidha S. OCT is an alternative to MRI for monitoring MS – YES. Mult Scler J. 2018;24:701–3.
129. Aboulenein-Djamshidian F, Serbecic N. OCT is an alternative to MRI for monitoring MS – NO. Mult Scler J. 2018;24:703–5.
130. Green AJ. OCT is an alternative to MRI for monitoring MS – Commentary. Mult Scler J. 2018;24:705–6.

131. Balcer LJ, Baier ML, Pelak VS, et al. New low-contrast vision charts: reliability and test characteristics in patients with multiple sclerosis. Mult Scler. 2000;6:163–71.
132. Balcer LJ, Frohman EM. Evaluating loss of visual function in multiple sclerosis as measured by low-contrast letter acuity. Neurology. 2010;74(Suppl 3):S16–23.
133. Talman LS, Bisker ER, Sackel DJ, et al. Longitudinal study of vision and retinal nerve fiber layer thickness in multiple sclerosis. Ann Neurol. 2010;67:749–60.
134. Schinzel J, Zimmermann H, Paul F, et al. Relations of low contrast visual acuity, quality of life and multiple sclerosis functional composite: a cross-sectional analysis. BMC Neurol. 2014;14:31.
135. Villoslada P, Cuneo A, Gelfand J, Hauser SL, Green A. Color vision is strongly associated with retinal thinning in multiple sclerosis. Mult Scler. 2012;18:991–9.
136. Harrison AC, Becker WJ, Stell WK. Colour vision abnormalities in multiple sclerosis. Can J Neurol Sci. 1987;14:279–85.
137. Martinez-Lapiscina EH, Ortiz-Perez S, Fraga-Pumar E, et al. Colour vision impairment is associated with disease severity in multiple sclerosis. Mult Scler. 2014;20:1207–16.
138. Henson DB. Visual fields. Oxford: Oxford University Press; 1993.
139. Castro SM, Damasceno A, Damasceno BP, et al. Visual pathway abnormalities were found in most multiple sclerosis patients despite history of previous optic neuritis. Arq Neuropsiquiatr. 2013;71:437–41.
140. Cheng H, Laron M, Schiffman JS, Tang RA, Frishman LJ. The relationship between visual field and retinal nerve fiber layer measurements in patients with multiple sclerosis. Invest Ophthalmol Vis Sci. 2007;48:5798–805.
141. Merle H, Olindo S, Donnio A, Richer R, Smadja D, Cabre P. Anatomic and functional correlation of frequency-doubling technology perimetry (FDTP) in multiple sclerosis. Int Ophthalmol. 2011;31:263–70.
142. Fisk JD, Pontefract A, Ritvo PG, Archibald CJ, Murray TJ. The impact of fatigue on patients with multiple sclerosis. Can J Neurol Sci. 1994;21:9–14.
143. McCulloch DL, Marmor MF, Brigell MG, et al. ISCEV standard for full-field clinical electroretinography (2015 update). Doc Ophthalmol. 2015;130:1–12.
144. Hood DC, Frishman LJ, Saszik S, Viswanathan S. Retinal origins of the primate multifocal ERG: implications for the human response. Invest Ophthalmol Vis Sci. 2002;43:1673–85.
145. Bearse MA Jr, Sutter EE. Imaging localized retinal dysfunction with the multifocal electroretinogram. J Opt Soc Am A Opt Image Sci Vis. 1996;13:634–40.
146. Luo X, Frishman LJ. Retinal pathway origins of the pattern electroretinogram (PERG). Invest Ophthalmol Vis Sci. 2011;52:8571–84.
147. Viswanathan S, Frishman LJ, Robson JG, Harwerth RS, Smith EL 3rd. The photopic negative response of the macaque electroretinogram: reduction by experimental glaucoma. Invest Ophthalmol Vis Sci. 1999;40:1124–36.
148. Klistorner AI, Graham SL, Grigg JR, Billson FA. Multifocal topographic visual evoked potential: improving objective detection of local visual field defects. Invest Ophthalmol Vis Sci. 1998;39:937–50.
149. Narayanan D, Cheng H, Tang RA, Frishman LJ. Reproducibility of multifocal visual evoked potential and traditional visual evoked potential in normal and multiple sclerosis eyes. Doc Ophthalmol. 2015;130:31–41.
150. Narayanan D, Cheng H, Tang RA, Frishman LJ. Longitudinal evaluation of visual function in multiple sclerosis. Optom Vis Sci. 2015;92:976–85.
151. Frohman AR, Schnurman Z, Conger A, et al. Multifocal visual evoked potentials are influenced by variable contrast stimulation in MS. Neurology. 2012;79:797–801.
152. Blanco R, Perez-Rico C, Puertas-Munoz I, Ayuso-Peralta L, Boquete L, Arevalo-Serrano J. Functional assessment of the visual pathway with multifocal visual evoked potentials, and their relationship with disability in patients with multiple sclerosis. Mult Scler. 2014;20:183–91.

153. Almarcegui C, Dolz I, Pueyo V, et al. Correlation between functional and structural assessments of the optic nerve and retina in multiple sclerosis patients. Neurophysiol Clin. 2010;40:129–35.
154. Rodriguez-Mena D, Almarcegui C, Dolz I, et al. Electropysiologic evaluation of the visual pathway in patients with multiple sclerosis. J Clin Neurophysiol. 2013;30:376–81.
155. Wang J, Cheng H, Hu YS, Tang RA, Frishman LJ. The photopic negative response of the flash electroretinogram in multiple sclerosis. Invest Ophthalmol Vis Sci. 2012;53:1315–23.
156. Robson AG, Nilsson J, Li S, et al. ISCEV guide to visual electrodiagnostic procedures. Doc Ophthalmol. 2018;136:1–26.
157. Gundogan FC, Demirkaya S, Sobaci G. Is optical coherence tomography really a new biomarker candidate in multiple sclerosis?--A structural and functional evaluation. Invest Ophthalmol Vis Sci. 2007;48:5773–81.
158. Fraser CL, Holder GE. Electroretinogram findings in unilateral optic neuritis. Doc Ophthalmol. 2011;123:173–8.
159. Ikeda H, Tremain KE, Sanders MD. Neurophysiological investigation in optic nerve disease: combined assessment of the visual evoked response and electroretinogram. Br J Ophthalmol. 1978;62:227–39.
160. Sutter EE, Bearse MA Jr. The optic nerve head component of the human ERG. Vis Res. 1999;39:419–36.
161. Schnurman ZS, Frohman TC, Beh SC, et al. Retinal architecture and mfERG: optic nerve head component response characteristics in MS. Neurology. 2014;82:1888–96.
162. Goldman D. Muller glial cell reprogramming and retina regeneration. Nat Rev Neurosci. 2014;15:431–42.
163. Saidha S, Sotirchos ES, Ibrahim MA, et al. Microcystic macular oedema, thickness of the inner nuclear layer of the retina, and disease characteristics in multiple sclerosis: a retrospective study. Lancet Neurol. 2012;11:963–72.
164. Gelfand JM, Nolan R, Schwartz DM, Graves J, Green AJ. Microcystic macular oedema in multiple sclerosis is associated with disease severity. Brain. 2012;135:1786–93.
165. Burggraaff MC, Trieu J, de Vries-Knoppert WA, Balk L, Petzold A. The clinical spectrum of microcystic macular edema. Invest Ophthalmol Vis Sci. 2014;55:952–61.
166. Sigler EJ. Microcysts in the inner nuclear layer, a nonspecific SD-OCT sign of cystoid macular edema. Invest Ophthalmol Vis Sci. 2014;55:3282–4.
167. Abegg M, Dysli M, Wolf S, Kowal J, Dufour P, Zinkernagel M. Microcystic macular edema: retrograde maculopathy caused by optic neuropathy. Ophthalmology. 2014;121:142–9.
168. Kaufhold F, Zimmermann H, Schneider E, et al. Optic neuritis is associated with inner nuclear layer thickening and microcystic macular edema independently of multiple sclerosis. PLoS One. 2013;8:e71145.
169. Gelfand JM, Cree BA, Nolan R, Arnow S, Green AJ. Microcystic inner nuclear layer abnormalities and neuromyelitis optica. JAMA Neurol. 2013;70:629–33.
170. Brandt AU, Oberwahrenbrock T, Kadas EM, Lagreze WA, Paul F. Dynamic formation of macular microcysts independent of vitreous traction changes. Neurology. 2014;83:73–7.
171. Balk LJ, Killestein J, Polman CH, Uitdehaag BM, Petzold A. Microcystic macular oedema confirmed, but not specific for multiple sclerosis. Brain. 2012;135:e226. Author reply e7.
172. Wolff B, Basdekidou C, Vasseur V, Mauget-Faysse M, Sahel JA, Vignal C. Retinal inner nuclear layer microcystic changes in optic nerve atrophy: a novel spectral-domain OCT finding. Retina. 2013;33:2133–8.
173. Hasegawa T, Akagi T, Yoshikawa M, et al. Microcystic inner nuclear layer changes and retinal nerve fiber layer defects in eyes with glaucoma. PLoS One. 2015;10:e0130175.
174. Barboni P, Carelli V, Savini G, Carbonelli M, La Morgia C, Sadun AA. Microcystic macular degeneration from optic neuropathy: not inflammatory, not trans-synaptic degeneration. Brain. 2013;136:e239.
175. Lujan BJ, Horton JC. Microcysts in the inner nuclear layer from optic atrophy are caused by retrograde trans-synaptic degeneration combined with vitreous traction on the retinal surface. Brain. 2013;136:e260.

176. Abegg M, Zinkernagel M, Wolf S. Microcystic macular degeneration from optic neuropathy. Brain. 2012;135:e225.
177. Kisimbi J, Shalchi Z, Mahroo OA, et al. Macular spectral domain optical coherence tomography findings in Tanzanian endemic optic neuropathy. Brain. 2013;136:3418–26.
178. Haldar S, Mukherjee R, Elston J. Microcystic macular edema in a case of tobacco-alcohol optic neuropathy. Can J Ophthalmol. 2017;52:e19–22.
179. Yoon DH, Kang DJ, Kim MJ, Kim HK. New observation of microcystic macular edema as a mild form of cystoid macular lesions after standard phacoemulsification: prevalence and risk factors. Medicine. 2018;97:e0355.
180. Sigler EJ, Randolph JC, Charles S. Delayed onset inner nuclear layer cystic changes following internal limiting membrane removal for epimacular membrane. Graefes Arch Clin Exp Ophthalmol. 2013;251:1679–85.
181. Petzold A. Retinal glymphatic system: an explanation for transient retinal layer volume changes? Brain. 2016;139:2816–9.
182. Veleri S, Lazar CH, Chang B, Sieving PA, Banin E, Swaroop A. Biology and therapy of inherited retinal degenerative disease: insights from mouse models. Dis Model Mech. 2015;8:109–29.
183. Dietrich M, Helling N, Hilla A, et al. Early alpha-lipoic acid therapy protects from degeneration of the inner retinal layers and vision loss in an experimental autoimmune encephalomyelitis-optic neuritis model. J Neuroinflammation. 2018;15:71.
184. Nishioka C, Liang HF, Barsamian B, Sun SW. Sequential phases of RGC axonal and somatic injury in EAE mice examined using DTI and OCT. Mult Scler Relat Disord. 2019;27:315–23.
185. Manogaran P, Walker-Egger C, Samardzija M, et al. Exploring experimental autoimmune optic neuritis using multimodal imaging. NeuroImage. 2018;175:327–39.
186. Hein K, Gadjanski I, Kretzschmar B, et al. An optical coherence tomography study on degeneration of retinal nerve fiber layer in rats with autoimmune optic neuritis. Invest Ophthalmol Vis Sci. 2012;53:157–63.
187. Enriquez-Algeciras M, Ding D, Chou TH, et al. Evaluation of a transgenic mouse model of multiple sclerosis with noninvasive methods. Invest Ophthalmol Vis Sci. 2011;52:2405–11.
188. Chu F, Shi M, Zheng C, et al. The roles of macrophages and microglia in multiple sclerosis and experimental autoimmune encephalomyelitis. J Neuroimmunol. 2018;318:1–7.
189. Robinson AP, Harp CT, Noronha A, Miller SD. The experimental autoimmune encephalomyelitis (EAE) model of MS: utility for understanding disease pathophysiology and treatment. Handb Clin Neurol. 2014;122:173–89.
190. Constantinescu CS, Farooqi N, O'Brien K, Gran B. Experimental autoimmune encephalomyelitis (EAE) as a model for multiple sclerosis (MS). Br J Pharmacol. 2011;164:1079–106.
191. Knier B, Rothhammer V, Heink S, et al. Neutralizing IL-17 protects the optic nerve from autoimmune pathology and prevents retinal nerve fiber layer atrophy during experimental autoimmune encephalomyelitis. J Autoimmun. 2015;56:34–44.
192. Zhang HK, Ye Y, Zhao ZN, et al. Neuroprotective effects of gypenosides in experimental autoimmune optic neuritis. Int J Ophthalmol. 2017;10:541–9.
193. Chen TC, Cense B, Miller JW, et al. Histologic correlation of in vivo optical coherence tomography images of the human retina. Am J Ophthalmol. 2006;141:1165–8.
194. Fischer MD, Huber G, Beck SC, et al. Noninvasive, in vivo assessment of mouse retinal structure using optical coherence tomography. PLoS One. 2009;4:e7507.
195. Beck RW, Cleary PA. Optic neuritis treatment trial. One-year follow-up results. Arch Ophthalmol. 1993;111:773–5.
196. Marracci GH, Jones RE, McKeon GP, Bourdette DN. Alpha lipoic acid inhibits T cell migration into the spinal cord and suppresses and treats experimental autoimmune encephalomyelitis. J Neuroimmunol. 2002;131:104–14.
197. Morini M, Roccatagliata L, Dell'Eva R, et al. Alpha-lipoic acid is effective in prevention and treatment of experimental autoimmune encephalomyelitis. J Neuroimmunol. 2004;148:146–53.

OCT in Parkinson's Disease and Related Disorders

12

Ivan Bodis-Wollner, Shahnaz Miri, Sofya Glazman,
Eric M. Shrier, and Reem Deeb

Abbreviations

AD	Alzheimer's disease
CS	Contrast sensitivity
HY scale	Hoehn and Yahr scale for staging PD
INL	Inner nuclear layer
IOA	Interocular asymmetry
IPL	The inner plexiform layer
IRL	Inner retinal layer
LBD	Lewy Body Disease
MMSE	Mini-mental status exam
MSA	Multisystem Atrophy
NDD	Neurodegenerative diseases
ONL	Outer nuclear layer
OPL	Outer plexiform layer
ORL	Outer retinal layer
PD	Parkinson's disease

I. Bodis-Wollner (✉)
Department of Neurology, SUNY Downstate Medical Center, Brooklyn, NY, USA

Department of Ophthalmology, SUNY Downstate Medical Center, Brooklyn, NY, USA
e-mail: ivan.bodis-wollner@downstate.edu

S. Miri
Department of Neurology, Medstar Georgetown University Hospital, Washington, DC, USA

S. Glazman · R. Deeb
Department of Neurology, SUNY Downstate Medical Center, Brooklyn, NY, USA
e-mail: sofya.glazman@downstate.edu; reem.deeb@downstate.edu

E. M. Shrier
Department of Ophthalmology, SUNY Downstate Medical Center, Brooklyn, NY, USA
e-mail: eric.shrier@downstate.edu

A. Grzybowski, P. Barboni (eds.), *OCT and Imaging in Central Nervous System Diseases*, https://doi.org/10.1007/978-3-030-26269-3_12

pRNFL	Peripapillar retinal nerve fiber layer
RF	Receptive field of retinal ganglion cells
SD-OCT	Spectral domain optical coherence tomography
UPDRS score	The score obtained using Unified Parkinson's Disease Rating Scale

Definitions

Contrast Sensitivity:	The inverse of the threshold contrast.
Spatial Frequency in cycles/degree (c/d):	The number of cycles of the visual pattern subtended in 1° of visual angle at the eye. In the studies here sinusoidal grating patterns are used as visual stimuli.
The UPDRS Score:	A numerical outcome of the rated PD examination by a certified rater. The subcomponent score of motor disability is most frequently used to assess the clinical status of a patient. The higher the score, the worse is the status.
HY scale:	A numerical scale used to define the disease stage in PD patients, I is mild disease, V represents the last stage of the disease.
DAT Scan:	A brain imaging technique using single photon emission computed tomography (SPECT) to visualize striatal dopamine transporter labeled by a radiopharmaceutical dye for diagnostic verification of patients with suspected Parkinsonism, who present with mild motor and early cognitive changes. Subjects for DAT Scan are selected because they are either Levodopa non-responders or subjects with typical PD cardinal motor symptoms who have visual hallucinations.
Pixel:	The size of each quadrangular element in a matrix.
Voxel:	The depth of the pixel. In the OCT the thickness of the retina is the equivalent term.
MMSE:	A scale for cognitive evaluation, with a total of 30 points. A score of 30 is normal. The cut-off commonly used is 24 (±2).

12.1 Introduction

The retina is a multilayered neural tissue with a diversity of neurons with distinct functions and different neurotransmitters. The outer nuclear layer (ONL) contains cell bodies of cones and rods photoreceptors; the inner nuclear layer (INL) includes cell bodies of bipolar, horizontal, and amacrine cells (Fig. 12.1) and the ganglion cell layer (GCL) contains ganglion cells and displaced amacrine cells [4]. The fovea is a highly specialized area of the retina, located at the temporal side of the optic disc. The foveal center contains the highest concentration of the cone photoreceptors, responsible for highest visual acuity. A Tyrosine Hydroxylase (TH) positive amacrine neuron is shown on the border of the inner nuclear and inner plexiform layer In Fig. 12.1b, c pathological alpha-synuclein (AS) immunostaining shows an individual neuron and fibers. The neuron corresponds in size and spatial frequency of a dopaminergic neuron with its extensive arborization in Fig. 12.2.

As cone density diminishes with distance from the center of the fovea, other retinal neurons successively emerge at the slope and at the edge of the foveal pit. It is called a pit because there are no inner layers which cover the central photoreceptors, hence the thickness of the retina is reduced here, compared to other sites in the retina. The neural layers and individual neurons are connected using lateral, forward and feedback paths. The interaction between receptors and their organization into a ganglion cell receptive field (RF) structure is responsible for high contrast

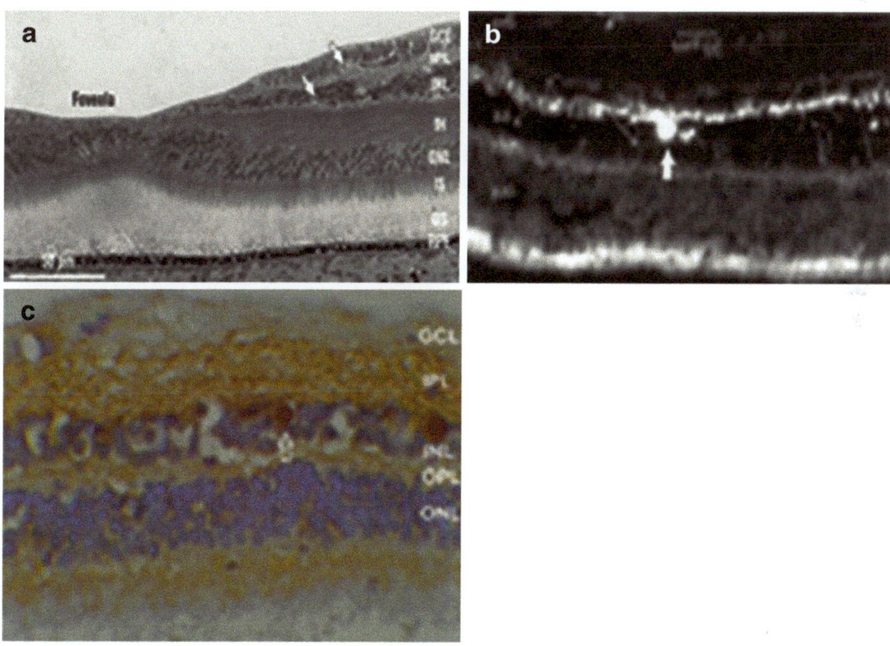

Fig. 12.1 (**a**) Histology of the foveal pit and retinal layers (After Provis and Hendrickson [1]). (**b**) Tyrosine-Hydroxylase staining of the retina demonstrating immunoreactivity in the inner plexiform layer. The *arrow* shows a dopaminergic amacrine cell on the border of the inner plexiform and inner nuclear layers (After Witkovsky [2]). (**c**) Postmortem slide of the PD retina with Alpha-Synuclein immunoreactivity (dark brown staining) in the inner retina [3]. GCL, IPL and the margin of INL reveal immunoreactivity with AS staining. The arrow shows a neuron with dense globular AS aggregation. *GCL* ganglion cell layer, *IPL* inner plexiform layer, *INL* inner plexiform layer, *fH* fiber layer of Henle, *OPL* outer plexiform layer, *ONL* outer nuclear layer, *IS* inner segment of the photoreceptors, *OS* outer segment of the photoreceptors, *RPE* retinal pigment epithelium

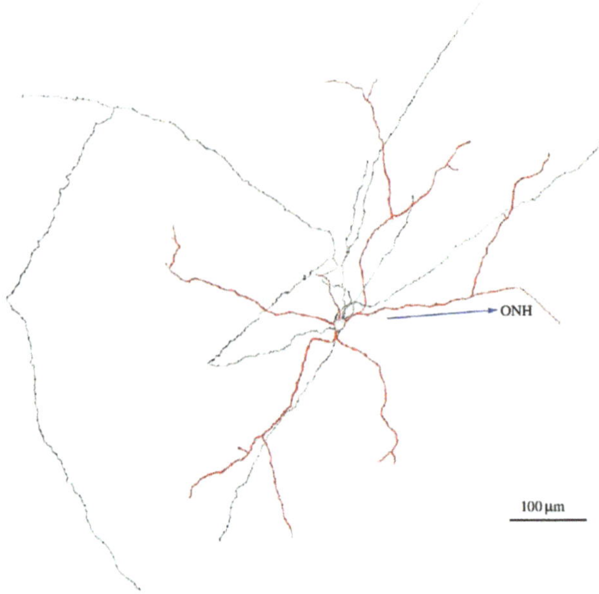

Fig. 12.2 A DA cell injected with neurobiotin was reconstructed from a montage of confocal images after treatment with a fluorescent antibody to the tracer. Only the cell body and the processes lying in stratum 1 of the inner plexiform layer are included in the figure. Dendrites and cell body are red, axons are black. The arrow points to the optic nerve head (ONH) (after Hirasawa et al. [5]). The figure illustrates that DA amacrines, although located at a distance from each other, cover a large interneuronal area

sensitivity [6–8]. The macular region, including the foveal region is the thickest part of the retina, due to increased density of photoreceptors (cones) and ganglion cells compared to the peripheral retina. There are abundant synaptic interactions in the central retina leading to a thick inner plexiform layer (IPL) [4]. The inner plexiform layer contains axons and dendrites of amacrine cells, including dopaminergic (DA) amacrine cells as shown in Fig. 12.2.

Dopaminergic amacrine cells in the human are relatively large and relatively infrequent, that is they are not spaced in close proximity to each other. However, their dendritic and axonal fields may span up to 2° of visual field size (Fig. 12.2) and establish a seamlessly connected network. Their activity is crucial for the structure of foveal ganglion cells in humans [6]. The Retinal Nerve Fiber Layer (RNFL) functions as the retinal output emanating from retinal ganglion cells. The nerve fibers are the axons of retinal ganglion cells and form the optic nerve behind the globe toward the lateral geniculate body and then onto the primary visual cortex [9]. Further visual processing takes place in other visual cortical areas [6].

The ten retinal layers are constant across the retina except at its center, the fovea [6, 10]. Here, individual layers emerge one by one, from the foveal pit which at its center contains the photoreceptors only.

Retinal involvement and ganglion cell receptive field re-organization in PD were described decades ago [11, 12]. Since then many studies put forward functional evidence that foveal vision is impaired in PD. Foveal visual deficits are manifested by decreased contrast sensitivity [13–17] and color vision abnormalities [13–16, 18]. Flash and pattern electroretinography demonstrated a decline in retinal bioelectrical activity [19–24]. The results of psychophysical and electrophysiological functional studies of pharmacological interventions in the dopaminergic system imply that impaired retinal processing in PD is caused by retinal dopaminergic deficiency [19–28] but deficit in dopaminergic transmission is not the only cause.

The cellular pathology of the retina in PD, as shown by intracellular alpha-synuclein aggregates at the border of INL in a typical position of dopaminergic amacrine cells, and also in the IPL and GCL [3, 29] (Fig. 12.1c) Recent studies have demonstrated that phosphorylated alpha-synuclein pathology correlates with the stage of brain pathology in PD and in incidental LBD [30].

In the last decades, OCT has emerged as a powerful tool for in-vivo imaging and in-depth quantification of structural properties of the retina, only seen until then using an ophthalmoscope (Fig. 12.3). OCT studies provided direct evidence of retinal structure abnormalities and retinopathy in PD [31, 32]. Peripapillary nerve fiber layer and the inner retina are thinned and the shape of the foveal pit is altered in PD [31] (Fig. 12.4).

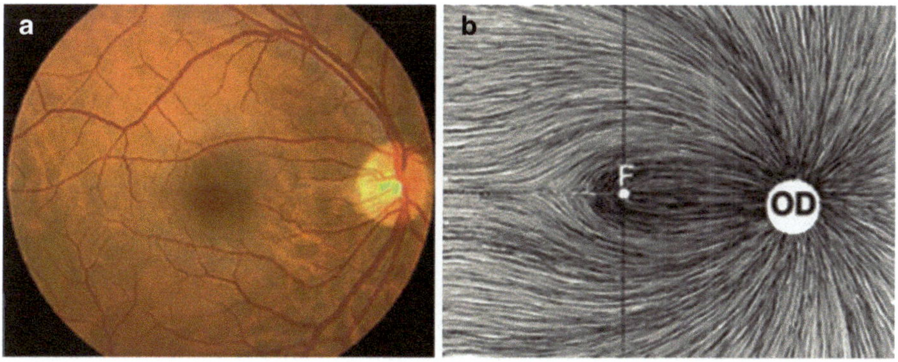

Fig. 12.3 Fundoscopic image of the retina which shows the peripapillary and the macular region, capillaries, the optic disc, and the retinal nerve fiber layer (After Bodis-Wollner et al. [31]). *OD* optic disc, *F* fovea

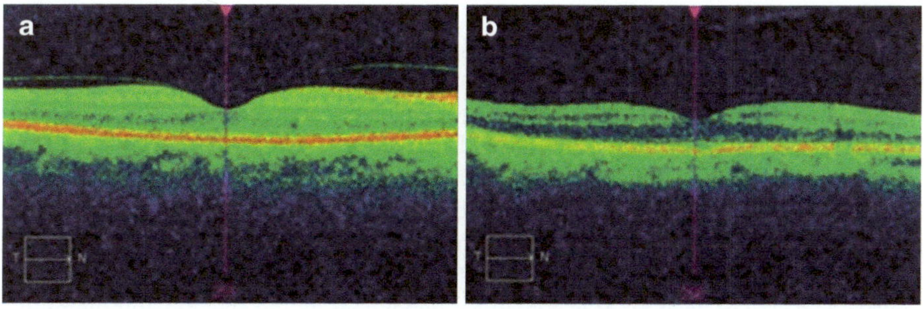

Fig. 12.4 OCT macular scan in a healthy control (**a**) and a PD patient (**b**). Notice the foveal thinning in the PD patient. Notice the thinning of the inner retina at the fovea and the flattening of the foveal pit in PD patient

Because treatment of NDD which affects several million people above the age of 55 is not very successful, a major goal of NDD research is to develop methods of precise diagnosis and to prevent disease progression in individual subjects. The eye is a magnificent gateway to the brain where exact structure/function relationships are established. In PD, LBD, MSA and AD select retinal neurons have the same proteomics pathology in the brain as in the retina.

12.2 The Public Health Relevance of Differential Diagnosis of NDD with OCT

Neurodegenerative Disorders (NDD) present socioeconomic burdens in all age groups although they are typically seen in adulthood. Among these are PD, LBD, MSA, and AD. They are progressive. Much current research is promising neuroprotective therapies. Unmet needs are early recognition and quantitative measures for follow-up progression and therapy. By targeting specific neurons retinal diagnosis has the power of an individual, rather than statistical group diagnosis and contribute a measuring device for the success of novel neuroimmunological therapies.

12.3 Optical Coherence Tomography: Data Acquisition

OCT was developed in 1991 [33] to obtain in-vivo two-dimensional images using low-coherence interferometry to measure the time delay of back-scattered light from different layers of tissue. It was first applied to in-vivo retinal imaging in 1993 [34]. OCT is a rapid, non-invasive method which provides high resolution cross-sectional and three-dimensional images of the retina. OCT has been applied to evaluate demyelinating diseases of the CNS including multiple sclerosis (MS), NDD of the retina such as glaucoma and in CNS NDD such as AD, PD, MSA, LBD which have all shown to affect differently the retina [31, 35–37].

The original OCT technology used time-domain OCT (TD-OCT) in which retinal thickness data were obtained through successive "slices" through the retina. TD-OCT takes time. Third-generation TD-OCT, Stratus OCT (Carl Zeiss Meditec AG, Jena, Germany), has been widely used with the scanning rate of 400 axial scans per second and 10 μm axial resolution [38]. The more recent introduction of Fourier-domain or spectral-domain OCT (SD-OCT) provides retinal imaging with faster scan rate and higher resolution, compared to older generation TD-OCT [39]. SD-OCT uses spectral interference and Fourier transform to extract the frequency spectrum of a signal. Fourier domain OCT can measure all light echoes with different delay time simultaneously which increase speed and sensitivity of detection. SD-OCT achieves an axial resolution of 5 μm and a scan velocity of 27,000 axial scans per second [40]. SD-OCT systems have a higher sensitivity, even in low light levels, with high-speed detection [38, 41]. Individual voxel data are anchored in a matrix. The size of each pixel is somewhat dependent on the specific commercially available OCT device. They have somewhat different data analysis algorithms and different sampling rate. The macular area is sampled at somewhat different resolution for each device [39, 42]. Within limits, the 20% pixel size difference (say between the Optovue and the Zeiss device), did not have any significant effect on the results.

The recently developed high-penetration OCT (HP-OCT) with a long wavelength (1050 nm, versus 840 nm in SD-OCT) provides deeper visualization of microstructures beneath the retinal pigmented epithelium. HP-OCT (Topcon, Tokyo, Japan) has a scanning rate of 100,000 per second [43].

Different sampling rate and retinal segmentation algorithms lead to the difference between macular thickness values obtained by different OCT equipment [44]. Matlach et al. [45], have demonstrated a high degree of repeatability for both Cirrus and RTvue-100 in measurements of peripapillary RNFL and inner retinal layer (IRL) thickness among idiopathic and atypical PD. Despite a high correlation between measurements of the two OCT devices and a high consistency in the measurements of the two devices, RTVue studies reported thicker macular RNFL-GCL-IPL and pRNFL thickness [45].

Device manufacturers supply automated measurements for macular thickness and for peripapillary nerve fiber layer thickness. The first program measures the foveal ganglion cell layer and the preganglionic layers' thickness, while the peripapillary program concentrates on the thickness of the retinal ganglion cell axons (Fig. 12.3).

12.4 Data Analysis

To visualize the three-dimensional retinal structure, cross-sectional OCT images in the 3D data set can be rendered volumetrically by the OCT software. The number of horizontal and vertical pixels obtained by OCT is different according to the company's scan protocols. The produced image is obtained over an area of 5 Å~5 or 6 Å~6 mm with 1 mm depth [46].

OCT image analysis is based on segmenting the retinal layers and measuring the distances between the layers. Image analysis starts with the correct detection of the Internal Limiting Membrane (ILM) [47]. Commercially available OCT devices use different layer segmentation algorithm based on quantification of the optical properties of the retinal layers [47, 48]. "Segmentation" refers to the establishment of the demarcation of different histological layers (Fig. 12.5a, b). Device dependent algorithm difference affects retinal thickness measures [49]. Accordingly, different sensitivities are reported for different OCT devices when the clinical results are compared in the same subjects. One of the critical variables is the estimation of the borders of different layers and the histological borders between layers is not a straight line. Hence thickness measurements idealized to a straight line approximation of the edges of different layers can suffer various inaccuracies.

As mentioned, the three-dimensional rendering of OCT images is acquired based on consecutive 2D OCT slices. Reconstructing methods are recently developed to

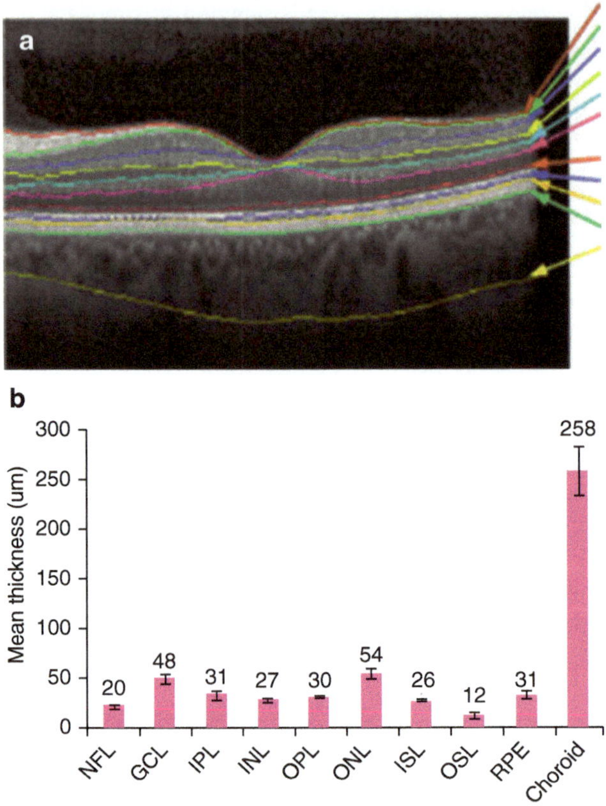

Fig. 12.5 (**a**) Layer segmentation of the retinal SD-OCT volume scans by the automated graph search algorithm to sequentially segment 11 retinal surfaces. (**b**) Average thickness of each individual retinal layer in total macular volume in healthy eyes (After Hu et al. [48]). This plot illustrates two pitfalls of comparing macular volumes. One, the percentage contribution of each layer to total macular volume is less than 10%. Thus, it is difficult to show statistical significance of a change in a single layer to the total volume. Secondly, several studies have shown that different diseases, for instance PD, affect more one, than another segment (temporal, nasal, superior, inferior) of the retina. Thus averaging the macular volume in NDD could yield spuriously insignificant change compared to HC

quantify raw voxel data from 2-D OCT slices and visualize them as 3D retinal images. These 3D rendering methods provide a more reliable segmentation and evaluation of volumetric images [50, 51].

Individual volumetric pixel data obtained from OCT can be imported into MATLAB software environment in order to analyze and reconstruct the data. This method, by not relying on straight line approximation in the segmentation method, minimizes analysis errors. Based on finely sampled volumetric data of perifoveolar raw thickness data, a mathematical equation for the foveal pit was developed [52]. This method does describe the shape of the fovea by "segmenting" at every 0.25 mm (RT-Vue) or 0.3 mm (Cirrus).

12.5 Novel Methods of OCT Data Analysis

Many of the devices supply data analysis in which depth of individual pixel values of the OCT are divided by the control (average pixel depth of an extended retinal volume) value to define the number and location of deviant voxels for each quadrant for each eye of each subject.

This is a computer time-consuming procedure, which has been developed in our facilities, working together with the Polytechnic Institute of NYU. The OCT voxel data formed the base for developing a mathematical formula for the healthy human foveal pit (SBD model: Symmetry, Breadth, and Depth) and its parameter changes in PD [52, 53]. At this point, NDD data have not been fitted with the model.

12.6 OCT Angiography

A recent OCT development is OCT angiography (OCTA) which provides three-dimensional quantification of the central retina capillaries. OCTA facilitates the study of neuronal and microvessels in neurodegenerative diseases. Quantification of the inner retinal capillary in PD has demonstrated microvascular remodeling in PD which correlates with the neuronal loss in the inner retina [54–56]. There are some inconsistencies in the studies on the choroidal vasculature (Fig. 12.5a) in PD (Table 12.1). Few studies have found the decreased thickness of choroid layer [59, 61], while another study has shown increased choroidal layer thickness [58] both in the peripapillary and macular area. Using different devices with different penetration depths and sensitivity, as well as, studying patients in different stages of the disease and on different medications can be a reason for the above discrepancy in the findings. Glumez Sevim et al. [60] has identified a decreased diameter of the superior temporal artery in PD patients on levodopa compared to other PD patients not using levodopa.

The inherent value in retinal capillary network studies in NDD is however in early infancy and will only be mentioned here en passant, concerning potential differential diagnostic value in PD and in AD [54, 56, 62, 63].

12.7 OCT Centered on the Fovea

The reason for focusing the OCT on the fovea (Fig. 12.3) in PD emanates from the results of visual processing studies in PD using electrophysiological (ERG, VEP) and psychophysical studies of color and contrast vision. Historically, the first evidence of visual deficits in PD was provided using visual evoked Potentials (VEP) [11]. However, the ERG [19–21] provided the first evidence in PD of foveal visual processing in the retina. OCT use in ND was first and consistently shown in PD subjects in 2004 [32]. OCT has confirmed the functional evidence of foveal impairment in PD. However the precise methods to quantify the changing thickness of individual retinal layers from the fovea is essential as shown in several studies in PD and other NDD [35–37, 64–66]. The precise quantitative methods applied for quantifying the foveal region are of crucial importance.

Table 12.1 A summary of studies on retinal microvasculature in PD

Study	Sample size	Device	Main finding
Miri et al. [54]	23 PD, 13 HC	RTVue	A smaller FAZ in PD associated with foveal thinning; no difference in macular capillary fractal dimensions
Kromer et al. [55]	49 PD, 49 HC	SD-OCT and SLO	A decreased contrast in the retinal vein in PD, no difference in vascular diameter
Eraslan et al. [57]	22 PD, 25 HC	RTVue	Decreased volume in lamina cribrosa and thinning of the choroid in PD
Satue et al. [58]	50 PD, 50 HC	Triton OCT (Topcon)	Increased Choroidal thickness both in macula and pRNFL in PD
Moschos and Chatziralli [59]	31 PD, 25 HC	Spectralis	Decreased choroidal thickness is all macular quadrants
Gulmez Sevim et al. [60]	41 PD, 35 HC	Spectralis	Decreased diameter of the superior temporal artery in PD patients on levodopa; no correlations between pRNFL thicknesses/disease duration with retinal vessel diameters
Kwapong et al. [56]	38 PD, 28 HC	RTVue	Reduced microvascular density in most of the areas of the macula, and in the superficial retinal capillary; correlated with thinning of the ganglion cell layer and inner plexiform layer

SLO scanning laser ophthalmoscope, *PD* Parkinson's disease, *HC* healthy controls, *pRNFL* peri-papillary retinal nerve fiber layer

12.8 OCT in the Study of NDD

The eye is a magnificent gateway to the brain. The retina is affected in several NDD [67, 68] not only in PD. OCT is increasingly applied in clinical ophthalmic care and also caught the interest researchers in NDD. Presently, treatment of NDD which affects several million people above the age of 55 is not very successful. Therefore, a major goal of NDD research is to develop methods of precise diagnosis and to prevent disease progression in individual subjects. Thus if in the retina, the exact cellular structure/function relationship is established, the eye can serve as a model for pathobiological studies in NDD. Select retinal neurons have the same distinct immunopathology in PD and LBD, in AD and MSA, as brain neurons. One goal of OCT research to distinguish retinal changes in NDD, has clinical and pathobiological merit.

12.9 OCT as a Potential Biomarker of NDD

One reason for developing OCT models for early NDD diagnosis is that OCT is a non-invasive, inexpensive and easily available quick tool and well suited to quantify retinal changes in NDD and importantly, in individual subjects. While this chapter is focused on PD, three related disorders (PDRD) will be also reflected on as the OCT may provide a differential diagnostic tool.

In this chapter, we focus on the foveal retina as seen and quantified by OCT. This foveal focus is partially because OCT is most accurate in quantifying the foveal structure, but most importantly, because foveal vision is commonly affected in PD. This is in contrast to the other NDD reviewed in this chapter.

A biomarker should reflect on the underlying neurobiopathology at the cellular level rather than relying on empirical correlation. In reflecting on cellular pathology the marker has a chance of being applicable to individual subjects for accurate diagnosis and differential diagnosis.

One of the compelling reason for differential diagnosis of NDD is the difference regarding their treatment. Several NDD share at the cellular level a burden of abnormal proteins [29, 69, 70]. For instance in PD, it is abnormally phosphorylated alpha-synuclein (AS) which interferes with the normal functioning of the cell [71] and this protein differs from the one which is characteristic of AD. Neuropathological findings can distinguish NDD, but from a therapy point of view, this is too late. Promising current treatments in NDD use immunological agents which target a specific protein, different in different diseases. Since neuroprotection via immunological techniques may slow down disease progression, early detection is important. This raises financial and logistical problems. We need easily accessible, inexpensive specific diagnostic tools which can be employed in suspect subjects. Our tools are just that: easily available, inexpensive, and non-invasive. The specificity of the diagnostic tool is particularly important in order to avoid treatment with an ineffective agent. Several biomarker tools provide good specificity in the spinal fluid; however, the technique is invasive and not easily applicable to subjects with suspected NDD. Brain imaging is invasive by the use of contrast agents, not easily available, and expensive. Some easily available tools such as tear analysis and olfactory testing are inexpensive but lack specificity.

One block in the way of developing biomarker tools is also the fact their value has been proven by correlating the results, empirically with a diagnostic entity. This approach works well for population studies, but for a biomarker to be useful for treating individuals, normative and deviant values derived from group averages provide less guidance for treatment of individual subjects.

Most clinical OCT studies report empirical correlations between the thickness of the nerve fiber layer, representing the axons of retinal ganglion cells and the clinical diagnosis. As valuable as this approach is for a general understanding of the effect of PD and other NDD on the retina, the results have limited value for classifying individual subjects.

12.10 Early Detection and Biomarkers

Due to the impact of NDD on society, researchers are evaluating methods to screen high-risk individuals. To be effective in a primary care setting, biomarker testing must be inexpensive, readily available, rapid, reproducible and well tolerated by the patient. The screening test must have a high sensitivity and specificity for the disease in question, particularly at its earliest manifestations.

In none of the NDD are there simple, inexpensive biomarkers to definitively diagnose a subject. Biomarker tests to support diagnosis include:

- Nuclear imaging tests such as single-photon emission computerized tomography (SPECT) and positron emission tomography (PET)
- Tests that measure nerve function of the heart's blood vessels (iodine-MIBG myocardial scintigraphy)
- Sleep studies that examine brain wave activity

Some of these tests are cumbersome, expensive, and not available except in tertiary centers. The allure of the specific retinal biomarker we have been developing is its low cost, simplicity, wide availability and the potential of yielding biologically relevant information. Precision retinal biomarkers give us a chance to identify individual subjects and gain new pathobiological knowledge.

From a clinical point of view and from exploring potential disease-modifying therapies To this aim the early recognition of individual subjects, not just groups is of outmost importance. We are not there yet but further research will answer whether specific NDD in early stages can be differentiated in individual subjects.

12.11 Biological Variables in Retinal Thickness

Gender or race is not factored into the research design in PD and NDD. However, studies on healthy eyes demonstrated a difference in retinal thickness between different races and genders [72]. It is reported that African-Americans have a decreased mean foveal thickness compared to Caucasians and Hispanics. Regardless of race, male gender is a predictor of increased mean foveal thickness. The difference between gender and race should be considered in the future studies of retinal thickness in NDD.

12.12 Foveal Vision in PD

Retinal involvement and ganglion cell receptive field re-organization in PD was described decades ago [11, 12]. Since then many studies put forward functional evidence that foveal vision is impaired in PD. Foveal visual deficits are manifested by decreased contrast sensitivity [13, 14, 16, 73] and color vision abnormalities [14, 16, 17, 74]. Flash and pattern electroretinography demonstrated a decline in retinal bioelectrical activity [19–24]. The specific deficit [21] in the pattern ERG was puzzling, as the pattern ERG relies on the activity of RGC [75] which are decidedly non-dopaminergic and the results of psychophysical and electrophysiological functional studies of pharmacological interventions in the dopaminergic system imply that impaired retinal processing in PD is caused by dopaminergic deficiency [20, 25–28]. AS stained human retina provided evidence that smallish ganglion cells are affected in the PD retina. Hence one must consider smallish retinal ganglion cells in the category of non-dopaminergic pathology of PD.

12.13 Macular and Peripapillary Nerve Fiber Layer OCT Studies in PD

OCT provides direct in-vivo visualization of retinal structure in the macular area and in the peripapillary area in PD [31, 32] (Fig. 12.4). A good number of OCT studies have shown the effects of PD in the retina. They can be grouped into two categories [31, 76]. Studies which quantified the thickness of the pRNFL and studies which quantified the thickness of the macular region (summarized in Table 12.2). In a meta-analysis by Yu et al. [76] for 13 case-control studies of pRNFL measurements in PD, a significant pRNFL thinning was reported in all quadrants in PD subjects compared to controls.

The rationale for sampling the macular area in PD is based on the localization of dopaminergic neurons and the nature of visual deficits in PD [20, 21]. There is a dopaminergic deficiency in the PD retina [27]. Dopaminergic neurons in the retina are located at the border of the inner nuclear layer and IPL and dopaminergic fibers are present in IPL [2]. Spatial geometry of the dopaminergic amacrine neurons is described in the foveal avascular zone (FAZ) (Fig. 12.6) [104]. Recent histopathological studies confirmed the pathognomonic involvement of the retina in PD by describing the presence of AS deposition in the inner retina [3, 29, 30] as it will be detailed later on.

Altintaş et al. [77] reported the first macular OCT study in PD. The results implied a decreased superior segment thickness of the IRL and a temporal, nasal, and inferior segment of the outer retinal layer (ORL). Hajee et al. reported a thinned inner [78] foveal retina in PD (Fig. 12.4) and the shape of the foveal pit is reported to be altered in these patients [51] (Fig. 12.6). Automated segmentation software recently has been developed to evaluate the specific layers involvement in PD compared to HC and other Parkinsonian syndromes (Fig. 12.7) [64]. However, the results of these studies [64, 94, 95] are difficult to compare due to the application of different algorithms and using different devices.

In the past, we studied the retinal ganglion cell complex of the central 5° of the fovea sampled in 207 PD eyes using OCT. The scans included grids of 5 × 5 mm (MM5 scan) or 6 × 6 mm (EMM5 scan) centered on the macula. In our study, the pixels have an edge of 0.25 mm and the foveal matrix is 6 × 6 mm. A 6 × 6 matrix corresponds to 24 × 24 pixels. Since 1° of visual angle corresponds to 0.287 mm on the retina [4] the matrix is 20.9 × 20.9°. Ding et al. [52] developed a mathematical equation of the foveal pit, based on finely sampled volumetric data of perifoveolar thickness to describe the foveal pit in PD and healthy eyes. Using this model, based on the RT-Vue 100 of the parameters foveal model had an over 70% discriminating power of PD.

Table 12.2 Investigations of macular and peripapillary nerve fiber layer thickness in PD compared to healthy controls

Study	Sample size	Device	Result
Inzelberg et al. [32]	10 PD, 10 HC	Not mentioned (NM)	**pRNFL**: ↓mean RNFL thickness, ↓inf, temp quad
Altintaş et al. [77]	17 PD, 11 HC	Stratus	**pRNFL**: ↓mean RNFL thickness, ↓sup, nasal quad **Macula**: ↓sup IRL; ↓temp, nasal, inf ORL; no difference in fovea
Hajee et al. [78]	24 PD, 17 HC	Optovue	**Macula**: ↓IRL in sup and inf quads; no change in ORL
Aaker et al. [50]	9 PD, 16 HC	Spectralis	**pRNFL**: No RNFL thickness difference **Macula**: No difference in IRL thickness; compared to published normal values, ↓ORL sup; ↑ORL nasal; ↑IRL inf quad
Cubo et al. [24]	9 PD, 9 HC	Spectralis	**Macula**: ↓foveal thickness; thinner fovea in the contralateral to the more affected side
Archibald et al. [79]	34 PD, 19 HC	Stratus	**Macula**: No difference in foveal thickness and macular volume
Moschos et al. [80]	16 PD, 20 HC	Stratus	**pRNFL**: No difference in mean RNFL thickness; ↓ thickness in inf, temp quad
Archibald et al. [79]	51 PD, 25 HC	Stratus	**pRNFL**: No RNFL thickness difference **Macula**: No difference in foveal thickness and macular volume
Tsironi et al. [81]	24 PD, 24 HC	Stratus	**pRNFL**: No RNFL thickness difference
Albrecht et al. [82]	40 PD, 35 HC	Spectralis	**pRNFL**: No RNFL thickness difference Macula: ↓INL especially in temp quad; no difference in other layers
Garcia-Martin et al. [83]	75 PD, 75 HC	Cirrus/ Spectralis	**pRNFL**: ↓RNFL thickness all quads, Spectralis more sensitive device than Cirrus
Shrier et al. [84]	23 PD, 18 HC	Optovue	**Macula**: ↓macular volume at 0.5–0.75 mm from the foveola; IOA in IRL
Spund et al. [51]	30 PD, 27 controls	Optovue	**Macula**: ↓IRL at 1–2 mm distance from the foveola
Adam et al. [85]	14 PD, 14 HC	Optovue	**Macula**: ↓IRL at radial distances (1–1.75 mm) form the foveola, especially sup quadrant
Rohani et al. [86]	27 PD, 27 HC	TOPCON, 3D-OCT Mark II	**pRNFL**: ↓RNFL thickness all quads, ↓inf, nasal quad more in akinetic-rigid PD type
Kirbas et al. [87]	42 PD, 40 HC	Cirrus	**pRNFL**: ↓mean RNFL thickness, ↓temp quad
La Morgia et al. [88]	43 PD, 86 HC	Stratus	**pRNFL**: No mean RNFL thickness difference, ↓temp quad, contralateral to d-side
Satue et al. [89]	100 PD, 100 HC	Cirrus/ Spectralis	**pRNFL**: ↓mean RNFL thickness, ↓inf-temp, sup-temp quad **Macula**: ↓mean macular, fovea, ORL inf quad

Table 12.2 (continued)

Study	Sample size	Device	Result
Moreno-Ramos et al. [90]	10 PD, 10 HC	NM	**pRNFL**: PD with dementia had ↓RNFL thickness compared to HC
Garcia-Martin et al. [91]	46 PD, 33 HC	Cirrus/ Spectralis	**pRNFL**: ↓mean RNFL thickness, ↓sup, temp, inf quad **Macula**: ↓fovea, IRL all quad; ↓inf ORL (Cirrus); ↓sup, nasal ORL (Spectralis)
Cubo et al. [24]	30 PD, 30 controls		**Macula**: No difference in full-thickness macular measures
Satue et al. [92]	153 PD, 242 HC	Cirrus	**Macula**: ↓fovea, ↓full thickness nasal and inf quads of outer macular ring
		Spectralis	**pRNFL**: ↓average RNFL thickness, and ↓RNFL thickness in sup, inf, and temp quads **Macula**: ↓in full macular thickness in all quads, no foveal thickness difference
Lee et al. [93]	56 PD, 30 HC	OPKO/OTI Spectral	**Macula**: ↓tem parafoveal INL, no difference in other layers; ↓sup outer segment of the total macular thickness
Roth et al. [94]	68 PD (114), 32 (63) HC	Cirrus	**pRNFL**: No difference in RNFL thickness **Macula**: ↓ONL/PRL, no difference in GCL + IPL, GCL + IPL + mRNLF, INL/OPL; no difference in macular volume
Garcia-Martin et al. [95]	129 (PD), 129 (HC)	Spectralis	**pRNFL**: ↓average RNFL thickness, and ↓RNFL thickness in sup, inf, sup-nasal, inf-nasal, inf-temp, sup-temp **Macula**: ↓in RNFL, GCL, IPL, OPL; ↑in INL
Jiménez et al. [96]	52 PD, 50 HC	Stratus	**pRNFL**: ↓average RNFL thickness and ↓RNFL thickness in all quads
Sen et al. [97]	18 PD, 11 HC	RTvue	**pRNFL**: ↓mean RNFL thickness, and ↓inf, sup-temp, inf-temp segment
Eraslan et al. [61]	25 PD and 23 controls	RTvue	**Macula**: Decreased mean RNFL thickness in PD
Quagliato et al. [98]	48 PD and 38 controls	RTvue	**pRNFL**: No difference in RNFL thickness **Macula**: No difference in macular thickness
Mailankody et al. [99]	30 PD and 30 controls	Spectralis	**Macula**: ↓central macular thickness in PD
Slotnick et al. [53]	72 PD and 24 controls	Cirrus and RTVue	**Macula**: ↓superior/inferior and to a lesser degree nasal-temporal foveal slope in PD
Eraslan et al. [57]	22 PD and 25 controls	RTVue	**RNFL**: No difference in ONH parameters in PD
Satue et al. [58]	50 PD and 50 controls	Triton OCT (Topcon)	**pRNFL**: ↓pRNFL thickness in all sectors in PD **Macula**: ↓GCL thickness in the inferotemporal sector; no difference in macular thickness

(continued)

Table 12.2 (continued)

Study	Sample size	Device	Result
Moschos and Chatziralli [59]	31 PD and 25 controls	Spectralis	**pRNFL**: Decreased average, superior, and temporal RNFL thickness **Macula**: ↓average GCC and choroidal thickness in PD
Unlu et al. [100]	58 PD and 30 controls	Spectralis	**Macula**: ↓IRL and ↓ORL, increased OPL volume
Aydin et al. [101]	25 PD and 29 controls	Spectralis	**pRNFL**: ↓nasal RNFL, ↓mean RNFL thickness
Gulmez Sevim et al. [60]	41 PD and 35 controls	Spectralis	**pRNFL**: ↓average pRNFL thickness
Uchida et al. [102]	24 AD, 22 amnestic MCI, 20 non-AD dementia, 22 PD, and 36 controls	Cirrus 4000 HD-OCT	**Macula**: No difference between macular thickness or volume between different groups
Sengupta et al. [103]	34 PD and 50 controls	Spectralis	**pRNFL**: ↓RNFL thickness in all quadrants **Macula**: ↓macular volume in both perifoveal and outer macular regions in all sectors
Kwapong et al. [56]	38 PD, 28 HC	RTVue	**Macula**: ↓total macular thickness; thinner in the sup, nasal, and Inf quadrants

OCT device: Carl Zeiss company: Cirrus, Stratus; Heidelberg company: Spectralis
Optovue, RTvue pRNFL peripapillary retinal nerve fiber layer, *IRL* inner retinal layer, *ORL* outer retinal layer thickness, *sup* superior quadrant, *inf* inferior quadrant, *temp* temporal quadrant, *INL* inner nuclear layer, ↓ a significant decrease in thickness, *IOA* interocular asymmetry

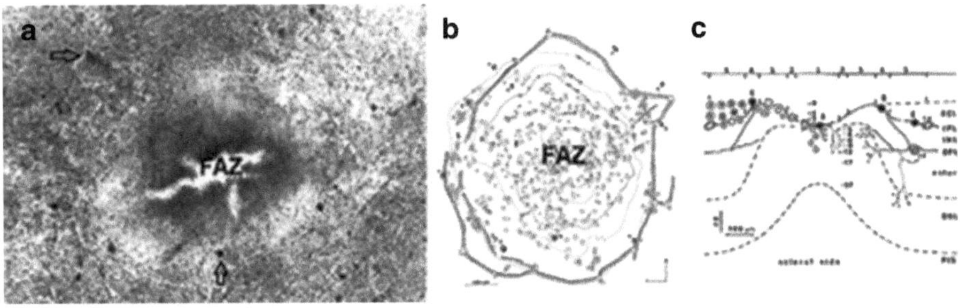

Fig. 12.6 (**a**) Tyrosine-Hydroxylase (TH) staining of dopaminergic neurons (arrows) in the human foveal avascular zone. Immunoreactivity is observed within the FAZ area, limited to the margin of the FAZ (After Savy et al. [104]). (**b**) Schematic view of spatial geometry of dopaminergic (DA) neurons in the FAZ within capillary borders. (**c**) The vertical profile view of the retina, showing the distribution of the DA neurons in the FAZ (After Savy et al. [104]). There is an insinuating spatial relationship of capillaries and TH labelled neurons in the human fovea

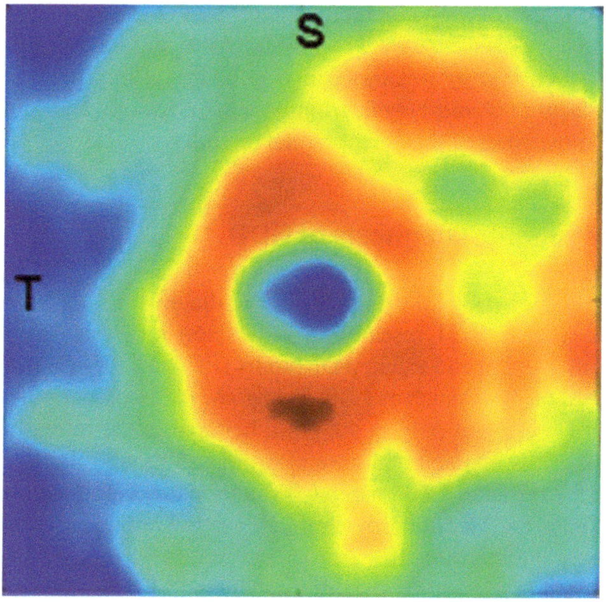

Fig. 12.7 Perifoveolar thickness attenuation in PD patients. This figure demonstrates mean foveal thickness difference between healthy controls and subjects. The reddish ring which is around 1–1.5 mm radial distance from the foveola, illustrates the zone of the largest difference of retinal thickness of PD and HC. Note: the course and distribution of the density of the NFL superior and inferior of the macula. This density contains the axons of the foveal ganglion cells. *S* superior, *T* temporal (After Spund et al. [51])

12.14 Does the OCT Correlate with Disease-Specific Neurobiopathology?

The number of OCT publications in NDD has been increasing year by year.

Some of these publications demonstrate success in showing empirical correlations of OCT and clinical features in PD and some other Related Disorders (PDRD). Some studies reveal correlations between retinal thinning and neuronal loss in select, disease specific brain areas. Behavioral correlates have also been shown: In PD, it is both motor and cognitive manifestations correlate with retinal pathology [91, 95, 96, 105]. There has been less progress in showing correlations of specific retinal and brain cell types in NDD. Such correlations would foster a very significant step toward understanding the neurobiopathology of different NDD. Such an understanding would be most helpful for developing novel rational NDD neuroprotective or disease retarding therapies. We shall discuss this vista of OCT studies in NDD later on in this chapter. Underlying such a biologically and not empirically based disease-modifying therapy is that the morphological diversity of retinal neurons is not random. Neuronal differences correlate with functional diversity. The functional differences correlational properties of individual retinal neurons and groups of neurons and their interconnections have been described by physiological and immunopharmacological methods. It is hoped that by obtaining in vivo neuronal information in the retina, NDD therapy research would benefit from detailed physiological, pharmacological and metabolic knowledge of the foveal retinal circuitry.

12.15 Early Specific Diagnosis of NDD

One goal for research is to develop OCT for diagnosing early on a suspected NDD. Another goal of OCT research is to develop a disease-specific biological marker for instance in PD and Related Disorders (PDRD). PDRD includes foremost AD and less frequent NDD such as LBD and MSA. Pathological proteins have been shown in each of these, not only in the brain but also in the retina [6, 29, 30, 106, 107]. In each, there is a specific abnormal protein, although there is overlap. The morphology of the retina in relationship to proteinopathy is not well defined, except perhaps n PD. Thus OCT could provide much needed retinal, cellular morphological correlate in each of-of these diseases.

The second goal to use retinal studies in NDD is to further the understanding of normal visual processing. This could be aided by quantifying changes in visual processing in conjunction with the precise morphological changes in these pathologies. In this research, the SBD model [52] and GCP [108] could serve useful tools. However, the effect of NDD on visual processing is not the focus of this chapter.

In a study by Kaur and colleagues [109], subclinical visual dysfunction in PD including impaired color vision and contrast sensitivity, as well as, pattern visual evoked response (VER) and multifocal ERG measures in PD patients correlated with retinal structural changes including ganglion cell layer loss captured on SD-OCT. According to these findings, GCL-IPL thinning may be a more reliable parameter than RNFL thickness for structural alterations of the retina in patients with PD. The GC-IPL complex was significantly thinner in PD cases in all 6 sectors. The average and minimum GCL-IPL values were also decreased in PD cases as compared with controls. A weak but significant correlation was also observed between structural changes on OCT (RNFL and GCL-IPL thickness) and functional changes on mfERG (RMS signal and P1 wave amplitude). Pattern VER latency correlated significantly with RNFL thickness but not with GCL-IPL thickness [109]. In another study, topographical assessment of retinal electrophysiological was performed using multifocal ERG in PD patients. The study showed inner and outer retinal layer and pRNFL were thinned in PD patients. Multifocal ERG findings suggest that delayed implicit times and decreased amplitudes in PD patients correlate with outer macular volumes and PR thicknesses [100].

What is unknown which cellular retinal structural changes correlate precisely with which visual processing deficits. OCT allows an analysis of the preganglionic layers of the retina and GCP [110]. A quantification of localized contrast processing deficits could be achieved by using Gabor Contrast Perimetry (GCP) [108] but has not been done so far.

12.16 OCT and Early Differential Diagnosis of PD and PD Related Disorders

OCT images the central retina and it is increasingly applied in clinical ophthalmic care. OCT has also caught the interest researchers in NDD. One reason is the hope to develop OCT for early diagnosis. OCT is a non-invasive, easily available quick tool and OCT angiography can quantify. The density and length of capillaries of the central retina OCT enables a short test that can be applied in a large population. Therefore, OCT could be useful for evaluating proposed new therapies in a large population where NDD is suspected.

The need for early diagnosis of NDD is linked to the availability of potential treatment for preventing disease progression. In that sense, OCT may play a pivotal role in developing disease retarding therapies. In most studies, PD is diagnosed using the UK Brain Bank Criteria [111] DAT scan is performed for diagnostic verification in subjects, who may have both mild motor and early cognitive changes, based on their neurological testing.

Subjects for DATscan are selected because they are either non Levodopa responders or subjects with typical PD cardinal motor symptoms who have visual hallucinations. In PD the OCT deficit is located in an annular zone about 0.075–1.25 mm from the fovea (Fig. 12.7).

Pathologically phosphorylated AS in PD affects specific amacrine cells which are located on the border of the inner extrasynaptic release of GABA and dopamine by retinal ganglionuclear and inner plexiform layers, judged by their large size and distribution are dopaminergic amacrines [5, 104] (Fig. 12.2).

A recent study by Ortuño-Lizarán et al. [30] demonstrated the correlation between phosphorylated AS pathology in the retina and the stage of brain pathology in PD. This study also revealed phosphorylated AS pathology in subjects with incidental Lewy body pathology with no history of clinical symptoms of Parkinsonism. This suggests that the retinal pathology can proceed clinical symptoms in PD and can be a suitable biomarker for early disease detection [30].

There is a functional diversity of retinal DA neurons [25]. Our focus is DA neurons primarily concerned with visual processing and controlling the center/surround organization of foveal ganglion cells [112, 113]. AS also marks non-dopaminergic, smallish ganglion cells of the central retina [3, 30].

LBD LBD is difficult to distinguish from PD. LBD subjects are generally diagnosed by Mayo Clinic criteria [69]. LBD subjects share with PD the typical cardinal symptoms but LBD manifests with a progressive decline in thinking. For a diagnosis of LBD two of the following core, symptoms must be present [114]: Fluctuating and unpredictable alertness and thinking (cognitive) function with repeated visual hallucinations [115–117]. Three cardinal Parkinsonian symptoms: REM sleep behavior disorder, in which people act out their dreams during sleep and autonomic dysfunction, which involves instability in blood pressure and heart rate, poor regulation of body temperature or sweating. The neural retina is affected in LBD and reveals intraneuronal pathological AS [116, 118–121].

AD Originally described by Hinton and Sadun [122, 123], there has been much retinal research and AD. Animal (transgenic) models became available and it was recently shown that retinal tau protein (the immunopathological hallmark of AD) precedes brain tau protein [118–121]. This result is promising for the development of an OCT biomarker in AD. Recent research significantly correlates retinal and brain changes in AD subjects [124, 125]. Quantification of central retinal neuronal and vascular remodeling could serve as a clinical biomarker [126].

One of the exciting findings of this study is the enlargement of the central avascular zone (FAZ) in AD. This finding is diametrically opposite of what was reported in PD [54]. Thus the size of the FAZ could be important for the specificity of the use of OCT in NDD.

MSA MSA is dominated by autonomic dysfunctions, however, PD "cardinal" symptoms such as rigidity, bradykinesia, tremor, and postural imbalance are also present. Since MSA immunopathology is also characterized by alpha-synuclein, a simple differential diagnostic tool to PD could be useful and the results instructive. The retina is affected in MSA. In a recent meta-analysis [127] the evidence was presented that AS in the brain is in the cytoplasm of oligodendrocytes as glial cytoplasmic inclusions [128, 129]. In addition to neuronal cytoplasmic inclusions [130].

OCT thus could make a contribution to the differential diagnosis of PD and MSA [131]. Mendoza-Santiesteban et al. [127] concluded that NFL losses in MSA represent a preferential damage to so-called magnocellular ganglion cells of the peripheral retina, as suggested by a postmortem study [127]. In fact, they suggest that MSA spares the central ganglion cells. This result does distinguish MSA and PD. In PD foveal vision and foveal ganglion cells are primarily affected. While the number of subjects who met the criteria for the meta-analysis is small the studies suggest that OCT may have a role in the differential diagnosis of PD and MSA.

12.17 Behavioral Correlates of OCT in NDD

Research studies show that retinal neuronal structures are affected in all NDD. Retinal thinning has been correlated with various visual and non-visual symptoms and with visual hallucinations in PD and LBD [115]. Retinal thinning correlates with the clinical score of motor impairment in PD [132] and with non-motor symptoms [133] LBD manifests with a progressive decline in thinking [133]. In a macular study of 124 participants with AD (24 eyes), mild cognitive impairment (22 eyes), non-AD dementia (20 eyes), PD (22 eyes), and controls (36 eyes), the volume of retinal pigment epithelium correlated with cognitive functional scores in all participants [102].

Disease duration is an important consideration: PD progresses at a faster rate than LBD. Significant other neurological impairment, such as stroke will complicate OCT results, especially OCTA. The main exclusion criterion is an ophthalmic pathology in many studies. A notable requirement for inclusion in that both the subject and caregiver must understand and agree with the purpose of the study and commit themselves to two visits. An MMS score below 22 excludes any subject.

In evaluating studies it is important to consider how the diagnosis of PD vs LBD was arrived Idiopathic PD is diagnosed by UK Bank Criteria. LBD subjects are diagnosed by modified Mayo Clinic criteria.

12.18 Potential Problems in Comparing OCT in PD and Related NDD

The major problem is to keep the GCP short within "ON" periods in PD in PD subjects with On and OFF stages. In LBD, sometimes fluctuations are unpredictable. In published research studies, these time constraints are rarely considered. For instance, one may have to repeat a short segment of the test the next day at the beginning of "ON" for the baseline and then conclude the test.

12.19 Concluding Remarks

The compelling pathological reason to quantify retinal changes in NDD is that phosphorylated (pathological) AS and tau protein are hallmarks of several of these diseases. They are present in PD and AD retina, respectively, in different neurons. In particular, it is the inner retina around the fovea which is affected in PD, while in AD the outer retina is more affected [134]. Furthermore, it has been shown in PD and also in LBD, that their retinal pathological proteins correlate with brain burden of the same proteins. These correlations are promising for developing a retinal biological marker. In this chapter we pointed out the promising research and also the lack of crucial studies in the field.

There are several essential open questions to be answered. Are the retinal markers specific for individual NDD? Are they robust enough that individual subjects, not just groups can be differentiated? If we had a precise cellular understanding of retinal changes in NDD, then we could develop the required specificity of a retinal biomarker of NDD.

References

1. Provis JM, Hendrickson AE. The foveal avascular region of developing human retina. Arch Ophthalmol. 2008;126:507–11.
2. Witkovsky P. Dopamine and retinal function. Doc Ophthalmol. 2004;108:17–40.
3. Bodis-Wollner I, Kozlowski PB, Glazman S, Miri S. α-Synuclein in the inner retina in Parkinson disease. Ann Neurol. 2014;75:964–6.
4. Kolb H. Simple anatomy of the retina. In: Kolb H, Fernandez E, Nelson R, editors. Webvision: the organization of the retina and visual system. Salt Lake City: University of Utah Health Sciences Center; 2005.

5. Hirasawa H, Contini M, Raviola E. Extrasynaptic release of GABA and dopamine by retinal dopaminergic neurons. Philos Trans R Soc Lond Ser B Biol Sci. 2015;370 https://doi.org/10.1098/rstb.2014.0186.
6. Bodis-Wollner I. Foveal vision is impaired in Parkinson's disease. Parkinsonism Relat Disord. 2013;19:1–14.
7. Bodis-Wollner I. Visual acuity and contrast sensitivity in patients with cerebral lesions. Science. 1972;178:769–71.
8. Bodis-Wollner I, Hendley CD. On the separability of two mechanisms involved in the detection of grating patterns in humans. J Physiol. 1979;291:251–63.
9. Berson DM. Retinal ganglion cell types and their central projections. In: Basbaum AI, Kaneko A, Shepherd GM, Westheimer G, editors. The senses: a comprehensive reference. San Diego: Academic; 2008. p. 491–519.
10. Polyak SL. The Retina, 4to. Pp. X and 607, plus 100 plates on 56 leaves. Chicago: The University of Chicago Press; 1941.
11. Bodis-Wollner I, Yahr MD. Measurements of visual evoked potentials in Parkinson's disease. Brain. 1978;101:661–71.
12. Bodis-Wollner I, Marx MS, Mitra S, Bobak P, Mylin L, Yahr M. Visual dysfunction in Parkinson's disease. Loss in spatiotemporal contrast sensitivity. Brain. 1987;110(Pt 6):1675–98.
13. Bulens C, Meerwaldt JD, van der Wildt GJ, Keemink CJ. Contrast sensitivity in Parkinson's disease. Neurology. 1986;36:1121.
14. Price MJ, Feldman RG, Adelberg D, Kayne H. Abnormalities in color vision and contrast sensitivity in Parkinson's disease. Neurology. 1992;42:887.
15. Rodnitzky RL. In: Pfeiffer RF, Bodis-Wollner I, editors. Parkinson's disease and nonmotor dysfunction. Basel: Springer; 2012. p. 305–15.
16. Pieri V, Diederich NJ, Raman R, Goetz CG. Decreased color discrimination and contrast sensitivity in Parkinson's disease. J Neurol Sci. 2000;172:7–11.
17. Haug BA, Kolle RU, Trenkwalder C, Oertel WH, Paulus W. Predominant affection of the blue cone pathway in Parkinson's disease. Brain. 1995;118(Pt 3):771–8.
18. Büttner T, Kuhn W, Müller T, Patzold T, Heidbrink K, Przuntek H. Distorted color discrimination in "de novo" parkinsonian patients. Neurology. 1995;45:386–7.
19. Gottlob I, Schneider E, Heider W, Skrandies W. Alteration of visual evoked potentials and electroretinograms in Parkinson's disease. Electroencephalogr Clin Neurophysiol. 1987;66:349–57.
20. Ikeda H, Head GM, Ellis CJK. Electrophysiological signs of retinal dopamine deficiency in recently diagnosed Parkinson's disease and a follow up study. Vis Res. 1994;34:2629–38.
21. Tagliati M, Bodis-Wollner I, Yahr MD. The pattern electroretinogram in Parkinson's disease reveals lack of retinal spatial tuning. Electroencephalogr Clin Neurophysiol. 1996;100:1–11.
22. Sartucci F, Orlandi G, Lucetti C, Bonuccelli U, Murri L, Orsini C, et al. Changes in pattern electroretinograms to equiluminant red-green and blue-yellow gratings in patients with early Parkinson's disease. J Clin Neurophysiol. 2003;20:375–81.
23. Nowacka B, Lubiński W, Karczewicz D. Ophthalmological and electrophysiological features of Parkinson's disease. Klin Ocz. 2010;112:247–52.
24. Cubo E, López Peña MJ, Diez-Feijo Varela E, Pérez Gil O, Garcia Gutierrez P, Araus González E, et al. Lack of association of morphologic and functional retinal changes with motor and non-motor symptoms severity in Parkinson's disease. J Neural Transm. 2014;121:139–45.
25. Nguyen-Legros J. Functional neuroarchitecture of the retina: hypothesis on the dysfunction of retinal dopaminergic circuitry in Parkinson's disease. Surg Radiol Anat. 1988;10:137–44.
26. Bodis-Wollner I. Visual deficits related to dopamine deficiency in experimental animals and Parkinson's disease patients. Trends Neurosci. 1990;13:296–302.
27. Harnois C, Di Paolo T. Decreased dopamine in the retinas of patients with Parkinson's disease. Invest Ophthalmol Vis Sci. 1990;31:2473–5.
28. Büttner T, Kuhn W, Patzold T, Przuntek H. L-Dopa improves colour vision in Parkinson's disease. J Neural Transm Park Dis Dement Sect. 1994;7:13–9.

29. Beach TG, Carew J, Serrano G, Adler CH, Shill HA, Sue LI, et al. Phosphorylated α-synuclein-immunoreactive retinal neuronal elements in Parkinson's disease subjects. Neurosci Lett. 2014;571:34–8.
30. Ortuño-Lizarán I, Beach TG, Serrano GE, Walker DG, Adler CH, Cuenca N. Phosphorylated α-synuclein in the retina is a biomarker of Parkinson's disease pathology severity. Mov Disord. 2018;33:1315–24.
31. Bodis-Wollner I, Miri S, Glazman S. Venturing into the no-man's land of the retina in Parkinson's disease. Mov Disord. 2013;29:15–22.
32. Inzelberg R, Ramirez JA, Nisipeanu P, Ophir A. Retinal nerve fiber layer thinning in Parkinson disease. Vis Res. 2004;44:2793–7.
33. Huang D, Swanson EA, Lin CP, Schuman JS, Stinson WG, Chang W, et al. Optical coherence tomography. Science. 1991;254:1178–81.
34. Swanson EA, Izatt JA, Hee MR, Huang D, Lin CP, Schuman JS, et al. In vivo retinal imaging by optical coherence tomography. Opt Lett. 1993;18:1864–6.
35. Cheung CY-L, Ong YT, Hilal S, Ikram MK, Low S, Ong YL, et al. Retinal ganglion cell analysis using high-definition optical coherence tomography in patients with mild cognitive impairment and Alzheimer's disease. J Alzheimers Dis. 2015;45:45–56.
36. Garcia-Martin E, Polo V, Larrosa JM, Marques ML, Herrero R, Martin J, et al. Retinal layer segmentation in patients with multiple sclerosis using spectral domain optical coherence tomography. Ophthalmology. 2014;121:573–9.
37. Ahn J, Lee J-Y, Kim TW. Retinal thinning correlates with clinical severity in multiple system atrophy. J Neurol. 2016;263:2039–47.
38. Lange AP, Sadjadi R, Saeedi J, Lindley J, Costello F, Traboulsee AL. Time-domain and spectral-domain optical coherence tomography of retinal nerve fiber layer in MS patients and healthy controls. J Ophthalmol. 2012;2012:1–7.
39. Sull AC, Vuong LN, Price LL, Srinivasan VJ, Gorczynska I, Fujimoto JG, et al. Comparison of spectral/Fourier domain optical coherence tomography instruments for assessment of normal macular thickness. Retina. 2010;30:235–45.
40. Leung CK-S, Cheung CY-L, Weinreb RN, Lee G, Lin D, Pang CP, et al. Comparison of macular thickness measurements between time domain and spectral domain optical coherence tomography. Invest Opthalmol Vis Sci. 2008;49:4893.
41. Leitgeb R, Hitzenberger C, Fercher A. Performance of Fourier domain vs. time domain optical coherence tomography. Opt Express. 2003;11:889–94.
42. Reznicek L, Dabov S, Kayat B, Liegl R, Kampik A, Ulbig M, et al. Scanning laser "en face" retinal imaging of epiretinal membranes. Saudi J Ophthalmol. 2014;28:134–8.
43. Sayanagi K, Gomi F, Ikuno Y, Akiba M, Nishida K. Comparison of spectral-domain and high-penetration OCT for observing morphologic changes in age-related macular degeneration and polypoidal choroidal vasculopathy. Graefes Arch Clin Exp Ophthalmol. 2014;252:3–9.
44. Wolf-Schnurrbusch UEK, Ceklic L, Brinkmann CK, Iliev ME, Frey M, Rothenbuehler SP, et al. Macular thickness measurements in healthy eyes using six different optical coherence tomography instruments. Invest Opthalmol Vis Sci. 2009;50:3432.
45. Matlach J, Wagner M, Malzahn U, Göbel W. Repeatability of peripapillary retinal nerve fiber layer and inner retinal thickness among two spectral domain optical coherence tomography devices. Invest Opthalmol Vis Sci. 2014;55:6536.
46. Wojtkowski M, Srinivasan V, Fujimoto JG, Ko T, Schuman JS, Kowalczyk A, et al. Three-dimensional retinal imaging with high-speed ultrahigh-resolution optical coherence tomography. Ophthalmology. 2005;112:1734–46.
47. Wieclawek W, Pietka E. Retina analysis in optical coherence tomography images. Inf Technol Biomed. 2014;3:247–58.
48. Hu Z, Wu X, Hariri A, Sadda SR. Multiple layer segmentation and analysis in three-dimensional spectral-domain optical coherence tomography volume scans. J Biomed Opt. 2013;18:76006.

49. Terasaki H, Shirasawa M, Yamashita T, Yamashita T, Yamakiri K, Sonoda S, et al. Comparison of foveal microstructure imaging with different spectral domain optical coherence tomography machines. Ophthalmology. 2012;119:2319–27.
50. Aaker GD, Myung JS, Ehrlich JR, Mohammed M, Henchcliffe C, Kiss S. Detection of retinal changes in Parkinson's disease with spectral-domain optical coherence tomography. Clin Ophthalmol. 2010;4:1427–32.
51. Spund B, Ding Y, Liu T, Selesnick I, Glazman S, Shrier EM, et al. Remodeling of the fovea in Parkinson disease. J Neural Transm. 2013;120:745–53.
52. Ding Y, Spund B, Glazman S, Shrier EM, Miri S, Selesnick I, et al. Application of an OCT data-based mathematical model of the foveal pit in Parkinson disease. J Neural Transm. 2014;121:1367–76.
53. Slotnick S, Ding Y, Glazman S, Durbin M, Miri S, Selesnick I, et al. A novel retinal biomarker for Parkinson's disease: quantifying the foveal pit with optical coherence tomography. Mov Disord. 2015;30:1692–5.
54. Miri S, Shrier EM, Glazman S, Ding Y, Selesnick I, Kozlowski PB, et al. The avascular zone and neuronal remodeling of the fovea in Parkinson disease. Ann Clin Transl Neurol. 2015;2:196–201.
55. Kromer R, Buhmann C, Hidding U, Keserü M, Keserü D, Hassenstein A, et al. Evaluation of retinal vessel morphology in patients with Parkinson's disease using optical coherence tomography. PLoS One. 2016;11:e0161136.
56. Kwapong WR, Ye H, Peng C, Zhuang X, Wang J, Shen M, et al. Retinal microvascular impairment in the early stages of Parkinson's disease. Invest Ophthalmol Vis Sci. 2018;59:4115–22.
57. Eraslan M, Cerman E, Yildiz Balci S, Celiker H, Sahin O, Temel A, et al. The choroid and lamina cribrosa is affected in patients with Parkinson's disease: enhanced depth imaging optical coherence tomography study. Acta Ophthalmol. 2016;94:e68–75.
58. Satue M, Obis J, Alarcia R, Orduna E, Rodrigo MJ, Vilades E, et al. Retinal and choroidal changes in patients with Parkinson's disease detected by swept-source optical coherence tomography. Curr Eye Res. 2018;43:109–15.
59. Moschos MM, Chatziralli IP. Evaluation of choroidal and retinal thickness changes in Parkinson's disease using spectral domain optical coherence tomography. Semin Ophthalmol. 2018;33:494–7.
60. Gulmez Sevim D, Unlu M, Sonmez S, Gultekin M, Karaca C, Ozturk Oner A. Retinal vessel diameter obtained by optical coherence tomography is spared in Parkinson's disease. Int Ophthalmol. 2018; https://doi.org/10.1007/s10792-018-0873-7.
61. Eraslan M, Balci SY, Cerman E, Temel A, Suer D, Elmaci NT. Comparison of optical coherence tomography findings in patients with primary open-angle glaucoma and Parkinson disease. J Glaucoma. 2016;25:e639–46.
62. Jiang H, Wei Y, Shi Y, Wright CB, Sun X, Gregori G, et al. Altered macular microvasculature in mild cognitive impairment and Alzheimer disease. J Neuroophthalmol. 2018;38:292–8.
63. Li Y, Choi WJ, Wei W, Song S, Zhang Q, Liu J, et al. Aging-associated changes in cerebral vasculature and blood flow as determined by quantitative optical coherence tomography angiography. Neurobiol Aging. 2018;70:148–59.
64. Schneider M, Müller H-P, Lauda F, Tumani H, Ludolph AC, Kassubek J, et al. Retinal single-layer analysis in Parkinsonian syndromes: an optical coherence tomography study. J Neural Transm. 2014;121:41–7.
65. Salobrar-Garcia E, Hoyas I, Leal M, de Hoz R, Rojas B, Ramirez AI, et al. Analysis of retinal peripapillary segmentation in early Alzheimer's disease patients. Biomed Res Int. 2015;2015:636548.
66. Lad EM, Mukherjee D, Stinnett SS, Cousins SW, Potter GG, Burke JR, et al. Evaluation of inner retinal layers as biomarkers in mild cognitive impairment to moderate Alzheimer's disease. PLoS One. 2018;13:e0192646.
67. Bodis-Wollner I, Hendley CD, Mylin LH, Thornton J. Visual evoked potentials and the visuogram in multiple sclerosis. Ann Neurol. 1979;5:40–7.

68. Bodis-Wollner I, Diamond SP. The measurement of spatial contrast sensitivity in cases of blurred vision associated with cerebral lesions. Brain. 1976;99:695–710.
69. Beach TG, Adler CH, Lue L, Sue LI, Bachalakuri J, Henry-Watson J, et al. Unified staging system for Lewy body disorders: correlation with nigrostriatal degeneration, cognitive impairment and motor dysfunction. Acta Neuropathol. 2009;117:613–34.
70. Lee H-J, Bae E-J, Lee S-J. Extracellular α--synuclein-a novel and crucial factor in Lewy body diseases. Nat Rev Neurol. 2014;10:92–8.
71. Maries E, Dass B, Collier TJ, Kordower JH, Steece-Collier K. The role of α-synuclein in Parkinson's disease: insights from animal models. Nat Rev Neurosci. 2003;4:727–38.
72. Kashani AH, Zimmer-Galler IE, Shah SM, Dustin L, Do DV, Eliott D, et al. Retinal thickness analysis by race, gender, and age using Stratus OCT. Am J Ophthalmol. 2010;149:496–502. e1.
73. Rodnitzky RL. Visual dysfunction in Parkinson's disease. Clin Neurosci. 1998;5:102–6.
74. Buttner T, Kuhn W, Muller T, Patzold T, Heidbrink K, Przuntek H. Distorted color discrimination in "de nova" parkinsonian patients. Neurology. 1995;45:386–7.
75. Maffei L, Fiorentini A, Bisti S, Holländer H. Pattern ERG in the monkey after section of the optic nerve. Exp Brain Res. 1985;59(2):423–5.
76. Yu J-G, Feng Y-F, Xiang Y, Huang J-H, Savini G, Parisi V, et al. Retinal nerve fiber layer thickness changes in Parkinson disease: a meta-analysis. PLoS One. 2014;9:e85718.
77. Altintaş Ö, Işeri P, Özkan B, Çağlar Y. Correlation between retinal morphological and functional findings and clinical severity in Parkinson's disease. Doc Ophthalmol. 2007;116:137–46.
78. Hajee ME, March WF, Lazzaro DR, Wolintz AH, Shrier EM, Glazman S, et al. Inner retinal layer thinning in Parkinson disease. Arch Ophthalmol. 2009;127:737–41.
79. Archibald NK, Clarke MP, Mosimann UP, Burn DJ. Retinal thickness in Parkinson's disease. Parkinsonism Relat Disord. 2011;17:431–6.
80. Moschos MM, Tagaris G, Markopoulos I, Margetis I, Tsapakis S, Kanakis M, et al. Morphologic changes and functional retinal impairment in patients with Parkinson disease without visual loss. Eur J Ophthalmol. 2011;21:24–9.
81. Tsironi EE, Dastiridou A, Katsanos A, Dardiotis E, Veliki S, Patramani G, et al. Perimetric and retinal nerve fiber layer findings in patients with Parkinson's disease. BMC Ophthalmol. 2012;12 https://doi.org/10.1186/1471-2415-12-54.
82. Albrecht P, Müller A-K, Südmeyer M, Ferrea S, Ringelstein M, Cohn E, et al. Optical coherence tomography in parkinsonian syndromes. PLoS One. 2012;7:e34891.
83. Garcia-Martin E, Satue M, Fuertes I, Otin S, Alarcia R, Herrero R, et al. Ability and reproducibility of Fourier-domain optical coherence tomography to detect retinal nerve fiber layer atrophy in Parkinson's disease. Ophthalmology. 2012;119:2161–7.
84. Shrier EM, Adam CR, Spund B, Glazman S, Bodis-Wollner I. Interocular asymmetry of foveal thickness in Parkinson disease. J Ophthalmol. 2012;2012:728457.
85. Adam CR, Shrier E, Ding Y, Glazman S, Bodis-Wollner I. Correlation of inner retinal thickness evaluated by spectral-domain optical coherence tomography and contrast sensitivity in Parkinson disease. J Neuroophthalmol. 2013;33:137–42.
86. Rohani M, Langroodi AS, Ghourchian S, Falavarjani KG, SoUdi R, Shahidi G. Retinal nerve changes in patients with tremor dominant and akinetic rigid Parkinson's disease. Neurol Sci. 2012;34:689–93.
87. Kirbas S, Turkyilmaz K, Tufekci A, Durmus M. Retinal nerve fiber layer thickness in Parkinson disease. J Neuroophthalmol. 2013;33:62–5.
88. La Morgia C, Barboni P, Rizzo G, Carbonelli M, Savini G, Scaglione C, et al. Loss of temporal retinal nerve fibers in Parkinson disease: a mitochondrial pattern? Eur J Neurol. 2012;20:198–201.
89. Satue M, Garcia-Martin E, Fuertes I, Otin S, Alarcia R, Herrero R, et al. Use of Fourier-domain OCT to detect retinal nerve fiber layer degeneration in Parkinson's disease patients. Eye. 2013;27:507–14.

90. Moreno-Ramos T, Benito-León J, Villarejo A, Bermejo-Pareja F. Retinal nerve fiber layer thinning in dementia associated with Parkinson's disease, dementia with Lewy bodies, and Alzheimer's disease. J Alzheimers Dis. 2013;34:659–64.
91. Garcia-Martin E, Rodriguez-Mena D, Satue M, Almarcegui C, Dolz I, Alarcia R, et al. Electrophysiology and optical coherence tomography to evaluate Parkinson disease severity. Invest Ophthalmol Vis Sci. 2014;55:696–705.
92. Satue M, Seral M, Otin S, Alarcia R, Herrero R, Bambo MP, et al. Retinal thinning and correlation with functional disability in patients with Parkinson's disease. Br J Ophthalmol. 2014;98:350–5.
93. Lee J-Y, Kim JM, Ahn J, Kim H-J, Jeon BS, Kim TW. Retinal nerve fiber layer thickness and visual hallucinations in Parkinson's disease. Mov Disord. 2013;29:61–7.
94. Roth NM, Saidha S, Zimmermann H, Brandt AU, Isensee J, Benkhellouf-Rutkowska A, et al. Photoreceptor layer thinning in idiopathic Parkinson's disease. Mov Disord. 2014;29:1163–70.
95. Garcia-Martin E, Larrosa JM, Polo V, Satue M, Marques ML, Alarcia R, et al. Distribution of retinal layer atrophy in patients with Parkinson disease and association with disease severity and duration. Am J Ophthalmol. 2014;157:470–8.e2.
96. Jiménez B, Ascaso FJ, Cristóbal JA, López del Val J. Development of a prediction formula of Parkinson disease severity by optical coherence tomography. Mov Disord. 2014;29:68–74.
97. Sen A, Tugcu B, Coskun C, Ekinci C, Nacaroglu SA. Effects of levodopa on retina in Parkinson disease. Eur J Ophthalmol. 2014;24:114–9.
98. Quagliato LB, Domingues C, Quagliato EMAB, de Abreu EB, Kara-Junior N. Applications of visual evoked potentials and Fourier-domain optical coherence tomography in Parkinson's disease: a controlled study. Arq Bras Oftalmol. 2014;77:238–42.
99. Mailankody P, Battu R, Khanna A, Lenka A, Yadav R, Pal PK. Optical coherence tomography as a tool to evaluate retinal changes in Parkinson's disease. Parkinsonism Relat Disord. 2015;21:1164–9.
100. Unlu M, Sevim DG, Gultekin M, Karaca C. Correlations among multifocal electroretinography and optical coherence tomography findings in patients with Parkinson's disease. Neurol Sci. 2018;39:533–41.
101. Aydin TS, Umit D, Nur OM, Fatih U, Asena K, Nefise OY, et al. Optical coherence tomography findings in Parkinson's disease. Kaohsiung J Med Sci. 2018;34:166–71.
102. Uchida A, Pillai JA, Bermel R, Bonner-Jackson A, Rae-Grant A, Fernandez H, et al. Outer retinal assessment using spectral-domain optical coherence tomography in patients with Alzheimer's and Parkinson's disease. Invest Opthalmol Vis Sci. 2018;59:2768.
103. Sengupta P, Dutta K, Ghosh S, Mukherjee A, Pal S, Basu D. Optical coherence tomography findings in patients of Parkinson's disease: an Indian perspective. Ann Indian Acad Neurol. 2018;21:150–5.
104. Savy C, Simon A, Nguyen-Legros J. Spatial geometry of the dopamine innervation in the avascular area of the human fovea. Vis Neurosci. 1991;7:487–98.
105. Miri S, Glazman S, Mylin L, Bodis-Wollner I. A combination of retinal morphology and visual electrophysiology testing increases diagnostic yield in Parkinson's disease. Parkinsonism Relat Disord. 2016;22(Suppl 1):S134–7.
106. Edwards MM, Rodríguez JJ, Gutierrez-Lanza R, Yates J, Verkhratsky A, Lutty GA. Retinal macroglia changes in a triple transgenic mouse model of Alzheimer's disease. Exp Eye Res. 2014;127:252–60.
107. Chiasseu M, Alarcon-Martinez L, Belforte N, Quintero H, Dotigny F, Destroismaisons L, et al. Tau accumulation in the retina promotes early neuronal dysfunction and precedes brain pathology in a mouse model of Alzheimer's disease. Mol Neurodegener. 2017;12 https://doi.org/10.1186/s13024-017-0199-3.
108. Bodis-Wollner I, Brannan JR, Storch RL, Hajee ME, Minko M. The effect of background spatial contrast on electroretinographic responses in the human retina. Vis Res. 2009;49:922–30.
109. Kaur M, Saxena R, Singh D, Behari M, Sharma P, Menon V. Correlation between structural and functional retinal changes in Parkinson disease. J Neuroophthalmol. 2015;35:254–8.

110. Bodis-Wollner I, Brannan JR. Hidden visual loss in optic neuropathy is revealed using Gabor patch contrast perimetry. Clin Neurosci. 1997;4:284–91.
111. Gibb WR, Lees AJ. The relevance of the Lewy body to the pathogenesis of idiopathic Parkinson's disease. J Neurol Neurosurg Psychiatry. 1988;51:745–52.
112. Bodis-Wollner I, Tzelepi A. The push-pull action of dopamine on spatial tuning of the monkey retina: the effects of dopaminergic deficiency and selective D1 and D2 receptor ligands on the pattern electroretinogram. Vis Res. 1998;38:1479–87.
113. Merigan WH, Eskin TA. Spatio-temporal vision of macaques with severe loss of P beta retinal ganglion cells. Vis Res. 1986;26:1751–61.
114. McKeith IG. Clinical diagnostic criteria for dementia with Lewy bodies. In: Dementia with Lewy bodies; 2016. p. 59–71.
115. Diederich NJ, Fénelon G, Stebbins G, Goetz CG. Hallucinations in Parkinson disease. Nat Rev Neurol. 2009;5:331–42.
116. Maurage C-A, Ruchoux M-M, de Vos R, Surguchov A, Destee A. Retinal involvement in dementia with Lewy bodies: a clue to hallucinations? Ann Neurol. 2003;54:542–7.
117. Lin W, Xie Y-C, Cheng P-Y, Dong L-Y, Hung G-U, Chiu P-Y. Association of visual hallucinations with very mild degenerative dementia due to dementia with Lewy bodies. PLoS One. 2018;13:e0205909.
118. Schön C, Herms J. In vivo imaging of tau aggregates in the mouse retina. Methods Mol Biol. 2016;1523:361–8.
119. Kayabasi UA, Rispoli M. Detection of tau tangles in the retina. Alzheimers Dement. 2017;13:P1535–6.
120. Kayabasi UA, Rose J. Importance of detecting tau protein in the retina. Alzheimers Dement. 2018;14:P840–1.
121. Ngolab J, Rockenstein E, Mante M, Florio JB, Masliah E, Rissman RA. Evaluating tau expression in the retina of triple repeat tau mice underperforming in visual-spatial test. Alzheimers Dement. 2018;14:P1139.
122. Hinton DR, Sadun AA, Blanks JC, Miller CA. Optic nerve degeneration in Alzheimer's disease. J Neuropathol Exp Neurol. 1986;45:340.
123. Blanks JC, Hinton DR, Sadun AA, Miller CA. Retinal ganglion cell degeneration in Alzheimer's disease. Brain Res. 1989;501:364–72.
124. den Haan J, Janssen SF, van de Kreeke JA, Scheltens P, Verbraak FD, Bouwman FH. Retinal thickness correlates with parietal cortical atrophy in early-onset Alzheimer's disease and controls. Alzheimers Dement. 2018;10:49–55.
125. Bulut M, Kurtuluş F, Gözkaya O, Erol MK, Cengiz A, Akıdan M, et al. Evaluation of optical coherence tomography angiographic findings in Alzheimer's type dementia. Br J Ophthalmol. 2017;102:233–7.
126. Gharbiya M, Trebbastoni A, Parisi F, Manganiello S, Cruciani F, D'Antonio F, et al. Choroidal thinning as a new finding in Alzheimer's disease: evidence from enhanced depth imaging spectral domain optical coherence tomography. J Alzheimers Dis. 2014;40:907–17.
127. Mendoza-Santiesteban CE, Palma J-A, Ortuño-Lizarán I, Cuenca N, Kaufmann H. Pathologic confirmation of retinal ganglion cell loss in multiple system atrophy. Neurology. 2017;88:2233–5.
128. Papp MI, Kahn JE, Lantos PL. Glial cytoplasmic inclusions in the CNS of patients with multiple system atrophy (striatonigral degeneration, olivopontocerebellar atrophy and Shy-Drager syndrome). J Neurol Sci. 1989;94:79–100.
129. Grazia Spillantini M, Spillantini MG, Anthony Crowther R, Jakes R, Cairns NJ, Lantos PL, et al. Filamentous α-synuclein inclusions link multiple system atrophy with Parkinson's disease and dementia with Lewy bodies. Neurosci Lett. 1998;251:205–8.
130. Cykowski MD, Coon EA, Powell SZ, Jenkins SM, Benarroch EE, Low PA, et al. Expanding the spectrum of neuronal pathology in multiple system atrophy. Brain. 2015;138:2293–309.
131. Fischer MD, Synofzik M, Heidlauf R, Schicks J, Srulijes K, Kernstock C, et al. Retinal nerve fiber layer loss in multiple system atrophy. Mov Disord. 2011;26:914–6.

132. Ahn J, Lee J-Y, Kim TW, Yoon EJ, Oh S, Kim YK, et al. Retinal thinning associates with nigral dopaminergic loss in de novo Parkinson disease. Neurology. 2018;91:e1003–12.
133. Biundo R, Weis L, Bostantjopoulou S, Stefanova E, Falup-Pecurariu C, Kramberger MG, et al. MMSE and MoCA in Parkinson's disease and dementia with Lewy bodies: a multicenter 1-year follow-up study. J Neural Transm. 2016;123:431–8.
134. La Morgia C, Di Vito L, Carelli V, Carbonelli M. Patterns of retinal ganglion cell damage in neurodegenerative disorders: parvocellular vs magnocellular degeneration in optical coherence tomography studies. Front Neurol. 2017;8:710. https://doi.org/10.3389/fneur.2017.00710. eCollection 2017.

Optical Coherence Tomography in Alzheimer's Disease

13

Gianluca Coppola, Vincenzo Parisi, Gianluca Manni, Francesco Pierelli, and Alfredo A. Sadun

Abbreviations

AD	Alzheimer's disease
ADAS-Cog	Alzheimer's disease assessment scale
aMCI	Amnestic type of mild cognitive impairment
APP	Beta-amyloid precursor protein
ERG	Electroretinogram
GCL	Ganglion cell layer
HRT	Heidelberg retina tomograph
IPL	Inner plexiform layer
OCT	Optical coherence tomography
ON	Optic nerve
PERG	Pattern electroretinogram
PS1	Presenilin 1
RBANS	Repeatable Battery for the Assessment of Neuropsychological Status
RNFL	Retina nerve fiber layer
VEP	Visual evoked potential

G. Coppola (✉) · F. Pierelli
Department of Medico-Surgical Sciences and Biotechnologies, Sapienza University of Rome Polo Pontino, Latina, Italy
e-mail: gianluca.coppola@uniroma1.it; francesco.pierelli@uniroma1.it

V. Parisi
IRCCS - Bietti Foundation, Research Unit of Neurophysiology of Vision and Neuroophthalmology, Rome, Italy

G. Manni
Department of Clinical Sciences and Translation Medicine, Tor Vergata University of Rome, Rome, Italy

A. A. Sadun
Doheny Eye Institute, Keck School of Medicine, Pasadena, CA, USA

A. Grzybowski, P. Barboni (eds.), *OCT and Imaging in Central Nervous System Diseases*, https://doi.org/10.1007/978-3-030-26269-3_13

13.1 Introduction

Alzheimer's disease (AD) is the most common cause of dementia with an incidence that increases with age exponentially. According to the World Health Organization the worldwide prevalence of Alzheimer' disease (AD) is increasing yearly and receives growing attention because it affects quality of life, and also because has a significant economic impact, being a major public-health problem [1] and a substantial financial burden on families [2]. The recent publication of the Global Burden of Disease survey 2016 shows that among neurological conditions, the global number of individuals who lived with dementia has doubled compared to 1990 and dementia was the fifth leading cause of death globally [3].

AD is a brain degenerative disorder, where inherited susceptibility and environmental factors are probably interrelated [4, 5]. The clinical evolution of AD is a slowly progressive and episodic memory loss as the predominant symptom, with various accompanying signs including aphasia, apraxia, and agnosia, and general cognitive symptomology, such as impaired judgement, decision-making, and orientation [4]. Because of the slowness of the disease's progression, the neurodegenerative processes are likely to start 20–30 years before the clinical manifestations of AD. This transitional phase is recognized as mild cognitive impairment (MCI), which has some memory deficit, preservation of general cognitive and functional abilities, and absence of diagnosed dementia as cardinal features [6]. The amnestic type of MCI (aMCI) shows the highest annual incidence conversion rate to AD [7]. Nonetheless MCI can be comorbid with other neurological disorders, such as nondemented Parkinson's disease (PD) patients and increased the risk of progressive cognitive decline and dementia [8].

Despite great advances in the understanding of AD pathophysiology in the last few years, the exact pathogenesis of AD and its precursor MCI is still not comprehensively understood.

At the histopathologic level, neuronal loss, beta-amyloid plaques, neurofibrillary tangles made of hyperphosphorylated tau and neuritic plaques, and granulovacuolar degeneration characterize the brain of AD [4]. These lesions have been seen in the hippocampus and other limbic structures, as well as in the visual associative areas [9, 10], the primary visual cortex [11, 12], and in subcortical structures including the lateral geniculate nuclei and the superior colliculi [13–15], and within the retina [16–18].

AD patients may be affected by various visual disturbances, such as deficits in contrast sensitivity [19–21], motion perception [22, 23], and color discrimination [24–26]. Historically, these visual dysfunctions in AD have been attributed to damage in the primary visual cortex and to degenerative processes in primary and associative visual cortical areas, but cortical dysfunction alone cannot explain the pattern of observed defects. Multiple forms of evidence points toward the involvement of retinal ganglion cells and their axons in the optic nerve as a basis of the visual dysfunction in AD [16, 27]. This peripheral involvement in AD and MCI could be independent from the central one [28].

In the last two decades, several studies have considered the retinal involvement in AD pathophysiology. Sophisticated imaging techniques have been used, such as optical coherence tomography (OCT), scanning laser polarimetry, and pattern electroretinography (PERG), to assess the morphologic and functional changes of the retina in AD [29].

Optical Coherence Tomography (OCT) permits the objective quantification *in vivo* of the retinal nerve fiber layer (RNFL) that consists of axons that form the optic nerve and contributes partially to the retinal thickness. This method consists of a non-invasive technology allowing cross-sectional imaging of the eye [30, 31]. The implementation of Spectral-Domain OCT provides advantages in signal-to-noise ratio, permitting faster signal acquisition [32, 33]. Taking in mind that the human eye is an embryological protrusion of the brain, and the nerves and axons of the retinal nerve fiber layer (RNFL) are similar to those in the brain, it is not surprising that OCT has been widely employed in assessing RNFL thickness in several neurologic as well as neuro-ophthalmologic disorders [34–38].

The intent of this chapter is to provide a comprehensive overview of the results provided by the OCT technique as used to understand morphological retinal changes that occur due to the degenerative processes associated with Alzheimer's disease and other dementing disorders.

13.2 Retina and Alzheimer's Disease

As an integrated part of the nervous system, the retina is physiologically under senescence processes, the majority of them still under intense scrutiny. Therefore, in order to better evaluating AD patients, it is important to quantify the degree of thinning arising with age in the absence of pathological processes. It is also important to determine whether age-related loss is uniformly distributed across the optic disc or has any tendency to be sectorial and might therefore be a confounding factor for a correct evaluation of disease-related processes.

In the quest for understanding the degenerative changes accompanying AD, researchers performed both histological and *in-vivo* studies on healthy subjects.

Using immunohistochemical techniques, Löffler and colleagues examined the presence and expression of amyloid-related proteins, the same that have been found in specimens of AD patients' brains, in the human retina collected from cadaver eyes at various ages [17]. They did not find any abnormal deposits or immunoreactivity changes in the outer neural retina. On the other hand, they demonstrated the presence of tau proteins and amyloid precursor protein in the inner retina layers, including retinal ganglion cells and nerve fiber layer, of the human retina in older persons. Small amounts of beta-amyloid were detected in the sub-retinal pigment epithelium space [17]. Intracellular and extracellular Aβ deposits were recently detected in immunoreactive melanopsin retinal ganglion cells (mRGC) in AD retinas with abnormal morphology [18].

The analysis of normal *in-vivo* human retinal nerve fiber layer thickness, as measured by time-domain OCT, has been repeatedly confirmed as an age-related reduction of RNFL thickness in normal subjects [39–42]. This thinning mainly involved the superior and inferior optic disc areas [43–45].

13.2.1 Animal Model of AD

One of the most recognised theories for the genesis of AD, the "amyloid cascade hypothesis", postulates that APP dysmetabolism and beta-amyloid deposition are the primary events that facilitate the disease process of AD [46].

In the past decade, through the use of genetic engineering techniques, transgenic (Tg) animal models over-expressing mutant forms of amyloid precursor protein (APP) and/or presenilin 1 (PS1) have been generated to mimic various aspects of AD pathology, including Aβ deposition, cognitive deficits, inflammation, and synaptic dysfunction, to test newly proposed therapeutic agents [47]. Recent publications have shown the accumulation of Aβ-plaques within the retina [48–51] and its microvasculature [52], retina ganglion cell death [53], and local neuroinflammation [52] in different Tg animal models. Nevertheless, these transgenic models only mimic part of the pathological features of AD.

An interesting Tg AD rat model, TgF344-AD, expressing mutant human amyloid precursor protein (APPsw) and presenilin 1 genes, seems to more faithfully encapsulate most of the features of AD. This animal model is characterized by an otherwise healthy long lifespan, but the rats suffer from later age cognitive decline, age-dependent cerebral amyloidosis, taupathy, gliosis, and frank neuronal loss that seems to parallel those in humans [54]. Tsai and colleagues investigated a group of TgF344-AD rats and age-matched wild type rats [55]. When compared with age-matched controls, the retinas of Tg rats demonstrated the presence of Aβ plaques, hypertrophic retinal pigment epithelial cells, signs of neuroinflammation, and a significant thinning of retinal choroid [55].

In mice models, non-mutant human Tau (hTau) gene expression may be sufficient to initiate AD and may thus be a more relevant model to study the disease [56]. In hTau mice at 5 and 17 months of age researchers examined functional, histological and molecular changes occurring in the visual system. They unexpectedly observed that hTau expression is not toxic for retinal cells at least in-so-far as the electroretinogram response was not altered in hTau compared with mTKO littermates, but even more pronounced in amplitude in hTau than in KO mice deprived of Tau retinae, suggesting a protective role of hTAU in visual physiology [57].

13.2.2 Histological Studies in Post-Mortem AD Eyes

In 1986, histological examination in a human post-mortem study revealed depletion of axons in the optic nerves from AD patients [16]. Sadun and colleagues were the first to demonstrate this primary AD-associated optic neuropathy and further, to characterize, by morphometric analysis, that the predominant effect was on the largest retinal ganglion cells (M-cells) that contribute their large caliber fibers to the optic nerve [27]. Other studies [58, 59] failed to confirm the selective large axon losses. This discrepancy has been attributed, at least in part, to methodological biases such as different *post-mortem* delays, different techniques in axonal counting and/or difficulties in obtaining well-preserved myelinated axons.

Extensive retinal ganglion cell loss in the central retina in AD was also observed in histological studies [16] or by other methods of evaluating the RNFL *in vitro*. Morphometric analysis of the central retina (fovea/foveola/parafoveal retina) in eyes from 9 AD and 11 age-matched controls revealing an overall decrease of 25% in total numbers of neurons in the ganglion cell layer (GCL) (fovea/parafoveal retina) in AD as compared with control eyes [60]. Moreover, the most severe decrease was observed in the foveal region (−43%) over the far temporal region. Similar results were obtained in AD patients with the evaluation of the peripheral retina: the neuronal loss was more pronounced in the superior and inferior quadrants (50–59%) and a significantly increased ratio of astrocytes to neurons was detected when compared with control eyes [61]. Moreover, histological signs of degeneration in the retinal ganglion cells (RGCs) were described to include a vacuolated, "frothy" appearance of the cytoplasm in the absence of neurofibrillary tangles within the RGCs, or of neuritic plaques or amyloid angiopathy in the retinas or optic nerves in AD [62].

Koronyo-Hamaoui and colleagues recently identified retinal Aβ plaques in *post-mortem* eyes from 8 AD patients and in 5 suspected early stage cases, but not in five age-matched non-AD individuals [50].

Plaque-like structures were seen in two retinas from two AD patients, with thickening of retinal choroid and no changes in the retinal pigment epithelial cells [55]. Fibrillar tau or Aβ aggregates were seen in *post-mortem* retinas from the same AD patients that had been previously observed by using an *in-vivo* imaging technique [63].

In a recent post-mortem study [18], researchers identified mRGCs with antibody targeting melanopsin from 14 AD patients with preserved retinal anatomy, and 13 controls. In AD patients, they revealed preserved retinal layers as compared to controls, but smaller somas and thinner dendrites, focal attenuations of melanopsin immunostaining, signs of optic neuropathy with axonal loss predominantly affecting the larger fibers in the superior quadrant. Melanopsin RGC number was significantly correlated with age in controls but not in AD patients, meaning that the degenerative processes at the basis of AD are, at least in part, independent from age related changes. Finally, in a subgroup of subjects, they found evidence of consistent accumulation of Aβ inside immunoreactive mRGCs soma and extracellular/abluminal areas in AD patients, while they were absent in controls [18].

13.2.3 Clinical Studies Based on the Subjective Evaluation of Fundus Photographs

The RNFL consists of the RNFL axons of retinal ganglion cells, converging at the optic disc forms the origin of the optic nerve.

That retinal ganglion cell degeneration occurs in AD is further evident by means of the use of a boundary-tracking program and RNFL photographs. A higher proportion of AD patients showed signs of optic neuropathy manifesting as optic disc atrophy, pathologic optic disc cupping, and thinning of the neuroretinal rim and of the RNFL [64, 65]. Tsai et al. [65] observed an increased cup-to-disc ratio, cup volume, and decreased optic disc rim area in AD patients by optic nerve analyser.

Analyzing mild to moderate AD patients with RNFL fundus photographs, Lu and colleagues found that all the AD patients had different types of RNFL abnormalities, including diffuse and wedge shape nerve fiber layer drop-out [66]. These abnormalities in AD patients were associated with a higher cup–disc ratio of 39–43% when compared to that in the control group.

However, these studies required the subjective evaluation of fundus photographs with the inherent observer bias.

13.3 *In-Vivo* Morphological Analysis in AD and MCI Patients

One confounding factor in analysing MCI and AD-related late-onset progressive changes is that there are anatomical and physiological changes normally found in aging eyes. In animal [67] and human [67, 68] studies, a physiological age-dependent progressive loss of optic nerve fibers, with progressive decrease of mean axonal diameter, has been demonstrated [69–71].

Optical coherence tomography (OCT) is a technique that can also be used in ophthalmology for the measurement of the macular thickness and volume. OCT can determine RNFL thickness of the peripapillary region reflecting axons and would allow quantification of axonal loss, measurement of macular thickness and volume would reflect retinal neurons, allowing quantification of neuronal loss [30].

Several previous studies using OCT techniques have examined the relationship between age and RNFL measurements. These have consistently shown that optic nerve, RNFL, and macular measurements with OCT all varied with age [41, 72], with the greatest decrease in mean RNFL occurring in the superior [44] and inferior quadrants [42], especially after age 50 years [43]. There was less loss in RNFL thickness in the nasal and temporal quadrants [73, 74]. This age-related decline in normal RNFL measurements needs to be considered when considering or monitoring ocular disease.

However, as described below, the reduction in RNFL thickness observed in most studies on AD patients was significantly greater than that observed in the age-matched controls and thus cannot be exclusively ascribed to aging (see some illustrative OCT imaging in Fig. 13.1 and a synopsis of published OCT studies in AD and MCI in Table 13.1).

Parisi and colleagues were the first who used OCT to study a group of 17 AD patients affected from mild severity cognitive impairment and compared them with a group of 14 age-matched controls. In AD patients, OCT results showed thinning of the average peripapillary RNFL and in all quadrants examined, showing the involvement of the neuroretinal tissue in AD [75, 76].

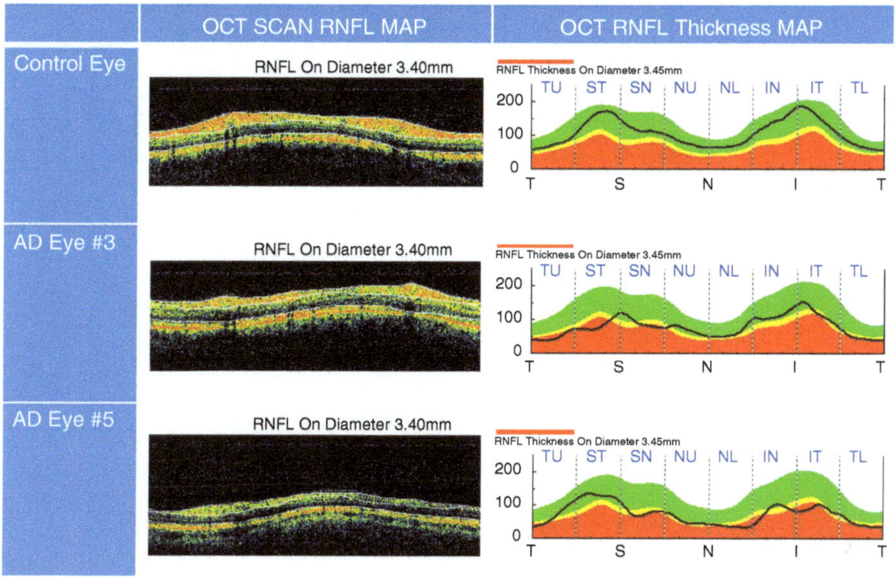

Fig. 13.1 Optical Coherence Tomography (OCT) imaging taken in cylindrical section of tissue surrounding the optic disc of a control eye and of 2 AD patients eyes. The images in the left panel are raw OCT data, while the maps in the right panel are quantitative data curve. In AD patients eyes OCT shows a decrease of RNFL reflection (reduced RNFL thickness) in each examined quadrant, with particular prevalence of the temporal ones

The mean RNFL thickness was corroborated to be reduced in AD patients by several independent groups [18, 66, 77–89]. Patients affected with MCI have also shown some RNFL thinning [81, 86, 88–90]. Individual examination of the quadrants was even more revealing. Most studies observed a significant reduction of RNFL thickness in the superior quadrant [18, 66, 75, 76, 79, 80, 83–88, 90–92], but for some also in the inferior quadrant [66, 75, 76, 79, 80, 84–88, 90–92], and for a less extent also in the nasal [75, 76, 80, 84, 86] and temporal [75–77, 79, 80, 84–86, 88] quadrants. In contradistinction, the preferential involvement of each quadrant is more inconsistent in MCI patients [86, 88, 90]. For the sake of completeness, some researchers did not observe reduced RNFL thickness both in AD [93–96] and MCI [87, 92–94, 96] patients in comparison with controls.

When assessed, the mean ganglion cell layer plus inner plexiform layer thickness (GCL-IPL) thickness was found to be reduced in AD eyes by several independent groups [77, 81, 87], and even in some patients affected with MCI [28]. In one study GCL-IPL thickness was reduced in moderate AD and in frontotemporal dementia, but not in MCI and mild AD patients [81].

Some researchers studied optic nerves of AD patients by using confocal scanning laser ophthalmoscopy (cSLO). Ophthalmoscopy in combination with cSLO, revealed an enlargement in the mean vertical cup-to-disc ratio (clinician and instrument derived), rim volume, rim area, and reduced RNFL thickness in patients with AD with respect to controls [97]. Compared with individuals in the lowest quarter

Table 13.1 Demographic data and RNFL thickness measurements in patients and controls as determined by OCT

Reference	No. of subjects and diagnosis	Mean MMSE/ AD stage	Mean age ± SD	OCT machine	Mean RNFL (μm)	Superior quadrant (μm)	Inferior quadrant (μm)	Nasal quadrant (μm)	Temporal quadrant (μm)	Note
Parisi et al. [75, 76]	17 AD 14 controls	/mild	70.37 ± 6.1	Humphrey	59.5 ± 16.70[a] 99.9 ± 8.95	72.1 ± 21.4[a] 104.6 ± 12.1	77.9 ± 26.4[a] 116.2 ± 9.87	50.4 ± 23.2[a] 93.4 ± 13.7	37.9 ± 17.60[a] 85.6 ± 8.21	RNFL overall values correlated with PERG
Iseri et al. [91]	14 AD 15 controls	18.5/mild to moderate 29.4	70.1 ± 9.7 65.1 ± 9.8	Carl Zeiss Meditec, Model 3000	87.4 ± 23.7[a] 113.1 ± 6.7	112.6 ± 35.3[a] 137.1 ± 16.4	103.1 ± 33.6[a] 141.5 ± 19.1	63.5 ± 19.1[a] 96.0 ± 34.4	64.9 ± 17.7 72.3 ± 16.4	Decline in both peripapillary and macular thickness and volume in AD eyes
Berisha et al. [101]	9 AD 8 HV	23.8/mild to moderate 29.5	74.3 ± 3.3 74.3 ± 5.8	Carl Zeiss Meditec, Model 3000		92.2 ± 21.6[a] 113.6 ± 10.8	117.0 ± 15.3 128.1 ± 11.4	67.0 ± 15.0 69.5 ± 11.1	65.7 ± 15.1 64.1 ± 7.3	Narrowing of the retinal microvasculature
Paquet et al. [82]	23 MCI 14 AD 12 AD 15 controls	28.8 22.6/mild 16.6/severe 28.9	78.7 ± 6.2 78.3 ± 5.1 78.8 ± 4.9 75.5 ± 5.1	Carl Zeiss Stratus OCT 3	89.3 ± 2.7[a] 89.2 ± 2.9[a] 76.6 ± 3.8[a] 102.2 ± 1.8					The involvement of retina is an early event in the course of this disorder
Lu et al. [66]	22 AD 22 controls		73 ± 8 68 ± 9	Carl Zeiss Meditec, Model 3000	90 ± 18[a, b] 98 ± 12	107 ± 30[a, b] 124 ± 16	116 ± 35[a, b] 128 ± 18	66 ± 26 70 ± 17	70 ± 20 71 ± 13	Enlarged optic cup to disc ratio in AD
Kesler et al. [90]	24 MCI 30 AD 24 controls	28.1 23.6	71.0 ± 10.0 73.7 ± 9.9 70.9 ± 9.2	Carl Zeiss Stratus OCT 3	85.8 ± 10.0[a] 84.7 ± 10.6[a] 94.3 ± 11.3	101.3 ± 15.2 99.0 ± 18.0[a] 110.0 ± 16.7	111.9 ± 16.1[a] 110.1 ± 19.1[a] 127.0 ± 15.5	65.9 ± 15.1 66.8 ± 14.5 76.4 ± 21.8	64.2 ± 13.9 61.7 ± 10.9 67.8 ± 15.1	RNFL thickness not correlated with MMSE
Kromer et al. [119, 120]	22 AD 22 controls	22.6/mild to moderate	75.9 ± 6.1 64.0 ± 8.2	Spectralis Heidelberg Engineering	80[b, c]	46[b, c]		47[b, c]		The RNFL of the AD patients did not correlate with pattern VEP latencies
Moreno-Ramos et al. [105]	10 AD 10 LB 10 PD 10 controls	16.4 14.9 16.4 29.2	73.0 ± 6.5 74.2 ± 5.1 74.3 ± 5.0 70.2 ± 5.5	TOPCON 3D OCT-1000	94.5 ± 2.2[a] 93.3 ± 1.5[a] 94.8 ± 2.0[a] 108.0 ± 2.2					Retinal involvement measured by OCT may also be present in non-AD dementias

Marziani et al. [84]	21 AD 21 controls	19.9/mild to moderate 27.9	79.3 ± 5.7 77.0 ± 4.2	(1) Optovue RTVue-100 and (2) Spectralis Heidelberg Engineering	244.1 ± 17.9^{1} 277.5 ± 21.7^{2} 252.3 ± 19.2^{1} 283.8 ± 27.3^{2} Central sector	274.8^{1a,d} 304.3^{2a,d} 288.9^{1d} 319.3^{2d}	273.25^{1a,d} 301.7^{2a,d} 286.25^{1d} 314.75^{2d}	278.4^{1a,d} 309.35^{2a,d} 290.85^{1d} 323.55^{2d}	271.8^{1a,d} 291.95^{2a,d} 286.25^{1d} 304.45^{2d}	Reduced RNFL in AD patients using 2 different OCT instruments
Kirbas et al. [83]	40 AD 40 controls	21.5	69.3 ± 4.9 68.9 ± 5.1	Spectral domain OCT	65 ± 6.2^{a} 75 ± 3.8	76 ± 6.7^{a} 105 ± 4.8	106 ± 11.5 108 ± 8.7	75 ± 2.8 76 ± 2.7	74 ± 6.7 77 ± 7.3	No correlation between MMSE and OCT results
Larrosa et al. [85]	151 AD 61 controls	18.31	75.29 74.87	(1) Carl Zeiss Meditec Cirrus and (2) Spectralis Heidelberg Engineering	97.5 ± 14.1^{1} 98.2 ± 17.1^{2a} 100.5 ± 13.0^{1} 102.7 ± 6.7^{2}	113.2 ± 18.7^{1a} 117.8 ± 19.0^{1a}	120.4 ± 20.1^{1a} 127.4 ± 21.0^{1}	72.7 ± 17.3^{1} 74.5 ± 17.2^{1}	64.5 ± 21.7^{1a} 67.8 ± 20.0^{1}	RNFL measurements were a very useful and precise tool for AD diagnosis.
Ascaso et al. [86]	21 aMCI 18 AD 41 controls	19.3 28.8	72.1 (AD + aMCI) 72.9	Stratus OCT 3	86.0 ± 7.2^{a} 64.7 ± 15.2^{a,e} 103.6 ± 8.9 (data showed from the right eye only)	96.7 ± 14.6^{a} 73.2 ± 22.0^{a,e} 126.6 ± 13.8	110.1 ± 17.7^{a} 86.2 ± 25.7^{a,e} 135.6 ± 17.6	71.0 ± 16.7^{a} 43.3 ± 20.4^{a,e} 77.8 ± 16.7	66.3 ± 12.1^{a} 56.7 ± 14.9^{a,e} 75.8 ± 16.6	A significant association between RNFL thickness in superior and nasal quadrants, and MMSE score
Cheung et al. [87]	41 MCI 100 AD 123 controls		70.4 ± 10.2^{a} 73.5 ± 6.23^{a} 65.7 ± 3.77	Carl Zeiss Meditec Cirrus HD-OCT	RNFL 89.21 86.83^{a} 90.37 GC-IPL 73.73^{a} 72.73^{a} 77.79	110.9 105.7^{a} 113.5 73.48^{a} 72.66^{a} 77.65	112.2 108.2^{a} 114.3 70.87^{a} 70.61^{a} 76.83	68.93 68.54 68.10 75.95^{a,f} 74.75^{a,f} 79.86^{f}	65.10 64.89 65.25 72.99^{a,f} 71.88^{a,f} 76.31^{f}	In the model adjusted for optic disc areas, hypertension, diabetes and, history of myocardial infarction, only superior quadrant reached the significance level

(continued)

Table 13.1 (continued)

Reference	No. of subjects and diagnosis	Mean MMSE/ AD stage	Mean age ± SD	OCT machine	Mean RNFL (μm)	Superior quadrant (μm)	Inferior quadrant (μm)	Nasal quadrant (μm)	Temporal quadrant (μm)	Note
Feke et al. [93]	21 MCI 10 AD 21 controls		74.3 ± 12.2 74.4 ± 10.5 69.1 ± 6.7	Stratus OCT 3000 (Carl Zeiss Meditec)		118.2 ± 13.4 108.8 ± 13.3 117.7 ± 15.2				No differences between the RNFL thicknesses measured in all retinal quadrants. Solely in AD patients, venous blood flow positively correlated with superior RNFL thickness
Gao et al. [88]	26 MCI 25 AD 21 controls	25.77 19.24 28.57	73.42 ± 1.54 74.72 ± 1.39 72.05 ± 1.02	Cirrus HD-OCT 4000, Carl Zeiss Meditec	92.38[a] 85.99[a] 98.60	112.12[a] 106.10[a] 122.25	123.87 108.64[a] 127.59	68.54 66.16 69.71	66.56[a] 63.14[a] 74.60	No correlation with MMSE test. AD data still significant after adjusting for age, sex, hypertension and diabetes
Oktem et al. [89]	35 MCI 35 AD 35 controls	28 18 29	74.1 ± 6.3 75.4 ± 6.9 70.2 ± 8.0	Zeiss Cirrus HD 5000 model OCT device	82.5 ± 7.3[a] 80.6 ± 9.6[a] 91.5 ± 7.1					In all study participants, a significant correlation was present between MMSE test and RNFL thickness

Garcia-Martin et al. [77]	150 AD 75 controls	18.35 29.78	75.33 74.79	Spectralis OCT	RNFL 95.67 ± 15.22[a] 99.23 ± 16.48 GC-IPL 6.27 ± 1.76[a] 6.45 ± 1.77			RNFL 77.02 ± 16.80 77.54 ± 18.88	RNFL 66.90 ± 15.34[a] 71.09 ± 15.52	The thickness of the RNFL, ganglion cell and inner plexiform layers were significantly decreased in AD patients with longer disease duration
Cunha et al. [79]	24 AD 24 controls	17.02 29.08	74.8 ± 6.25 72.25 ± 7.31	3D OCT-2000, Topcon Corp	93.75 ± 13.42[a] 102.96 ± 9.19	110.88 ± 19.76[a] 122.12 ± 15.55	112.38 ± 23.25[a] 130.10 ± 12.78	82.64 ± 17.82[a] 86.46 ± 13.61	66.91 ± 16.66 72.69 ± 9.16	Significant correlation between most OCT parameters and MMSE scores
Pillai et al. [94]	21 aMCI 21 AD 20 non-AD 20 PD 34 controls		68.2 ± 6.7 65.8 ± 11.1 68.7 ± 8.4 62.6 ± 9.5 65.1 ± 8.3	Cirrus 4000 HD-OCT (Zeiss)	89.9 ± 2.1 88.9 ± 2.1 89.9 ± 2.1 88.5 ± 2.1 85.3 ± 1.6	109.3 ± 3.2 107.2 ± 3.3 111.9 ± 3.4 110.1 ± 3.4 106.0 ± 2.6	117.0 ± 3.6 114.4 ± 3.6 114.3 ± 3.7 111.9 ± 3.7 108.7 ± 2.8	69.8 ± 2.5 72.5 ± 2.5 73.8 ± 2.6 72.9 ± 2.5 66.9 ± 2.0	63.4 ± 2.5 61.8 ± 2.5 59.5 ± 2.6 59.2 ± 2.6 59.1 ± 2.0	No retinal involvement in AD and non-AD dementias
Trebbastoni et al. [95]	36 AD 36 controls	22.7 28.6	72.0 ± 7.3 71.7 ± 6.0	Heidelberg Spectralis (Heidelberg Engineering)	96.7 ± 6.3 97.6 ± 8.3	114.6 ± 11.2 118.5 ± 13.1	126.3 ± 11.7 125.1 ± 11.6	74.1 ± 8.9 76.3 ± 10.9	71.9 ± 9.8 70.9 ± 12.5	After 12 months AD patients had a significant reduction of the total RNFL thickness, as well as the RNFL thickness of the inferior and superior quadrants

(continued)

Table 13.1 (continued)

Reference	No. of subjects and diagnosis	Mean MMSE/ AD stage	Mean age ± SD	OCT machine	Mean RNFL (μm)	Superior quadrant (μm)	Inferior quadrant (μm)	Nasal quadrant (μm)	Temporal quadrant (μm)	Note
Liu et al. [28]	50 CIND 27 AD 47 controls	25.2 16.6 27.4	69.7 ± 8.2 75.2 ± 7.8 67.3 ± 6.2	Cirrus HD-OCT (Carl Zeiss Meditec)	GC-IPL 76.92 ± 6.29[a] 78.41 ± 5.85 80.19 ± 5.89					Correlation was observed between GC-IPL thickness and WM microstructure and GMV of healthy controls in several brain area. This correlation was absent both in CIND and in AD patients
La Morgia et al. [18]	21 AD 74 controls	18.3	71.2 ± 10.5 69.1 ± 8.1		88.8 ± 8.4[a] 95.8 ± 12.3	104.4 ± 13.4[a] 117.1 ± 17.6	116.5 ± 15.5 122.4 ± 18.1	66.6 ± 13.9 74.3 ± 15.3	67.2 ± 10.4 69.3 ± 10.5	Inverse correlation between average RNFL thickness and age
Cunha et al. [80]	50 AD 152 controls		73.1 ± 5.36 71.0 ± 4.62	SD-OCT (Spectralis Heidelberg Engineering)	85.72 ± 14.42[a] 96.51 ± 9.36	114.44[a, f] 133.14[f]	96.27[a, f] 106.75[f]	68.76 ± 16.99[a] 74.77 ± 13.73	64.22 ± 13.01[a] 71.38 ± 12.66	AD patients showed thickness reduction in global and temporal quadrants in the peripapillary RNFL and in the superior sector of the macula

Ferrari et al. [81]	27 MCI 20 mild AD 17 moderate AD 17 FTD 49 controls	26.62 23.0 16.59 21.64	70.45 ± 5.51 69.75 ± 7.51 71.23 ± 6.95 65.59 ± 6.89 68.32 ± 6.96	Fourier-domain OCT Heidelberg Spectralis™	RNFL 92.79 ± 10.31[a] 94.55 ± 6.84 91.33 ± 13.16[a] 87.47 ± 7.34[a] 97.49 ± 8.52 GCL-IPL 55.61 ± 8.17 57.52 ± 0.27 50.07 ± 7.21[a] 51.83 ± 7.48[a] 58.18 ± 7.94					GCL-IPL was significantly correlated with raw MMSE in AD
Kwon et al. [92]	30 MCI 30 AD 30 controls	24.17 17.2 27.47	72.17 ± 4.98 73.60 ± 3.67 70.93 ± 4.68	Carl Zeiss Meditec cirrus HD-OCT	46.31 ± 4.85 42.75 ± 4.53 44.83 ± 4.24	115.0 ± 13.19 106.78 ± 13.5[e] 115.30 ± 14.78	120.84 ± 17.59 113.82 ± 16.14[a] 113.70 ± 12.02	68.22 ± 9.40 64.47 ± 7.75 66.40 ± 7.22	68.75 ± 9.79 63.71 ± 9.91 66.23 ± 12.98	
Golzan et al. [96]	23 pre-AD 28 AD 50 controls		80 ± 4 70 ± 9 79 ± 5		RNFL 101.15 99.17 93.18 GLC-IPL 98 ± 9 91 ± 2 96 ± 9[a, e]					The association between RNFL and RGCL thickness and neocortical Aβ standardized uptake value ratio in the grouped control and preclinical cohort

AD Alzheimer's disease, *aMCI* amnestic mild cognitive impairment, *CIND* patients with cognitive impairment but no dementia, *FTD* frontotemporal dementia, *GC-IPL* ganglion cell-inner plexiform layer, *LB* dementia with Lewy bodies, *MCI* mild cognitive impairment, *MMSE* mini mental state examination, *pre-AD* preclinical AD, *RNFL* retinal nerve fiber layer, *PD* dementia associated with Parkinson's disease

[a]Significantly different from controls

[b]Data extrapolated from the bar chart

[c]Statistics do not clearly show

[d]Mean of internal plus external sectors

[e]Significantly different from MCI

[f]Mean of supero-nasal or temporal plus infero-nasal or temporal sectors

[1]Optovue RT Vue-100 and

[2]Spectralis Heidelberg Engineering

of values of cup-to-disc ratios, those with higher values generally had an increased risk of AD [97]. Lu et al. [66] also observed an enlarged cup-to-disc ratio and a thinner RNFL thickness in their 22 mild to moderate AD patients. In contrast, Kergoat et al. [98] found no differences in the regional distribution of RNFL thickness between patients with mild to moderate AD and healthy controls evaluated with scanning laser polarimetry. The same researchers did not observed optic nerve head structural abnormalities in AD by using real-time topographical images obtained with a Heidelberg retina tomograph (HRT) from individuals in the early stages of AD compared with age-matched controls [98]. The same negative results were obtained by Kurna and coworkers in a group of patients with mild to moderate AD [99]. Despite that, Csincsik et al. [100] used ultra-widefield (UWF) scanning laser ophthalmoscope of the retina to determine phenotypic variations in 59 patients with AD and 48 healthy controls and found significantly higher prevalence of a hard drusen phenotype in the periphery of AD patients compared to controls, as well as changes to the arterial and venular vasculature beyond the posterior pole. The number of optic nerve head drusen increased at the 2 years follow-up measurement in AD patients [100].

Berisha et al. [101] tried to determine whether regional thinning of the RNFL occurred in the nine patients with mild to moderate AD and to determine whether the retinal circulation was abnormal in these patients. AD patients showed a marked narrowing of the retinal venous blood column diameter and a reduction in retinal blood flow rate compared with eight age-matched control subjects. OCT data confirmed a significant thinning of the peripapillary RNFL that was most pronounced in the superior quadrant, which did not correlate with the retinal blood flow [101]. They argued that the mechanisms producing reduced blood flow in the retina are related to those that produce cerebral blood flow abnormalities, which are known to occur in AD, such as increased venous wall thickness due to collagen and β-amyloid deposition [102].

In a cross-sectional study on 150 patients with low-to-moderate dementia and 61 controls, researchers compared the parameters provided by two commercially available spectral domain OCT devices, the Cirrus and the Spectralis OCT instruments [85]. With both devices, they confirmed retinal thinning in AD patients, and they found that the best parameter for distinguishing AD patients from healthy controls using OCT measurements was the Spectralis looking at RNFL [85]. Along these lines, Marziani et al. [84] used both Optovue RTVue-100 and Spectralis instruments to evaluate retinal thickness in 21 patients affected by AD in comparison with 21 healthy controls. Both instruments showed a significant difference in full retinal thickness between patients and controls in all the macular sectors except in the central sector and for the superior external sector [84].

In order to verify whether involvement of the retina is an early event in the course of AD, a few studies compared MCI versus AD patients and healthy aged people. Paquet and coworkers [82] enrolled 23 MCI patients, 14 mild AD, 12 moderate to severe AD patients, and 15 healthy subjects. Overall, mean RNFL thickness was reduced in all patient groups in respect to controls. The subgroup analyses revealed no difference between the results observed in MCI and in mild AD patients, whereas

RNFL thickness assessed in moderate to severe AD patients was significantly reduced in respect with that assessed in MCI patients [82]. Kesler et al. [90] obtained similar results finding that the mean RNFL was significantly thinner in both AD and MCI patients groups compared to controls, and that the MCI group fell in between the other two groups. This difference was particularly prominent in the inferior quadrant, whereas the AD patients had significantly thinner retinal NFL values also in the superior quadrant [90].

Some investigators attempted to identify individuals who might be at a high risk of developing AD, and observed that, despite the reduction in peripapillary RNFL thickness, central 1-mm foveal thickness and macular volume were significantly increased in aMCI patients, but not in AD patients, when compared with age-matched controls. The authors argued that retinal swelling might be the first sign of macular retinal ganglion cell degeneration probably due to inflammation and/or gliosis in the early stages of AD [86]. Other independent research groups found decreased thickness of the RNFL in MCI patients, with values sometime equal to [81, 89] or in between [88] the control and AD groups, sometimes accompanied by a reduced macular volume [88]. However, we noticed that 5 studies were unable to find differences between MCI patients and controls [87, 92–94, 96] challenging the utility of OCT in differentiation MCI from mild-to-moderate AD.

Two studies, relying both on cross-sectional and longitudinal data, recruited individuals in the preclinical stage of the disease to perform a correlation analysis between retinal structural measurements and positron emission tomography (PET) Aβ binding in the neocortex. In adults with preclinical AD, the Aβ positive group of participants showed higher volume in the IPL in comparison with the Aβ negative group [103]. The same research group found that the mean RNFL volume reduction over 27 months was linearly related to neocortical Aβ accumulation, after controlling for normal aging [104].

Finally, it is worth noting that thinning of RNFL is also present in other types of dementia, such as frontotemporal dementia [81], dementia with Lewy bodies, dementia associated with Parkinson's disease [105] and with cerebral autosomal dominant arteriopathy with subcortical infarcts and leuco-encephalopathy (CADASIL) [106] challenging the specificity of OCT findings in AD patients.

13.4 Structural-Functional Correlations

The functional activity of the visual system can be dissected by the use of electrophysiological techniques such as pattern electroretinogram (PERG) and visual evoked potentials (VEPs) that have the capability of assessing, respectively, the bioelectrical activity of retinal ganglion cells and their fibers, and the functional integrity of the entire visual pathways from retina to the visual cortex.

The implicit times were delayed and/or the amplitudes reduced [75, 76, 107–110] in most of the PERG studies performed in AD patients at various stages, reflecting retinal ganglion cell dysfunction. However, in some studies PERG parameters were within the range of normality [111, 112]. In one study luminance pattern

ERGs were delayed and amplitudes reduced, whereas isoluminant chromatic ERGs were always within the normal ranges [110].

The implicit time of patterned VEP was normal in some studies [107, 110, 113, 114] and in others delayed [109, 112, 115, 116], with the amplitudes within the range of normality. A delayed P2 component of the flash VEP is a common finding across studies in AD patients [107, 113, 117, 118], with one exception [115].

Taken as a whole, these electrophysiological results are consistent with the early histological studies showing retinal ganglion cell dysfunction in AD [25, 118] and supports the notion that this damage in AD preferentially affects the larger, faster-conducting retinal ganglion cells and their retinocortical projections.

Parisi and coworkers [75, 76] used OCT and PERG in a group of 17 mild severity AD patients compared with a group of 14 healthy controls. They observed that the general reduction of peripapillary RNFL thickness was accompanied with delayed N35, P50 and N95 implicit times and reduced N35-P50 and P50-N95 amplitudes in their AD patients. More interestingly, in AD eyes, the RNFL overall values were positively correlated to the PERG P50 and N95 implicit times and PERG P50-N95 amplitude. This was not so in controls [75, 76]. However, Iseri et al. [91] did not find significant differences in VEP P100 implicit times and N75-P100 amplitudes recorded at high spatial frequency in a group of 14 mild to moderate AD patients when compared with a group of 15 controls. Moreover, they saw no correlation between any of the abnormally in RNFL and macular OCT thickness and VEP in AD [91]. This negative correlation, between VEPs parameters recorded at both high and low spatial frequency and OCT peripapillary scans, was later corroborated [119].

Liu et al. [28] for the first time observed that thinner macular GC-IPL is associated with lower integrity of the white matter microstructure, as verified using MRI diffusion tension imaging, in healthy controls in fronto-parieto-occipital and cingulate regions, as well as with lower grey matter volume in occipital pole and cerebellum. These results in controls were contrast with those obtained in AD and MCI patients where these relationships between macula and brain microstructure and volume were not detectable. The authors suggested that neurodegenerative processes related to the AD and MCI pathology can disrupt the physiological retina-brain coupling [28].

13.5 Correlations with Psychometric Measures

Along with personal history, physical examination and laboratory tests, questionnaires are often used to help test a range of everyday mental skills of persons with symptoms of dementias. Widely used tests include the mini mental state examination (MMSE), the Alzheimer's disease assessment scale- (ADAS-Cog), clinical dementia rating (CDR) score, and the Repeatable Battery for the Assessment of Neuropsychological Status (RBANS).

The previously mentioned parameters of increased cup-to-disc ratio, cup volume, and decreased optic disc rim area, all found in AD patients by optic nerve analyser, positively correlated with ADAS-Cog scores and disease's duration [65]. In AD patients, a significant relationship between inferior RNFL thickness change and ADAS-Cog scores change as well as CDR scores at 12 months follow-up was observed. Interestingly, the linear regression model revealed that for every 10 μm decrease of RNFL thickness, there was an accompanying ADAS-Cog increase of 5 units [95].

Moreover, the reduced total macular volume in patients with AD was positively correlated with the severity of the disease as assessed by the MMSE [79, 89, 91, 95, 105]. Other studies failed to find the same associations [82, 83, 90, 119, 120]. However, some authors observed that the thinner the RNFL, ganglion cell and inner plexiform layers the longer the AD disease duration, even if the latter were not significantly related to severity of the disease (assessed with MMSE score) [77]. Nonetheless, RNFL thickness of AD or MCI patients was not associated with other patient demographic features, such as age [82, 85], gender, and AD stage [120]. In another study assessing the association between macular GC-IPL and peripapillary RNFL thicknesses with disease progression in MCI and AD, the CDR scale score exhibited significant negative relationships with the average GC-IPL thickness and GC-IPL thickness in the supero-temporal, supero-nasal, and infero-nasal sectors [121]. Furthermore, the composite memory score exhibited significant positive association with the average GC-IPL thickness and the GCIPL thickness in the supero-temporal, inferonasal, and inferotemporal sectors. A positive association between the central macular thickness and the MMSE score was also observed [121].

More recently, La Morgia et al. [18] with the scope to verify the integrity of a subpopulation of retinal ganglion cells expressing the photopigment melanopsin, observed that clinical parameters (age, age at onset, disease duration, and MMSE score) and OCT data were not correlated to AD patients actigraphic data assessing rest–activity circadian rhythms. There may have been a minimum threshold such that relatively few melanopsin retinal ganglion cells sufficed to maintain circadian rhythms.

In AD patients, but not in aMCI, multiple linear regression models showed a strong association between overall RNFL thickness and MMSE score. The same association was found between MMSE and RNFL thickness in superior and nasal quadrants. Macular thickness and volume were not associated with MMSE score either in aMCI or in AD patients [86].

A prospective study attempted to determine whether deterioration of patients' cognitive functions, as verified with the RBANS test, correlated to specific OCT findings [122–124]. These investigators followed, for a period of 25 months, two groups of subjects: 82 participants with a normal cognitive status and 22 MCI patients. The participants who completed the observational period were further categorized as 60 participants experiencing a stable cognitive status and 18 participants who experienced a worsening of their cognitive status. The investigators found that in those participants who remained stable, greater attenuation of RNFL in the superior quadrant could predict specific cognitive deteriorations. In contradistinction, in participants who worsened, less attenuation of RNFL in the inferior quadrant could predict greater cognitive deterioration [122–124]. These findings suggest that patients who have less reduction in the thickness of the inferior quadrant of RNFL over time may have a higher risk of developing MCI and dementia, leading the authors to put forward RNFL thickness as a potential biomarker of dementia.

13.6 Conclusions

The diagnosis of AD is often based on psychometric assessments by a multidisciplinary team (neurologists, psychiatrists, and psychologist) and a neurological examination. Because of inter- and intra-individual variability, neurophysiological and neuroimaging tests have not yet been considered as criteria on which to base a diagnosis. In fact, neurophysiological as well as other paraclinical tests are recommended only on suspicion of secondary causes of dementia as part of the differential diagnosis of AD. The AD diagnosis is confirmed only with *post mortem* histopathology. Nonetheless, the last few decades have seen the use of structural and functional techniques as potential biomarkers that might also identify factors that may predispose individuals to AD. The optical coherence tomography (OCT) technique for the measurement of the peripapillary RNFL, the macular thickness and volume, has been demonstrated as useful for the demonstration of significant retinal changes in patients that roughly correlate with the severity of the disease (Fig. 13.2).

Particularly intriguing results of recent experiments include:

- In animal models, expressing mutant forms of amyloid precursors, and histological studies on *post mortem* AD eyes, researchers have observed various retinal pathological changes, such as accumulation of Aβ aggregates within the retina and its microvasculature, retina ganglion cell death and signs of neuroinflammation.
- In evaluations with the optic nerve analyser, a higher proportion of AD patients show signs of optic neuropathy manifesting as optic disc atrophy, pathologic optic disc cupping, and thinning of the neuroretinal rim and of the RNFL.
- In agreement with *post mortem* studies, OCT data studies indicate a significant decline in peripapillary RNFL and also changes in macular thickness and volume that is progressive from MCI to AD eyes.
- Electrophysiological and OCT studies in AD patients show RNFL thickness reduction that is related to neuronal degeneration in the retinal ganglion cell layer that is not a consequence of retrograde degeneration from the post-chiasmatic visual pathway.
- The acquisition in the same patients of OCT and objective measurements of brain microstructure and volume shows that RNFL cannot be used as a surrogate for magnetic resonance imaging measurements of the brain.
- The correlations between morphological and clinical features tend to suggest a potential role for optic nerve head analysis in monitoring the progression of AD and as outcome measures in the assessment of any purported AD treatments.

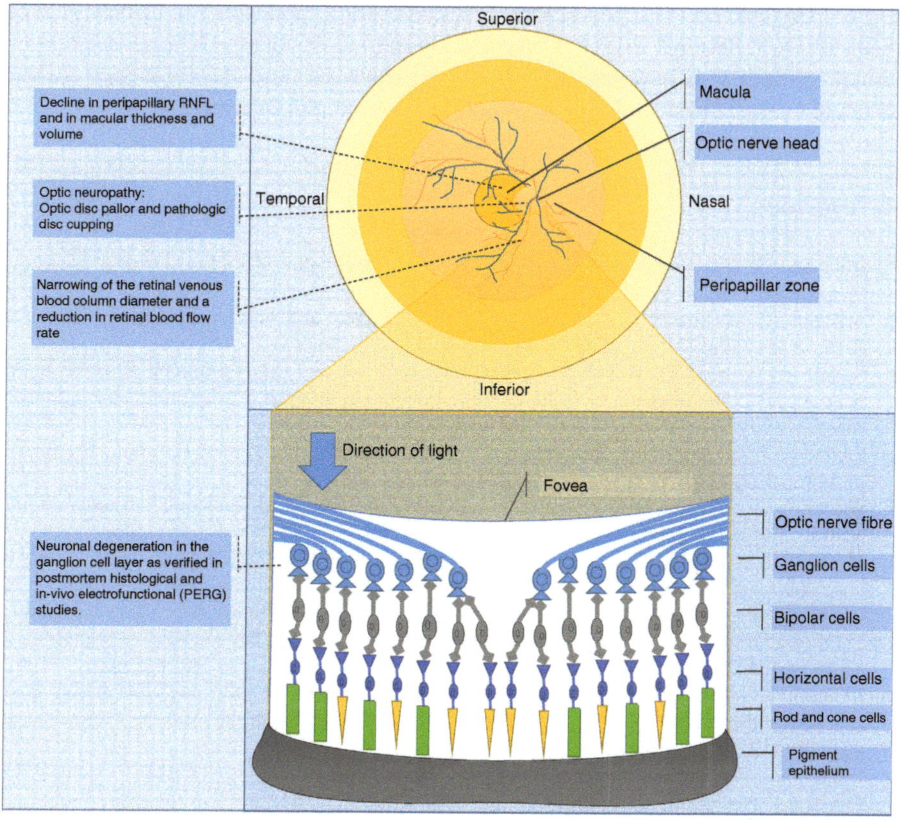

Fig. 13.2 Schematic representation of an entire retina with superimposed anatomic zones (upper panel **a**) and a schematic enlargement of a portion of the retina with the main cell classes (lower panel **b**). On the left panel (**c**) are summarized the findings from the OCT and electrophysiological studies in AD

Overall, these results suggest that degeneration of the retinal ganglion cells should be added to the constellation of neuropathologic changes found in patients with Alzheimer's disease.

Other neurodegenerative disorders, like Parkinson's disease and glaucoma, may enter in the differential diagnosis of RNFL thinning [125]. A particular mention merits the controversial association between primary open angle glaucoma (POAG) and AD. This is based on various indirect evidence of some shared genetic, histopathological and functional features [126, 127]. The association of AD and POAG is poorly supported by epidemiological studies [128, 129]. Nonetheless, for some authors glaucoma could be, in a subgroup of patients, the expression of a neurodegenerative process of the CNS that may be partially influenced by the risk factor of intraocular pressure (IOP) [130, 131]. However, the link between AD and the risk of developing glaucoma persists even without elevated IOP levels [78].

Future research in OCT as a biomarker of AD requires establishing a better specificity of OCT findings in AD. These and similar studies using OCT parameters of retinal changes will be important as objective in vivo outcome measures against which to evaluate new molecules purported to help in the treatment of AD.

References

1. Stefanacci R. The costs of Alzheimer's disease and the value of effective therapies. Am J Manag Care. 2011;13:S356–62.
2. Alzheimer's Association. 2016 Alzheimer's disease facts and figures. Alzheimers Dement. 2016;12:459–509.
3. Nichols E, Szoeke CEI, Vollset SE, et al. Global, regional, and national burden of Alzheimer's disease and other dementias, 1990–2016: a systematic analysis for the Global Burden of Disease Study 2016. Lancet Neurol. 2019;18:88–106.
4. Blennow K, de Leon MJ, Zetterberg H. Alzheimer's disease. Lancet (London, England). 2006;368:387–403.
5. Waring S, Rosenberg RN. Genome-wide association studies in Alzheimer disease. Arch Neurol. 2008;65:329–34.
6. Morris J, Storandt M, Miller JP, McKeel DW, Price JL, Rubin EH, Berg L. Mild cognitive impairment represents early-stage Alzheimer disease. Arch Neurol. 2001;58:397–405.
7. Winblad B, Palmer K, Kivipelto M, et al. Mild cognitive impairment--beyond controversies, towards a consensus: report of the International Working Group on Mild Cognitive Impairment. J Intern Med. 2004;256:240–6.
8. Litvan I, Goldman JG, Tröster AI, et al. Diagnostic criteria for mild cognitive impairment in Parkinson's disease: Movement Disorder Society Task Force guidelines. Mov Disord. 2012;27:349–56.
9. Whitehouse PJ, Price DL, Clark AW, Coyle JT, DeLong MR. Alzheimer disease: evidence for selective loss of cholinergic neurons in the nucleus basalis. Ann Neurol. 1981;10:122–6.
10. van de Nes JAP, Nafe R, Schlote W. Non-tau based neuronal degeneration in Alzheimer's disease—an immunocytochemical and quantitative study in the supragranular layers of the middle temporal neocortex. Brain Res. 2008;1213:152–65.
11. Leuba G, Kraftsik R. Visual cortex in Alzheimer's disease: occurrence of neuronal death and glial proliferation, and correlation with pathological hallmarks. Neurobiol Aging. 1994;15:29–43.
12. Armstrong RA. Is there a spatial association between senile plaques and neurofibrillary tangles in Alzheimer's disease? Folia Neuropathol. 2005;43:133–8.
13. Leuba G, Saini K. Pathology of subcortical visual centres in relation to cortical degeneration in Alzheimer's disease. Neuropathol Appl Neurobiol. 1995;21:410–22.
14. Baloyannis S, Mauroudis I, Manolides SL, Manolides LS. Synaptic alterations in the medial geniculate bodies and the inferior colliculi in Alzheimer's disease: a Golgi and electron microscope study. Acta Otolaryngol. 2009;129:416–8.
15. Dugger B, Tu M, Murray ME, Dickson DW. Disease specificity and pathologic progression of tau pathology in brainstem nuclei of Alzheimer's disease and progressive supranuclear palsy. Neurosci Lett. 2011;491:122–6.
16. Hinton DR, Sadun AA, Blanks JC, Miller CA. Optic-nerve degeneration in Alzheimer's disease. N Engl J Med. 1986;315:485–7.
17. Löffler K, Edward DP, Tso MO. Immunoreactivity against tau, amyloid precursor protein, and beta-amyloid in the human retina. Invest Ophthalmol Vis Sci. 1995;36:24–31.
18. La Morgia C, Ross-Cisneros FN, Koronyo Y, et al. Melanopsin retinal ganglion cell loss in Alzheimer disease. Ann Neurol. 2016;79:90–109.

19. Hutton J, Morris JL, Elias JW, Poston JN. Contrast sensitivity dysfunction in Alzheimer's disease. Neurology. 1993;43:2328–30.
20. Gilmore G, Whitehouse PJ. Contrast sensitivity in Alzheimer's disease: a 1-year longitudinal analysis. Optom Vis Sci. 1995;72:83–91.
21. Crow R, Levin LB, LaBree L, Rubin R, Feldon SE. Sweep visual evoked potential evaluation of contrast sensitivity in Alzheimer's dementia. Invest Ophthalmol Vis Sci. 2003;44:875–8.
22. Gilmore G, Wenk HE, Naylor LA, Koss E. Motion perception and Alzheimer's disease. J Gerontol. 1994;49:P52–7.
23. Rizzo M, Nawrot M. Perception of movement and shape in Alzheimer's disease. Brain. 1998;121:2259–70.
24. Wijk H, Berg S, Sivik L, Steen B. Colour discrimination, colour naming and colour preferences among individuals with Alzheimer's disease. Int J Geriatr Psychiatry. 1999;14:1000–5.
25. Wijk H, Berg S, Bergman B, Hanson AB, Sivik L, Steen B. Colour perception among the very elderly related to visual and cognitive function. Scand J Caring Sci. 2002;16:91–102.
26. Salamone G, Di L, Mosti S, Lupo F, Cravello L, Palmer K, Musicco M, Caltagirone C. Color discrimination performance in patients with Alzheimer's disease. Dement Geriatr Cogn Disord. 2009;27:501–7.
27. Sadun A, Bassi CJ. Optic nerve damage in Alzheimer's disease. Ophthalmology. 1990;97:9–17.
28. Liu S, Ong Y-T, Hilal S, Loke YM, Wong TY, Chen CL-H, Cheung CY, Zhou J. The association between retinal neuronal layer and brain structure is disrupted in patients with cognitive impairment and Alzheimer's disease. J Alzheimers Dis. 2016;54:585–95.
29. Coppola G, Di Renzo A, Ziccardi L, Martelli F, Fadda A, Manni G, Barboni P, Pierelli F, Sadun AA, Parisi V. Optical coherence tomography in Alzheimer's disease: a meta-analysis. PLoS One. https://doi.org/10.1371/journal.pone.0134750.
30. Huang D, Swanson EA, Lin CP, et al. Optical coherence tomography. Science (New York, NY). 1991;254:1178–81.
31. Puliafito C, Hee MR, Lin CP, Reichel E, Schuman JS, Duker JS, Izatt JA, Swanson EA, Fujimoto JG. Imaging of macular diseases with optical coherence tomography. Ophthalmology. 1995;102:217–29.
32. Yaqoob Z, Wu J, Yang C. Spectral domain optical coherence tomography: a better OCT imaging strategy. BioTechniques. 2005;39:S6–13.
33. Kiernan D, Mieler WF, Hariprasad SM. Spectral-domain optical coherence tomography: a comparison of modern high-resolution retinal imaging systems. Am J Ophthalmol. 2010;149:18–31.
34. Schuman JS, Hee MR, Puliafito CA, Wong C, Pedut-Kloizman T, Lin CP, Hertzmark E, Izatt JA, Swanson EA, Fujimoto JG. Quantification of nerve fiber layer thickness in normal and glaucomatous eyes using optical coherence tomography. Arch Ophthalmol. 1995;113:586–96.
35. Parisi V, Manni G, Gandolfi SA, Centofanti M, Colacino G, Bucci MG. Visual function correlates with nerve fiber layer thickness in eyes affected by ocular hypertension. Invest Ophthalmol Vis Sci. 1999;40:1828–33.
36. Parisi V, Manni G, Spadaro M, Colacino G, Restuccia R, Marchi S, Bucci MG, Pierelli F. Correlation between morphological and functional retinal impairment in multiple sclerosis patients. Invest Ophthalmol Vis Sci. 1999;40:2520–7.
37. Parisi V, Manni G, Centofanti M, Gandolfi SA, Olzi D, Bucci MG. Correlation between optical coherence tomography, pattern electroretinogram, and visual evoked potentials in open-angle glaucoma patients. Ophthalmology. 2001;108:905–12.
38. Kardon RH. Role of the macular optical coherence tomography scan in neuro-ophthalmology. J Neuroophthalmol. 2011;31:353–61.
39. Sung K, Wollstein G, Bilonick RA, Townsend KA, Ishikawa H, Kagemann L, Noecker RJ, Fujimoto JG, Schuman JS. Effects of age on optical coherence tomography measurements of healthy retinal nerve fiber layer, macula, and optic nerve head. Ophthalmology. 2009;116:1119–24.
40. Mwanza J, Durbin MK, Budenz DL, Girkin CA, Leung CK, Liebmann JM, Peace JH, Werner JS, Wollstein G. Profile and predictors of normal ganglion cell-inner plexiform layer thickness

measured with frequency-domain optical coherence tomography. Invest Ophthalmol Vis Sci. 2011;52:7872–9.
41. Girkin C, McGwin G, Sinai MJ, et al. Variation in optic nerve and macular structure with age and race with spectral-domain optical coherence tomography. Ophthalmology. 2011;118:2403–8.
42. Alasil T, Wang K, Keane PA, Lee H, Baniasadi N, de Boer JF, Chen TC. Analysis of normal retinal nerve fiber layer thickness by age, sex, and race using spectral domain optical coherence tomography. J Glaucoma. 2013;22:532–41.
43. Parikh R, Parikh SR, Sekhar GC, Prabakaran S, Babu JG, Thomas R. Normal age-related decay of retinal nerve fiber layer thickness. Ophthalmology. 2007;114:921–6.
44. Feuer W, Budenz DL, Anderson DR, Cantor L, Greenfield DS, Savell J, Schuman JS, Varma R. Topographic differences in the age-related changes in the retinal nerve fiber layer of normal eyes measured by Stratus optical coherence tomography. J Glaucoma. 2011;20:133–8.
45. Lee J, Hwang YH, Lee SM, Kim YY. Age and retinal nerve fiber layer thickness measured by spectral domain optical coherence tomography. Korean J Ophthalmol. 2012;26:163–8.
46. Hardy J, Allsop D. Amyloid deposition as the central event in the aetiology of Alzheimer's disease. Trends Pharmacol Sci. 1991;12:383–8.
47. Braidy N, Muñoz P, Palacios AG, Castellano-Gonzalez G, Inestrosa NC, Chung RS, Sachdev P, Guillemin GJ. Recent rodent models for Alzheimer's disease: clinical implications and basic research. J Neural Transm. 2012;119:173–95.
48. Ning A, Cui J, To E, Ashe KH, Matsubara J. Amyloid-beta deposits lead to retinal degeneration in a mouse model of Alzheimer disease. Invest Ophthalmol Vis Sci. 2008;49:5136–43.
49. Perez S, Lumayag S, Kovacs B, Mufson EJ, Xu S. Beta-amyloid deposition and functional impairment in the retina of the APPswe/PS1DeltaE9 transgenic mouse model of Alzheimer's disease. Invest Ophthalmol Vis Sci. 2009;50:793–800.
50. Koronyo-Hamaoui M, Koronyo Y, Ljubimov AV, Miller CA, Ko MK, Black KL, Schwartz M, Farkas DL. Identification of amyloid plaques in retinas from Alzheimer's patients and noninvasive in vivo optical imaging of retinal plaques in a mouse model. NeuroImage. 2011;1:S204–17.
51. Koronyo Y, Salumbides BC, Black KL, Koronyo-Hamaoui M. Alzheimer's disease in the retina: imaging retinal Aß plaques for early diagnosis and therapy assessment. Neurodegener Dis. 2012;10:285–93.
52. Liu B, Rasool S, Yang Z, Glabe CG, Schreiber SS, Ge J, Tan Z. Amyloid-peptide vaccinations reduce {beta}-amyloid plaques but exacerbate vascular deposition and inflammation in the retina of Alzheimer's transgenic mice. Am J Pathol. 2009;175:2099–110.
53. Cordeiro M, Guo L, Coxon KM, et al. Imaging multiple phases of neurodegeneration: a novel approach to assessing cell death in vivo. Cell Death Dis. 2010;1:10.
54. Cohen R, Rezai-Zadeh K, Weitz TM, et al. A transgenic Alzheimer rat with plaques, tau pathology, behavioral impairment, oligomeric aβ, and frank neuronal loss. J Neurosci. 2013;33:6245–56.
55. Tsai Y, Lu B, Ljubimov AV, Girman S, Ross-Cisneros FN, Sadun AA, Svendsen CN, Cohen RM, Wang S. Ocular changes in TgF344-AD rat model of Alzheimer's disease. Invest Ophthalmol Vis Sci. 2014;55:523–34.
56. Andorfer C, Acker CM, Kress Y, Hof PR, Duff K, Davies P. Cell-cycle reentry and cell death in transgenic mice expressing nonmutant human tau isoforms. J Neurosci. 2005;25:5446–54.
57. Rodriguez L, Mdzomba JB, Joly S, Boudreau-Laprise M, Planel E, Pernet V. Human tau expression does not induce mouse retina neurodegeneration, suggesting differential toxicity of tau in brain vs. retinal neurons. Front Mol Neurosci. 2018;11:293.
58. Curcio C, Drucker DN. Retinal ganglion cells in Alzheimer's disease and aging. Ann Neurol. 1993;33:248–57.
59. Davies D, McCoubrie P, McDonald B, Jobst KA. Myelinated axon number in the optic nerve is unaffected by Alzheimer's disease. Br J Ophthalmol. 1995;79:596–600.
60. Blanks J, Torigoe Y, Hinton DR. Blanks RH retinal pathology in Alzheimer's disease. I. Ganglion cell loss in foveal/parafoveal retina. Neurobiol Aging. 1996;17:377–84.

61. Blanks JC, Schmidt SY, Torigoe Y, Porrello KV, Hinton DR. Blanks RHI retinal pathology in Alzheimer's disease. II. Regional neuron loss and glial changes in GCL. Neurobiol Aging. 1996;17:385–95.
62. Blanks J, Hinton DR, Sadun AA, Miller CA. Retinal ganglion cell degeneration in Alzheimer's disease. Brain Res. 1989;501:364–72.
63. Schön C, Hoffmann NA, Ochs SM, et al. Long-term in vivo imaging of fibrillar tau in the retina of P301S transgenic mice. PLoS One. 2012;7:10.
64. Hedges TR, Perez G, Speigelman D, Barbas NR, Peli E, Yardley CJ. Retinal nerve fiber layer abnormalities in Alzheimer's disease. Acta Ophthalmol Scand. 1996;74:271–5.
65. Tsai C, Ritch R, Schwartz B, Lee SS, Miller NR, Chi T, Hsieh FY. Optic nerve head and nerve fiber layer in Alzheimer's disease. Arch Ophthalmol. 1991;109:199–204.
66. Lu Y, Li Z, Zhang X, Ming B, Jia J, Wang R, Ma D. Retinal nerve fiber layer structure abnormalities in early Alzheimer's disease: evidence in optical coherence tomography. Neurosci Lett. 2010;480:69–72.
67. Balazsi AG, Rootman J, Drance SM, Schulzer M, Douglas GR. The effect of age on the nerve fiber population of the human optic nerve. Am J Ophthalmol. 1984;97:760–6.
68. Fortune B, Reynaud J, Cull G, Burgoyne CF, Wang L. The effect of age on optic nerve axon counts, SDOCT scan quality, and peripapillary retinal nerve fiber layer thickness measurements in rhesus monkeys. Transl Vis Sci Technol. 2014;3:2.
69. Johnson BM, Miao M, Sadun AA. Age-related decline of human optic nerve axon populations. Age (Omaha). 1987;10:5–9.
70. Repka M, Quigley HA. The effect of age on normal human optic nerve fiber number and diameter. Ophthalmology. 1989;96:26–32.
71. Sadun AA. Discussion of the effect of age on normal human optic nerve fiber number and diameter. Ophthalmology. 1989;96:31–2.
72. Bowd C, Zangwill LM, Blumenthal EZ, Vasile C, Boehm AG, Gokhale PA, Mohammadi K, Amini P, Sankary TM, Weinreb RN. Imaging of the optic disc and retinal nerve fiber layer: the effects of age, optic disc area, refractive error, and gender. J Opt Soc Am Opt Image Sci Vision. 2002;19:197–207.
73. Leung C, Yu M, Weinreb RN, Ye C, Liu S, Lai G, Lam DS. Retinal nerve fiber layer imaging with spectral-domain optical coherence tomography: a prospective analysis of age-related loss. Ophthalmology. 2012;119:731–7.
74. Celebi A, Mirza GE. Age-related change in retinal nerve fiber layer thickness measured with spectral domain optical coherence tomography. Invest Ophthalmol Vis Sci. 2013;54:8095–103.
75. Parisi V, Restuccia R, Fattapposta F, Mina C, Bucci MG, Pierelli F. Morphological and functional retinal impairment in Alzheimer's disease patients. Clin Neurophysiol. 2001;112:1860–7.
76. Parisi V. Correlation between morphological and functional retinal impairment in patients affected by ocular hypertension, glaucoma, demyelinating optic neuritis and Alzheimer's disease. Semin Ophthalmol. 2003;18:50–7.
77. Garcia-Martin E, Bambo MP, Marques ML, Satue M, Otin S, Larrosa JM, Polo V, Pablo LE. Ganglion cell layer measurements correlate with disease severity in patients with Alzheimer's disease. Acta Ophthalmol. 2016;94:e454–9.
78. Cesareo M, Martucci A, Ciuffoletti E, Mancino R, Cerulli A, Sorge RP, Martorana A, Sancesario G, Nucci C. Association between Alzheimer's disease and glaucoma: a study based on Heidelberg retinal tomography and frequency doubling technology perimetry. Front Neurosci. 2015;9:479.
79. Cunha LP, Lopes LC, Costa-Cunha LVF, Costa CF, Pires LA, Almeida ALM, MLR M. Macular thickness measurements with frequency domain-OCT for quantification of retinal neural loss and its correlation with cognitive impairment in Alzheimer's disease. PLoS One. 2016;11:e0153830.
80. Cunha JP, Proença R, Dias-Santos A, Almeida R, Águas H, Alves M, Papoila AL, Louro C, Castanheira-Dinis A. OCT in Alzheimer's disease: thinning of the RNFL and superior hemiretina. Graefes Arch Clin Exp Ophthalmol. 2017;255:1827–35.

81. Ferrari L, Huang S-C, Magnani G, Ambrosi A, Comi G, Leocani L. Optical coherence tomography reveals retinal neuroaxonal thinning in frontotemporal dementia as in Alzheimer's disease. J Alzheimers Dis. 2017;56:1101–7.
82. Paquet C, Boissonnot M, Roger F, Dighiero P, Gil R, Hugon J. Abnormal retinal thickness in patients with mild cognitive impairment and Alzheimer's disease. Neurosci Lett. 2007;420:97–9.
83. Kirbas S, Turkyilmaz K, Anlar O, Tufekci A, Durmus M. Retinal nerve fiber layer thickness in patients with Alzheimer disease. J Neuroophthalmol. 2013;33:58–61.
84. Marziani E, Pomati S, Ramolfo P, Cigada M, Giani A, Mariani C, Staurenghi G. Evaluation of retinal nerve fiber layer and ganglion cell layer thickness in Alzheimer's disease using spectral-domain optical coherence tomography. Invest Ophthalmol Vis Sci. 2013;54:5953–8.
85. Larrosa J, Garcia-Martin E, Bambo MP, Pinilla J, Polo V, Otin S, Satue M, Herrero R, Pablo LE. Potential new diagnostic tool for Alzheimer's disease using a linear discriminant function for Fourier domain optical coherence tomography. Invest Ophthalmol Vis Sci. 2014;55:3043–51.
86. Ascaso F, Cruz N, Modrego PJ, Lopez-Anton R, Santabárbara J, Pascual LF, Lobo A, Cristóbal JA. Retinal alterations in mild cognitive impairment and Alzheimer's disease: an optical coherence tomography study. J Neurol. 2014;261:1522–30.
87. Cheung C, Ong Y, Hilal S, et al. Retinal ganglion cell analysis using high-definition optical coherence tomography in patients with mild cognitive impairment and Alzheimer's disease. J Alzheimers Dis. 2015;45:45–56.
88. Gao L, Liu Y, Li X, Bai Q, Liu P. Abnormal retinal nerve fiber layer thickness and macula lutea in patients with mild cognitive impairment and Alzheimer's disease. Arch Gerontol Geriatr. 2015;60:162–7.
89. Oktem EO, Derle E, Kibaroglu S, Oktem C, Akkoyun I, Can U. The relationship between the degree of cognitive impairment and retinal nerve fiber layer thickness. Neurol Sci. 2015;36:1141–6.
90. Kesler A, Vakhapova V, Korczyn AD, Naftaliev E, Neudorfer M. Retinal thickness in patients with mild cognitive impairment and Alzheimer's disease. Clin Neurol Neurosurg. 2011;113:523–6.
91. Iseri P, Altinaş O, Tokay T, Yüksel N. Relationship between cognitive impairment and retinal morphological and visual functional abnormalities in Alzheimer disease. J Neuroophthalmol. 2006;26:18–24.
92. Kwon JY, Yang JH, Han JS, Kim DG. Analysis of the retinal nerve fiber layer thickness in Alzheimer disease and mild cognitive impairment. Korean J Ophthalmol. 2017;31:548.
93. Feke GT, Hyman BT, Stern RA, Pasquale LR. Retinal blood flow in mild cognitive impairment and Alzheimer's disease. Alzheimer's Dement (Amsterdam, Netherlands). 2015;1:144–51.
94. Pillai JA, Bermel R, Bonner-Jackson A, Rae-Grant A, Fernandez H, Bena J, Jones SE, Ehlers JP, Leverenz JB. Retinal nerve fiber layer thinning in Alzheimer's disease. Am J Alzheimers Dis Other Dement. 2016;31:430–6.
95. Trebbastoni A, D'Antonio F, Bruscolini A, Marcelli M, Cecere M, Campanelli A, Imbriano L, de Lena C, Gharbiya M. Retinal nerve fibre layer thickness changes in Alzheimer's disease: results from a 12-month prospective case series. Neurosci Lett. 2016;629:165–70.
96. Golzan SM, Goozee K, Georgevsky D, et al. Retinal vascular and structural changes are associated with amyloid burden in the elderly: ophthalmic biomarkers of preclinical Alzheimer's disease. Alzheimers Res Ther. 2017;9:13.
97. Danesh-Meyer H, Birch H, Ku JY, Carroll S, Gamble G. Reduction of optic nerve fibers in patients with Alzheimer disease identified by laser imaging. Neurology. 2006;67:1852–4.
98. Kergoat H, Kergoat MJ, Justino L, Chertkow H, Robillard A, Bergman H. An evaluation of the retinal nerve fiber layer thickness by scanning laser polarimetry in individuals with dementia of the Alzheimer type. Acta Ophthalmol Scand. 2001;79:187–91.
99. Kurna SA, Akar G, Altun A, Agirman Y, Gozke E, Sengor T. Confocal scanning laser tomography of the optic nerve head on the patients with Alzheimer's disease compared to glaucoma and control. Int Ophthalmol. 2014;34:1203–11.

100. Csincsik L, MacGillivray TJ, Flynn E, et al. Peripheral retinal imaging biomarkers for Alzheimer's disease: a pilot study. Ophthalmic Res. 2018;59:182–92.
101. Berisha F, Feke GT, Trempe CL, McMeel JW, Schepens CL. Retinal abnormalities in early Alzheimer's disease. Invest Ophthalmol Vis Sci. 2007;48:2285–9.
102. Jellinger KA. Alzheimer disease and cerebrovascular pathology: an update. J Neural Transm. 2002;109:813–36.
103. Snyder PJ, Johnson LN, Lim YY, Santos CY, Alber J, Maruff P, Fernández B. Nonvascular retinal imaging markers of preclinical Alzheimer's disease. Alzheimers Dement. 2016;4:169–78.
104. Santos CY, Johnson LN, Sinoff SE, Festa EK, Heindel WC, Snyder PJ. Change in retinal structural anatomy during the preclinical stage of Alzheimer's disease. Alzheimers Dement. 2018;10:196–209.
105. Moreno-Ramos T, Benito-León J, Villarejo A, Bermejo-Pareja F. Retinal nerve fiber layer thinning in dementia associated with Parkinson's disease, dementia with Lewy bodies, and Alzheimer's disease. J Alzheimers Dis. 2013;34:659–64.
106. Parisi V, Pierelli F, Coppola G, Restuccia R, Ferrazzoli D, Scassa C, Bianco F, Parisi L, Fattapposta F. Reduction of optic nerve fiber layer thickness in CADASIL. Eur J Neurol. 2007;14:627–31.
107. Katz B, Rimmer S, Iragui V, Katzman R. Abnormal pattern electroretinogram in Alzheimer's disease: evidence for retinal ganglion cell degeneration? Ann Neurol. 1989;26:221–5.
108. Trick G, Barris MC, Bickler-Bluth M. Abnormal pattern electroretinograms in patients with senile dementia of the Alzheimer type. Ann Neurol. 1989;26:226–31.
109. Krasodomska K, Lubiński W, Potemkowski A, Honczarenko K. Pattern electroretinogram (PERG) and pattern visual evoked potential (PVEP) in the early stages of Alzheimer's disease. Doc Ophthalmol. 2010;121:111–21.
110. Sartucci F, Borghetti D, Bocci T, Murri L, Orsini P, Porciatti V, Origlia N, Domenici L. Dysfunction of the magnocellular stream in Alzheimer's disease evaluated by pattern electroretinograms and visual evoked potentials. Brain Res Bull. 2010;82:169–76.
111. Strenn K, Dal-Bianco P, Weghaupt H, Koch G, Vass C, Gottlob I. Pattern electroretinogram and luminance electroretinogram in Alzheimer's disease. J Neural Transm. 1991;33:73–80.
112. Kergoat H, Kergoat MJ, Justino L, Chertkow H, Robillard A, Bergman H. Visual retinocortical function in dementia of the Alzheimer type. Gerontology. 2002;48:197–203.
113. Philpot M, Amin D, Levy R. Visual evoked potentials in Alzheimer's disease: correlations with age and severity. Electroencephalogr Clin Neurophysiol. 1990;77:323–9.
114. Justino L, Kergoat M, Bergman H, Chertkow H, Robillard A, Kergoat H. Neuroretinal function is normal in early dementia of the Alzheimer type. Neurobiol Aging. 2001;22:691–5.
115. Pollock V, Schneider LS, Chui HC, Henderson V, Zemansky M, Sloane RB. Visual evoked potentials in dementia: a meta-analysis and empirical study of Alzheimer's disease patients. Biol Psychiatry. 1989;25:1003–13.
116. Partanen J, Hartikainen P, Könönen M, Jousmäki V, Soininen H, Riekkinen P. Prolonged latencies of pattern reversal visual evoked early potentials in Alzheimer disease. Alzheimer Dis Assoc Disord. 1994;8:250–8.
117. Coburn K, Ashford JW, Moreno MA. Visual evoked potentials in dementia: selective delay of flash P2 in probable Alzheimer's disease. J Neuropsychiatry Clin Neurosci. 1991;3:431–5.
118. Moore N, Tucker KA, Jann MW, Hostetler RM, Coburn KL. Flash P2 delay in primary degenerative dementia of the Alzheimer type. Prog Neuro-Psychopharmacol Biol Psychiatry. 1995;19:403–10.
119. Kromer R, Serbecic N, Hausner L, Froelich L, Beutelspacher S. Comparison of visual evoked potentials and retinal nerve fiber layer thickness in Alzheimer's disease. Front Neurol. 2013;4:203.
120. Kromer R, Serbecic N, Hausner L, Froelich L, Aboul-Enein F, Beutelspacher S. Detection of retinal nerve fiber layer defects in Alzheimer's disease using SD-OCT. Front Psych. 2014;5:22.

121. Choi SH, Park SJ, Kim NR. Macular ganglion cell-inner plexiform layer thickness is associated with clinical progression in mild cognitive impairment and Alzheimers disease. PLoS One. 2016;11:e0162202.
122. Shen Y, Shi Z, Jia R, Zhu Y, Cheng Y, Feng W, Li C. The attenuation of retinal nerve fiber layer thickness and cognitive deterioration. Front Cell Neurosci. 2013;7:142.
123. Shen Y, Liu L, Cheng Y, Feng W, Shi Z, Zhu Y, Wu W, Li C. Retinal nerve fiber layer thickness is associated with episodic memory deficit in mild cognitive impairment patients. Curr Alzheimer Res. 2014;11:259–66.
124. Shi Z, Wu Y, Wang M, Cao J, Feng W, Cheng Y, Li C, Shen Y. Greater attenuation of retinal nerve fiber layer thickness in Alzheimer's disease patients. J Alzheimers Dis. 2014;40:277–83.
125. Yu J, Feng Y, Xiang Y, Huang J, Savini G, Parisi V, Yang W, Fu X. Retinal nerve fiber layer thickness changes in Parkinson disease: a meta-analysis. PLoS One. 2014;9:10.
126. Janssen S, Gorgels TG, Ramdas WD, Klaver CC, van Duijn CM, Jansonius NM, Bergen AA. The vast complexity of primary open angle glaucoma: disease genes, risks, molecular mechanisms and pathobiology. Prog Retin Eye Res. 2013;37:31–67.
127. Ghiso JA, Doudevski I, Ritch R, Rostagno AA. Alzheimer's disease and glaucoma: mechanistic similarities and differences. J Glaucoma. 2013;22(Suppl 5):S36–8.
128. Tamura H, Kawakami H, Kanamoto T, Kato T, Yokoyama T, Sasaki K, Izumi Y, Matsumoto M, Mishima HK. High frequency of open-angle glaucoma in Japanese patients with Alzheimer's disease. J Neurol Sci. 2006;246:79–83.
129. Ou Y, Grossman DS, Lee PP, Sloan FA. Glaucoma, Alzheimer disease and other dementia: a longitudinal analysis. Ophthalmic Epidemiol. 2012;19:285–92.
130. Nucci C, Martucci A, Cesareo M, Mancino R, Russo R, Bagetta G, Cerulli L, Garaci FG. Brain involvement in glaucoma: advanced neuroimaging for understanding and monitoring a new target for therapy. Curr Opin Pharmacol. 2013;13:128–33.
131. Nucci C, Martucci A, Cesareo M, Garaci F, Morrone LA, Russo R, Corasaniti MT, Bagetta G, Mancino R. Links among glaucoma, neurodegenerative, and vascular diseases of the central nervous system. Prog Brain Res. 2015;221:49–65.

Friedreich's Ataxia and More: Optical Coherence Tomography Findings in Rare Neurological Syndromes

14

Chiara La Morgia and Michele Carbonelli

14.1 Friedreich's Ataxia

Friedreich's ataxia (FA) is an autosomal recessive slowly progressive neurodegenerative disorder starting usually in young adulthood or childhood [1]. FA is characterized by spinocerebellar and sensory ataxia with absence of deep tendon reflexes, dysarthria, hypertrophic cardiomyopathy and scoliosis [2]. FA is due to a GAA triplet expansion in the first intron of the frataxin gene (FXN) on chromosome 9q13-q21.1. A minority of FRDA patients are compound heterozygotes for the GAA triplet expansion and a point mutation [3].

Frataxin is a mitochondrial protein with a crucial role in the insertion of Fe-S cluster in different enzymes of the mitochondrial respiratory chain and in particular complex I, II and III and aconitase [4, 5]. The abnormal function of FXN leads to dysregulation of cellular iron metabolism with mitochondrial accumulation [6]. Evidence of mitochondrial defective respiration has been demonstrated in the heart and muscle of FA patients [7, 8]. Recent studies demonstrated that mitochondrial dysfunction induced by frataxin is also related to abnormal calcium handling in the mitochondria leading to increased autophagy [9]. Overall, frataxin deficiency leads to abnormal iron homeostasis [10] and increased oxidative stress [11, 12].

C. La Morgia (✉)
UOC Clinica Neurologica, IRCCS Istituto delle Scienze Neurologiche di Bologna, Bologna, Italy

Dipartimento di Scienze Biomediche e Neuromotorie, Università di Bologna, Bologna, Italy
e-mail: chiara.lamorgia@unibo.it

M. Carbonelli
UOC Clinica Neurologica, IRCCS Istituto delle Scienze Neurologiche di Bologna, Bologna, Italy

A. Grzybowski, P. Barboni (eds.), *OCT and Imaging in Central Nervous System Diseases*, https://doi.org/10.1007/978-3-030-26269-3_14

Visual system involvement is well characterized in FA [13]. In particular, abnormalities of the visual efferent system such as fixation instability (square wave jerks), saccadic dysmetria, disrupted pursuit, and vestibular abnormalities have been reported [13]. Moreover, optic neuropathy, optic radiation abnormalities and retinitis pigmentosa have been described in FA patients [14–19].

The optic neuropathy described in FA is usually asymptomatic and does not affect central vision [16]. The most severe visual phenotype has been associated with large GAA expansion of the FTX gene and with compound heterozygous mutations [16]. Visual evoked potentials demonstrated delayed latency and reduced amplitude of the cortical responses [15, 16]. Visual field defects may vary from small paracentral or arcuate to diffuse and generalized defects [16]. Only rarely FA patients present an acute loss of visual acuity, which resembles Leber's hereditary optic neuropathy (LHON) [16].

A few optical coherence tomography (OCT) studies are available for FA. These described a diffuse reduction of the retinal nerve fiber layer (RNFL) thickness without a preferential involvement of the temporal quadrant [16–19], unlike mitochondrial optic neuropathies [20]. The severity of optic atrophy can be variable and usually is not associated with a subjective visual complaint [15, 16]. Specifically, time-domain OCT studies reported a generalized RNFL thinning in FA patients [16–18]. Interestingly, in the largest OCT series (63 FA patients) available to now, the only sector with a significant RNFL thinning was the superior [18] (Table 14.1).

Retinal nerve fiber layer thinning significantly correlated with age at onset and International Cooperative Ataxia Rating Scale (ICARS) in the series (n = 26) by Fortuna and coauthors [16]; with ICARS score, disease duration, visual acuity (VA) and low-contrast letter VA in the series (n = 23) by Noval and coauthors [17] and with VA, GAA repeat length, Friedreich's Ataxia Rating Scale (FARS) and age at onset in the series (n = 63) by Seyer and coauthors [18] (Table 14.1).

The only spectral domain (SD) OCT study available to date documented a reduction of the average RNFL thickness and in all four optic disc sectors in 10 FA patients [19]. Moreover, ganglion cell thickness was significantly reduced in superior and inferior macula [19] (Table 14.1).

Macular thickness has been reported as normal in one study [17], significantly reduced [19] and below the 1st percentile of controls in 20.7% of the FA patients examined in another series [18] (Table 14.1).

Correlation of OCT measurement with VA is not consistent across the studies and the degree of VA loss is reported as variable, but usually not clinically significant [16, 17]. Differently, low contrast visual acuity is significantly reduced in FA

Table 14.1 OCT findings in Friedreich's ataxia

	OCT	N. of pts	Main findings	Correlations
Fortuna et al. [16]	TD-Stratus	26	↓ avg RNFL ↓ RNFL in all 4 sectors	ICARS, age at onset
Noval et a. [17]	TD-Stratus	17	↓ avg RNFL in 75% Temporal RNFL thickness normal Normal Macular morphology and thickness	ICARS, disease duration, VA, low-contrast VA
Seyer et al. [18]	TD-Stratus	63	↓ RNFL (52.7% of eyes below 5th percentile of controls) Only superior thickness significantly lower	VA, GAA expansion, age at onset, FARS
Seyer et al. [18]	SD-Cirrus	23	Macular thickness below the 1st percentile of controls in 20.7%	Not significant
Dağ et al. [19]	SD	10	↓ avg RNFL ↓ RNFL in all 4 quadrants ↓ Peripapillary and foveal retinal thickness Choroidal thickness not significant ↓ GC thickness in superior and inferior macula	VA, ICARS (RNFL thickness) Disease duration (foveal thickness)

RNFL retinal nerve fiber layer, *avg* average, *ICARS* International Cooperative Ataxia Rating Scale, *FARS* Friedreich's Ataxia Rating Scale, *VA* visual acuity

patients [17]. Fundus oculi abnormalities are detected only in a small percentage of the FA subjects with loss of retinal nerve fibers documented by OCT [17].

Overall, OCT measurements in FA are able to detect subclinical optic neuropathy in the large majority of FA cases (about 70%) being a more sensible measure of optic nerve degeneration than other metrics (visual acuity, visual fields and/or fundus examination). It is not clear yet why the papillomacular bundle is not primarily affected in FA, even if a mitochondrial dysfunction is well known in FA.

In line with OCT data, visual evoked potentials (VEPs) documented an increased P100 latency and reduced amplitude of cortical responses [15, 16] in the large majority of patients. These electrophysiological and anatomical data suggest a slowly progressive degeneration of the anterior and posterior optic pathway, as proved also by the increased diffusion in optic radiations demonstrated in FA patients by magnetic resonance imaging studies [16].

Examples of swept-source OCT images and fundus oculi pictures are provided for two FA patients presenting, respectively a mild and severe optic atrophy (Fig. 14.1).

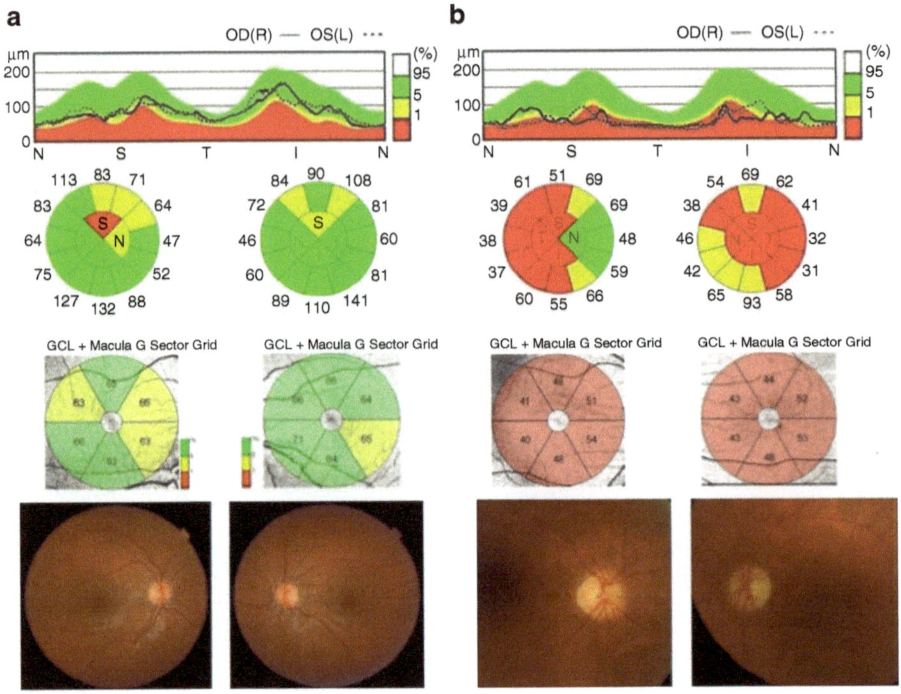

Fig. 14.1 (Friedreich) (**a**) This is a 20 year-old female who suffered ataxic gait since she was 15 years. She does not complain specific visual disturbances. Her visual acuity is 12/10 bilaterally and visual fields showed a small nasal step in the RE and a small superior defect in the LE. OCT shows a mild superior RNFL thinning and a small GCC defect. Fundus oculi showed mild temporal pallor bilaterally. (**b**) This is a 43 year-old female who presented gait ataxia since she was 13 years old. She started complaining visual loss since she was 38 years and her visual acuity progressively worsened over time. Her visual acuity is now 1.6/10 in the RE and 0.5/10 in the LE. Visual fields showed generalized defect with relative central sparing bilaterally. OCT shows generalized RNFL thinning with relative nasal sparing and diffuse GCC loss. Fundus oculi showed diffuse pallor more evident on the temporal sector

14.2 Jansky-Bielschowsky Disease (CLN2)

Jansky-Bielschowsky disease (JBD) is a late infantile neuronal ceroid lipofuscinosis (LINCL) disorder due to mutation of the *CLN2* gene (cr 11p15), which encodes for the tripetidylpeptidase 1 protein [21, 22]. Similarly to other Neuronal Ceroid Lipofuscinosis (NCL) JBD is a lysosomal storage disease characterized by the accumulation of autofluorescent material in the cytoplasm of neurons [23]. JBD disease is characterized by mental and motor retardation, psychomotor regression, ataxia, seizures and visual dysfunction [23].

Visual dysfunction is common in NCL and usually manifests early in juvenile forms and later in the LINCL [24]. The typical ocular manifestation of NCL is retinal degeneration of variable severity (from mild pigmentary changes to Bull's eye maculopathy to severe outer retina atrophy) [24]. Retinal changes in LINCL have been documented by fundus oculi examination, histopathology and electrophysiological studies [24–27]. Furthermore, the presence of inner retina and optic nerve degeneration has been demonstrated in different animal models of NCL [28–31]. Besides outer retina degeneration, optic atrophy is a frequent finding in LINCL [25, 32]. The only OCT study available to now in JBD applied a comprehensive ophthalmologic evaluation in 25 LINCL patients with mutations in the *CLN2* gene [33]. The protocol included fundus oculi, spectral domain macula OCT, fluorangiography (FA) and indocyanine green angiography (IGA) and was carried out under anesthesia. The results obtained were used to generate a Weill Cornell LINCL Ophthalmologic Severity Scale score. According to the degree of pigmentary changes at fundus oculi examination, FA and IGA and the severity of outer retina degeneration documented by OCT the patients were graded as score 0–5 (from normal to severe changes). The average score in this case series was 2.6. This score correlated strongly with the neurological score suggesting that the retinal involvement is parallel to the neurological deterioration. Interestingly, the authors failed to document any abnormality in the anterior segment, at difference with other lysosomal storage diseases. The posterior segment showed variable degrees of optic nerve and retinal atrophy. In particular, retinal degeneration typically starts from the fovea in which the first pigmentary changes are visible expanding to the far periphery [33]. The OCT was able, in this case series, to detect subtle abnormalities not visible at fundus examination or with FA. The OCT changes documented by Orlin and coauthors for the 5 stages were: *Stage 1*: normal; *Stage 2*: Normal retinal layers immediately adjacent at fovea; immediately outside fovea, outer retinal/photoreceptor atrophy; *Stage 3*: Outer retinal atrophy/photoreceptor loss extending to 1.0 disc diameter from fovea; retinal layers appear normal outside fovea; *Stage 4*: Early buildup of outer retinal hyper-reflective material in macula; more extensive outer retinal abnormalities extending 1.0–2.0 disc diameters from fovea; beyond 2.0 disc diameters, outer retina appears normal; *Stage 5*: Severe retinal thinning with generalized loss of photoreceptors and outer retina, involving the entire macula; extensive clumps of outer retinal hyper-reflective material; thickness map shows central thinning with paracentral thickening, with outer ring of further thinning (with bull's eye appearance); outer retinal changes also found outside the macula [33]. The majority of patients in this case series presented normal or mildly abnormal ocular findings (32% stage 0, 24% stage 1, 8% stage 3, 24% stage 4 and 12% stage 5) [33].

14.3 Juvenile Neuronal Ceroid Lipofuscinosis-Batten Disease (CLN3)

Juvenile neuronal ceroid lipofuscinosis (JNCL) is the most frequent form of the NCL disorders due to biallelic mutations in the *CLN3* gene [34]. Visual loss is usually the earliest symptom of the disease manifesting between 4 and 8 years of age. The ophthalmological features of CLN3 patients include optic nerve pallor, bull's-eye maculopathy, and intraretinal pigmentation, associated with abnormalities at electrophysiological testing. Neurological features include mental retardation, extrapyramidal symptoms and seizures.

Ku and coauthors extensively investigated the clinical phenotype of retinal degeneration in CLN3 patients [35]. In this case series OCT demonstrated in patients with preserved visual acuity and late-onset disease a focal preservation of the ellipsoid zone and outer nuclear layer in the fovea, despite the presence of macular edema. At difference, in patients with decreased visual acuity and early-onset disease, a moderate-severe foveal outer nuclear layer and ellipsoid zone loss were evident, in association in some patients with hyperreflective deposits at the level of the retinal pigment epithelium. Electroretinography showed a rod-cone pattern of dysfunction in 6 patients and were completely undetectable in 2 patients [35]. Ophthalmoscopic findings included macular edema, mild intraretinal bone spicule migration, and significant macular atrophy. Fundus autofluorescence imaging showed central retinal hypoautofluorescence.

In CLN2 the opthalmological findings include a complete retinal atrophy starting from bull's eye maculopathy and optic nerve pallor. OCT show a centripetal degeneration of the outer layers starting from the parafoveal region in the ellipsoid zone and developing into the fovea and outward to the periphery. In CLN3 patients with relatively short disease duration, Preising and coauthors [36] described by SD-OCT a general reduction of the entire retinal thickness resulting mostly from photoreceptor-associated and the inner nuclear layers (first and second neurons). At difference, the retinal nerve fiber layer (RNFL) and the ganglion cell layer (GCL+) were described as within normal thickness values, even though the presence of gliosis and irregular inner limiting membrane (ILM) suggest a degeneration of retinal ganglion cells (RGCs) constituting the optic nerve. The retinal pigmented epithelium (RPE) layer thickness is described as within normal values. This pattern is different from macular dystrophies like ABCA4-associated cone-rode dystrophy (CRD) where the first neuron layer is affected before the second neuron layer and the third neuron is preserved. The preservation of the first neuron outside the macula suggests in the youngest CLN3 case a centrifugal progression of the retinal degeneration, which corresponds to the later stages of CLN2 retinal degeneration. In the later stages of the disease, also the optic nerve is affected showing neuronal loss [37].

14.4 DNMT1 Disease

DNA (cytosine-5)-methyltransferase 1 (DNMT1) disease is a complex neurodegenerative disorder due to autosomal dominant mutations in the *DNMT1* gene (DNA-methyltransferase 1) [38].

Two distinct phenotypes have been described in association with mutations in the *DNMT1* gene: the autosomal dominant cerebellar ataxia, deafness and narcolepsy (ADCA-DN) [39] associated with mutations in exon 21 of the *DNMT1* gene and the hereditary sensory autonomic neuropathy with dementia and hearing loss type IE (HSAN IE), described in association with mutations in exon 20 [38]. Recently, our group demonstrated that the boundaries between these two distinct entities are less pronounced [40]. In fact, both diseases share the presence of narcolepsy as a prominent feature [40]. Moreover, we demonstrated that subclinical optic atrophy is a common finding to both phenotypes [40].

Visual acuity was normal in all five DNMT1 patients included in the study (two with the ADCA-DN and three with the HSAN IE phenotype). Fundus oculi disclosed temporal pallor in one ADCA-DN case, diffuse pallor in the other ADCA-DN and mild temporal pallor of the optic disc in all three HSAN IE subjects. Pattern VEPs were abnormal in both ADCA-DN probands, showing increased latency and decreased amplitude of cortical responses, whereas they were normal in HSAN IE patients [40]. OCT showed reduction of the RNFL thickness more evident in the temporal than in the superior and inferior quadrants with nasal sparing in one ADCA-DN patient, more diffuse in the other ADCA-DN patient with nasal sparing. In the HSAN IE cases OCT disclosed a diffuse reduction of retinal nerve fiber layer thickness in one case, a diffuse reduction with nasal sparing in the second case, and temporal and less evident superior/inferior quadrants thinning in the third case.

Macular ganglion cell layer (GCL) analysis disclosed diffuse atrophy in both ADCA-DN probands and diffuse thinning in all three HSAN IE subjects [40].

Examples of swept-source OCT (RNFL and macular GCL) and fundus oculi images are reported for two DNMT1 patients carrying respectively the p.Glu575Lys mutation at exon 21 and the p.Pro507Arg mutation at exon 20 [40] (Fig. 14.2).

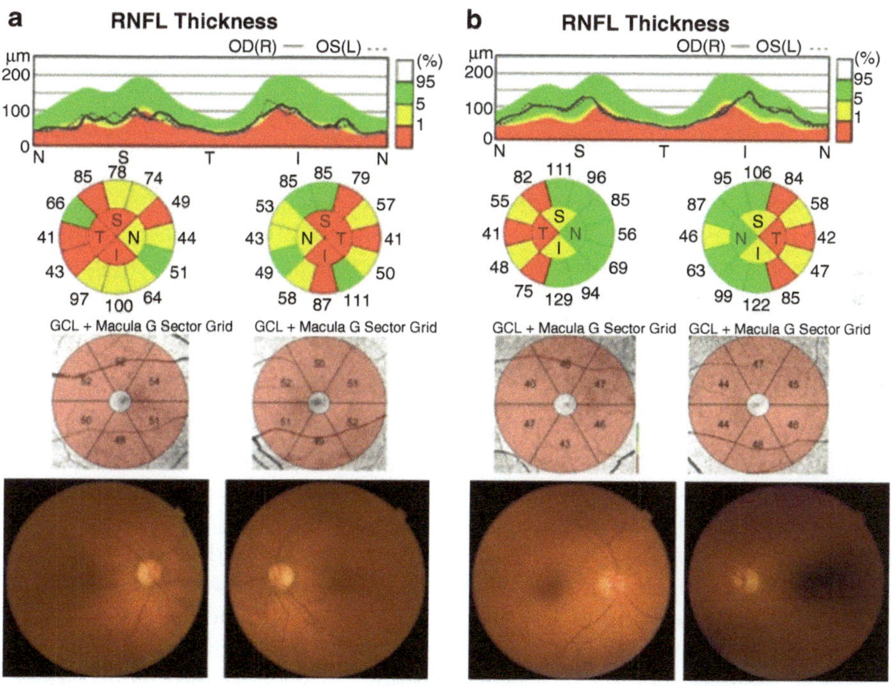

Fig. 14.2 DNMT1. (**a**) This is a 49-year old female carrying the p.Glu575Lys mutation at exon 21 in the DNMT1 gene. Visual acuity is 10/10 bilaterally. OCT shows a diffuse optic nerve fiber thinning, as demonstrated also by the diffuse GCC defect. Fundus oculi image show increased optic disc excavation and mild temporal pallor. (**b**) This is a 38-year old male carrying the p. pro-507Arg mutation at exon 20. Visual acuity is 12/10 bilaterally. OCT shows temporal RNFL thinning, as well as fundus oculi reveals a mild temporal pallor

Interestingly, optic atrophy was previously reported in the ADCA-DN phenotype [41, 42] but never described in the HSAN IE phenotype. OCT investigation in our DNMT1 case series revealed a subclinical optic nerve involvement in all cases with a prevalent involvement of the temporal sector and relative nasal sparing that resembles the pattern observed in mitochondrial optic neuropathies [20]. The mitochondrial pattern of optic nerve degeneration may be explained by the possible effect of defective methylation of nuclear DNA on nuclear encoded mitochondrial proteins [43] or a direct effect on DNA methylation of the mitochondrial-targeted isoform of DNMT1 [44, 45]. At this regard, interestingly DNMTs including DNMT1, through epigenetic regulation, may play a role in the development and homeostasis of photoreceptors and other retinal neurons within the mammalian retina [46].

14.5 Hereditary Spastic Paraplegia Due to SPG7 Mutations

Hereditary spastic paraplegias (HSP) are a heterogeneous group of neurodegenerative disorders characterized by a variable phenotypic expression, which includes a pure spastic paraparesis or "uncomplicated" and a "complicated" form. The genetic basis of HSP is heterogeneous including autosomal dominant, autosomal recessive, X-linked, or maternally inherited (mitochondrial) inheritance [47].

More than 56 HSP loci and 41HSP-related genes have been identified [47].

Mutations in the *SPG7* gene are responsible for autosomal recessive SPG7-HSP. The first *SPG7* mutation was identified in 1998 [48, 49]. *SPG7* gene encodes for paraplegin, which is a metalloprotease protein belonging to the AAA (ATPase associated with various cellular activities) proteins. Paraplegin is a mitochondrial protein localized to the inner mitochondrial membrane and it assembles with the paralogous AFG3L2 protein in the mAAA protease complex [50–53]. Mitochondrial dysfunction has been described in SPG7 pedigrees including OXPHOS defects in muscle biopsy [48]. Interestingly, mAAA protease like paraplegin plays also a role in the processing of the OPA1 protein [54]. Given the mitochondrial pathogenesis of SPG7 HSP, the presence of optic atrophy is expected, but not systematically investigated. Optic atrophy has been reported in the first identified pedigrees [48, 49, 53]. Klebe and coauthors extensively described the phenotype of 23 SPG7 families [55]. In a subgroup (n = 10) investigated by OCT, RNFL thinning was detected in 100% of cases even if it was symptomatic only in one case, associated with reduced visual acuity in 40% and with optic disc pallor at fundus examination in 50% of cases. These data suggest that the OCT investigation may detect subtle abnormalities in SPG7 patients and the presence of optic atrophy in the context of an autosomal recessive spastic paraplegia should point to the *SPG7* gene. In this case series one French pedigree positive for the *SPG7* mutation presented with an isolated autosomal dominant early onset (first decade of life) progressive optic atrophy. Electroneurography disclosed in this pedigree also the presence of mixed peripheral polyneuropathy [55].

On the basis of the clinical findings of this cohort the authors proposed that *SPG7* gene should be screened in autosomal recessive or sporadic HSP patients with middle-age onset particularly if spastic paraplegia is associated with cerebellar atrophy/signs and/or optic neuropathy (also if detected only with OCT).

Van Gassen and coauthors, in another large SPG7 Dutch case-series (n = 49), demonstrated the presence of a severe optic atrophy with childhood onset in two siblings carrying a homozygous missense mutation (p.Arg470Gln, exon 10) *SPG7* mutation and in one case with compound heterozygous (p.Arg485_Glu487 and p.Leu706fs) *SPG7* mutation. For one of the p.Arg470Gln mutation carriers, postmortem tissues including the optic nerve were available. In this case a severe optic atrophy was documented. Interestingly, the p.Arg470Gln mutation was located in the ATPase AAA core domain and the authors hypothesized that the severe optic nerve involvement can be explained by a possible deleterious interaction of SPG7 with OPA1. Unfortunately, for these patients OCT data were not available [56].

Moreover, Marcotulli and coauthors have recently described a 43-year-old male SPG7 case presenting with severe congenital optic atrophy. This patient developed spastic paraparesis at 30 years of age. OCT documented reduced RNFL and macular thickness [57].

Overall, these data suggest that optic neuropathy is a common finding in SPG7-related HSP and the use of OCT screening in large cohort of HSP patients might be a useful tool to reveal subclinical optic atrophy and guide the diagnostic process.

Interestingly, Wiethoff and coauthors conducted an OCT study on 28 HSP patients including "pure" (n = 22) and "complicated" (n = 6) HSP demonstrating a significant reduction of the RNFL only in the "complicated" group. The case series included also 3 SPG7 cases and two of them, presenting a complicated phenotype, manifested a global RNFL thickness reduction, especially in the temporal quadrant [58].

We recently had the opportunity to diagnose the presence of compound heterozygous SPG7 mutations in a 24 year-old female who presented ophthalmological features (Fig. 14.3) indistinguishable from OPA1 patients. Neurological examination was unremarkable except for the presence of optic nerve temporal pallor and specifically did not reveal any sign of spastic paraparesis. This case highlights the possibility that SPG7 mutations might be associated to pure optic atrophy cases.

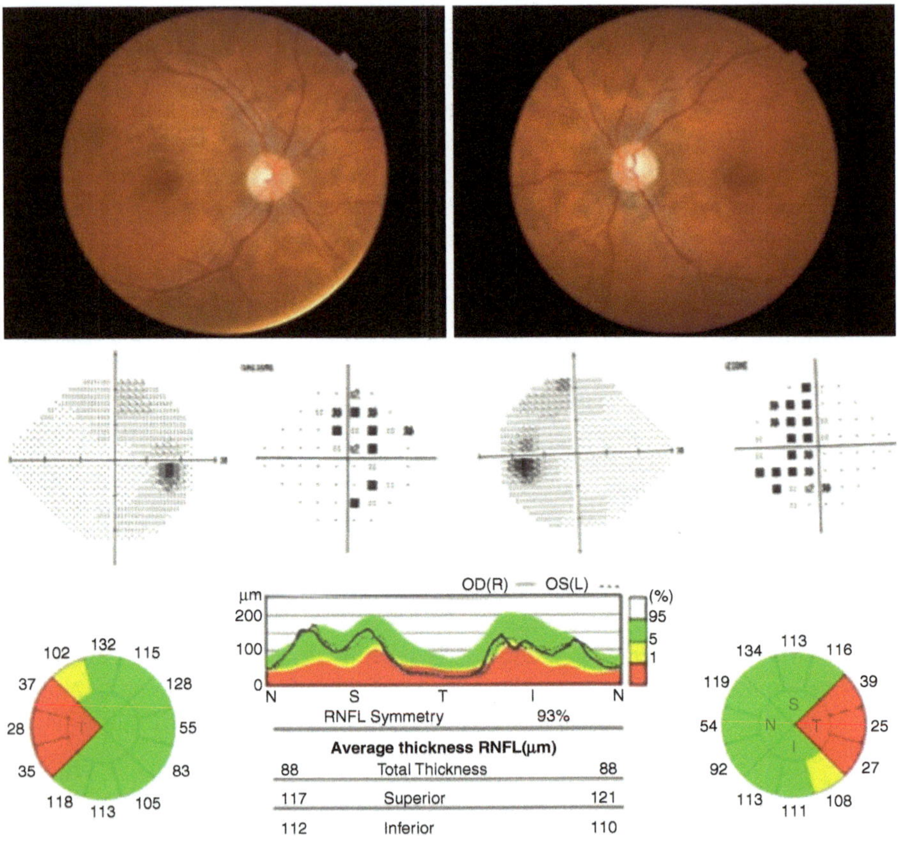

Fig. 14.3 SPG7. 24 year female carrying compund heterozygous mutations- c.524T>C (p.LI75P) + c1968_69 ins A (p.165NfsX22) in the SPG7 gene. Visual acuity is 20/32 (0.63). Fundus oculi reveals bilateral temporal optic nerve pallor. Visual fields showed small central scotoma bilaterally and OCT demonstrated temporal RNFL thinning bilaterally. Brain MRI, somatosensory and motor evoked potentials were normal. Neurological examination did not show the presence of spastic paraparesis

14.6 CADASIL

Cerebral autosomal dominant arteriopathy with subcortical infarcts and leukoencephalopathy (CADASIL) is an autosomal dominant disorder characterized by the occurrence of juvenile subcortical ischemic events, migraine, epilepsy, psychiatric disturbances and cognitive impairment in variable combinations [59]. Brain MRI typically shows T2 hyperintensity involving the white matter of the temporal pole and/or the external capsulae, but the severity of white matter involvement can be highly variable evolving into most cases to a diffuse bilateral subcortical leukoencephalopathy [60].

CADASIL is due to mutations of the *NOTCH3 (Neurogenic locus notch homolog protein 3)* gene, located on chromosome 19 [61]. Notch3 is a protein mainly expressed in vascular smooth cells with a crucial role in the control of vascular tone [62]. Cerebral vasculopathy is the main hallmark of the disease, due to the degeneration of the vascular smooth muscle cells with deposition of granular osmiophilic material, but also retinal vascular changes have been described in CADASIL [63–65]. These changes include retinal arteriolar narrowing, arteriovenous nicking and arteriolar sheating [64, 66]. Moreover, electrophysiological [67], histological [68] and OCT studies [66, 69, 70] documented a specific neurodegeneration of the neuroretina in CADASIL. In particular, Parisi and coauthors demonstrated by time-domain OCT a diffuse reduction of the RNFL thickness involving all the quadrants in 6 CADASIL patients (three asymptomatic mutation carriers) [69]. The authors interpreted these findings as secondary to the chronic vascular changes characterizing the disease. Similarly, Rufa and coauthors demonstrated with time-domain OCT a diffuse RNFL thinning in all optic nerve quadrants except the nasal one in 17 CADASIL patients. In particular, this thinning was more evident in the superior sector [70]. Fundus oculi examination revealed neuroretinal rim pallor in 41% and a crowded optic disc in 18% of the 34 CADASIL patients described by Pretegiani and coauthors [66]. The optic nerve involvement in CADASIL is also confirmed by histological findings in a postmortem study, which demonstrated diffuse demyelination in the optic nerve and chiasm with loss of nerve fibers [68]. The loss of fibers in the optic nerve is usually not associated with a reduction of the visual acuity and can be associated with variable visual field defects [66].

OCT studies are also particularly relevant for highlighting the vascular component of retinal changes in CADASIL patients. In particular, OCT-angiography studies demonstrated reduced vessel density in the deep retinal plexus (DRP) of CADASIL patients [71]. These abnormalities may reflect pericyte dysfunction in retinal capillaries secondary to NOTCH3 mutations and hypoperfusion in the DRP may cause nutritional deficiency in the synaptic connections of the retinal elements. In this case series choroidal vessels are affected in CADASIL patients [71]. These results are in line with previous OCT studies demonstrating increased wall thicknesses and outer diameters of arterial and venous retinal vessels [72]. Interestingly, retinal vessel changes may be correlated to brain MRI findings, highlighting the possible role of retinal changes as biomarker of the disease [73]. These results, pointing to a reduced retinal vessel density in CADASIL, are a confirmation of previous studies demonstrating by fractal analysis a reduced retinal vessel branching in CADASIL [74].

14.7 Wolfram Syndrome

Wolfram syndrome (WS) was first described in 1938 [75]. It is a rare neurodegenerative disorder characterized by the occurrence of diabetes mellitus and optic atrophy starting in childhood and a variable association of diabetes insipidus, other endocrinopathies, deafness, cerebellar ataxia, neurogenic bladder, cardiomyopathy and psychiatric disturbances [76]. In fact, it is also known as DIDMOAD (Diabetes Insipidus, Diabetes Mellitus, Optic Atrophy) [77, 78]. Usually diabetes is the first sign of the disease. Optic atrophy appears in the first-second decade of life and it is in most cases severe [77, 79]. Wolfram's disease is due to mutations in the wolframin gene (*WFS1*) [80] and in the large majority of cases is inherited in an autosomal recessive fashion, but autosomal dominant inheritance has also been reported [81]. In these latter cases optic atrophy can be milder [81] and can be associated with deafness without diabetes [82]. Autosomal dominant mutations in the *WFS1* gene have been associated also with non-syndromic deafness [83], diabetes [84] and cataract [85]. Neuropathological studies reported atrophy of the optic nerve, chiasm, lateral geniculate nucleus, optic tracts and occipital cortex in WS [86–90].

A few OCT studies are available for WS. In a case report, spectral domain OCT documented a diffuse optic atrophy more evident in the superior and inferior quadrants in a 21 year-old male [91]. Bucca and coauthors reported time-domain findings in a 13 year-old female showing loss of retinal nerve fibers in the temporal quadrant [92]. More recently, Grenier and coauthors reported OCT findings in a case series of 15 WS cases carrying both autosomal recessive-ar (11 cases, 8 with diabetes and 3 without diabetes) and 4 autosomal dominant-ad *WFS1* mutations with hearing loss. Using SD-OCT, the authors showed that RNFL loss was more profound in the group with syndromic ar-WS compared to the WS cases without diabetes, especially in the inferior sectors. The comparison of ar-WS cases with ad-WS cases by time-domain OCT revealed a more severe RNFL thinning in the ar-WS group in both the superior and inferior quadrants [93].

In a pediatric case series of 12 genetically confirmed WS cases, the authors reported a significant reduction in the WS cases compared with individual with type 1 diabetes and controls of OCT parameters (including average and single quadrants RNFL thickness, macular full-thickness and macular ganglion cell layer/inner plexiform layer) especially in the superior and inferior sectors and brain MRI visual pathway measurements (intraorbital and intracranial thickness of the optical nerve, as well as the optic chiasm and visual tracts). Interestingly, in this case series some optic nerve parameters measured by MRI such as the thickness of the intraorbital parts of the optic nerves in WS cases correlated with superior RNFL thickness of the optic nerve evaluated by OCT [94].

Another interesting OCT finding in 8 ad-WS cases compared to 6 ar-WS cases is the presence of an abnormal reflectivity (lamination) of the outer plexiform layer, which may be related to the high wolframin expression in the retinal Müller cells [95]. This finding needs to be confirmed by larger clinical series.

Moreover, OCT parameters can be used as a marker of disease progression, as showed by a recent paper evaluating OCT changes over time in a group of 12 WS cases compared to type 1 diabetes patients. In this paper the WS cases were re-evaluated after a follow-up period of about 2 years and OCT measurements, including total thickness of the RNFL, average retinal thickness and total retinal volume, significantly decreased compared to the baseline investigation [96].

Finally, a postmortem study documented a specific pattern of optic atrophy predominantly involving the temporal and inferior quadrants, i.e. the papillomacular

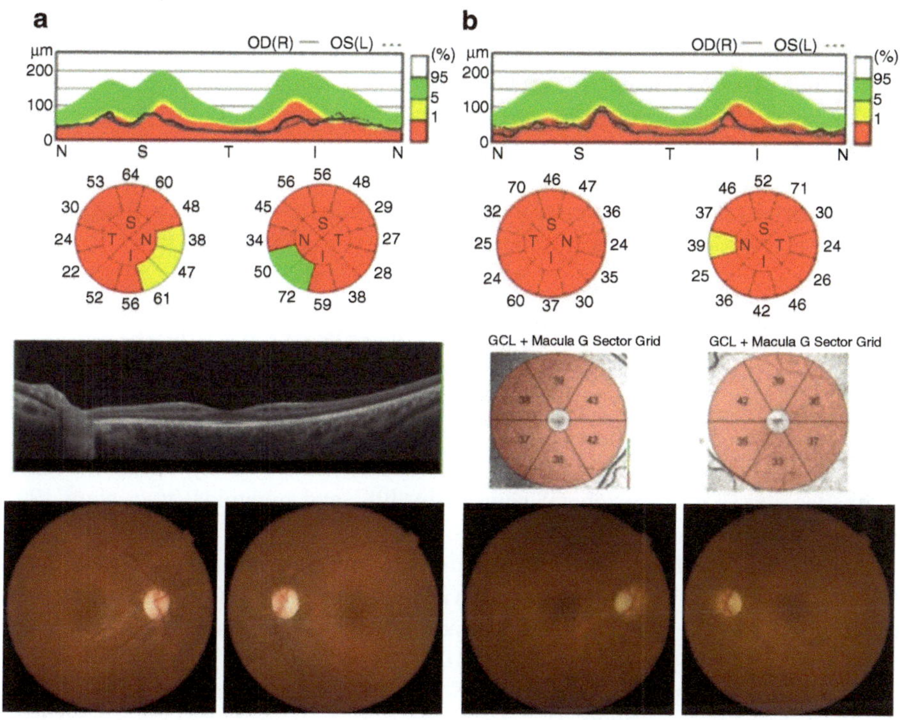

Fig. 14.4 (Wolfram) (**a**) This is a 18 year-old female, born from consanguineous parents, started complaining visual loss during childhood. She did not suffer diabetes. Visual acuity is 4/10 in RE and 3.2/10 in LE. Visual fields show a generalized defect (inf > nasal). OCT reveals diffuse RNFL thinning with relative nasal sparing and perimacular inner nuclear layer cysts. Fundus oculi images show a diffuse optic nerve pallor. (**b**) This is a 27-year-old female. She suffered diabetes mellitus since she was 10 year now on insulin therapy. Optic atrophy was noticed when she was 15 years. Visual acuity is 2.5/10 in the RE and 4/10 in the LE. OCT demonstrates diffuse RNFL thinning, as evident also at GCC. Fundus oculi images show bilateral temporal pallor

bundle of the optic nerve, in a WS case. This pattern resembles that described in mitochondrial optic neuropathies [90].

We here show the OCT findings of two WS patients (Fig. 14.4). A brief summary of their clinical history is reported below and ophthalmological findings are illustrated in Fig. 14.4.

14.7.1 Case 1

This is a 18 year-old female, born from consanguineous parents, started complaining visual loss during childhood. She did not suffer diabetes. Genetic analysis revealed the presence of the homozygous c.1553T>A mutation (p.M518K) in the *WFS1* gene. Lactic acid levels after standardized exercise were abnormally elevated. Muscle biopsy was histologically normal. Brain MRI and spectroscopy were normal.

14.7.2 Case 2

This is a 27 year-old female. She presented growth hormone deficiency at 8 years of age and diabetes mellitus at 10 year-old. She suffered from migraine since the age of 17. Genetic analysis showed the presence of compound heterozygous mutations c.409_426dup16 and c.2104 G>A in the *WFS1* gene. Brain MRI at 22 years showed microstructural degenerative cerebellar changes (middle cerebellar peduncles and emispheres). Optic atrophy was noticed when she was 15 years.

14.8 Autosomal Recessive Spastic Ataxia of Charlevoix-Saguenay (ARSACS)

Autosomal recessive spastic ataxia of Charlevoix-Saguenay (ARSACS) is a complex hereditary neurodegenerative disorder characterized by early childhood-onset cerebellar ataxia [97], peripheral neuropathy [98] and pyramidal tract signs [99, 100].

The name of the disease derives from its high prevalence, as a result of a founder effect, in the French-Canadian population of the Charlevoix-Saguenay region in the northeast of Quebec. After these initial reports ARSACS was also described in other countries and ethnic groups worldwide [101, 102].

ARSACS is due to mutations in the *SACS* gene, which were first identified by Engert and coauthors in 2000. The *SACS* gene is located on chromosome 13q12.12 and encodes the protein sacsin with a chaperone activity [102–105]. Sacsin is required for normal mitochondrial dynamics, and loss of function of this protein can result in an altered balance between mitochondrial fusion and fission [105, 106].

Furthermore, a recent study on a sacsin-knockout mouse model described a disruption of mitochondrial fission/fusion dynamics [106].

The majority of ARSACS patients show early ocular signs including the alteration of smooth ocular pursuit (horizontal gaze-evoked nystagmus) and the presence of prominent myelinated fibers radiating from the optic disc. These myelinated fibers are visible ophthalmoscopically and were considered the main clinical manifestations of ARSACS. However, there is phenotypic variability and the presence of myelinated fibers was rarely described in non-Quebec patients [107–114].

In the original characterization of ARSACS the authors described yellow streaks of hypermyelinated fibers that focally embed the retinal vessels, emanating radially from the edges of the optic disc [101]. In recent years, with the advent of new and more sophisticated quantitative retinal imaging technologies, the nature of the myelinated fibers in ARSACS has been debated.

In 2011, different OCT studies demonstrated that the typical ophthalmoscopic appearance in ARSACS patients is due to the increased hyper-reflectivity and thickness of the peripapillary RNFL and not to the presence of myelinated fibers [115–117]. Vingolo and coauthors [115] showed that the absence of shadowing behind the fibers in the OCT of ARSACS patients differentiates them from subjects with persistent myelinated fibers. In the latter, in fact, OCT clearly revealed a posterior

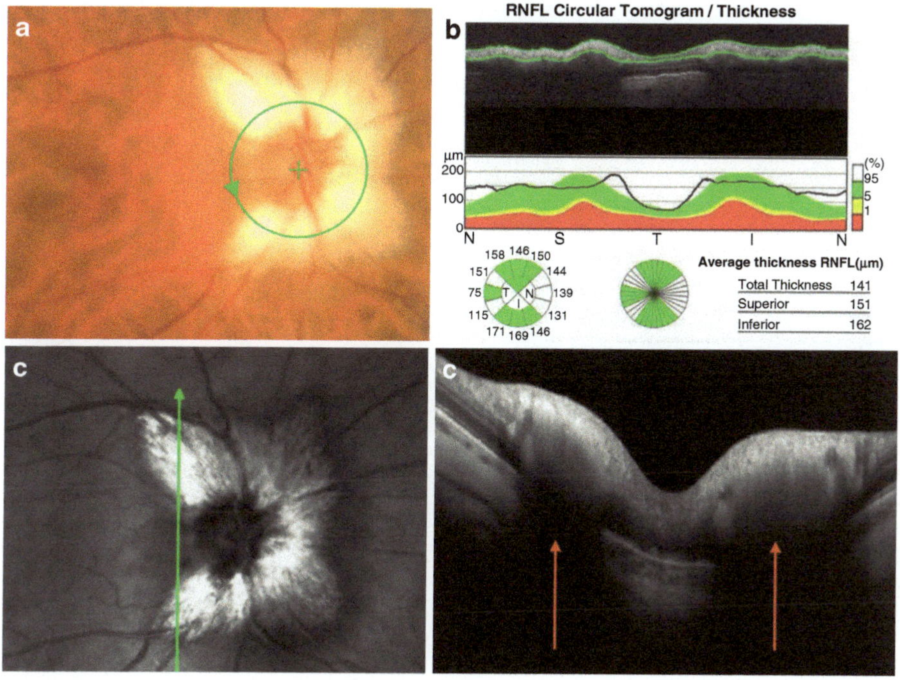

Fig. 14.5 OCT findings in persistent myelinated fibers. (**a**) Fundus photography of peripapillar myelin fibers. (**b**, **c**) Thickening of the peripapillar retinal fibers hiding the deep layers of retina (red arrow)

shadowing, due to the hyper-reflectivity and consequent "shield-effect" of the myelinated areas, which does not allow the OCT infrared laser to enter into the retina (Fig. 14.5).

The thickening of the retinal fibers can overcome the peripapillary region and reach the macula. Thus, the average macular thickness (mainly in nasal quadrant) and the average foveolar thickness may be increased in ARSACS patients [117]. Moreover, in 2016, by means of Spectral Domain-OCT (SD-OCT), Shah and coauthors, describing the characteristics of the fovea in an ARSAC patient, detected the incursion of inner retinal layers upon the foveal region leading to the lost of pit, exactly resembling the abnormality of development as seen in grade 2 foveal hypoplasia [118] (Fig. 14.6).

Also the OCT Angiography (Angio-OCT) of the ONH highlights the increase of vessel density in the radial peripapillary capillary plexus (RPC) probably due to the increased metabolic demand of the hypertrophic fibers (Fig. 14.7).

Recently Parkinson and coauthor, studying a large cohort of ARSACS patients found an inverse correlation between peripapillary RNFL thickness and both age at examination and age at onset; however, a significant correlation between the average peripapillary RNFL thickness and disease duration was not found [119].

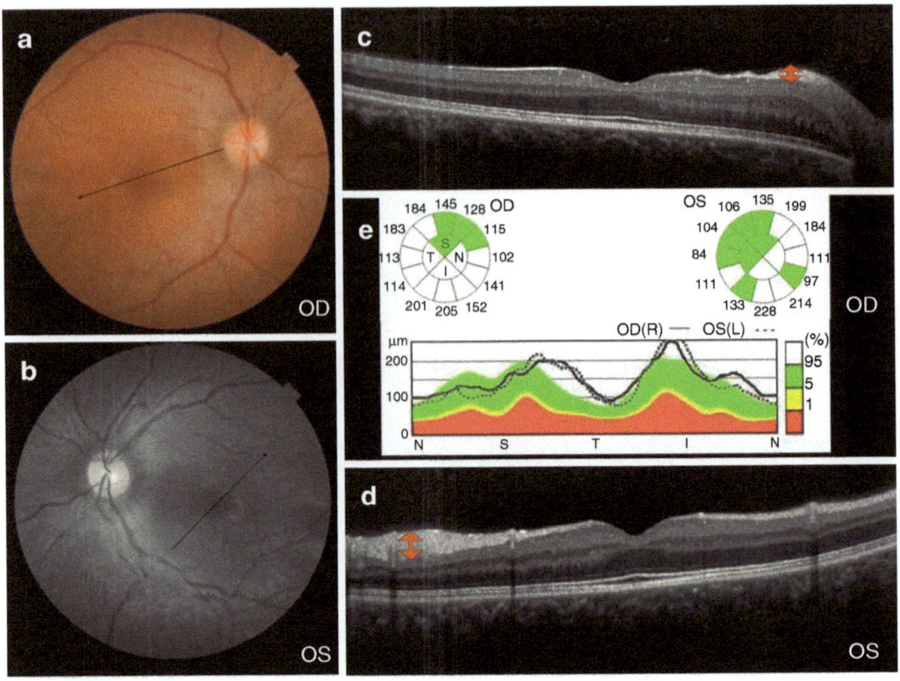

Fig. 14.6 OCT findings in a ARSACS patient. This is a 25-year old female carrying mutations in the *SACS* gene located on chromosome 13q12.12p. Visual acuity is 10/10 bilaterally. (**a**, **b**) Color and red-free fundus photograph. (**c**, **d**) OCT scans through the fovea reveal the hypertrophia of the nerve fiber layer (red arrows) and the incursion of inner retinal layers upon the foveal region as seen in grade 2 foveal hypoplasia (**e**) Increased thickness of peripapillar RNFL predominant in upper and lower temporal sectors

Typically, visual acuity is normal or rarely slightly reduced, without any central visual field defects (only mild and peripheral visual defects are reported). These findings overall support the absence of myelin deposition in the retina of these patients, given that the presence of myelin, would have caused more evident visual field defects as blind spot enlargement [120].

Concerning the ARSACS asymptomatic carriers, the results of two recent studies have been inconsistent and it is unclear whether or not there is some degree of RNFL hypertophy in individuals carrying heterozygous SACS gene mutations [119, 121].

Thus, it is preferable to use the term "retinal nerve fiber hypertrophy" [116] to define the retinal aspect of patients with ARSACS. In fact, the recent OCT findings, at least among non-Quebec patients, suggest that retinal hypermyelination has been used inappropriately to describe the striated appearance of a thickened RNFL around the optic discs in ARSACS patients [122]. Yu-Wai-Man and coauthors in 2013 have proposed the speculative hypothesis that the RNFL thickening in ARSACS could be related to the axoplasmic stasis within the long axons of the retinal ganglion cells as they converge to form the optic nerve in the anatomically tight region of the lamina cribrosa [122].

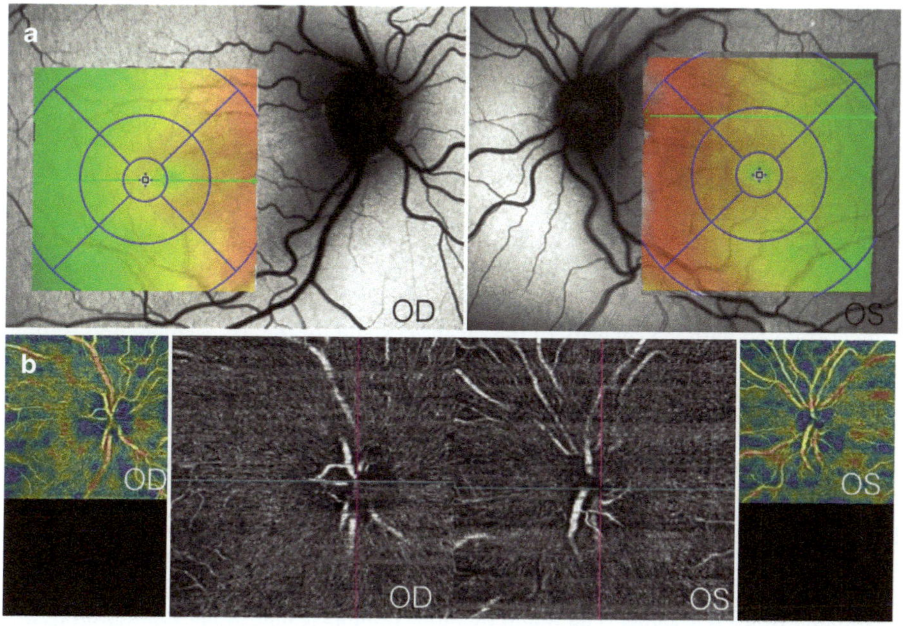

Fig. 14.7 AF and Angio-OCT findings in a ARSACS patient. (same patient as in Fig. 14.6). (**a**) Fundus autofluorescence with superimposed the ETDR thickness map shows a shadowing of the AF signal and a thickening in the OCT map in the area of the RNFL hypertrophy. (**b**) Angio-OCT of the ONH shows an increase of the numbers of the radial peripapillary capillaries (RPC)

14.9 Spinocerebellar Ataxias (SCAs)

Spinocerebellar ataxias (SCAs) are a genetically heterogeneous group of autosomal dominant neurodegenerative disorders characterized by ataxia, ocular motor abnormalities, and variable other neurological features, such as pyramidal tract, basal ganglia or brainstem dysfunction [123, 124]. The SCAs are classified on the basis of the genotype and currently include up to 40 genetically distinct entities [125]. SCA1, 2, 3, and 6, the most common ones, are caused by a trinucleotide CAG repeat expansion encoding glutamine in four unrelated proteins. SCA1, 2, and 3 are characterized by cerebellar degeneration and variable degrees of involvement of other central nervous system regions, whereas SCA6 is associated with a nearly pure cerebellar atrophy [123].

Abnormal afferent visual testing and optic atrophy have been described as a feature of SC1, SCA2 and SCA3 [126, 127]. Rarely, SCA2 is also associated with retinitis pigmentosa, most notably in the infantile form with extremely expanded CAG repeats [128], and pigmentary retinopathy has been reported in a patient homozygous for a pathological repeat expansion in the SCA6 gene [129].

Unlike other SCAs, patients with SCA7 exhibit a spectrum of severity of retinal disease from mild to severe dysfunction. Early functional abnormalities occur in both cones and rods, but greater centrally than peripherally [130, 131].

14.10 Spinocerebellar Ataxia Type 2-3-6 (SCA2-3-6)

Pula et al. in a spectral-domain OCT study reported in 29 SCA and cerebellar multisystem atrophy patients (SCA1-2-3-6 and MSA-C) a significant reduction of the peripapillar RNFL thickness for SCA2 and SCA3 patients only. This RNFL thinning correlated with the severity of the disease (Scale for the Assessment and Rating of Ataxia, SARA score) [132].

Another study by Alvarez and colleagues [133] demonstrated a significant reduction of the average RNFL thickness in nine SCA3 patients compared to age- and sex-matched controls. There was a reduction in the RNFL thickness in all quadrants except the temporal one, preserved in all eyes. Therefore, papillomacular bundle probably is not primarily involved in SCA-3 and consequently visual acuity is preserved in these patients (mean BCVA 20/25 and normal colour vision in all patients, except for the one with congenital dyscromatopsia). RNFL thickness was inversely correlated to SARA score. The mean macular thickness was lower compared to the control group only in two eyes (11.11%). In four patients, (eight eyes) OCT studies were performed with an average follow-up of 14.25 months, and in five eyes (62.50%) there was a trend towards a RNFL thickness reduction. Thus, the authors concluded that the pattern of the optic nerve involvement in SCA-3 is more similar to that observed in Alzheimer's and Parkinson's disease than to SCA-1 and toxic or mitochondrial optic nerve diseases where there is a preferential involvement of the papillo-macular bundle [133].

14.11 Spinocerebellar Ataxia Type 1 (SCA1)

Spinocerebellar ataxia type 1 (SCA1) is an autosomal dominantly inherited, late-onset neurodegenerative disease primarily affecting the cerebellar cortex and brainstem. Affected patients suffer from disturbed motor coordination, slurred speech, dysphagia, spasticity, extrapyramidal movements such as dystonia or chorea, cerebellar oculomotor disturbances, ophthalmoparesis, saccade slowing and cognitive impairment [134].

SCA1 is due to a CAG-repeat expansion of variable length reaching between 39 and 83 repeats encoding for a prolonged polyglutamine chain in the *ATXN1* gene on chromosome 6p23 encoding for the ataxin1 protein [134].

In SCA1 patients, besides the well-described cerebellar oculomotor abnormalities, there is also evidence of ocular pathology. There is evidence of visual acuity reduction, color vision impairment and central scotoma or contraction of visual fields [135, 136]. In some case series there is evidence of worsening of ocular symptoms with disease duration [137, 138]. The reduced visual acuity in SCA1 has been attributed to optic atrophy, which was first described at fundus examination [138]. Optic nerve involvement was also suggested by abnormal VEP findings in SCA1 patients [139, 140]. However, VEPs were normal in 40–50% of SCA1 patients and retinal or optic nerve pathology was not consistently reported in SCA1 [141].

Stricker et al. [142], in a series of 9 SCA1 subjects compared to age- and sex-matched controls, demonstrated with OCT a pattern of temporal atrophy of the RNFL in most of the patients, suggesting a preferential involvement of the papillomacular bundle. Segmentation analysis of the retina confirmed temporal RNFL thickness reduction whereas there was no significant difference in the average ganglion cell layer, inner and outer plexiform layer, photoreceptor layer and pigment epithelium. SCA1 patients showed a reduction in visual acuity and average RNFL thickness compared to healthy controls (84.0 μm vs. 97.2 μm). RNFL thinning was predominant and significant in temporal sectors ($p < 0.001$,) and was not found in nasal sectors. OCT findings were correlated with disease duration and disease severity measured by SARA score. The patient with the longest disease duration and highest SARA score showed additional severe macular atrophy, indicating that, at a later disease stage, nerve fiber atrophy could lead to ganglion cell degeneration and consecutively to macular volume reduction. Differently, VEP P100 latencies were not significantly different between SCA1 patients and controls [142].

The authors speculated that the selective temporal RNFL involvement could be explained by a differential vulnerability of the parvocellular axons to mutated ataxin1. In fact, the pattern of temporal RNFL thinning seen in these SCA1 patients could be due to localized oxidative dysfunction, which does not involve the magnocellular ganglion cell axons and the photoreceptors [142].

In 2013, two different groups [135, 136] simultaneously described a case series of six SCA1 patients presenting with progressive maculopathy and retinal dysfunction. The patients exhibited bilateral, progressive painless visual loss with macular drusen and mild pigmentary alterations at fundus examination.

In particular, Vaclavik and coauthors [136] showed two genetically confirmed SCA1 patients with bilateral areas of hypopigmented retinal pigment epithelium within the macula. Autofluorescence imaging revealed a central macular hyperautofluorescence surrounded by a ring of hypoautofluorescence. Spectral-domain OCT disclosed bilateral hyporeflective "foveal cavitation" corresponding to loss of the highly reflective inner segment/outer segment junction, as well as thinning of the outer nuclear layer. Outside the macula, the retina was within normal range. Fluorescein angiography showed small areas of patchy hyperfluorescence in the macula, corresponding to areas of depigmented retinal pigment epithelium without any leakage at later stages. Goldmann kinetic manual perimetry revealed a relative central scotoma bilaterally. The retinal function was tested using full-field ERG which was within normal limits under photopic and scotopic conditions. Multifocal electroretinography (mfERG) was not performed [136].

Two other patients with bilateral foveal cavities had OCT features similar to those reported previously in achromatopsia [143], and cone dystrophy [144], whereas RNFL thickness was not evaluated. Similarly, Lebranchu and coauthors reported a SCA1 family with maculopathy [135]. Four SCA1 patients showed central scotoma in most of the eyes at visual field examination and visual acuities ranged between 20/20 and 20/200. Central retinal thinning with disorganized photoreceptor layers or foveal cavitation were found at OCT. Two patients showed mild temporal optic disc pallor at fundoscopy and thinning of the temporal RNFL at OCT, confirming the involvement of the papillomacular bundle [135]. In one patient, multifocal electroretinography (mfERG) revealed central retinal dysfunction. In these patients, OCT demonstrated alterations of the external layers of the fovea, suggesting a loss of structural integrity of the photoreceptors. The authors suggested that foveolar cavitation associated with the thinning of the whole macular area (including the surrounding perifoveolar retina) could be related to a cone dystrophy, as supported by the fact that a cluster of genes (*GUCA1A, PRPH2*) involved in macular diseases is located in a chromosome region (6p21.1) near the *SCA1* gene [135].

14.12 Spinocerebellar Ataxia Type 7 (SCA7)

Spinocerebellar ataxia type 7 (SCA7) is a progressive ataxia that is characterized by a high prevalence of retinal photoreceptor abnormalities. Recent studies suggest that the retinopathy of SCA7 is a cone-rod dystrophy [130, 131]. This degenerative retinopathy initially affects cones, and then progresses to cone–rod dystrophy [130]. Fundus examination demonstrates macular pigmentary changes, sometimes associated with mild temporal optic disc pallor [145]. The gene encodes for a protein (ataxin-7) widely expressed in the human retina [146]. This protein may interact with the function of CRX (cone–rod homeobox), a known transcription factor implicated in human cone–rod dystrophy [147].

In the last 10 years, with the advent of high-resolution spectral domain optical coherence tomography (SD-OCT), many studies demonstrated the presence of different grade of outer retinal atrophy with loss of the outer nuclear layer and ellipsoid zone in the central macula in SCA7 patients. Thus, the loss of the subfoveal ellipsoid zone corresponds to loss of cone photoreceptor cells which may be the earliest clinical sign of cone-rod dystrophy associated with SCA7 [148–152].

Manrique et al. [150] have described a case series of 7 patients with SCA7 in which the subjects with mild disease showed retinal thinning only at the fovea and subjects with more advanced disease tended to present retinal thinning also in the outer zone of the macula. Mean peripapillary RNFL thickness was decreased in all patients with sparing of the temporal quadrant until the advanced phases of the disease.

Furthermore, another study by Ahn et al. [151], using OCT and mfERG, revealed that retinal thinning extended outside the visible atrophic lesions and that the areas of functional deficits were greater than those of anatomic deficits.

Additionally, at a later stage of disease the maculopathy can evolve into a “bull’s eye” pattern [149]. The sparing of the temporal sector has been discussed as a possible result of the relative sparing of the inner macula around the central fovea associated with normal ganglion cell layer thickness at an earlier disease stage [151, 153].

14.13 Spinocerebellar Ataxia Type 10 (SCA10)

SCA 10 is caused by a pentanucleotide (ATTCT) repeat expansion on chromosome 22q13-qter. The SCA10 patients can present a purely cerebellar syndrome or a cerebellar syndrome concomitantly with epilepsy, polyneuropathy, and hematologic heart and liver conditions [154]. SCA10 shows a less aggressive clinical course than SCA3.

In 2017, Spina Tensini and coauthors used OCT to compare peripapillary RNFL and macular GCL thickness in patients with SCA3 and those with SCA10. They confirmed the reduction of the RNFL thickness in all quadrants but the temporal one in SCA3 patients and moreover they found RNFL thicker in SCA10 ($p > 0.05$) without any correlation between size of expansion, Scale for the Assessment and Rating of Ataxia (SARA), and RNFL or GCL thickness in SCA10 patients. These OCT structural findings are in accordance with the clinical course of SCA10, less aggressive than other SCAs [155].

14.14 Conclusions

In summary, OCT is a useful tool for investigating optic nerve and retinal involvement in many rare neurological disorders. Up to now, only a limited number of diseases have been extensively studied, as reported in this chapter. Single case reports with OCT findings are available for other rare neurological disorders such as Charcot-Marie-Tooth type 2A [156], and the X-linked adrenoleukodystrophy [157]. Thus, the application of this technique to larger case series will allow a better characterization of the ocular phenotype in these and other neurological diseases.

References

1. Collins A. Clinical neurogenetics: friedreich ataxia. Neurol Clin. 2013;31:1095–120.
2. Parkinson MH, Boesch S, Nachbauer W, Mariotti C, Giunti P. Clinical features of Friedreich's ataxia: classical and atypical phenotypes. J Neurochem. 2013;126(Suppl 1):103–17.
3. Campuzano V, Montermini L, Moltò MD, Pianese L, Cossée M, Cavalcanti F, et al. Friedreich's ataxia: autosomal recessive disease caused by an intronic GAA triplet repeat expansion. Science. 1996;271:1423–7.
4. Tan G, Napoli E, Taroni F, Cortopassi G. Decreased expression of genes involved in sulfur amino acid metabolism in frataxin-deficient cells. Hum Mol Genet. 2003;12:1699–711.
5. Shan Y, Napoli E, Cortopassi G. Mitochondrial frataxin interacts with ISD11 of the NFS1/ISCU complex and multiple mitochondrial chaperones. Hum Mol Genet. 2007;16:929–41.
6. Martelli A, Puccio H. Dysregulation of cellular iron metabolism in Friedreich ataxia: from primary iron-sulfur cluster deficit to mitochondrial iron accumulation. Front Pharmacol. 2014;5:130.
7. Rötig A, de Lonlay P, Chretien D, Foury F, Koenig M, Sidi D, et al. Aconitase and mitochondrial iron-sulphur protein deficiency in Friedreich ataxia. Nat Genet. 1997;17:215–7.
8. Lodi R, Cooper JM, Bradley JL, Manners D, Styles P, Taylor DJ, et al. Deficit of in vivo mitochondrial ATP production in patients with Friedreich ataxia. Proc Natl Acad Sci U S A. 1999;96:11492–5.

9. Bolinches-Amorós A, Mollá B, Pla-Martín D, Palau F, González-Cabo P. Mitochondrial dysfunction induced by frataxin deficiency is associated with cellular senescence and abnormal calcium metabolism. Front Cell Neurosci. 2014;8:124.
10. Babcock M, de Silva D, Oaks R, Davis-Kaplan S, Jiralerspong S, Montermini L, et al. Regulation of mitochondrial iron accumulation by Yfh1p, a putative homolog of frataxin. Science. 1997;276:1709–12.
11. Wong A, Yang J, Cavadini P, Gellera C, Lonnerdal B, Taroni F, et al. The Friedreich's ataxia mutation confers cellular sensitivity to oxidant stress which is rescued by chelators of iron and calcium and inhibitors of apoptosis. Hum Mol Genet. 1999;8:425–30.
12. Gomes CM, Santos R. Neurodegeneration in Friedreich's ataxia: from defective frataxin to oxidative stress. Oxidative Med Cell Longev. 2013;2013:487534.
13. Kersten HM, Roxburgh RH, Danesh-Meyer HV. Ophthalmic manifestations of inherited neurodegenerative disorders. Nat Rev Neurol. 2014;10:349–62.
14. Andermann E, Remillard GM, Goyer C, Blitzer L, Andermann F, Barbeau A. Genetic and family studies in Friedreich's ataxia. Can J Neurol Sci. 1976;3:287–301.
15. Carroll WM, Kriss A, Baraitser M, Barrett G, Halliday AM. The incidence and nature of visual pathway involvement in Friedreich's ataxia. A clinical and visual evoked potential study of 22 patients. Brain. 1980;103:413–34.
16. Fortuna F, Barboni P, Liguori R, Valentino ML, Savini G, Gellera C, et al. Visual system involvement in patients with Friedreich's ataxia. Brain. 2009;132:116–23.
17. Noval S, Contreras I, Sanz-Gallego I, Manrique RK, Arpa J. Ophthalmic features of Friedreich ataxia. Eye. 2012;26:315–20.
18. Seyer LA, Galetta K, Wilson J, Sakai R, Perlman S, Mathews K, et al. Analysis of the visual system in Friedreich ataxia. J Neurol. 2013;260:2362–9.
19. Dağ E, Örnek N, Örnek K, Erbahçeci-Timur IE. Optical coherence tomography and visual field findings in patients with Friedreich ataxia. J Neuroophthalmol. 2014;34:118–21.
20. Barboni P, Carbonelli M, Savini G, Ramos Cdo V, Carta A, Berezovsky A, et al. Natural history of Leber's hereditary optic neuropathy: longitudinal analysis of the retinal nerve fiber layer by optical coherence tomography. Ophthalmology. 2010;117:623–7.
21. Cotman SL, Karaa A, Staropoli JF, Sims KB. Neuronal ceroid lipofuscinosis: impact of recent genetic advances and expansion of the clinicopathologic spectrum. Curr Neurol Neurosci Rep. 2013;13:366.
22. Wheeler RB, Schlie M, Kominami E, Gerhard L, Goebel HH. Neuronal ceroid lipofuscinosis: late infantile or Jansky Bielschowsky type--re-revisited. Acta Neuropathol. 2001;102:485–8.
23. Bennett MJ, Rakheja D. The neuronal ceroid-lipofuscinoses. Dev Disabil Res Rev. 2013;17:254–9.
24. Hainsworth DP, Liu GT, Hamm CW, Katz ML. Funduscopic and angiographic appearance in the neuronal ceroid lipofuscinoses. Retina. 2009;29:657–68.
25. Worgall S, Kekatpure MV, Heier L, Ballon D, Dyke JP, Shungu D, et al. Neurological deterioration in late infantile neuronal ceroid lipofuscinosis. Neurology. 2007;69:521–35.
26. Goebel HH, Zeman W, Damaske E. An ultrastructural study of the retina in the Jansky-Bielschowsky type of neuronal ceroid-lipofuscinosis. Am J Ophthalmol. 1977;83:70–9.
27. Weleber RG. The dystrophic retina in multisystem disorders: the electroretinogram in neuronal ceroid lipofuscinoses. Eye. 1998;12:580–90.
28. Sappington RM, Pearce DA, Calkins DJ. Optic nerve degeneration in a murine model of juvenile ceroid lipofuscinosis. Invest Ophthalmol Vis Sci. 2003;44:3725–31.
29. Weimer JM, Custer AW, Benedict JW, Alexander NA, Kingsley E, Federoff HJ, et al. Visual deficits in a mouse model of Batten disease are the result of optic nerve degeneration and loss of dorsal lateral geniculate thalamic neurons. Neurobiol Dis. 2006;22:284–93.
30. Mahmood F, Fu S, Cooke J, Wilson SW, Cooper JD, Russell C. A zebrafish model of CLN2 disease is deficient in tripeptidyl peptidase 1 and displays progressive neurodegeneration accompanied by a reduction in proliferation. Brain. 2013;136:1488–507.
31. Groh J, Stadler D, Buttmann M, Martini R. Non-invasive assessment of retinal alterations in mouse models of infantile and juvenile neuronal ceroid lipofuscinosis by spectral domain optical coherence tomography. Acta Neuropathol Commun. 2014;2:54.

32. Nardocci N, Verga ML, Binelli S, Zorzi G, Angelini L, Bugiani O. Neuronal ceroid-lipofuscinosis: a clinical and morphological study of 19 patients. Am J Med Genet. 1995;57:137–41.
33. Orlin A, Sondhi D, Witmer MT, Wessel MM, Mezey JG, Kaminsky SM, et al. Spectrum of ocular manifestations in CLN2-associated batten (Jansky-Bielschowsky) disease correlate with advancing age and deteriorating neurological function. PLoS One. 2013;8:e73128.
34. Wisniewski KE, Zhong N, Philippart M. Pheno/genotypic correlations of neuronal ceroid lipofuscinoses. Neurology. 2001;57(4):576–81.
35. Ku CA, Hull S, Arno G, Vincent A, Carss K, Kayton R, Weeks D, Anderson GW, Geraets R, Parker C, Pearce DA, Michaelides M, MacLaren RE, Robson AG, Holder GE, Heon E, Raymond FL, Moore AT, Webster AR, Pennesi ME. Detailed clinical phenotype and molecular genetic findings in CLN3-associated isolated retinal degeneration. JAMA Ophthalmol. 2017;135(7):749–60.
36. Preising MN, Abura M, Jäger M, Wassill KH, Lorenz B. Ocular morphology and function in juvenile neuronal ceroid lipofuscinosis (CLN3) in the first decade of life. Ophthalmic Genet. 2017;38(3):252–9.
37. Dulz S, Wagenfeld L, Nickel M, et al. Novel morphological macular findings in juvenile CLN3 disease. Br J Ophthalmol. 2016;100:824–8.
38. Klein CJ, Botuyan MV, Wu Y, Ward CJ, Nicholson GA, Hammans S, et al. Mutations in DNMT1 cause hereditary sensory neuropathy with dementia and hearing loss. Nat Genet. 2011;43:595–600.
39. Winkelmann J, Lin L, Schormair B, Kornum BR, Faraco J, Plazzi G, et al. Mutations in DNMT1 cause autosomal dominant cerebellar ataxia, deafness and narcolepsy. Hum Mol Genet. 2012;21:2205–10.
40. Moghadam KK, Pizza F, La Morgia C, Franceschini C, Tonon C, Lodi R, et al. Narcolepsy is a common phenotype in HSAN IE and ADCA-DN. Brain. 2014;137:1643–55.
41. Melberg A, Hetta J, Dahl N, Nennesmo I, Bengtsson M, Wibom R, et al. Autosomal dominant cerebellar ataxia deafness and narcolepsy. J Neurol Sci. 1995;134:119–29.
42. Lundberg PO, Wranne I, Brun A. Family with optic atrophy and neurological symptoms. Acta Neurol Scand. 1967;43:87–105.
43. Takasugi M, Yagi S, Hirabayashi K, Shiota K. DNA methylation status of nuclear-encoded mitochondrial genes underlies the tissue-dependent mitochondrial functions. BMC Genomics. 2010;11:481.
44. Shock LS, Thakkar PV, Peterson EJ, Moran RG, Taylor SM. DNA methyltransferase 1, cytosine methylation, and cytosine hydroxymethylation in mammalian mitochondria. Proc Natl Acad Sci U S A. 2011;108:3630–5.
45. Bellizzi D, D'Aquila P, Scafone T, Giordano M, Riso V, Riccio A, et al. The control region of mitochondrial DNA shows an unusual CpG and non-CpG methylation pattern. DNA Res. 2013;20:537–47.
46. Singh RK, Mallela RK, Hayes A, Dunham NR, Hedden ME, Enke RA, Fariss RN, Sternberg H, West MD, Nasonkin IO. Dnmt1, Dnmt3a and Dnmt3b cooperate in photoreceptor and outer plexiform layer development in the mammalian retina. Exp Eye Res. 2017;159:132–46.
47. Lo Giudice T, Lombardi F, Santorelli FM, Kawarai T, Orlacchio A. Hereditary spastic paraplegia: clinical-genetic characteristics and evolving molecular mechanisms. Exp Neurol. 2014;261C:518–39.
48. Casari G, De Fusco M, Ciarmatori S, Zeviani M, Mora M, Fernandez P, et al. Spastic paraplegia and OXPHOS impairment caused by mutations in paraplegin, a nuclear-encoded mitochondrial metalloprotease. Cell. 1998;93:973–83.
49. De Michele G, De Fusco M, Cavalcanti F, Filla A, Marconi R, Volpe G, et al. A new locus for autosomal recessive hereditary spastic paraplegia maps to chromosome 16q24.3. Am J Hum Genet. 1998;63:135–9.
50. Rugarli EI, Langer T. Translating m-AAA protease function in mitochondria to hereditary spastic paraplegia. Trends Mol Med. 2006;12:262–9.

51. Nolden M, Ehses S, Koppen M, Bernacchia A, Rugarli EI, Langer T. The m-AAA protease defective in hereditary spastic paraplegia controls ribosome assembly in mitochondria. Cell. 2005;123:277–89.
52. Atorino L, Silvestri L, Koppen M, Cassina L, Ballabio A, Marconi R, et al. Loss of m-AAA protease in mitochondria causes complex I deficiency and increased sensitivity to oxidative stress in hereditary spastic paraplegia. J Cell Biol. 2003;163:777–87.
53. McDermott CJ, Dayaratne RK, Tomkins J, Lusher ME, Lindsey JC, Johnson MA, et al. Paraplegin gene analysis in hereditary spastic paraparesis (HSP) pedigrees in Northeast England. Neurology. 2001;56:467–71.
54. Ehses S, Raschke I, Mancuso G, Bernacchia A, Geimer S, Tondera D, et al. Regulation of OPA1 processing and mitochondrial fusion by m-AAA protease isoenzymes and OMA1. J Cell Biol. 2009;187:1023–36.
55. Klebe S, Depienne C, Gerber S, Challe G, Anheim M, Charles P, et al. Spastic paraplegia gene 7 in patients with spasticity and/or optic neuropathy. Brain. 2012;135:2980–93.
56. van Gassen KL, van der Heijden CD, de Bot ST, den Dunnen WF, van den Berg LH, Verschuuren-Bemelmans CC, et al. Genotype-phenotype correlations in spastic paraplegia type 7: a study in a large Dutch cohort. Brain. 2012;135:2994–3004.
57. Marcotulli C, Leonardi L, Tessa A, De Negris AM, Cornia R, Pierallini A, et al. Early-onset optic neuropathy as initial clinical presentation in SPG7. J Neurol. 2014;261:1820–1.
58. Wiethoff S, Zhour A, Schöls L, Fischer MD. Retinal nerve fibre layer loss in hereditary spastic paraplegias is restricted to complex phenotypes. BMC Neurol. 2012;12:143.
59. Chabriat H, Joutel A, Dichgans M, Tournier-Lasserve E, Bousser MG. Cadasil. Lancet Neurol. 2009;8:643–53.
60. O'Sullivan M, Jarosz JM, Martin RJ, Deasy N, Powell JF, Markus HS. MRI hyperintensities of the temporal lobe and external capsule in patients with CADASIL. Neurology. 2001;56:628–34.
61. Joutel A, Corpechot C, Ducros A, Vahedi K, Chabriat H, Mouton P, et al. Notch3 mutations in cerebral autosomal dominant arteriopathy with subcortical infarcts and leukoencephalopathy (CADASIL), a mendelian condition causing stroke and vascular dementia. Ann N Y Acad Sci. 1997;826:213–7.
62. Belin de Chantemèle EJ, Retailleau K, Pinaud F, Vessières E, Bocquet A, Guihot AL, et al. Notch3 is a major regulator of vascular tone in cerebral and tail resistance arteries. Arterioscler Thromb Vasc Biol. 2008;28:2216–24.
63. Robinson W, Galetta SL, McCluskey L, Forman MS, Balcer LJ. Retinal findings in cerebral autosomal dominant arteriopathy with subcortical infarcts and leukoencephalopathy (cadasil). Surv Ophthalmol. 2001;45:445–8.
64. Roine S, Harju M, Kivelä TT, Pöyhönen M, Nikoskelainen E, Tuisku S, et al. Ophthalmologic findings in cerebral autosomal dominant arteriopathy with subcortical infarcts and leukoencephalopathy: a cross-sectional study. Ophthalmology. 2006;113:1411–7.
65. Haritoglou C, Rudolph G, Hoops JP, Opherk C, Kampik A, Dichgans M. Retinal vascular abnormalities in CADASIL. Neurology. 2004;62:1202–5.
66. Pretegiani E, Rosini F, Dotti MT, Bianchi S, Federico A, Rufa A. Visual system involvement in CADASIL. J Stroke Cerebrovasc Dis. 2013;22:1377–84.
67. Parisi V, Pierelli F, Fattapposta F, Bianco F, Parisi L, Restuccia R, et al. Early visual function impairment in CADASIL. Neurology. 2003;60:2008–10.
68. Rufa A, Malandrini A, Dotti MT, Berti G, Salvadori C, Federico A. Typical pathological changes of CADASIL in the optic nerve. Neurol Sci. 2005;26:271–4.
69. Parisi V, Pierelli F, Coppola G, Restuccia R, Ferrazzoli D, Scassa C, et al. Reduction of optic nerve fiber layer thickness in CADASIL. Eur J Neurol. 2007;14:627–31.
70. Rufa A, Pretegiani E, Frezzotti P, De Stefano N, Cevenini G, Dotti MT, et al. Retinal nerve fiber layer thinning in CADASIL: an optical coherence tomography and MRI study. Cerebrovasc Dis. 2011;31:77–82.
71. Nelis P, Kleffner I, Burg MC, Clemens CR, Alnawaiseh M, Motte J, Marziniak M, Eter N, Alten F. OCT-angiography reveals reduced vessel density in the deep retinal plexus of CADASIL patients. Sci Rep. 2018;8(1):8148.

72. Alten F, Motte J, Ewering C, Osada N, Clemens CR, Kadas EM, Eter N, Paul F, Marziniak M. Multimodal retinal vessel analysis in CADASIL patients. PLoS One. 2014;9(11):e112311.
73. Fang XJ, Yu M, Wu Y, Zhang ZH, Wang WW, Wang ZX, Yuan Y. Study of enhanced depth imaging optical coherence tomography in cerebral autosomal dominant arteriopathy with subcortical infarcts and leukoencephalopathy. Chin Med J. 2017;130(9):1042–8.
74. Cavallari M, Falco T, Frontali M, Romano S, Bagnato F, Orzi F. Fractal analysis reveals reduced complexity of retinal vessels in CADASIL. PLoS One. 2011;6(4):e19150.
75. Wolfram D, Wagener HP. Diabetes mellitus and simple optic atrophy among siblings: report of four cases. Proc Staff Meet Mayo Clin. 1938;13:715–8.
76. Rigoli L, Di Bella C. Wolfram syndrome 1 and Wolfram syndrome 2. Curr Opin Pediatr. 2012;24:512–7.
77. Barrett TG, Poulton K, Bundey S. DIDMOAD syndrome; further studies and muscle biochemistry. J Inherit Metab Dis. 1995;18:218–20.
78. Barrett TG, Bundey SE. Wolfram (DIDMOAD) syndrome. J Med Genet. 1997;34:838–41.
79. Barrett TG, Bundey SE, Fielder AR, Good PA. Optic atrophy in Wolfram (DIDMOAD) syndrome. Eye. 1997;11:882–8.
80. Inoue H, Tanizawa Y, Wasson J, Behn P, Kalidas K, Bernal-Mizrachi E, et al. A gene encoding a transmembrane protein is mutated in patients with diabetes mellitus and optic atrophy (Wolfram syndrome). Nat Genet. 1998;20:143–8.
81. Eiberg H, Hansen L, Kjer B, Hansen T, Pedersen O, Bille M, et al. Autosomal dominant optic atrophy associated with hearing impairment and impaired glucose regulation caused by a missense mutation in the WFS1 gene. J Med Genet. 2006;43:435–40.
82. Rendtorff ND, Lodahl M, Boulahbel H, Johansen IR, Pandya A, Welch KO, et al. Identification of p.A684V missense mutation in the WFS1 gene as a frequent cause of autosomal dominant optic atrophy and hearing impairment. Am J Med Genet A. 2011;155A:1298–313.
83. Bai X, Lv H, Zhang F, Liu J, Fan Z, Xu L, et al. Identification of a novel missense mutation in the WFS1 gene as a cause of autosomal dominant nonsyndromic sensorineural hearing loss in all-frequencies. Am J Med Genet A. 2014;164:3052–60.
84. Bonnycastle LL, Chines PS, Hara T, Huyghe JR, Swift AJ, Heikinheimo P, et al. Autosomal dominant diabetes arising from a Wolfram syndrome 1 mutation. Diabetes. 2013;62:3943–50.
85. Berry V, Gregory-Evans C, Emmett W, Waseem N, Raby J, Prescott D, et al. Wolfram gene (WFS1) mutation causes autosomal dominant congenital nuclear cataract in humans. Eur J Hum Genet. 2013;21:1356–60.
86. Carson MJ, Slager UT, Steinberg RM. Simultaneous occurrence of diabetes mellitus, diabetes insipidus, and optic atrophy in a brother and sister. Am J Dis Child. 1977;131:1382–5.
87. Jackson MJ, Bindoff LA, Weber K, Wilson JN, Ince P, Alberti KG, et al. Biochemical and molecular studies of mitochondrial function in diabetes insipidus, diabetes mellitus, optic atrophy, and deafness. Diabetes Care. 1994;17:728–33.
88. Shannon P, Becker L, Deck J. Evidence of widespread axonal pathology in Wolfram syndrome. Acta Neuropathol. 1999;98:304–8.
89. Hilson JB, Merchant SN, Adams JC, Joseph JT. Wolfram syndrome: a clinicopathologic correlation. Acta Neuropathol. 2009;118:415–28.
90. Ross-Cisneros FN, Pan BX, Silva RA, Miller NR, Albini TA, Tranebjaerg L, et al. Optic nerve histopathology in a case of Wolfram syndrome: a mitochondrial pattern of axonal loss. Mitochondrion. 2013;13:841–5.
91. Bababeygy SR, Wang MY, Khaderi KR, Sadun AA. Visual improvement with the use of idebenone in the treatment of Wolfram syndrome. J Neuroophthalmol. 2012;32:386–9.
92. Bucca BC, Klingensmith G, Bennett JL. Wolfram syndrome: a rare optic neuropathy in youth with type 1 diabetes. Optom Vis Sci. 2011;88:E1383–90.
93. Grenier J, Meunier I, Daien V, Baudoin C, Halloy F, Bocquet B, Blanchet C, Delettre C, Esmenjaud E, Roubertie A, Lenaers G, Hamel CP. WFS1 in optic neuropathies: mutation findings in nonsyndromic optic atrophy and assessment of clinical severity. Ophthalmology. 2016;123(9):1989–98.

94. Zmyslowska A, Waszczykowska A, Baranska D, Stawiski K, Borowiec M, Jurowski P, Fendler W, Mlynarski W. Optical coherence tomography and magnetic resonance imaging visual pathway evaluation in Wolfram syndrome. Dev Med Child Neurol. 2019;61: 359–65.
95. Majander A, Bitner-Glindzicz M, Chan CM, Duncan HJ, Chinnery PF, Subash M, Keane PA, Webster AR, Moore AT, Michaelides M, Yu-Wai-Man P. Lamination of the outer plexiform layer in optic atrophy caused by dominant WFS1 mutations. Ophthalmology. 2016;123(7):1624–6.
96. Zmyslowska A, Fendler W, Waszczykowska A, Niwald A, Borowiec M, Jurowski P, Mlynarski W. Retinal thickness as a marker of disease progression in longitudinal observation of patients with Wolfram syndrome. Acta Diabetol. 2017;54(11):1019–24.
97. Bouhlal Y, Amouri R, El Euch-Fayeche G, Hentati F. Autosomal recessive spastic ataxia of Charlevoix-Saguenay: an overview. Parkinsonism Relat Disord. 2011;17:418–22.
98. Berciano J, García A, Infante J. Peripheral nerve involvement in hereditary cerebellar and multisystem degenerative disorders. Handb Clin Neurol. 2013;115:907–32.
99. Duquette A, Brais B, Bouchard JP, Mathieu J. Clinical presentation and early evolution of spastic ataxia of Charlevoix-Saguenay. Mov Disord. 2013;28:2011–4.
100. Baets J, Deconinck T, Smets K, Goossens D, Van den Bergh P, Dahan K, et al. Mutations in SACS cause atypical and late-onset forms of ARSACS. Neurology. 2010 28;75:1181–8.
101. Bouchard JP, Barbeau A, Bouchard R, Bouchard RW. Autosomal recessive spastic ataxia of Charlevoix-Saguenay. Can J Neurol Sci. 1978;5:61e9.
102. De Braekeleer M, Giasson F, Mathieu J, Roy M, Bouchard JP, Morgan K. Genetic epidemiology of autosomal recessive spastic ataxia of Charlevoixe-Saguenay in northeastern Quebec. Genet Epidemiol. 1993;10:17e25.
103. Engert JC, Bérubé P, Mercier J, Doré C, Lepage P, Ge B, Bouchard JP, Mathieu J, et al. ARSACS, a spastic ataxia common in northeastern Québec, is caused by mutations in a new gene encoding an 11.5-kb ORF. Nat Genet. 2000;24:120e5.
104. Cheetham ME, Caplan AJ. Structure, function and evolution of DnaJ: conservation and adaptation of chaperone function. Cell Stress Chaperones. 1998;3:28e36.
105. Parfitt DA, Michael GJ, Vermeulen EG, Prodromou NV, Webb TR, Gallo JM, et al. The ataxia protein sacsin is a functional co-chaperone that protects against polyglutamine-expanded ataxin-1. Hum Mol Genet. 2009;18:1556e65.
106. Girard M, Larivière R, Parfitt DA, Deane EC, Gaudet R, Nossova N, et al. Mitochondrial dysfunction and Purkinje cell loss in autosomal recessive spastic ataxia of Charlevoix-Saguenay (ARSACS). Proc Natl Acad Sci U S A. 2012;109:1661–6.
107. El Euch-Fayache G, Lalani I, Amouri R, Turki I, Ouahchi K, Hung WY, et al. Phenotypic features and genetic findings in sacsin-related autosomal recessive ataxia in Tunisia. Arch Neurol. 2003;60:982e8.
108. Grieco GS, Malandrini A, Comanducci G, Leuzzi V, Valoppi M, Tessa A, et al. Novel SACS mutations in autosomal recessive spastic ataxia of Charlevoixe-Saguenay type. Neurology. 2004;62:103e6.
109. Criscuolo C, Banfi S, Orio M, Gasparini P, Monticelli A, Scarano V, et al. A novel mutation in SACS gene in a family from southern Italy. Neurology. 2004;62:100e2.
110. Takiyama Y. Autosomal recessive spastic ataxia of Charlevoixe-Saguenay. Neuropathology. 2006;26:368e75.
111. Bouhlal Y, Zouari M, Kefi M, Ben Hamida C, Hentati F, Amouri R. Autosomal recessive ataxia caused by three distinct gene defects in a single consanguineous family. J Neurogenet. 2008;22:139e48.
112. Vermeer S, Meijer RP, Pijl BJ, Timmermans J, Cruysberg JR, Bos MM, et al. ARSACS in the Dutch population: a frequent cause of early-onset cerebellar ataxia. Neurogenetics. 2008;10:87.
113. Bouhlal Y, El Euch-Fayeche G, Hentati F, Amouri R. A novel SACS gene mutation in a Tunisian family. J Mol Neurosci. 2009;39:333e6.
114. Takiyama Y. Sacsinopathies: sacsin-related ataxia. Cerebellum. 2007;6:353–9.

115. Vingolo EM, Di Fabio R, Salvatore S, Greco G, Bertini E, Lezzi V, et al. Myelinated retinal fibers in autosomal recessive spastic ataxia of Charlevoix-Saguenay. Eur J Neurol. 2011;18:1187–90.
116. Pablo LE, Garcia-Martin E, Gazulla J, Larrosa JM, Ferreras A, Santorelli FM, et al. Retinal nerve fiber hypertrophy in ataxia of Charlevoix-Saguenay patients. Mol Vis. 2011;17:1871–6.
117. Desserre J, Devos D, Sautière BG, Debruyne P, Santorelli FM, Vuillaume I, et al. Thickening of peripapillar retinal fibers for the diagnosis of autosomal recessive spastic ataxia of Charlevoix-Saguenay. Cerebellum. 2011;10:758–62.
118. Shah CT, Ward TS, Matsumoto JA, et al. Foveal hypoplasia in autosomal recessive spastic ataxia of Charlevoix-Saguenay. J AAPOS. 2016;20(1):81–3.
119. Parkinson MH, Bartmann AP, Clayton LMS, et al. Optical coherence tomography in autosomal recessive spastic ataxia of Charlevoix-Saguenay. Brain. 2018;141(4):989–99.
120. Gazulla J, Benavente I, Vela AC, Marín MA, Pablo LE, Tessa A, Barrena MR, et al. New findings in the ataxia of Charlevoix-Saguenay. J Neurol. 2012;259:869–78.
121. Van Lint M, Hoornaert K, Ten Tusscher MPM. Retinal nerve fiber layer thickening in ARSACS carriers. J Neurol Sci. 2016;370:119–22.
122. Yu-Wai-Man P, Pyle A, Griffin H, Santibanez-Korev M, Chinnery PF. Abnormal retinal thickening is a common feature among patients with ARSACS-related phenotypes. Br J Ophthalmol. 2014;98:711–3.
123. Koeppen AH. The pathogenesis of spinocerebellar ataxia. Cerebellum. 2005;4:62–73.
124. Durr A. Autosomal dominant cerebellar ataxias: polyglutamine expansions and beyond. Lancet Neurol. 2010;9:885–94.
125. Mudwiler A, Shakkottai VG. Autosomal-dominant cerebellar ataxias. Handb Clin Neurol. 2018;147:173–85.
126. Pula JH, Gomez CM, Kattah JC. Ophthalmologic features of the common spinocerebellar ataxias. Curr Opin Ophthalmol. 2010;21:447–53.
127. Newman NJ, Biousse V. Hereditary optic neuropathies. Eye. 2004;18(11):1144–60.
128. Rufa A, Dotti MT, Galli L, Orrico A, Sicurelli F, Federico A. Spinocerebellar ataxia type 2 (SCA2) associated with retinal pigmentary degeneration. Eur Neurol. 2002;47:128–9.
129. Fukutake T, Kamitsukasa I, Arai K, Hattori T, Nakajima T. A patient homozygous for the SCA6 gene with retinitis pigmentosa. Clin Genet. 2002;61:375–9.
130. Aleman TS, Cideciyan AV, Volpe NJ, Stevanin G, Brice A, Jacobson SG. Spinocerebellar ataxia type 7 (SCA7) shows a cone-rod dystrophy phenotype. Exp Eye Res. 2002;74:737–45.
131. Abe T, Tsuda T, Yoshida M, Wada Y, Kano T, Itoyama Y, et al. Macular degeneration associated with aberrant expansion of trinucleotide repeat of the SCA7 gene in 2 Japanese families. Arch Ophthalmol. 2000;118:1415–21.
132. Pula JH, Towle VL, Staszak VM, Cao D, Bernard JT, Gomez CM. Retinal nerve fibre layer and macular thinning in spinocerebellar ataxia and cerebellar multisystem atrophy. Neuroophthalmology. 2011;35(3):108–14.
133. Alvarez G, Rey A, Sanchez-Dalmau FB, Muñoz E, Ríos J, Adán A. Optical coherence tomography findings in spinocerebellar ataxia-3. Eye. 2013;27:1376–81.
134. Schöls L, Bauer P, Schmidt T, Schulte T, Riess O. Autosomal dominant cerebellar ataxias: clinical features, genetics, and pathogenesis. Lancet Neurol. 2004;3:291–304.
135. Lebranchu P, Le Meur G, Magot A, David A, Verny C, Weber M, et al. Maculopathy and spinocerebellar ataxia type 1: a new association? J Neuroophthalmol. 2013;33:225–31.
136. Vaclavik V, Borruat FX, Ambresin A, Munier FL. Novel maculopathy in patients with spinocerebellar ataxia type 1 autofluorescence findings and functional characteristics. JAMA Ophthalmol. 2013;131:536–8.
137. Abe T, Abe K, Tsuda T, Itoyama Y, Tamai M. Ophthalmological findings in patients with spinocerebellar ataxia type 1 are not correlated with neurological anticipation. Graefes Arch Clin Exp Ophthalmol. 2001;239:722–8.
138. Abe T, Abe K, Aoki M, Itoyama Y, Tamai M. Ocular changes in patients with spinocerebellar degeneration and repeated trinucleotide expansion of spinocerebellar ataxia type 1 gene. Arch Ophthalmol. 1997;115:231–6.

139. Abele M, Bürk K, Andres F, Topka H, Laccone F, Bösch S, et al. Autosomal dominant cerebellar ataxia type I. Nerve conduction and evoked potential studies in families with SCA1, SCA2 and SCA3. Brain. 1997;120:2141–8.
140. Perretti A, Santoro L, Lanzillo B, Filla A, De Michele G, Barbieri F, et al. Autosomal dominant cerebellar ataxia type I: multimodal electrophysiological study and comparison between SCA1 and SCA2 patients. J Neurol Sci. 1996;142:45–53.
141. Robitaille Y, Schut L, Kish SJ. Structural and immunocytochemical features of olivopontocerebellar atrophy caused by the spinocerebellar ataxia type 1 (SCA-1) mutation define a unique phenotype. Acta Neuropathol. 1995;90:572–81.
142. Stricker S, Oberwahrenbrock T, Zimmermann H, Schroeter J, Endres M, Brandt AU, et al. Temporal retinal nerve fiber loss in patients with spinocerebellar ataxia type 1. PLoS One. 2011;6:e23024.
143. Varsányi B, Somfai GM, Lesch B, Vámos R, Farkas A, et al. Optical coherence tomography of the macula in congenital achromatopsia. Invest Ophthalmol Vis Sci. 2007;48:2249–53.
144. Birch DG, Wen Y, Locke K, Hood DC. Rod sensitivity, cone sensitivity, and photoreceptor layer thickness in retinal degenerative diseases. Invest Ophthalmol Vis Sci. 2011;52:7141–7.
145. Aleman TS, Cideciyan AV, Volpe NJ, Stevanin G, Brice A, Jacobson SG. Spinocerebellar ataxia type 7 (SCA7) shows a cone-rod dystrophy phenotype. Exp Eye Res. 2002;74:737e45.
146. Gouw LG, Digre KB, Harris CP, Haines JH, Ptacek LJ. Autosomal dominant cerebellar ataxia with retinal degeneration: clinical, neuropathologic, and genetic analysis of a large kindred. Neurology. 1994;44:1441–7.
147. Cancel G, Duyckaerts C, Holmberg M, Zander C, Yvert G, Lebre AS, et al. Distribution of ataxin-7 in normal human brain and retina. Brain. 2000;123:2519–30.
148. La Spada AR, Fu Y, Sopher BL, Libby RT, Wang X, Li LY, et al. Polyglutamine-expanded ataxin-7 antagonizes CRX function and induces cone-rod dystrophy in a mouse model of SCA7. Neuron. 2001;31:913–27.
149. Kumar N, Pulido JS. High-definition spectral domain optical coherence tomography in the evaluation of ataxia with visual impairment. Br J Ophthalmol. 2011;95:591–8.
150. Manrique RK, Noval S, Aguilar-Amat MJ, Arpa J, Rosa I, Contreras I. Ophthalmic features of spinocerebellar ataxia type 7. J Neuroophthalmol. 2009;29:174–9.
151. Ahn JK, Seo JM, Chung H, Yu HG. Anatomical and functional characteristics in atrophic maculopathy associated with spinocerebellar ataxia type 7. Am J Ophthalmol. 2005;139:923–5.
152. McLaughlin ME. Dryja TP ocular findings in spinocerebellar ataxia 7. Arch Ophthalmol. 2002;120:655–9.
153. Levinson JD, Yan J, Lambert SR, Shankar SP. Multimodal imaging of a family with spinocerebellar ataxia type 7 demonstrating phenotypic variation and progression of retinal degeneration. Retin Cases Brief Rep. 2016;10(3):267–72.
154. Teive HAG, Munhoz RP, Arruda WO, et al. Spinocerebellar ataxia type 10 - a review. Parkinsonism Relat Disord. 2011;17:655–61.
155. Spina Tensini F, Sato MT, Shiokawa N, Ashizawa T, Teive HAG. A comparative optical coherence tomography study of spinocerebellar ataxia types 3 and 10. Cerebellum. 2017;16(4):797–801.
156. Gowrisankaran S, Anastasakis A, Fishman GA, Alexander KR. Structural and Functional Measures of Inner Retinal Integrity Following Visual Acuity Improvement in a Patient with Hereditary Motor and Sensory Neuropathy Type VI. Ophthalmic Genetics 2011;32 (3):188–92.
157. Grainger BT, Papchenko TL, Danesh-Meyer HV. Optic nerve atrophy in adrenoleukodystrophy detectable by optic coherence tomography. J Clini Neurosci. 2010;17(1):122–4.

Other Neurological Disorders: Migraine, Neurosarcoidosis, Schizophrenia, Obstructive Sleep Apnea-Hypopnea Syndrome and Bipolar Disorder

15

Francisco J. Ascaso, Javier Mateo, Laura Cabezón, Paula Casas, and Andrzej Grzybowski

15.1 Optical Coherence Tomography in Migraine Patients

Migraine, one of the most frequent debilitating disorders in the world [1], is a chronic and episodic neurovascular disease presenting with recurrent attacks of typically unilateral, moderate-to severe headaches which produce significant dysfunction [2, 3]. The prevalence of chronic migraine ranges between 1 and 3% of the general population [4]. The pain is generally aggravated by physical activity and is often associated with a number of autonomic nervous system symptoms, such as nausea and vomiting [5]. There are two types of migraine: migraine with aura (MwA), namely classic migraine, and migraine without aura (MwoA) or common migraine [6]. The MwA is a combination of focal neurological disturbances which are seen prior to, during, and rarely following an attack [7]. It usually lasts for less

F. J. Ascaso
Department of Ophthalmology, Hospital Clínico Universitario "Lozano Blesa", Zaragoza, Spain

School of Medicine, University of Zaragoza, Zaragoza, Spain

Aragon Health Research Institute (IIS Aragon), Zaragoza, Spain

J. Mateo · P. Casas
Department of Ophthalmology, Hospital Clínico Universitario "Lozano Blesa", Zaragoza, Spain

Aragon Health Research Institute (IIS Aragon), Zaragoza, Spain

L. Cabezón
Department of Ophthalmology, Hospital Clínico Universitario "Lozano Blesa", Zaragoza, Spain

A. Grzybowski (✉)
University of Warmia and Mazury, Olsztyn, Poland

Institute for Research in Ophthalmology, Poznań, Poland

A. Grzybowski, P. Barboni (eds.), *OCT and Imaging in Central Nervous System Diseases*, https://doi.org/10.1007/978-3-030-26269-3_15

than 1 h. In up to one-third of migraneurs the headache is preceded by transient neurological and sensory symptoms, most frequently visual [8]. Accompanying ocular symptoms may include periorbital pain, photophobia, or other visual complaints. Because of this, ophthalmologists are usually the first doctors to evaluate migraine patients. Furthermore, migraine is a well-known risk factor for developing glaucoma [9].

Although its pathophysiology is not completely understood [10, 11], migraine is a multifactorial syndrome precipitated by intrinsic or extrinsic factors in individuals with a genetic predisposition [12]. Several mechanisms have been proposed, including the vasogenic, neurogenic, hormonal and genetic hypotheses [12–14]. A prolonged vasospasm in the occipital hemisphere followed by vasodilation, detected by transcranial Doppler ultrasound in migraine patients, is the most accepted theory in the explanation of migraine attacks with visual aura [1, 8, 15]. In certain patients, the reduction in brain blood flow secondary to cerebral vasospasm has been shown to start from other parts of brain or even in tissues located outside the brain, especially in the retina [16–18]. Ocular blood flow can be estimated by colour duplex imaging, Doppler flowmetry and laser speckle contrast imaging. Improvements in optical coherence tomography (OCT) software, like the "enhanced depth imaging OCT" (EDI-OCT), have provided the method to explore the choroidal structure [5]. Besides an increased risk for ischemic stroke [19, 20], local infarctions caused by retinal artery occlusions have been reported in migraine patients with aura [16, 17]. Moreover, in chronic migraine, the altered perfusion in retinal microcirculation would cause ganglion cell death, leading to permanent structural abnormalities of the retina [10].

OCT is a relatively recent, reliable, reproducible, noninvasive, noncontact in vivo imaging technique similar to ultrasonography except that it uses infrared wavelengths of 820 nm and has a sensitivity of 8–10 μm. Numerous studies have demonstrated a thinning in retinal nerve fiber layer (RNFL) measurements in neurodegenerative disorders such as multiple sclerosis, Alzheimer's disease, and Parkinson's disease [21–24].

OCT has been used as an imaging technique for evaluating the RNFL, ganglion cell layer (GCL), and choroid in various neuro-ophthalmological disorders [25]. Thus, the peripapillary RNFL thickness can be used as a biomarker to assess GCL and RNFL alterations [6]. Moreover, the new-generation spectral domain OCT (SD-OCT) devices use special software techniques, such as EDI program, to acquire high-resolution OCT images and effectively evaluate the choroidal thickness [26, 27].

A few studies have investigated the RNFL thickness in patients who have migraine with and without aura by using scanning laser polarimetry [10, 11, 28, 29]. Thus, Tan et al. did not find differences in RNFL thickness between patients with migraine and healthy controls [10]. On the contrary, Martínez et al., with the same imaging technique, suggested a significant difference between the migraine patients with aura and those without aura [28]. There are also numerous studies with OCT on the thickness of the RNFL, macula, and choroid in migraine patients and the results show certain discrepancies (Table 15.1). In this sense, Martínez et al.

Table 15.1 Published studies on optical coherence tomography (OCT) in migraine patients

Author (year)	No. migraine patients/HC	OCT type	OCT measurements	Type of study	Results
Martínez et al. (2008) [10]	70/53	TD-OCT	RNFL thickness	Case-control	Thinner RNFL in the temporal sector in migraine patients. Migraine severity is associated with RNFL measurements
Sorkhabi et al. (2013) [6]	60/30	TD-OCT	RNFL thickness	Case-control	RNFL thinner in nasal quadrant in migraineurs
Kirbas et al. (2013) [2]	49 CM/40 HC	SD-OCT	RNFL and FT	Case-control	Superior quadrant RNFL thickness was thinner in CM patients. No macular changes in CM
Gipponi et al. (2013) [29]	24/16	SD-OCT	RNFL thickness	Case-control	Reduced RNFL thickness in the superior retinal quadrant in migraine patients. No influence of illness duration or frequency. No changes in macular parameters were found
Ekinci et al. (2014) [7]	90 (45 MwA, 45 MwoA)/30	SD-OCT	RNFL, GCL, and CT	Case-control	Reduced RNFL, GCL, and CT in individuals with MwA
Yülek et al. (2015) [30]	50 (30 MwA, 20 MwoA)/50	SD-OCT	RNFL, GCL, and FT	Case-control	Average RNFL thickness in migraine patients thinner than in HC. No correlation between length of migraine history and RNFL thickness
Demircan et al. (2015) [31]	76 (36 MwA, 40 MwoA)/38	SD-OCT	RNFL and CT	Case-control	Decreased thickness of RNFL in nasal sectors and foveal CT in migraineurs. Macular and choroidal thicknesses were not significantly different between the MwA and MwoA subgroups
Simsek (2016) [32]	40 (with and without WML)/40	SD-OCT	RNFL, GCL, and CT	Case-control	Diminished RNFL thickness in migraine patients with WML

(continued)

Table 15.1 (continued)

Author (year)	No. migraine patients/HC	OCT type	OCT measurements	Type of study	Results
Gunes et al. (2016) [33]	58/58	SD-OCT	RNFL	Case-control	Thinner RNFL thickness on the side of headache and on the contralateral side compared with control eyes
Colak et al. (2016) [34]	45/45	SD-OCT	RNFL, GCL, and CT	Case-control	Reduced RNFL in the superior and inferior quadrants of migraineurs compared to HC. Subfoveal, temporal, and nasal CT lower in the migraine group than in HC
Feng et al. (2016) [35]	432/281	SD-OCT	RNFL	Meta-analysis	Decreased RNFL thickness in the migraine patients
Cankaya and Tecellioglu (2016) [36]	39 (28 MwA, 40 MwA)/40	SD-OCT	RNFL	Case-control	Reduced FT values in MwA
Reggio et al. (2017) [37]	72 (12 MwA, 21 MwoA, 44 CM)/42	SD-OCT	RNFL, GCL, FT, CT, and TMV	Case-control	Thinner RNFL, GCL and CT in migraineurs, especially in CM. RNFL thickness is inversely associated with the frequency of migraine attacks
Acer et al. (2017) [38]	38 MwoA/44	SD-OCT	RNFL, GCL, and FT	Case-control	Sectorial RNFL thinning in MwoA patients. No significant changes in the macular area in MwoA
El-Shazly et al. (2017) [40]	60/30	SD-OCT	RNFL	Case-control	RNFL thickness thinner in patients during the aura compared to controls. It increased significantly post-aura but remained lower than the controls
Chang et al. (2017) [43]	27 (15 MwA, 12 MwoA)/22	OCTA	FAZ area and vessel density	Case-control	Enlarged FAZ area in migraineurs when compared with HC. Superficial foveal vessel density was decreased in MwA patients when compared with MwoA participants and HC

Table 15.1 (continued)

Author (year)	No. migraine patients/HC	OCT type	OCT measurements	Type of study	Results
Tunç et al. (2017) [44]	60 (19 MwA, 41 MwoA)/60		RNFL, GCL and macular changes	Case-control	There were significant differences between MwA and HC regarding average, superior and inferior quadrant RNLF thickness. There were significant differences between MwoA and the HC regarding average and inferior faces
Nalcacioglu et al. (2017) [56]	40/40	SD-OCT	RNFL, GCL, IPL, FT, and CT	Case-control	FT, GCL, IPL, peripapillary RNFL, and CT were not significantly different during an attack-free period in pediatric migraine patients than in healthy subjects
Gunes et al. (2018) [39]	47/34	SD-OCT	RNFL, GCL, and CT	Case-control	CM has no effect on RNFL thickness. Increases in CT and decreases in GCL thickness were observed in migraine patients
Tak et al. (2018) [41]	77 CM (39 with WML and 38 without WML)/43 HC	SD-OCT	RNFL, GCL, IPL, and CT	Case control	Thinner RNFL in migraine patients. IPL, GCL, and CT were similar between patients and controls
Abdellatif and Fouad (2018) [42]	90/40	SD-OCT	RNFL, GCL, and CT	Case control	GCL, RNFL, and CT are significantly thinner in patients with migraine

CM chronic migraine, *MwA* migraine with aura, *MwoA* migraine without aura, *HC* healthy controls, *TD-OCT* time domain optical coherence tomography, *SD-OCT* spectral domain optical coherence tomography, *OCTA* optical coherence tomography angiography, *RNFL* retinal nerve fiber layer thickness, *GCL* ganglion cell layer thickness, *IPL* inner plexiform layer, *FT* foveal thickness, *TMV* total macular volume, *CT* choroidal thickness, *FAZ* foveal avascular zone, *WML* white matter lesions detected using magnetic resonance imaging

evaluated 70 patients with migraine and 53 controls by using OCT. The mean RNFL thickness in migraineurs was similar to that of controls, but RNFL thickness in temporal quadrant was thinner in patients compared to normal people [10]. Gipponi et al. found no significant differences in foveal thickness and total macular volume in female migraine patients compared to healthy women, but demonstrated a significant thinning in the RNFL thickness in the superior quadrant in the female migraine patients [29]. However, they did not classify the patients according to the presence of aura. Sorkhabi et al. demonstrated that nasal quadrant RNFL thickness was significantly thinner in migraine patients compared with that of age-matched healthy individuals [6]. Ekinci et al. detected a thinning of the RNFL and GCL only in patients who had MwA [7]. According to these authors, the RNFL thinning would be secondary to the neurodegenerative changes in the central nervous system (CNS) after ischemia in the migraine patients with aura. Yulek et al. [30] found an average RNFL thickness in migraine patients thinner than in healthy controls, but no relationship between length of migraine history and RNFL thickness. Demircan et al. [31] observed decreased thickness of RNFL in nasal sectors and foveal choroidal thickness in migraineurs. Macular and choroidal thicknesses were not significantly different between the MwA and MwoA subgroups. Using magnetic resonance imaging, Simsek [32] observed that in migraine patients with white matter lesions (WML), RNFL was thinner than in controls and migraine patients with no WML. Further research should analyze the relationship between brain WML and retinal damage to clarify whether there is a common pathogenic mechanism. A thinner RNFL thickness was reported by Gunes et al. [33] on the side of headache and on the contralateral side compared with control eyes. Colak et al. [34] described a reduced RNFL in the superior and inferior quadrants of migraineurs compared to controls. Subfoveal, temporal, and nasal choroidal thickness was lower in the migraine group than in healthy subjects. Feng et al. [35] reported significant changes in RNFL based on the length of the history of migraine. Thus, mean RNFL thickness was decreased when migraine history was longer than 15 years. While controversial, this finding could be associated with glaucoma. Cankaya and Tecellioglu [36] found reduced foveal thickness in MwA. Thinner RNFL, GCL and choroidal thickness in migraineurs, especially in chronic migraine were reported by Reggio et al. [37]. Moreover, according to these authors, RNFL thickness is inversely associated with the frequency of migraine attacks. Acer et al. [38] observed a sectorial RNFL thinning but no significant changes in the macular area in MwoA. Recently, Gunes et al. [39] found migraine to be correlated with GCL and choroidal thickness. Nevertheless, chronic migraine did not have any effect on peripapillary RNFL thickness. According to El-Shazly et al. [40], migraine attacks impose both functional and structural retinal changes. Thus, RNFL thickness was found to be thinner in patients during the aura compared with controls. It increased significantly post-aura but remained lower than the controls. Therefore, structural changes are not fully reversible after the aura and vigorous prevention of migraine attacks would protect the retina. Tak et al. [41] reported thinner RNFL in migraine patients when they compared with controls but inner plexiform layer (IPL), GCL, and choroid layer values were similar. Also, all parameters were similar between patients with or without WML. Abdellatif and Fouad [42] concluded that GCL, RNFL, and choroidal thickness are significantly thinner in patients with migraine. However, whereas the severity of migraine has more significant influence in the thinning of GCL and RNFL, the duration of the disease affected the choroidal thickness more. Chang et al. [43] used optical coherence tomography angiography (OCTA) to assess perfusion of the macula and optic nerve in migraine patients. They observed that migraine with, but not without, aura was associated with foveal and peripapillary vascular decrements, which may possibly mediate increased risk of ocular and systemic vascular complications in these patients. OCTA could potentially be useful as a biomarker for MwA. Tunç et al. [44] found significant differences between MwA and healthy individuals regarding average, superior and inferior quadrant RNLF thickness. They also found significant differences between MwoA and the controls regarding average and inferior faces.

The choroid is the vascular compartment of the eye and is directly influenced by intraocular and perfusion pressures [5]. It supplies oxygen and nutrients to the outer retina [7]. The major blood supply to the retina is the choroid, especially in darkness, where 90% of the oxygen comes from choroidal circulation [45]. In term of accuracy of measuring choroidal thickness, SD-OCT is even better than histology, as this cannot estimate the thickness of the living choroid [46]. Nevertheless, although it is not clear the relationship between choroidal thickness and choroidal blood flow and further prospective studies are required to clarify it, changes in choroidal thickness were recently described as a consequence of the vasodilatory effect on choroidal circulation of certain drugs, including sildenafil and cigarette smoking [47, 48]. Likewise, choroidal thickness has been reported to be reduced in high myopia, retinal dystrophy and age-related choroidal atrophy, whereas increased choroidal thickness was reported in Vogt-Koyanagi-Harada disease and central serous chorioretinopathy [48–50]. According to the above-mentioned articles, migraine seems to be a neurovascular disorder in which there is a reduction in the central retinal artery and posterior ciliary artery blood flow; the choroidal thinning would be an expected clinical outcome in patients with migraine. Likewise, a thinning of the choroidal layer is observed in migraine patients both with aura and without aura [7]. Dadaci et al. were the first authors to estimate the changes in the choroidal thickness during the attack episode in migraine patients using EDI-OCT [3]. They observed a significant increase in the choroidal thickness during the migraine attack. Ekinci et al. reported a significant thinning of the RNLF, GCL and choroid in migraine patients with aura, but no significant differences in RNFL and GCL measurements between migraine patients without aura and healthy individuals [7]. Zengin et al. [5] evaluated choroidal thickness by using SD-OCT in patients who had migraine and compared the results with healthy subjects. To avoid the possible effects of systemic drugs, only recently diagnosed migraine patients who were not using any medication and were non-smokers were included. The difference in choroidal thickness between migraineurs (276.8 ± 37.8 μm) and controls (300.4 ± 24.9 μm) was significant ($p = 0.001$). Although it is not easy to obtain OCT images during a painful episode, an acute decrease in choroidal thickness of approximately 45 μm was reported during the attack period when compared to basal levels in a group of five patients [5]. Nevertheless, there was no correlation between severity and type of migraine with choroidal thickness. This decrease in mean choroidal thickness may be related to the vasogenic etiology of migraine. Autonomic nervous system dysfunctions are often reported in migraine patients and related to trigeminovascular pain pathway activation. They are commonly ipsilateral to the headache and provide another explanation for the increased choroidal thickness during the migraine attack [51–53]. The reproducibility of this technique is high, although the relatively long duration of manual measuring of choroidal thickness (5 min per scan), may lead to observe fatigue and increase the possibility of false measurements [54]. Furthermore, it has been suggested that menstrual cycle and pregnancy status of the female participants, smoking, alcohol consumption, drinking caffeinated beverages, body mass index, systemic blood pressure, and environmental lighting conditions, which significantly affect choroidal thickness, should be addressed in these studies [55].

Nalcacioglu et al. [56] found that total macular thickness, GCL, IPL, peripapillary RNFL, and choroidal thickness were not significantly different during an attack-free period in pediatric migraine patients than in healthy subjects.

In conclusion, although several factors should be considered, it is important to underline that peripapillary RNFL thickness and choroidal thickness measurement by using SD-OCT could be a new interesting method to evaluate the migraine patients, identifying localized neuronal loss.

15.2 Optical Coherence Tomography in Neurosarcoidosis

Sarcoidosis is a granulomatous disease of unknown origin that can affect most of the organs of the body; although the lungs, skin, lymph nodes—mainly thoracic—liver and the eyes, are more frequently affected. The non-caseating granulomas are formed by macrophages, epithelioid cells and lymphocytes, and can be found in different organs after an abnormal immune response [57, 58]. Its incidence is low in people from countries such as Japan or Spain (0.2–2 out of 100,000), but is very high in Scandinavian and African origin patients (5–82 out of 100,000). It usually appears before 50 years of age; however, the incidence is higher between 20 and 39 years [57–60].

Sarcoidosis is diagnosed after radiologic, clinical and histologic findings. Differential diagnosis includes other granulomatous diseases, lymphoma, adverse reactions to certain drugs or infections such as tuberculosis or fungal infections [59].

Although often asymptomatic, sarcoidosis can show various clinical signs, depending on the organs that are affected. Common symptoms include fatigue, weakness, asthenia, dry cough, dyspnea, weight loss, fever, erythema nodosum, joint pain, as well as the presence of lymph nodes and night sweating [58, 59].

Sarcoidosis can affect the CNS in 5% of cases, thus being called neurosarcoidosis [56, 61, 62]. Basal leptomeninges are usually affected, causing cranial polyneuropathies, aseptic meningitis, hydrocephalus and polyradiculopathy. Cranial neuropathies are also frequently present, mainly showing facial palsy, but also alteration of the cranial nerve VIII and, less commonly, nerves V, VI, IX and X. Other possible neurologic symptoms are seizures, fever, headaches or dysfunction of the hypothalamic-pituitary axis [61–63].

The most frequent ophthalmologic finding in sarcoidosis is anterior granulomatous uveitis with mutton-fat endothelial precipitates. Less common ocular manifestations include conjunctival nodules, dry eye, iris nodules, cataract, vitritis, intermediate uveitis with aggregates of inflammatory cells in the vitreous (snowballs), posterior segment uveitis with associated macular edema, epiretinal membrane, branch retinal vein occlusion, choroiditis and perivascular sheathing [57, 59, 64, 65]. Nevertheless, in neurosarcoidosis, even though anterior uveitis is still the most common alteration, other important signs that can be found include optic neuropathy, followed by cranial nerve involvement (mainly diplopia caused by common ocular motor nerve palsy) [66–69].

OCT, and especially SD-OCT, is an excellent noninvasive and noncontact technique, which can be very useful for studying the optic neuropathy present in some cases of neurosarcoidosis. As well as in other neurologic disorders, the measurement of the RNFL thickness can be used to detect structural damage of the optic nerve [21–24, 70]. Other way of studying the optic neuropathy would be the segmentation of the GCL in the macular area [71–73]. Macular thickness study is also important to evaluate the cystoid macular edema (CME), present in patients with sarcoidosis who develop posterior segment uveitis [57, 59] (Fig. 15.1). Likewise, choroidal structure can be studied with EDI-OCT, showing a thickening of the choroid during active posterior uveitis, mainly involving Sattler's medium-sized vessel layer, and a thinning of it during inactive phases [74–76].

Some articles have studied choroidal, retinal and optic nerve granulomas in sarcoidosis. They are described as hypo or hyperreflective homogeneous choroidal thickening with thinning of the overlying choriocapillaris and intrarretinal hyperreflective inflammatory lesions. Following treatment with corticosteroids, the granulomas significantly decreased their size or even disappeared and, sometimes, subretinal fibrosis and alterations of outer retina and choroid appeared [77–88].

A few case reports of CME in patients with posterior uveitis or panuveitis and sarcoidosis can also be found. In these cases, OCT helped to make the diagnosis of sarcoidosis and to make a detailed study of the macular edema and its favorable evolution following therapy [89–91].

As in other neurologic diseases, OCT can demonstrate alteration of the optic nerve in sarcoidosis. Peripapillary abnormalities of the RNFL could be detected

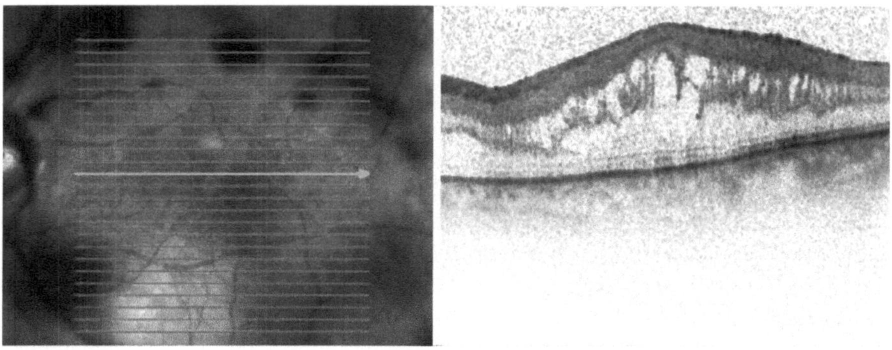

Fig. 15.1 Spectral-domain OCT showing a macular edema in a patient with sarcoidosis

and, even when the patients showed no ophthalmologic clinical signs, the RNFL was thinner when compared with healthy controls, likely being a consequence of previous optic neuropathy. Macular thickness had decreased in numerous patients, probably as a result of neuropathy and/or repeated CME in uveitis. Increased RNFL thickness was found in some patients, probably as a manifestation of optic neuritis [91].

Recently, OCTA has shown to be a very useful complementary examination to fluorescein angiography in patients with ocular sarcoidosis. This technique evaluates the superficial and deep capillary plexuses in the fovea, as well as the choriocapillaris. It shows that the capillary vessels density in the fovea is below normal in eyes affected by sarcoidosis. Other alterations found include capillary dropout and hypoperfusion usually in the superficial plexus, and capillary abnormalities most frequently in the deep plexus [92, 93].

OCT and its features, including OCTA, EDI-OCT and GCL segmentation, has become an essential part of the ophthalmological examination in disorders like sarcoidosis, that can affect the optic nerve, the retina and the choroid. It can detect abnormalities in these structures, even if the patient has shown no ophthalmologic symptoms, being also very useful for the follow-up of the disease and its response to the treatment.

15.3 Optical Coherence Tomography in Schizophrenic Patients

Schizophrenia is a devastating mental condition which involves one of the most important psychiatric disorders from the viewpoint of public health [94]. The course of the disease is often chronic and highly variable, causing a great loss of quality of life of patients and their families, as well as a high cost to society. Only in the US up to two million people are affected by this disease [95].

Schizophrenia is a clinical syndrome with a variable psychopathology that affects cognition, emotion, perception, and other aspects of human behavior. The expression of these manifestations is different in each patient and varies with time [96, 97]. However, schizophrenia lacks a clearly defined or diagnostic neuropathological signature and its etiology remains poorly understood. The diagnosis of schizophrenia is still based on clinical history and symptoms observed and reported by the patient [98, 99].

The best validated neuropathological abnormalities include possible reductions of neuronal density in the thalamus, reductions in the number of some interneurons and in the number and function of oligodendrocytes [100]. Neuroimaging techniques such as structural magnetic resonance imaging (sMRI) and functional magnetic resonance imaging (fMRI) have been extensively studied in recent years aiming at developing new diagnostic biomarkers for schizophrenia. These studies have been very important to try to understand the biological substrate of the disease. The most striking abnormal findings include white and gray matter abnormalities [101–103]. Nevertheless, it is difficult to establish solid conclusions regarding the precise neuropathological changes that underlie these neuroimaging findings [104, 105].

One of the difficulties in measuring brain volumes in schizophrenic patients with MRI is that the volumetric loss is less than 4% per year, which may be near the limit of detection by MRI, known the precision of the volumetric methods [106, 107]. In the search for new biomarkers in schizophrenia, which may be obtained quickly, non-invasively and with less cost than MRI, lie the observable changes in the retina, as this through the optic nerve is not more than a projection of CNS. Jindahra et al. [108] reviewed the utility of OCT in clinical practice of neurological diseases such as multiple sclerosis, neuromyelitis, Alzheimer's disease and Parkinson's disease. The decrease of RGCs observed in these disorders can reflect degenerative changes in the brain. Therefore, they proposed RNFL thickness as a biological marker in these disorders. Similarly, it was thought that measurement of macular thickness and volume by OCT could reflect neuronal cell bodies and allow to quantify the neuronal loss [109].

In 2010, we published the first preliminary study relating the schizophrenic disease with RNFL thickness changes measured by OCT [110]. This study showed that patients with schizophrenia have a decreased peripapillary RNFL thickness. This reduction was statistically significant, both in terms of value average (in all four quadrants) RNFL thickness as in relation to nasal quadrant (Fig. 15.2).

Posterior studies have supported these findings, Yilmaz et al. reported a reduction in average and nasal RNFL thicknesses in schizophrenic patients, as well as macular thicknesses of nasal outer and inferior outer quadrants [111].

A similar research has been carried out by Chu et al. in patients with schizophrenia [112]. In this study, which included 38 patients with schizophrenia and 11 patients with schizo-affective disorder, no statistically significant differences were found in the RNFL thickness globally and individually in each of its quadrants between

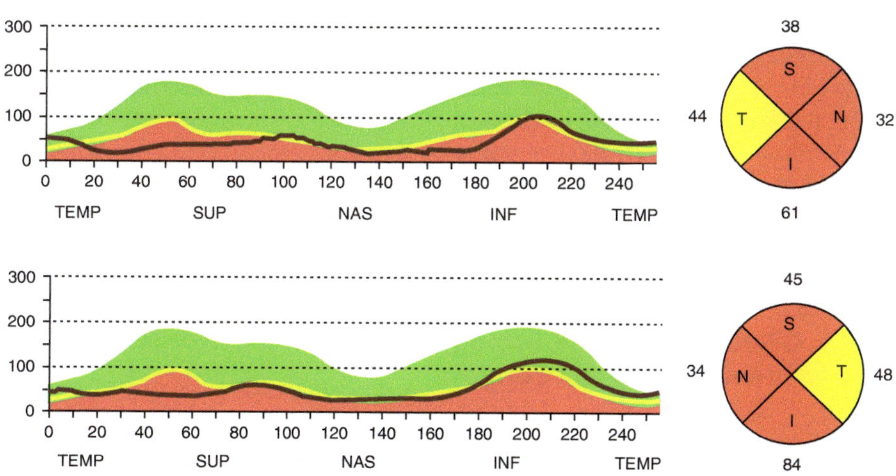

Fig. 15.2 OCT showing decreased peripapillary RNFL thickness specifically in nasal quadrant in a patient with schizophrenia

healthy controls and patients. However, it was observed that patients with schizo-affective disorder had RNFL nasal quadrant thickness of the right eye statistically decreased than those patients with schizophrenia. This difference from the previous study may be due to these authors recruited patients with first episode of psychosis and included in their sample not only patients with schizophrenia, but also patients with schizo-affective disorder. Moreover, an inverse and significant association was found between the values of macular volume in patients with schizophrenia and schizo-affective disorder and the severity of positive symptomatology. Also, if the analysis took into account only the patients with schizophrenia this association between macular volume and severity of positive symptoms was stronger [112].

A posterior study that uses SD-OCT for retina segmentation reports that the GCL and IPL volumes were decreased in the patients with schizophrenia compared with the controls. In addition, the GCL and IPL volumes were lower in the treatment-refractory patients with schizophrenia compared to the treatment responsive patients. They found higher correlations of these two measurements with disease parameters than RNFL thickness [113].

Recently, Silverstein et al. refuted the "decreased RNFL in schizophrenic patients" approach, they concluded that thinning of RNFL, macula, or ganglion cell-inner plexiform layer may be artifacts of medical comorbidity that is over-represented in schizophrenia, as diabetes or hypertension [114].

Lee et al. reported that schizophrenic patients showed a statistically significant reduction in overall peripapillary RNFL thickness, macular thickness, as well as macular volume. Furthermore, the degree of thinning and reduction was more significant in the chronic phase of the disease and correlated with the duration of illness [115]. This correlation between illness duration and retinal measurements was not supported by Ascaso et al. [116]. However, they found reduced RNFL measurements only in patients with non-recent illness episodes.

Respect to choroidal thickness, there is just one small study in which six psychotic patients showed a decreased choroidal thickness compared to age- and sex-matched healthy controls [117].

There is still the controversy in schizophrenia in relation to neurodegenerative model, that begins at about the time of symptoms onset and manifests as progressive volumetric loss thereafter, and neurodevelopmental model that results in abnormal brain volume beginning at an early age [118], so that only longitudinal studies using OCT may help to clarify the underlying neurobiological processes in both models [119, 120].

15.4 Optical Coherence Tomography in Obstructive Sleep Apnea–Hypopnea Patients

Obstructive sleep apnea-hypopnea syndrome (OSAHS) is part of a broad group of disorders known as "sleep-related breathing disorders". OSAHS is characterized by brief episodes of complete or partial upper airway collapse during sleep, causing an increased thoraco-abdominal effort and decreased arterial oxygen saturation, leading to an arousal response which takes the form of apneas and periodic hypopneas during sleep [121]. This fact produces an excessive daytime sleepiness. Local and systemic inflammation play an important role in the pathogenesis of OSAHS, contributing to anatomic narrowing of the upper airway, increased collapsibility of the airway tissues, and abnormalities in reflexes that affect upper respiratory tract caliber and pharyngeal inspiratory muscle function [122]. In OSAHS, balance between vasodilators, such as nitric oxide, and vasoconstrictors such as endothelin, is disturbed [123]. As well as hypoxia-reoxygenation pattern contributes to the activation of sympathetic system [124]. Moreover, there is some evidence that OSAHS is a risk factor for neurovascular and cardiovascular diseases. Arterial hypertension, cardiac arrhythmia and/or ischemia, congestive heart failure, and cerebrovascular disease are events more likely in the presence of the obstructive sleep disturbance [125, 126].

Clinical features of OSAHS have inspired studies about brain structural abnormalities in this disease. MRI studies have reported a loss of gray and white matter in certain brain areas, suggesting a premature degeneration of CNS in patients suffering from OSAHS [127, 128].

In the last few years, multiple investigators have studied the relationship between the apneic syndrome and some ophthalmological disorders such as floppy eyelid syndrome [129–133], retinal vein occlusion [134], central serous chorioretinopathy [135–138], diabetic retinopathy [139, 140] and certain optic nerve dysfunctions. Thus, papilledema and increased intracranial pressure have been reported in OSAHS patients [141, 142], improving after continuous positive airway pressure (CPAP) treatment [143, 144]. It was postulated that non-arteritic anterior ischemic optic neuropathy has a higher incidence in patients with the apneic dysfunction [145]. Likewise, an increased frequency of normal and high tension glaucoma in patients with OSAHS was shown [146–153].

15.4.1 Peripapillary RNFL Findings in Apneic Disorder

The latest research reveals a diffuse loss of ganglion cells in the optic nerve of patients with apnea, without the characteristics of glaucomatous neuropathy, including generalized/focal enlargement of the cup, usually at superior and inferior poles, accompanied of visual field defects as nasal step, paracentral or arcuate scotomas, or arcuate blind spot enlargement [154]. Kargi et al. [155] published a diffuse loss of RNFL thickness measured with GDx polarimetry. Sagiv et al. [156] and Lin et al. [157] detected a decreased RNFL thickness in the superior, inferior and temporal quadrants compared with a control group. Reduction in the peripapillary RNFL thickness was also confirmed by Moghimi et al. [158] (with laser polarimetry GDX®), Lin et al. [159], Xin et al. [152], and Gutiérrez-Díaz [160]. Nevertheless, they did not exclude patients with glaucoma, what could have influenced their results. All these studies suggest a diffuse loss in the RNFL without any preferential location. On the other hand, Casas et al. [161] found a localized RNFL reduction in nasal sector of optic nerve in OSAHS patients (Fig. 15.3).

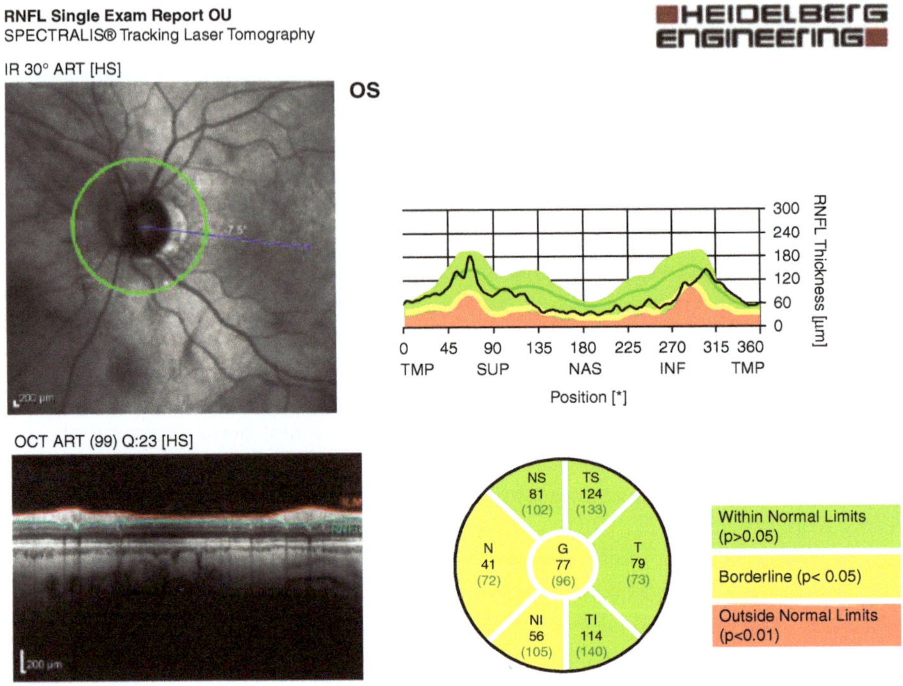

Fig. 15.3 Spectral-domain OCT showing a reduction of the peripapillary RNFL thickness in the nasal quadrant and nasal-inferior sector of the left eye in an OSAHS patient

Ozge et al. [162] and Yazgan et al. [163] found a diffuse decrease in RNFL of OSAHS patients, once glaucoma was excluded of the sample. Zengin et al. [164] described in OSAHS patients a progressive thinning of RNFL thickness, over 1 year-follow up, in spite using CPAP device. In addition, severe OSAHS patients showed a greater decrease of RNFL thickness compared with mild-moderate OSAHS and controls [157, 165]. Furthermore, certain studies have found a significant negative correlation between the RNFL thickness and apnea-hypopnea index (AHI) [155, 164–166].

Despite these promising impressions, opposing results have also been published. Thus, several authors have found no significant difference between OSAHS and controls regarding the average RNFL thickness [167–170]. Salzgeber et al. [171] found no differences in RNFL and optic nerve morphological parameters in their study with laser polarimetry GDX® and confocal laser scanning HRT II®. Yuvaci et al. [172] did not report any differences between OSAHS and controls, but they detected a reduction in RNFL after CPAP treatment in patients with severe OSAHS. Therefore, there is no consensus about whether the severity of OSAHS reflects the RNFL thickness.

Although several theories have been proposed, the pathogenesis of optic nerve damage is complex and remains still unknown. Thus, recurrent episodes of nocturnal hypoxia during apnea may result in direct anoxic damage, or in an indirect effect on optic nerve head blood flow, vascular dysregulation of the optic nerve by OSAHS could result from hypoxia-induced imbalance between nitric oxide and endothelin [173]. Another presumption is the recurrent papilledema, which would be secondary to a hypoxemic cerebral vasodilation phenomenon. The perpetuation of RNFL swelling could lead to a cellular loss, with the consequent thinning of RNFL as the disease progresses [161]. Based on this idea, Huseyinoglu et al. [165] do not approve OCT to demonstrate neurodegeneration in OSAHS patients, considering that different confusing data such as normal or increased RNFL thickness as a result of optic nerve subtle edema, could mask possible peripapillary axonal loss.

15.4.2 Macular and Choroidal Findings in Apneic Disorder

Regarding macular thickness, Casas et al. [161] reported that temporal inner macular thickness was significantly higher in mild–moderate OSAHS compared to severe patients and controls. When SD-OCT segmentation was applied, Ferrandez et al. [174] not described any difference between controls and OSAHS in macular GCL and ganglion cell-inner plexiform layer (GC-IPL) thicknesses. Nevertheless, Kara et al. [170] reported that average GC-IPL and minimum GC-IPL thicknesses were significantly lower in severe OSAHS group than in healthy controls. Moreover, there was a significant negative correlation between AHI and both average GCL and IPL.

Xin et al. [175] found that macular and foveal thickness in nasal area of healthy individuals were significantly thinner than those in OSAHS patients with severe disorder, whereas subfoveal and nasal choroid were thinner in severe OSAHS comparing to controls. They suggested that a sympathetic nervous regulation disorder exists in OSAHS patients because of chronic intermittent hypoxia, which is followed by changes in the structure of the normal retina and choroid. However, the authors did not exclude the subjects having systemic diseases, such as arterial hypertension, what could be a possible error source. Nevertheless, Bayhan et al. [176] and Yazgan et al. [163] confirm the difference in choroidal thickness between severe OSAHS versus moderate-controls in a group of patients without systemic pathologies. Yuvaci et al. [177] observed a thinning in the central subfoveal choroidal thickness in severe OSAHS cases in which treatment was administered, although subjective clinical recovery of the apneic disorder was observed.

The proposed hypothesis for these findings is in relation with the double retinal blood supply from the central retinal artery and the choroid. The inner retina is provided by retinal blood vessels and is sensitive to tissue oxygen partial pressure changes. Thus, anoxia may result in an increased blood flow to the retina [178]. On the other hand, outer retina and choroid is supplied by choroidal system. The adaptation of choroidal resistance is achieved through the sympathetic nervous system [179]. The hypoxia-reoxygenation pattern and sleep fragmentation associated with OSAHS contribute to the activation of sympathetic system. Thus, expecting choroidal structural changes is reasonable.

There are also studies presenting no macular and choroidal disturbances in apneic patients [157, 180–182]. Zengin et al. [180] and Karaca et al. [181]

compared choroidal thickness in patients recently diagnosed with OSAS and healthy controls and found that the difference in mean choroidal thickness was not statistically significant. Furthermore, choroidal thickness did not significantly differ among the mild, moderate, and severe OSAHS groups and no correlation between AHI and choroidal thickness was found [180, 181]. Khayi et al. [182] did not found any differences in choroidal vascular responses to posture and exercise between healthy control subjects and healthy OSAHS patients. Similar results were reported by Lin et al. [157] regarding to macular thickness in OSAHS patients and controls.

Tonini et al. [183] studied vascular choroidal reactivity during hyperoxia and hypercapnia with choroidal laser Doppler flowmetry. Patients with OSAHS without comorbidities and control subjects exhibited similar choroidal reactivity during hyperoxia and hypercapnia. The author suggested that other microvascular comorbidities as atherosclerosis or arterial hypertension have an important role in the choroidal vascular regulation and healthy individuals with OSAHS have long-term adaptive mechanisms active in ocular microcirculation.

With the recent arrival of the OCTA two articles have been published on the retinal microvasculature in patients with OSAHS, getting different results. On one hand, Yu et al. [184] found a decreased vessel density in peripapillary and parafoveal arcas, which were negatively correlated with AHI. Thus, the retinal vessel density decreased with greater severity of OSAHS. On the other hand, Moyal et al. [185], in a sample of 53 eyes with OSAHS, did not find differences when the macular, optic nerve head and radial peripapillary capillaries vessel density were compared to healthy control eyes.

15.5 Optical Coherence Tomography in Bipolar Disorder Patients

Bipolar disorder (BD) is a chronic psychiatric disease that alternates episodes of mania with episodes of depression. It is a major public health problem, with an estimated prevalence ranging from 1 to 6% of the general population [186, 187].

There are only four published articles on OCT reporting retinal axonal loss in these patients. However, the results are contradictory. Thus, Kalenderoglu et al. [188] compared the GCL volume and RNFL thickness in 43 BD patients and 43 healthy subjects by using SD-OCT. Patients showed a lower RNFL thickness compared with controls at all measured regions, and this reduction was statistically significant for the global RNFL value. The GCL volume was also significantly lower in the patient group. A negative correlation between some disorder parameters, such as duration of the disease and number of hospitalizations, and GCL volume. According to the authors, these findings would reflect that neurodegeneration occurs during the course of BD. This degeneration may be demonstrated by reduced GCL at early phases, and as the disorder progresses, involvement of other retinal layers, such as the RNFL and IPL, may be observed. Khalil et al. [189] compared 40 inpatients with BD to 40 matched healthy controls. BD patients showed thinning of RNFL and reduced GCC in comparison with control individuals. Age at onset, number of episodes, and disease severity did not significantly correlate with SD-OCT measurements. Furthermore, Mehraban et al. [190], by using SD-OCT, compared the peripapillary RNFL thickness in 60 eyes corresponding to 30 patients with BD and 60 eyes of 30 age-matched controls. Reduction of peripapillary RNFL thickness was reported in BD patients, and is related to the duration of disorder. They conclude that RNFL thickness might be a beneficial biomarker for studying neurodegenerative changes over time to detect the severity and duration of the disease. Finally, Polo et al. [191] have used the recent swept source (SS) technology for OCT in the study of retinal changes in 23 patients with BD and 23 healthy subjects. They reported that BD patients were shown to have significant thinning of full retinal thickness and the GCL in the macular area, as well as a peripapillary reduction of the RNFL and GCL thickness. The authors state that the analysis of the retinal sublayers with SS-OCT might be a useful marker to demonstrate degeneration and monitor disease progression in BD.

In conclusion, research in BD suggests the presence of structural brain alterations. Nevertheless, it is not clear if these changes might be trait markers or operate with the onset and progress with duration and disease severity.

References

1. Friberg L, Olesen J, Lassen NA, Olsen TS, Karle A. Cerebral oxygen extraction, oxygen consumption, and regional cerebral blood flow during the aura phase of migraine. Stroke. 1994;25:974–9.
2. Kirbas S, Tufekci A, Turkyilmaz K, Kirbas A, Oner V, Durmus M. Evaluation of the retinal changes in patients with chronic migraine. Acta Neurol Belg. 2013;113:167–72.
3. Dadaci Z, Doganay F, Acir NO, Aydin HD, Borazan M. Enhanced depth imaging optical coherence tomography of the choroid in migraine patients: implications for the association of migraine and glaucoma. Br J Ophthalmol. 2014;98:972–5.
4. Carod-Artal FJ, Irimia P, Ezpeleta D. Chronic migraine: definition, epidemiology, risk factors and treatment. Rev Neurol. 2012;54:629–37.
5. Zengin MO, Elmas Z, Cinar E, Kucukerdonmez C. Choroidal thickness changes in patients with migraine. Acta Neurol Belg. 2015;115:33–7.
6. Sorkhabi R, Mostafaei S, Ahoor M, Talebi M. Evaluation of retinal nerve fiber layer thickness in migraine. Iran J Neurol. 2013;12:51–5.
7. Ekinci M, Ceylan E, Çağatay HH, Keleş S, Hüseyinoğlu N, Tanyildiz B, Çakici O, Kartal B. Retinal nerve fibre layer, ganglion cell layer and choroid thinning in migraine with aura. BMC Ophthalmol. 2014;14:75.
8. Lipton R, Bigal M, Diamond M, Freitag F, Reed M, Stewart W. Migraine prevalence, disease burden and the need for preventive therapy. Neurology. 2007;68:343–9.
9. Worley A, Grimmer-Somers K. Risk factors for glaucoma: what do they really mean? Aust J Prim Health. 2011;17:233–9.
10. Martínez A, Proupim N, Sánchez M. Retinal nerve fiber layer thickness measurements using optical coherence tomography in migraine patients. Br J Ophthalmol. 2008;92:1069–75.
11. Tan FU, Akarsu C, Güllü R. Retinal nerve fiber layer thickness is unaffected in migraine patients. Acta Neurol Scand. 2005;112:19–23.
12. Bolay H, Moskowitz MA. The neurobiology of migraine and transformation of headache therapy. In: Waxman S, editor. From neuroscience to neurology: neuroscience, molecular medicine, and the therapeutic transformation of neurology. San Diego: Elsevier; 2004. p. 107–23.

13. Panconesi A, Bartolozzi ML, Guidi L. Migraine pain: reflections against vasodilatation. J Headache Pain. 2009;10:317–25.
14. Totan Y, Çekiç O. Görme ile ilgili elektrofizyolojik testler ve klinik uygulamaları (Vision-related electrophysiological tests and their clinical applications). MN Oftalmol. 1996;3:195–8.
15. Thie A, Spitzer K, Lachenmayer L, Kunze K. Prolonged vasospasm in migraine detected by noninvasive transcranial Doppler ultrasound. Headache J Head Face Pain. 1988;8:183–6.
16. Killer HE, Forrer A, Flammer J. Retinal vasospasm during an attack of migraine. Retina. 2003;23:253–4.
17. Beversdof D, Stommel E, Allen C, Stevens R, Lessel S. Recurrent branch retinal infarcts in association with migraine. Headache. 1997;37:396–9.
18. Abdul-Rahman AM, Gilhotra JS, Selva D. Dynamic focal retinal arteriolar vasospasm in migraine. Indian J Ophthalmol. 2011;59:51–3.
19. Kurth T, Slomke MA, Kase CS, Cook NR, Lee IM, Gaziano JM, Diener HC, Buring JE. Migraine, headache, and the risk of stroke in women: a prospective study. Neurology. 2005;64:1020–6.
20. Sacco S, Ricci S, Carolei A. Migraine and vascular diseases: a review of the evidence and potential implications for management. Cephalalgia. 2012;32:785–95.
21. Frohman E, Costello F, Zivadinov R, Stuve O, Conger A, Winslow H, Trip A, Frohman T, Balcer L. Optical coherence tomography in multiple sclerosis. Lancet Neurol. 2006;5:853–63.
22. Galetta KM, Calabresi PA, Frohman EM, Balcer LJ. Optical coherence tomography (OCT): imaging the visual pathway as a model for neurodegeneration. Neurotherapeutics. 2011;8:117–32.
23. Ascaso FJ, Cruz N, Modrego PJ, López-Antón R, Santabárbara J, Pascual LF, Lobo A, Cristóbal JA. Retinal alterations in mild cognitive impairment and Alzheimer's disease: an optical coherence tomography study. J Neurol. 2014;261:1522–30.
24. Jiménez B, Ascaso FJ, Cristóbal JA, López del Val J. Development of a prediction formula of Parkinson disease severity by optical coherence tomography. Mov Disord. 2014;29:68–74.
25. Xu W, Yao K, Shentu X. The comparison of two methods to predict the postoperative visual acuity of cataractous patients. Zhonghua Yan Ke Za Zhi. 2001;37:121–4.
26. Branchini L, Regatieri CV, Flores-Moreno I, et al. Reproducibility of choroidal thickness measurements across three spectral domain optical coherence tomography systems. Ophthalmology. 2012;119:119–23.
27. Manjunath V, Taha M, Fujimoto JG, Duker JS. Choroidal thickness in normal eyes measured using Cirrus-HD optical coherence tomography. Am J Ophthalmol. 2010;150:325–9.
28. Martínez A, Proupim N, Sánchez M. Scanning laser polarimetry with variable corneal compensation in migraine patients. Acta Ophthalmol. 2009;87:746–53.
29. Gipponi S, Scaroni N, Venturelli E, Forbice E, Rao R, Liberini P, Padovani A, Semeraro F. Reduction in retinal nerve fiber layer thickness in migraine patients. Neurol Sci. 2013;34:841–5.
30. Yülek F, Dirik EB, Eren Y, Simavlı H, Ugurlu N, Cagil N, et al. Macula and retinal nerve fiber layer in migraine patients: analysis by spectral domain optic coherence tomography. Semin Ophthalmol. 2015;30:124–8.
31. Demircan S, Ataş M, Arık Yüksel S, Ulusoy MD, Yuvacı İ, et al. The impact of migraine on posterior ocular structures. J Ophthalmol. 2015;2015:868967.
32. Simsek IB. Retinal nerve fibre layer thickness of migraine patients with or without white matter lesions. Neuroophthalmology. 2016;41:7–11.
33. Gunes A, Demirci S, Tok L, Tok O, Demirci S, Kutluhan S. Is retinal nerve fiber layer thickness change related to headache lateralization in migraine? Korean J Ophthalmol. 2016;30:134–9.
34. Colak HN, Kantarcı FA, Tatar MG, Eryilmaz M, Uslu H, Goker H, et al. Retinal nerve fiber layer, ganglion cell complex, and choroidal thicknesses in migraine. Arq Bras Oftalmol. 2016;79:78–81.
35. Feng YF, Guo H, Huang JH, Yu JG, Yuan F. Retinal nerve fiber layer thickness changes in migraine: a meta-analysis of case-control studies. Curr Eye Res. 2016;41:814–22.

36. Cankaya C, Tecellioglu M. Foveal thickness alterations in patients with migraine. Med Arch. 2016;70:123–6.
37. Reggio E, Chisari CG, Ferrigno G, Patti F, Donzuso G, Sciacca G, et al. Migraine causes retinal and choroidal structural changes: evaluation with ocular coherence tomography. J Neurol. 2017;264:494–502.
38. Acer S, Oğuzhanoğlu A, Çetin EN, Ongun N, Pekel G, Kaşıkçı A, et al. Ocular pulse amplitude and retina nerve fiber layer thickness in migraine patients without aura. BMC Ophthalmol. 2016;16:1.
39. Gunes A, Karadag AS, Yazgan S, Celik HU, Simsek A. Evaluation of retinal nerve fibre layer, ganglion cell layer and choroidal thickness with optical coherence tomography in migraine patients: a case-control study. Clin Exp Optom. 2018;101:109–15.
40. El-Shazly AAE, Farweez YA, Hamdi MM, El-Sherbiny NE. Pattern visual evoked potential, pattern electroretinogram, and retinal nerve fiber layer thickness in patients with migraine during and after aura. Curr Eye Res. 2017;42:1327–32.
41. Tak AZA, Sengul Y, Bilak S. Evaluation of white matter hyperintensities and retinal fiber layer, ganglion cell layer, inner plexiform layer, and choroidal layer in migraine patients. Neurol Sci. 2018;39:489–96.
42. Abdellatif MK, Fouad MM. Effect of duration and severity of migraine on retinal nerve fiber layer, ganglion cell layer, and choroidal thickness. Eur J Ophthalmol. 2018;28:714–21.
43. Chang MY, Phasukkijwatana N, Garrity S, Pineles SL, Rahimi M, Sarraf D, Johnston M, Charles A, Arnold AC. Foveal and peripapillary vascular decrement in migraine with aura demonstrated by optical coherence tomography angiography. Invest Ophthalmol Vis Sci. 2017;58:5477–84.
44. Tunç A, Güngen BD, Evliyaoğlu F, Aras YG, Tekeşin AK. Evaluation of retinal nerve fiber layer, ganglion cell layer and macular changes in patients with migraine. Acta Neurol Belg. 2017;117:121–9.
45. Linsenmeier RA, Braun RD. Oxygen distribution and consumption in the cat retina during normoxia and hypoxia. J Gen Physiol. 1992;99:177–97.
46. Maul EA, Friedman DS, Chang DS, et al. Choroidal thickness measured by spectral domain optical coherence tomography: factors affecting thickness in glaucoma patients. Ophthalmology. 2011;118:1571–9.
47. Sizmaz S, Küçükerdönmez C, Pinarci EY, Karalezli A, Canan H, Yilmaz G. The effect of smoking on choroidal thickness measured by optical coherence tomography. Br J Ophthalmol. 2013;97:601–4.
48. Fujiwara T, Imamura Y, Margolis R, Slakter JS, Spaide RF. Enhanced depth imaging optical coherence tomography of the choroid in highly myopic eyes. Am J Ophthalmol. 2009;148:445–50.
49. Ikuno Y, Tano Y. Retinal and choroidal biometry in highly myopic eyes with spectral-domain optical coherence tomography. Invest Ophthalmol Vis Sci. 2009;50:3876–80.
50. Yeoh J, Rahman W, Chen F, et al. Choroidal imaging in inherited retinal disease using the technique of enhanced depth imaging optical coherence tomography. Graefes Arch Clin Exp Ophthalmol. 2010;248:1719–28.
51. Peroutka SJ. Migraine: a chronic sympathetic nervous system disorder. Headache. 2004;44:53–64.
52. Drummond PD. The effect of sympathetic blockade on facial sweating and cutaneous vascular responses to painful stimulation of the eye. Brain J Neurol. 1993;116(Pt 1):233–41.
53. Gupta R, Bhatia MS. A report of cranial autonomic symptoms in migraineurs. Cephalalgia. 2007;27:22–8.
54. Karaca EE, Ozdek S, Yalçin NG, et al. Reproducibility of choroidal thickness measurements in healthy Turkish subjects. Eur J Ophthalmol. 2014;24:202–8.
55. Uzun S, Pehlivan E. Retinal nerve fiber layer, ganglion cell complex, and choroidal thicknesses in migraine. Arq Bras Oftalmol. 2016;79:352.
56. Nalcacioglu P, Taslipinar Uzel AG, Uzel MM, Cagil N, Citak Kurt AN. Are there any changes in posterior ocular structure parameters in pediatric migraine patients? Eur J Ophthalmol. 2017;27:495–501.

57. Whitcup SM. Sarcoidosis. In: Nussenblatt RB, Whitcup SM, editors. Uveitis. Fundamentals and clinical practice. 3rd ed. Philadelphia: Mosby; 2004. p. 301–10.
58. Ianuzzi MC, Rybicki BA, Teirstein AS. Sarcoidosis. N Engl J Med. 2007;357:2153–65.
59. Nunes H, Bouvry D, Valeyre D. Sarcoidosis. Orphanet J Rare Dis. 2007;2:46.
60. Reich JM. A critical analysis of sarcoidosis incidence assessment. Multidiscip Respir Med. 2013;8:57.
61. Hoyle JC, Jablonski C, Newton HB. Neurosarcoidosis: clinical review of a disorder with challenging inpatient presentations and diagnostic considerations. Neurohospitalist. 2014;4:94–101.
62. Nowak DA, Widenka DC. Neurosarcoidosis: a review of its intracranial manifestation. J Neurol. 2001;248:363–72.
63. Titlic M, Bradic-Hammoud M, Miric L, Punda A. Clinical manifestations of neurosarcoidosis. Bratisl Lek Listy. 2009;110:576–9.
64. Bezo C, Majzoub S, Nochez Y, Leruez S, Charlin JF, Milea D, Pisella PJ. Sarcoïdose oculaire et neuro-ophtalmologique: étude retrospective sur 30 cas. J Fr Ophtalmol. 2013;36:473–80.
65. Hickman SJ, Quhill F, Pepper M. The evolution of an optic nerve head granuloma due to sarcoidosis. Neuro-Ophthalmology. 2016;40:59–68.
66. Koczman JJ, Rouleau J, Gaunt M, Kardon RH, Wall M, Lee AG. Neuro-ophthalmic sarcoidosis: the University of Iowa experience. Semin Ophthalmol. 2008;23:157–68.
67. Menezo V, Lobo A, Yeo TK, du Bois RM, Lightman S. Ocular features in neurosarcoidosis. Ocul Immunol Inflamm. 2009;17:170–8.
68. Frohman LP, Guirgis M, Turbin RE, Bielory L. Sarcoidosis of the anterior visual pathway: 24 new cases. J Neuroophthalmol. 2003;23:190–7.
69. Beardsley TL, Brown SV, Sydnor CF, Grimson BS, Klintworth GK. Eleven cases of sarcoidosis of the optic nerve. Am J Ophthalmol. 1984;97:62–77.
70. Frohman EM, Fujimoto JG, Frohman TC, Calabresi PA, Cutter G, Balcer LJ. Optical coherence tomography: a window into the mechanisms of multiple sclerosis. Nat Clin Pract Neurol. 2008;4:664–75.
71. Rebolleda G, Muñoz-Negrete FJ. Macular segmentation in neuroophthalmology: descriptive or predictive? Arch Soc Esp Oftalmol. 2013;88:289–90.
72. Syc SB, Saidha S, Newsome SD, Ratchford JN, Levy M, Ford E, Crainiceanu CM, Durbin MK, Oakley JD, Meyer SA, Frohman EM, Calabresi PA. Optical coherence tomography segmentation reveals ganglion cell layer pathology after optic neuritis. Brain. 2012;135:521–33.
73. Kardon R. The role of the macula OCT scan in neuro-ophthalmology. J Neuroophthalmol. 2011;31:353–61.
74. Baltmr A, Lightman S, Tomkins-Netzer O. Examining the choroid in ocular inflammation: a focus on enhanced depth imaging. J Ophthalmol. 2014;2014:459136.
75. Mehta H, Sim DA, Keane PA, Zarranz-Ventura J, Gallagher K, Egan CA, Westcott M, Lee RWJ, Tufail A, Pavesio CE. Structural changes of the choroid in sarcoid and tuberculosis related granulomatous uveitis. Eye. 2015;29:1060–8.
76. Güngör SG, Akkoyun I, Reyhan HN, Yesilirmak N, Yilmaz G. Choroidal thickness in ocular sarcoidosis during quiescent phase using enhanced depth imaging optical coherence tomography. Ocul Immunol Inflamm. 2014;22:287.
77. Modi YS, Epstein A, Bhaleeya S, Harbour JW, Albini T. Multimodal imaging of sarcoid choroidal granulomas. J Ophthalmic Inflamm Infect. 2013;3:58.
78. Wong M, Javowicz M, Tessler HH, Goldstein DA. High-resolution optical coherence tomography of presumed sarcoid retinal granulomas. Retina. 2009;29:1545–6.
79. Rostaqui O, Querques G, Haymann P, Fardeau C, Coscas G, Souied EH. Visualization of sarcoid choroidal granuloma by enhanced depth imaging optical coherence tomography. Ocul Immunol Inflamm. 2014;22:239–41.
80. Papavasileiou E, Miller JB, Sobrin L. Swept-source optical coherence tomography findings in convalescent phase of treated sarcoid choroidal granulomas. Retin Cases Brief Rep. 2016;10:32–6.

81. Pichi F. Vascularized sarcoid granuloma complicated by placoid disease in a pediatric patient. Retin Cases Brief Rep. 2018; https://doi.org/10.1097/ICB.0000000000000806.
82. Turkoglu EB, Lally SE, Shields CL. Choroidal sarcoid granuloma simulating prostate carcinoma metastasis. Retin Cases Brief Rep. 2017;11:S226–8.
83. Inverzzini A, Agarwal A, Mapelli C, Nguyen QD, Staurenghi G, Viola F. Longitudinal follow-up of choroidal granulomas using enhanced depth imaging optical coherence tomography. Retina. 2017;37:144–53.
84. Qu-Knafo L, Auregan-Giocanti A. Granulome papillair sarcoïdosique. J Fr Ophtalmol. 2017;40:115–7.
85. Goldberg NR, Jabs DA, Busingye J. Optical coherence tomography image of presumed sarcoid retinal and optic nerve nodules. Ocul Immunol Inflamm. 2016;24:293–6.
86. Inverzzini A, Mapelli C, Viola F, Cigada M, Cimino L, Ratiglia R, Staurenghi G, Gupta A. Choroidal granulomas visualized by enhanced depth imaging optical coherence tomography. Retina. 2015;35:525–31.
87. Isihara M, Shibuya E, Tanaka S, Mizuki N. Diagnostic and therapeutic evaluation of multiple choroidal granulomas in a patient with confirmed sarcoidosis using enhanced depth imaging optic coherence tomography. Int Ophthalmol. 2017; https://doi.org/10.1007/s10792-017-0720-2.
88. McMahon JF, Adam MK, Dunn JP. Optical coherence tomography and management of retinal granuloma in presumed ocular sarcoidosis. Ocul Immunol Inflamm. 2018; https://doi.org/10.1080/09273948.2018.1497662.
89. Cabrillo-Estévez L, Juan-Marcos LD, Kyriakou D, Hernández-Galilea E. Cistoid macular edema as first manifestation of sarcoidosis. Int Ophthalmol. 2014;34:961–5.
90. Simmons-Rear A, Yeh S, Chan-Kai BT, Lauer AK, Flaxel CJ, Smith JR, Rosenbaum JT, Suhler EB. Characterization of serous retinal detachments in uveitis patients with optical coherence tomography. J Ophthalm Inflamm Infect. 2012;2:191–7.
91. Eckstein C, Saidha S, Sotirchos ES, Byraiah G, Seigo M, Stankiewicz A, Syc SB, Ford E, Sharma S, Calabresi PA, Pardo CA. Detection of clinical and subclinical retinal abnormalities in neurosarcoidosis with optical coherence tomography. J Neurol. 2012;259:1390–8.
92. Cerquaglia A, Iaccheri B, Fiore T, Fruttini D, Belli FB, Khairallah M, Lupidi M, Cagini C. New insights on ocular sarcoidosis: an optical coherence tomography angiography study. Ocul Immunol Inflamm. 2018; https://doi.org/10.1080/09273948.2018.1497665.
93. Abucham-Neto JZ, Miranda Torriceli AA, Fioravanti Lui AC, Napoli Guimaraes S, Nascimento H, Regatieri CV. Comparison between optical coherence tomography angiography and fluorescein angiography findings in retinal vasculitis. Int J Ret Vit. 2018;4:15.
94. Mueser KT, McGurk SR. Schizophrenia. Lancet. 2004;363:2063–72.
95. Wu EQ, Birnbaum HG, Shi L, et al. The economic burden of schizophrenia in the United States in 2002. J Clin Psychiatry. 2005;66:1122–9.
96. Sadock B, Sadock V. Sinopsis de Psiquiatría. Kaplan and Sadock. 10th ed. Madrid: Wolters Kluwer; 2008.
97. Svensson AC, Lichtenstein P, Sandin S, Öberg S, Sullivan PF, Hultman CM. Familial aggregation of schizophrenia: the moderating effect of age at onset, parental immigration, paternal age and season of birth. Scand J Public Health. 2012;40:43–50.
98. Steen RG, Mull C, McClure R, Hamer RM, Lieberman JA. Systematic review and meta-analysis of magnetic resonance imaging studies. Br J Psychiatry. 2006;188:510–8.
99. Siever LJ, Davis KL. The pathophysiology of schizophrenia disorders: perspectives from the spectrum. Am J Psychiatry. 2004;161:398–413.
100. Harrison PJ, Weinberger DR. Schizophrenia genes, gene expression, and neuropathology: on the matter of their convergence. Mol Psychiatry. 2005;10:40–68.
101. Bracht T, Horn H, Strik W, et al. White matter pathway organization of the reward system is related to positive and negative symptoms in schizophrenia. Schizophr Res. 2014;153:136–42.
102. Takayanagi M, Wentz J, Takayanagi Y, et al. Reduced anterior cingulate gray matter volume and thickness in subjects with deficit schizophrenia. Schizophr Res. 2013;150:484–90.

103. Glahn DC, Laird AR, Ellison-Wright I, et al. Meta-analysis of gray matter anomalies in schizophrenia: application of anatomic likelihood estimation and network analysis. Biol Psychiatry. 2008;64:774–81.
104. Arnone D, Cavanagh J, Gerber D, Lawrie SM, Ebmeier KP, Mcintosh AM. Magnetic resonance imaging studies in bipolar and schizophrenia: meta-analysis. Br J Psychiatry. 2009;195:194–201.
105. Fornito A, Yücel M, Dean B, Wood SJ, Pantelis C. Anatomical abnormalities of the anterior cingulate cortex in schizophrenia: bridging the gap between neuroimaging and neuropathology. Schizophr Bull. 2009;35:973–93.
106. Howard MA, Roberts N, García-Fiñana M, Cowell PE. Volume estimation of prefrontal cortical subfields using MRI and stereology. Brain Res Brain Res Protoc. 2003;10:125–38.
107. MacFall JR, Payne ME, Krishnan KRR. MR scanner geometry changes: phantom measurements compared to intracranial contents calculations. Proc Int Soc Magn Reson Med. 2004;11:2182.
108. Jindahra P, Hedges TR, Mendoza-Santiesteban CE, Plant GT. Optical coherence tomography of the retina: applications in neurology. Curr Opin Neurol. 2010;23:16–23.
109. Lamirel C, Newman N, Biousse V. The use of optical coherence tomography in neurology. Rev Neurol Dis. 2009;6:E105–20.
110. Ascaso FJ, Cabezón L, Quintanilla MA, Gutiérrez-Galve L, López-Antón R, Cristóbal JA, Lobo A. Retinal nerve fiber layer thickness measured by optical coherence tomography in patients with schizophrenia: a short report. Eur J Psychiat. 2010;24:227–35.
111. Yılmaz U, Küçük E, Ülgen A, Özköse A, Demircan S, Ulusoy DM, Zararsız G. Retinal nerve fiber layer and macular thickness measurement in patients with schizophrenia. Eur J Ophthalmol. 2016;26:375–8.
112. Chu EM, Kolappan M, Barnes TR, Joyce EM, Ron MA. A window into the brain: an in vivo study of the retina in schizophrenia using optical coherence tomography. Psychiatry Res. 2012;203:89–94.
113. Celik M, Kalenderoglu A, Sevgi Karadag A, Bekir Egilmez O, Han-Almis B, Şimşek A. Decreases in ganglion cell layer and inner plexiform layer volumes correlate better with disease severity in schizophrenia patients than retinal nerve fiber layer thickness: findings from spectral optic coherence tomography. Eur Psychiatry. 2016;32:9–15.
114. Silverstein SM, Paterno D, Cherneski L, Green S. Optical coherence tomography indices of structural retinal pathology in schizophrenia. Psychol Med. 2018;48:2023–33.
115. Lee WW, Tajunisah I, Sharmilla K, Peyman M, Subrayan V. Retinal nerve fiber layer structure abnormalities in schizophrenia and its relationship to disease state: evidence from optical coherence tomography. Invest Ophthalmol Vis Sci. 2013;54:7785–92.
116. Ascaso FJ, Rodriguez-Jimenez R, Cabezón L, López-Antón R, Santabárbara J, De la Cámara C, Modrego PJ, Quintanilla MA, Bagney A, Gutierrez L, Cruz N, Cristóbal JA, Lobo A. Retinal nerve fiber layer and macular thickness in patients with schizophrenia: influence of recent illness episodes. Psychiatry Res. 2015;229:230–6.
117. Joe P, Ahmad M, Riley G, Weissman J, Smith RT, Malaspina D. A pilot study assessing retinal pathology in psychosis using optical coherence tomography: choroidal and macular thickness. Psychiatry Res. 2018;263:158–61.
118. Maynard TM, Sikich L, Lieberman JA, LaMantia AS. Neural development, cell-cell signaling, and the 'two-hit' hypothesis of schizophrenia. Schizophr Bull. 2001;27:457–76.
119. Kochunov P, Hong LE. Neurodevelopmental and neurodegenerative models of schizophrenia: white matter at the center stage. Schizophr Bull. 2014;40:721–8.
120. Pantelis C, Yücel M, Wood SJ, et al. Structural brain imaging evidence for multiple pathological processes at different stages of brain development in schizophrenia. Schizophr Bull. 2005;31:672–96.
121. Guilleminault C. Clinical features and evaluation of obstructive sleep apnea syndrome. In: Kryger MH, Roth T, Dement WC, editors. Principles and practice of sleep medicine. Philadelphia: WB Saunders; 1994. p. 667–77.

122. Hatipoğlu U, Rubinstein I. Inflammation and obstructive sleep apnea syndrome pathogenesis: a working hypothesis. Respiration. 2003;70:665–71.
123. Lavie L, Hefetz A, Luboshitzky R, Lavie P. Plasma levels of nitric oxide and L-arginine in sleep apnea patients: effects of nCPAP treatment. J Mol Neurosci. 2003;21:57–63.
124. Grover DP. Obstructive sleep apnea and ocular disorders. Curr Opin Ophthalmol. 2010;21:454–8.
125. Shahar E, Whitney CW, Redline S, Lee ET, Newman AB, Javier Nieto F, O'Connor GT, Boland LL, Schwartz JE, Samet JM. Sleep-disordered breathing and cardiovascular disease: cross sectional results of the Sleep Heart Health Study. Am J Respir Crit Care Med. 2001;163:19–25.
126. Rudnicka A, Pływaczewski R, Jończak L, Górecka D, Sliwiński P. Prevalence of stroke in patients with obstructive sleep apnoea. Pneumonol Alergol Pol. 2010;78:121–5.
127. Macey PM, Henderson LA, Macey KE, Alger JR, Frysinger RC, Woo MA, Harper RK, Yan-Go FL, Harper RM. Brain morphology associated with obstructive sleep apnea. Am J Respir Crit Care Med. 2002;166:1382–7.
128. Kumar R, Birrer BV, Macey PM, Woo MA, Gupta RK, Yan-Go FL, Harper RM. Reduced mammillary body volume in patients with obstructive sleep apnea. Neurosci Lett. 2008;438:330–4.
129. McNab AA. Floppy eyelid syndrome and obstructive sleep apnea. Ophthal Plast Reconstr Surg. 1997;13:98–114.
130. Woog JJ. Obstructive sleep apnea and the floppy eyelid syndrome. Am J Ophthalmol. 1990;110:314–5.
131. Karger RA, White WA, Park WC, et al. Prevalence of floppy eyelid syndrome in obstructive sleep apnea-hypopnea syndrome. Ophthalmology. 2006;113:1669–74.
132. Muniesa M, Sánchez-de-la-Torre M, Huerva V, Lumbierres M, Barbé F. Floppy eyelid syndrome as an indicator of the presence of glaucoma in patients with obstructive sleep apnea. J Glaucoma. 2014;23:81–5.
133. Pedrotti E, Demasi CL, Bruni E, Bosello F, Di Sarro PP, Passilongo M, Fasolo A, Gennaro N, De Gregorio A, Ferrari M, Marchini G. Prevalence and risk factors of eye diseases in adult patients with obstructive sleep apnoea: results from the SLE.E.P.Y cohort study. BMJ Open. 2017;7:e016142.
134. Leroux les Jardins G, Glacet-Bernard A, Lasry S, Housset B, Coscas G, Soubrane G. Retinal vein occlusion and obstructive sleep apnea syndrome. J Fr Ophtalmol. 2009;32:420–4.
135. Kloos P, Laube I, Thoelen A. Obstructive sleep apnea in patients with central serous chorioretinopathy. Graefes Arch Clin Exp Ophthalmol. 2008;246:1225–8.
136. Jain AK, Kaines A, Schwartz S. Bilateral central serous chorioretinopathy resolving rapidly with treatment for obstructive sleep apnea. Graefes Arch Clin Exp Ophthalmol. 2010;248:1037–9.
137. Chatziralli I, Kabanarou SA, Parikakis E, Chatzirallis A, Xirou T, Mitropoulos P. Risk factors for central serous chorioretinopathy: multivariate approach in a case-control study. Curr Eye Res. 2017;42:1069–73.
138. Wu CY, Riangwiwat T, Rattanawong P, Nesmith BLW, Deobhakta A. Association of obstructive sleep apnea with central serous chorioretinopathy and choroidal thickness: a systematic review and meta-analysis. Retina. 2018 (in press).
139. Chang AC, Fox TP, Wang S, Wu AY. Relationship between obstructive sleep apnea and the presence and severity of diabetic retinopathy. Retina. 2017 (in press).
140. Vié AL, Kodjikian L, Agard E, Voirin N, El Chehab H, Denis P, Coste O, Dot C. Evaluation of obstructive sleep apnea syndrome as a risk factor for diabetic macular edema in patients with type II diabetes. Retina. 2017 (in press).
141. Purvin VA, Kawasaki A, Yee RD. Papilledema and obstructive sleep apnea syndrome. Arch Ophthalmol. 2000;118:1626–30.
142. Franklin KA. Cerebral haemodynamics in obstructive sleep apnoea and Cheyne–Stokes respiration. Sleep Med Rev. 2002;6:429–41.

143. Lee AG, Golnik K, Kardon R, Wall M, Eggenberger E, Yedavally S. Sleep apnea and intracranial hypertension in men. Ophthalmology. 2002;109:482–5.
144. O'Donoghue FJ, Briellmann RS, Rochford PD, Abbott DF, Pell GS, Chan CH, Tarquinio N, Jackson GD, Pierce RJ. Cerebral structural changes in severe obstructive sleep apnea. Am J Respir Crit Care Med. 2005;171:1185–90.
145. Hayreh SS, Zimmerman MB, Podhajsky P, Alward WL. Nocturnal arterial hypotension and its role in optic nerve head and ocular ischemic disorders. Am J Ophthalmol. 1994;17:603–24.
146. Mojon DS, Hess CW, Goldblum D, Fleischhauer J, Koerner F, Bassetti C, Mathis J. High prevalence of glaucoma in patients with sleep apnea syndrome. Ophthalmology. 1999;106:1009–12.
147. Mojon DS, Hess CW, Goldblum D, Böhnke M, Körner F, Mathis J. Primary open-angle glaucoma is associated with sleep apnea syndrome. Ophthalmologica. 2000;214:115–8.
148. Bendel RE, Kaplan J, Heckman M, Fredrickson PA, Lin SC. Prevalence of glaucoma in patients with obstructive sleep apnoea—a cross-sectional case-series. Eye (Lond). 2008;22:1105–9.
149. Faridi O, Park SC, Liebmann JM, Ritch R. Glaucoma and obstructive sleep apnoea syndrome. Clin Exp Ophthalmol. 2012;40:408–19.
150. Sergi M, Salerno DE, Rizzi M, Blini M, Andreoli A, Messenio D, Pecis M, Bertoni G. Prevalence of normal tension glaucoma in obstructive sleep apnea syndrome patients. J Glaucoma. 2007;16:42–6.
151. Bilgin G. Normal-tension glaucoma and obstructive sleep apnea syndrome: a prospective study. BMC Ophthalmol. 2014;14:27.
152. Xin C, Zhang W, Wang L, Yang D, Wang J. Changes of visual field and optic nerve fiber layer in patients with OSAS. Sleep Breath. 2015;19:129–34.
153. Friedlander AH, Graves LL, Chang TI, Kawakami KK, Lee UK, Grabich SC, Fang ZT, Zeidler MR, Giaconi JA. Prevalence of primary open-angle glaucoma among patients with obstructive sleep apnea. Oral Surg Oral Med Oral Pathol Oral Radiol. 2018 (in press).
154. Examen del paciente. Campo visual. In: European Glaucoma Society, editor. Terminología y pautas para el glaucoma. 3rd ed. Savona: Dogma; 2009. p. 61–89.
155. Kargi SH, Altin R, Koksal M, Kart L, Cinar F, Ugurbas SH, Ayoglu F. Retinal nerve fibre layer measurements are reduced in patients with obstructive sleep apnoea syndrome. Eye (Lond). 2005;19:575–9.
156. Sagiv O, Fishelson-Arev T, Buckman G, Mathalone N, Wolfson J, Segev E, Peled R, Lavi I, Geyer O. Retinal nerve fiber layer thickness measurements by optical coherence tomography in patients with sleep apnea syndrome. Clin Exp Ophthalmol. 2014;42:132–8.
157. Lin PW, Friedman M, Lin HC, Chang HW, Pulver TM, Chin CH. Decreased retinal nerve fiber layer thickness in patients with obstructive sleep apnea/hypopnea syndrome. Graefes Arch Clin Exp Ophthalmol. 2011;249:585–93.
158. Moghimi S, Ahmadraji A, Sotoodeh H, Sadeghniat K, Maghsoudipour M, Fakhraie G, Latifi G, Nassiri N, Giaconi JA. Retinal nerve fiber thickness is reduced in sleep apnea syndrome. Sleep Med. 2013;14:53–7.
159. Lin PW, Friedman M, Lin HC, Chang HW, Wilson M, Lin MC. Normal tension glaucoma in patients with obstructive sleep apnea/hypopnea syndrome. J Glaucoma. 2011;20:553–8.
160. Gutiérrez-Díaz E, Pérez-Rico C, de Atauri MJ, Mencía-Gutiérrez E, Blanco R. Evaluation of the visual function in obstructive sleep apnea syndrome patients and normal-tension glaucoma by means of the multifocal visual evoked potentials. Graefes Arch Clin Exp Ophthalmol. 2012;250:1681–8.
161. Casas P, Ascaso FJ, Vicente E, Tejero-Garcés G, Adiego MI, Cristóbal JA. Retinal and optic nerve evaluation by optical coherence tomography in adults with obstructive sleep apnea-hypopnea syndrome (OSAHS). Graefes Arch Clin Exp Ophthalmol. 2013;251:1625–34.
162. Ozge G, Dogan D, Koylu MT, Ayyildiz O, Akincioglu D, Mumcuoglu T, Mutlu FM. Retina nerve fiber layer and choroidal thickness changes in obstructive sleep apnea syndrome. Postgrad Med. 2016;128:317–22.

163. Yazgan S, Erboy F, Celik HU, Ornek T, Ugurbas SH, Kokturk F, Ayar O, Akdemir MO, Celik E. Peripapillary choroidal thickness and retinal nerve fiber layer in untreated patients with obstructive sleep apnea-hypopnea syndrome: a case-control study. Curr Eye Res. 2017;42:1552–60.
164. Zengin MO, Tuncer I, Karahan E. Retinal nerve fiber layer thickness changes in obstructive sleep apnea syndrome: one year follow-up results. Int J Ophthalmol. 2014;7:704–8.
165. Huseyinoglu N, Ekinci M, Ozben S, Buyukuysal C, Kale MY, Sanivar HS. Optic disc and retinal nerve fiber layer parameters as indicators of neurodegenerative brain changes in patients with obstructive sleep apnea syndrome. Sleep Breath. 2014;18:95–102.
166. Shiba T, Takahashi M, Sato Y, Onoda Y, Hori Y, Sugiyama T, Bujo H, Maeno T. Relationship between severity of obstructive sleep apnea syndrome and retinal nerve fiber layer thickness. Am J Ophthalmol. 2014;157:1202–8.
167. Nowak MS, Jurowski P, Gos R, Prost ME, Smigielski J. Pulsatile ocular blood flow in subjects with sleep apnoea syndrome. Arch Med Sci. 2011;7:332–6.
168. Adam M, Okka M, Yosunkaya S, Bozkurt B, Kerimoğlu H, Turan M. The evaluation of retinal nerve fiber layer thickness in patients with obstructive sleep apnea syndrome. J Ophthalmol. 2013;2013:292158.
169. Ferrandez B, Ferreras A, Calvo P, Abadia B, Marin JM, Pajarin AB. Assessment of the retinal nerve fiber layer in individuals with obstructive sleep apnea. BMC Ophthalmol. 2016;16:40.
170. Kara N, Sayin N, Bayramoglu SE, Savas AU. Peripapillary retina nerve fiber layer thickness and macular ganglion cell layer thickness in patients with obstructive sleep apnea syndrome. Eye (Lond). 2018;32:701–6.
171. Salzgeber R, Iliev ME, Mathis J. Do optic nerve head and visual field parameters in patients with obstructive sleep apnea syndrome differ from those in control individuals? Klin Monatsbl Augenheilkd. 2014;231:340–3.
172. Yuvacı İ, Pangal E, Bayram N, Yüksel SA, Alabay B, Ağadayı A, Sırakaya E, Gülhan A. Evaluation of posterior ocular changes using enhanced depth imaging-optical coherence tomography in patients with obstructive sleep apnea syndrome. Arq Bras Oftalmol. 2016;79:247–52.
173. Kato M, Roberts-Thomson P, Phillips BG, Haynes WG, Winnicki M, Accurso V, Somers VK. Impairment of endothelium dependent vasodilation of resistance vessels in patients with obstructive sleep apnea. Circulation. 2000;102:2607–10.
174. Ferrandez B, Ferreras A, Calvo P, Abadia B, Pajarin AB, Marin JM, Iester M. Macular retinal ganglion cell layer thickness is not reduced in patients with obstructive sleep apnea. Ophthalmic Res. 2016;56:85–91.
175. Xin C, Wang J, Zhang W, Wang L, Peng X. Retinal and choroidal thickness evaluation by SD-OCT in adults with obstructive sleep apnea-hypopnea syndrome (OSAS). Eye (Lond). 2014;28:415–21.
176. Bayhan HA, Bayhan SA, Intepe YS, Muhafız E, Gurdal C. Evaluation of the macular choroidal thickness using spectral optical coherence tomography in patients with obstructive sleep apnea syndrome. Clin Exp Ophthalmol. 2014 (in press).
177. Yuvaci İ, Pangal E, Bayram N, Yüksel SA, Alabay B, Ağadayı A, Sırakaya E, Gülhan A. Evaluation of posterior ocular changes using enhanced depth imaging-optical coherence tomography in patients with obstructive sleep apnea syndrome. Arq Bras Oftalmol. 2016;79:247–52.
178. Frayser R, Gray GW, Houston CS. Control of the retinal circulation at altitude. J Appl Physiol. 1974;37:302–4.
179. Delaey C, Van De Voorde J. Regulatory mechanisms in the retinal and choroidal circulation. Ophthalmic Res. 2000;32:249–56.
180. Zengin MÖ, Oz T, Baysak A, Cinar E, Küçükerdönmez C. Changes in choroidal thickness in patients with obstructive sleep apnea syndrome. Ophthalmic Surg Lasers Imaging Retina. 2014;45:298–304.
181. Karaca EE, Ekici F, Yalçin NG, Ciftçi TU, Ozdek S. Macular choroidal thickness measurements in patients with obstructive sleep apnea syndrome. Sleep Breath. 2015;19:335–41.

182. Khayi H, Pepin JL, Geiser MH, Tonini M, Tamisier R, Renard E, Baguet JP, Levy P, Romanet JP, Chiquet C. Choroidal blood flow regulation after posture change or isometric exercise in men with obstructive sleep apnea syndrome. Invest Ophthalmol Vis Sci. 2011;52:9489–96.
183. Tonini M, Khayi H, Pepin JL, Renard E, Baguet JP, Lévy P, Romanet JP, Geiser MH, Chiquet C. Choroidal blood-flow responses to hyperoxia and hypercapnia in men with obstructive sleep apnea. Sleep. 2010;33:811–8.
184. Yu J, Xiao K, Huang J, Sun X, Jiang C. Reduced retinal vessel density in obstructive sleep apnea syndrome patients: an optical coherence tomography angiography study. Invest Ophthalmol Vis Sci. 2017;58:3506–12.
185. Moyal L, Blumen-Ohana E, Blumen M, Blatrix C, Chabolle F, Nordmann JP. Parafoveal and optic disc vessel density in patients with obstructive sleep apnea syndrome: an optical coherence tomography angiography study. Graefes Arch Clin Exp Ophthalmol. 2018;256:1235–43.
186. Kessler RC, Bergland P, Demler O, et al. Lifetime prevalence and age-of-onset distributions of DSM-IV disorders in the National Comorbidity Survey Replication. Arch Gen Psychiatry. 2005;62:593–602.
187. Akiskal HS, Bourgeois ML, Angst J, Post R, Möller H, Hirschfeld R. Re-evaluating the prevalence of and diagnostic composition within the broad clinical spectrum of bipolar disorders. J Affect Disord. 2000;59:S5–30.
188. Kalenderoglu A, Sevgi-Karadag A, Celik M, Egilmez OB, Han-Almis B, Ozen ME. Can the retinal ganglion cell layer (GCL) volume be a new marker to detect neurodegeneration in bipolar disorder? Compr Psychiatry. 2016;67:66–72.
189. Khalil MA, Saleh AA, Gohar SM, Khalil DH, Said M. Optical coherence tomography findings in patients with bipolar disorder. J Affect Disord. 2017;218:115–22.
190. Mehraban A, Samimi SM, Entezari M, Seifi MH, Nazari M, Yaseri M. Peripapillary retinal nerve fiber layer thickness in bipolar disorder. Graefes Arch Clin Exp Ophthalmol. 2016;254:365–71.
191. Polo V, Satue M, Gavin A, Vilades E, Orduna E, Cipres M, Garcia-Campayo J, Navarro-Gil M, Larrosa JM, Pablo LE, Garcia-Martin E. Ability of swept source OCT to detect retinal changes in patients with bipolar disorder. Eye (Lond). 2019;33(4):549–56.

Hereditary Optic Neuropathies

16

Piero Barboni, Nicole Balducci, and Alfredo A. Sadun

Hereditary optic neuropathies are diseases affecting the optic nerve. They may occur as isolated optic neuropathies or in association with systemic diseases. The minimum point prevalence of hereditary optic neuropathies is 1 per 10,000 subjects [1]. The most common isolated optic neuropathies are Leber's Hereditary Optic Neuropathy (LHON) and Dominant Optic Atrophy (DOA). They both share a defect of the mitochondria function that leads to the selective loss of retinal ganglion cells (RGC) and axons, in particular of the papillo-macular bundle (PMB), which requires great energy for its high demanding activity. Consequently to the PMB involvement, the main symptoms are related to loss of central vision and color vision defects. Over the last decade optical coherence tomography (OCT) has been extensively used to investigate the changes occurring in optic nerve and macular areas in these diseases.

16.1 Leber's Hereditary Optic Neuropathy

LHON is a maternally inherited genetic disorder due to mitochondrial DNA (mtDNA) mutations and predominantly affects men. The three most frequent pathogenic mutations affect nucleotide positions 11778, 3460, and 14484, respectively, in ND4, ND1, and ND6 subunit genes of complex I [2, 3]. The mtDNA mutation is

P. Barboni (✉)
Studio Oculistico d'Azeglio, Bologna, Italy

Scientific Institute San Raffaele, Milan, Italy
e-mail: p.barboni@studiodazeglio.it

N. Balducci
IRCCS-Fondazione Bietti, Rome, Italy

A. A. Sadun
Doheny Eye Institute, UCLA, Los Angeles, CA, USA

A. Grzybowski, P. Barboni (eds.), *OCT and Imaging in Central Nervous System Diseases*, https://doi.org/10.1007/978-3-030-26269-3_16

necessary, but not sufficient, to induce the disease. Other, still poorly defined, genetic and environmental factors may be implicated [4]. Thus, penetrance in LHON is not complete and may vary even in different sub-branches of the same family harboring a homoplasmic mtDNA mutation [5].

LHON usually leads to a subacute, large bilateral centrocecal scotomas in otherwise healthy young adults [2, 3]. The smaller-caliber fibers of the PMB are selectively lost at a very early stage of the pathologic process, which eventually extends to the rest of the nerve, leading to optic atrophy [6–9].

Clinically, most patients with LHON go through pre-symptomatic ophthalmoscopic changes before the acute phase, characterized by visual loss, develops.

Recently, four clinical stages of LHON have been defined by an International LHON consensus statement [10], according to time from symptoms onset and clinical investigations:

0. Asymptomatic (mutation carriers).
1. Subacute (<6 months from onset).
2. Dynamic (6–12 months).
3. Chronic (>12 months).

Ophthalmoscopic features, already present at the **asymptomatic stage**, include peripapillary microangiopathy, small vessel tortuosity, mild swelling of the retinal nerve fiber layer (RNFL) and lack of vessel leakage at fluorescein angiography [11, 12]. These characteristics may wax and wane throughout life in many carrier subjects. Once the disease becomes symptomatic and the patient experiences loss of central vision during the **subacute stage**, the vascular changes increase with swelling of the superior and inferior fiber arcades and rapid loss of the papillomacular bundle [12, 13]. As the pathologic process progresses, temporal pallor become evident. Then nerve fiber swelling decreases concomitantly with the extension of optic disc pallor toward complete atrophy during the **dynamic stage**. By 6 months after onset, optic atrophy is usually evident, and visual loss stabilizes, having reached the nadir [14, 15]. The **chronic stage** is universally reached by 1 year after onset. Rare reports described a stepwise worsening of visual acuity, whereas some individuals may recover different degrees of visual acuity [2, 3, 15].

16.1.1 Retinal Nerve Fiber Layer Analysis

OCT has been used to investigate the RNFL of LHON asymptomatic carriers [16], as well as LHON affected patients in the early and atrophic stages of the disease [17, 18].

As regards LHON asymptomatic carriers, a significant thickening has been observed in the temporal RNFL quadrant and, in males, also in the inferior quadrant (Fig. 16.1) [16]. This finding confirms that in asymptomatic LHON, the PMB is selectively involved. This preferential involvement of the PMB has been linked to the disadvantageous energetic conditions of small axons from macular parvocellular retinal ganglion cells. These small fibers have a high firing rate and are thought to be very energy dependent [8]. RNFL thickening seems mostly

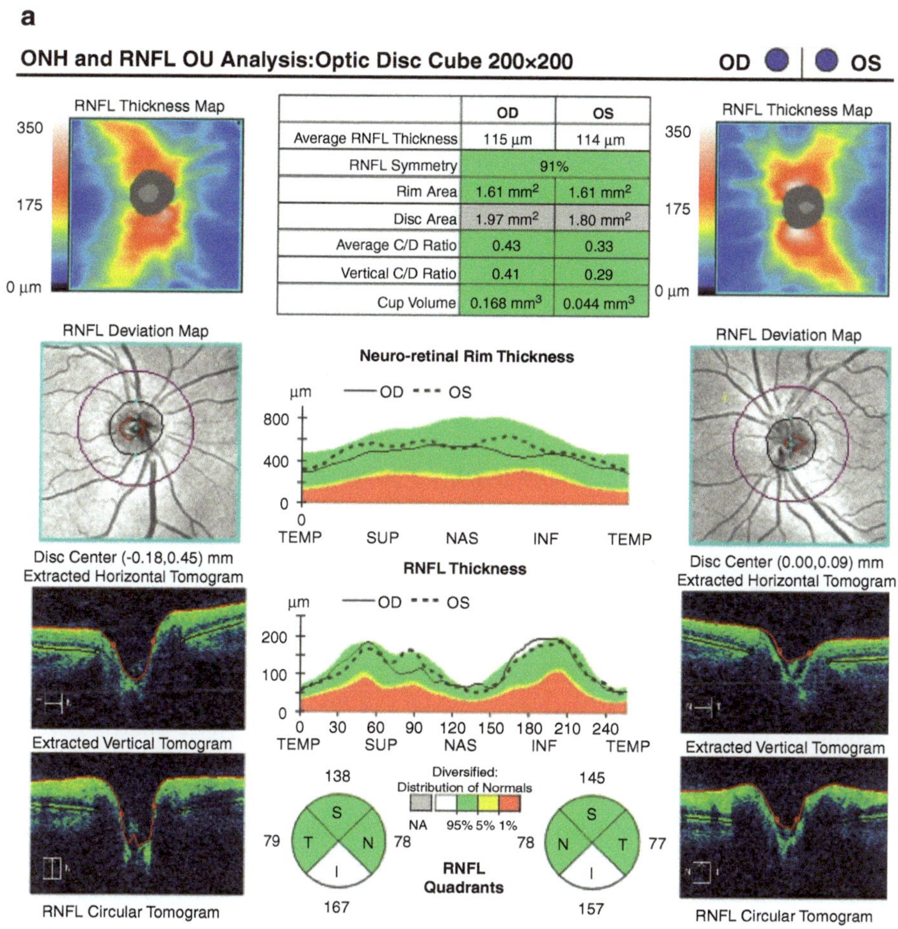

Fig. 16.1 (**a**) Peripapillary RNFL thickening more evident in the inferior quadrant of an unaffected LHON-carrier; (**b**) The left optic disc of the same patient

Fig. 16.1 (continued)

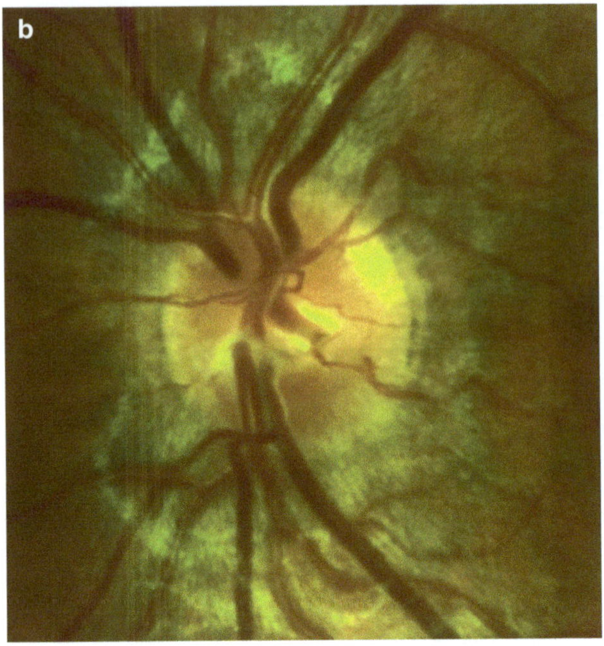

related to axonal swelling, which has been proposed to be a sign of impaired axonal transport, with redistribution of mitochondria within the dysfunctional retinal ganglion cells, particularly affecting the prelaminar, unmyelinated portion of the axons at the optic nerve head [8, 19]. Moreover, the peripapillary RNFL in LHON carriers showed higher thickness variability compared to controls, when measured at different time points [20]. The explanation of the RNFL variability could be either a compensatory mechanism (due to increased mitochondrial biogenesis) or an axonal stasis preceding the RGCs loss [8]. Another subclinical factor, which may cause RNFL variability, is LHON microangiopathy [20]. It is important to note that OCT measures the fiber layers that contain both retinal ganglion cell axons and vessels, so we cannot quantitatively differentiate the contribution of fiber swelling from microangiopathy.

In the subacute phase, RNFL analysis shows thickening in the superior and inferior quadrants, whereas the temporal quadrant shows no significant differences or reduction compared to the controls (Fig. 16.2a, b) [17, 21–23]. In fact, the PMB shows marked swelling at the time of visual loss, but its thickness starts decreasing soon due to early atrophy. A simultaneous thickening takes place in

Fig. 16.2 (**a**) Acute stage of LHON with (**a**) peripapillary RNFL thickening, (**b**) early ganglion cell thinning, (**c**) temporal pallor of the optic disc and (**d**), central scotoma in the visual field. (**b**) (**a**) RNFL thickness and deviation maps (top) RNFL progression analysis (bottom); (**b**) Progressive RNFL thinning in LHON from acute (top) to the chronic (bottom) stage; (**c**) RNFL thickness profile

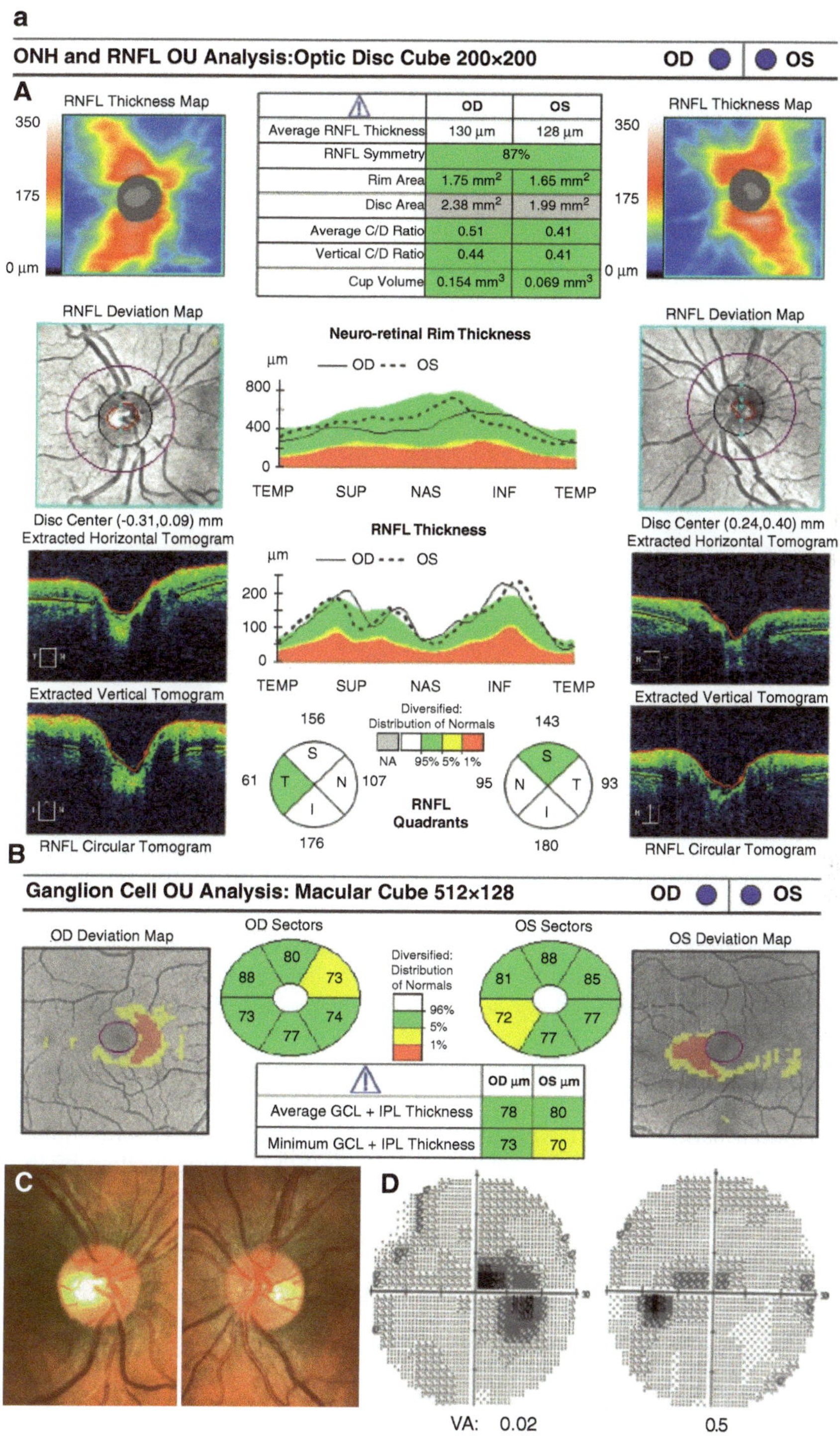
a
ONH and RNFL OU Analysis:Optic Disc Cube 200×200
OD
OS
A
RNFL Thickness Map
350
175
0 µm
OD
OS
Average RNFL Thickness
130 µm
128 µm
RNFL Symmetry
87%
Rim Area
1.75 mm²
1.65 mm²
Disc Area
2.38 mm²
1.99 mm²
Average C/D Ratio
0.51
0.41
Vertical C/D Ratio
0.44
0.41
Cup Volume
0.154 mm³
0.069 mm³
RNFL Deviation Map
Neuro-retinal Rim Thickness
µm
OD
OS
800
400
0
TEMP
SUP
NAS
INF
TEMP
Disc Center (-0.31,0.09) mm
Disc Center (0.24,0.40) mm
Extracted Horizontal Tomogram
RNFL Thickness
200
100
Extracted Vertical Tomogram
Diversified: Distribution of Normals
NA
95%
5%
1%
156
61
107
176
S
T
N
I
143
95
93
180
RNFL Quadrants
RNFL Circular Tomogram
B
Ganglion Cell OU Analysis: Macular Cube 512×128
OD Deviation Map
OD Sectors
80
88
73
73
74
77
OS Sectors
88
81
85
72
77
77
Diversified: Distribution of Normals
96%
5%
1%
OS Deviation Map
OD µm
OS µm
Average GCL + IPL Thickness
78
80
Minimum GCL + IPL Thickness
73
70
C
D
VA: 0.02
0.5

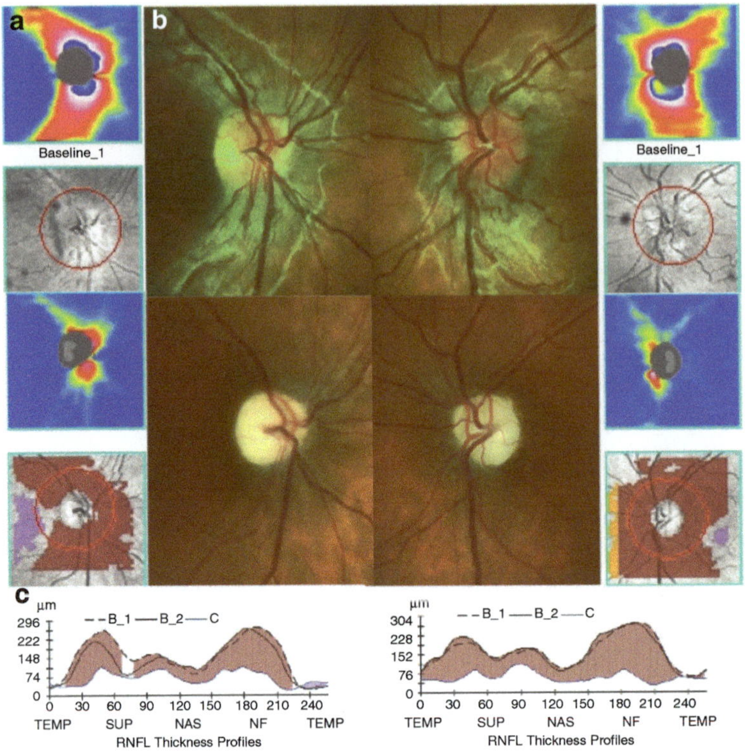

Fig. 16.2 (continued)

the inferior RNFL sectors for the first 3 months, after which the fibers begin to thin [21]. The superior and nasal sector are involved in a subsequent stage and show thickening after 3 months, when the other sectors are already in the atrophic phase [21]. The subacute phase of LHON has proven to be a progressive phase, being characterized by a series of events lasting at least 3 months (Fig. 16.3a, b) [21].

A study on RNFL pattern of swelling and subsequent atrophy, hypothesized a different natural course between patients carrying 11778/ND4 vs 14484/ND6 mutations [24]. The RNFL thickening in the subacute stage and thinning in the dynamic stage was significant greater in 11778/ND4 patients than in 14484/ND6 [24]. These results could explain the different visual prognosis between mutations and establish a correlation between the initial swelling of RNFL and visual prognosis [24].

Finally, once the optic nerve is atrophic, all quadrants of the peripapillary RNFL show a thinning of the fibers. In the chronic stage, patients with visual recovery maintain a thicker RNFL than the subgroup without visual recovery in all quadrants, but the temporal one [17]. The three primary mtDNA mutations have different visual prognosis: worst for 3460/ND1, intermediate for 11778/ND4, and better for 14484/ND6 [14]. OCT studies did not show any difference in RNFL thickness between chronic patients without visual recovery carrying 11778/ND4 and 3460/ND1 mutations [17]. The rare LHON mtDNA 3890/ND1 mutation is associated with a bad visual prognosis and a severe thinning of the peripapillary RNFL [25]. A study in a large cohort of Korean LHON patients demonstrated a similar pattern of RNFL thinning in patients carrying primary and secondary mtDNA mutations, despite the better visual prognosis in patients with secondary mutation [26].

OCT analysis of the RNFL in classical **childhood LHON** (defined as children with subacute disease presentation before the age of 12 years) [10] shows diffuse

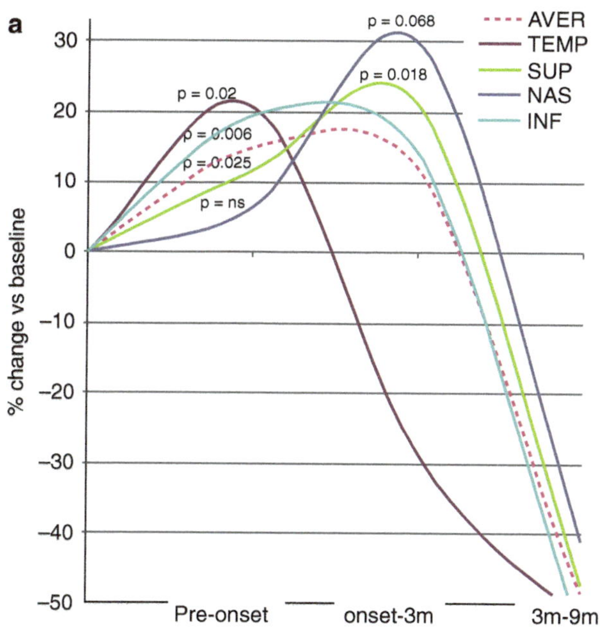

Fig. 16.3 (**a**) Longitudinal RNFL changes from the onset of visual symptoms to the chronic stage of LHON. The temporal quadrant reveals early thickening, whereas the remaining quadrants undergo later thickening up to 3 months. The RNFL thickness changes are expressed as percent with respect to baseline (asymptomatic stage). *AVER* average, *INF* inferior, *NAS* nasal, *SUP* superior, *TEMP* temporal (reproduced with permission from: Barboni et al. [20]) (**b**) Example of progressive RNFL thinning in a patient with LHON from the subacute stage to the chronic stage. Note that the OCT software fails to detect temporal thinning in the late stages as the RNFL thickness is too low, producing a floor effect

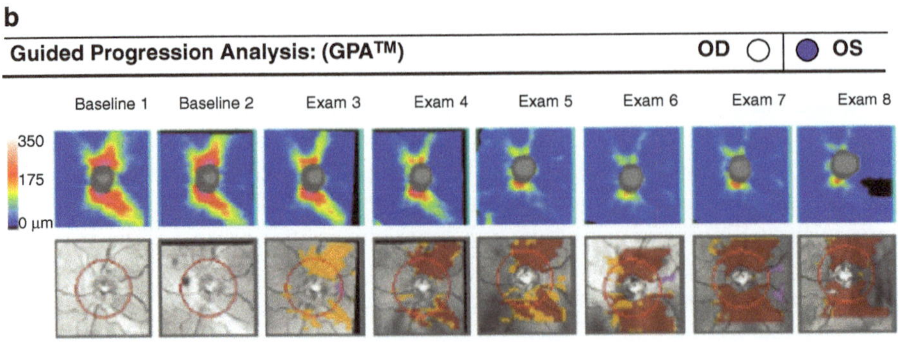

RNFL and ONH Summary Parameters

		Exam Date/Time	Serial Number	Registration Method	SS	Avg RNFL Thickness (µm)	Inf Quadrant RNFL (µm)	Sup Quadrant RNFL (µm)	Rim Area (mm²)	Average Cup-to-Disc Ratio	Vertical Cup-to-Disc Ratio	Cup Volume (mm³)
Baseline 1:	1	12/16/2010 1:16:30 PM	4000-2487		9/10	105	144	130	1.76	0.46	0.37	0.136
Baseline 2:	2	1/20/2011 12:40:56 PM	4000-2487	R2	7/10	96	136	125	1.86	0.46	0.37	0.142
	3	6/27/2011 1:38:32 PM	4000-2487	R2	8/10	80	116	91	1.54	0.54	0.45	0.193
	4	9/29/2011 1:31:33 PM	4000-2487	R2	7/10	70	99	79	1.36	0.60	0.50	0.231
	5	3/16/2012 3:06:54 PM	4000-2487	R1	7/10	61	76	66	1.23	0.67	0.56	0.273
	6	11/26/2012 1:31:48 PM	4000-2487	R1	7/10	59	69	64	1.18	0.69	0.60	0.304
	7	4/16/2013 1:18:51 PM	4000-2487	R1	8/10	58	68	57	1.18	0.69	0.60	0.287
Current:	8	11/25/2013 1:09:17 PM	4000-2487	R1	6/10	55	66	58	1.31	0.72	0.63	0.350

Fig. 16.3 (continued)

fiber atrophy affecting all quadrants (Fig. 16.4) [27]. The classical bilateral childhood presentation does not differ from adult-onset one. In children, other presentations can be more frequently found like *subclinical, slowly progressive* or *atypical unilateral presentation*. Subclinical and slowly progressive forms show a significant fiber reduction in the temporal quadrant, which extends, albeit mildly, to the inferior quadrant, with relative preservation of fibers in the other sectors [27].

16.1.2 Retinal Ganglion Cell Analysis

The macular retinal ganglion cell layer (GCL) is diffusely thinner in LHON affected patients [28, 29]. The early and preferential involvement of RGCs, which precedes RNFL thinning, has been demonstrated by OCT in the subacute stage of the disease [18, 23, 28–30].

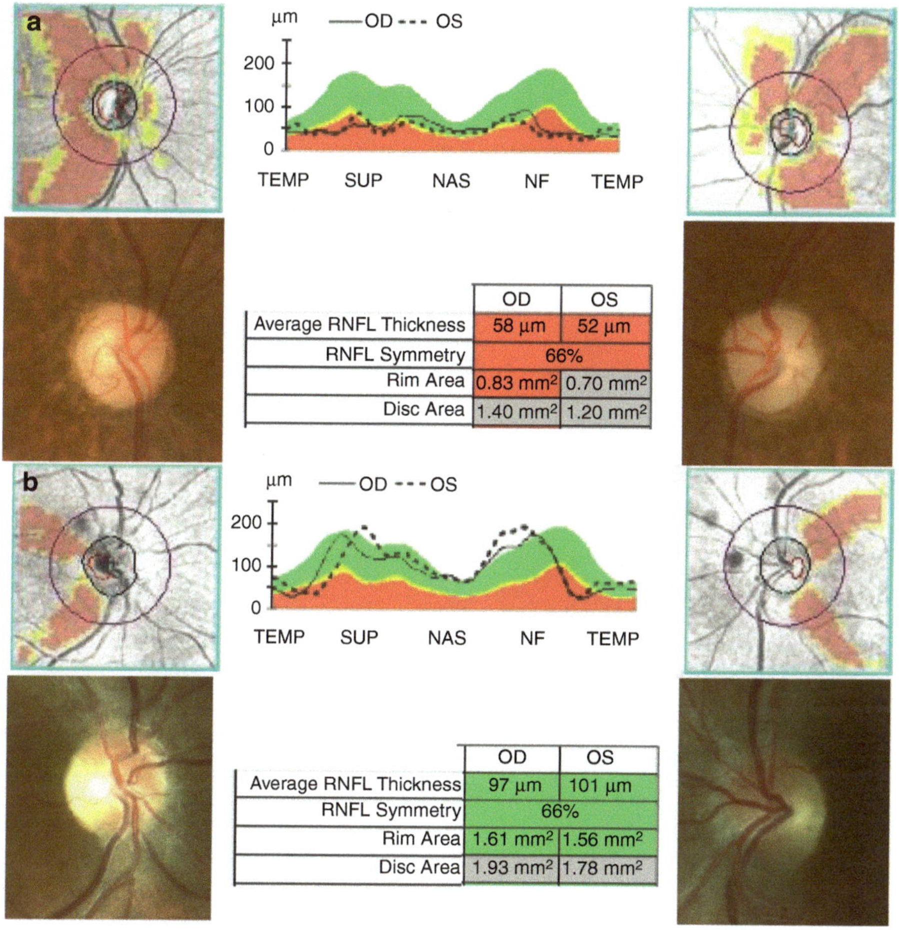

	OD	OS
Average RNFL Thickness	58 µm	52 µm
RNFL Symmetry	66%	
Rim Area	0.83 mm²	0.70 mm²
Disc Area	1.40 mm²	1.20 mm²

	OD	OS
Average RNFL Thickness	97 µm	101 µm
RNFL Symmetry	66%	
Rim Area	1.61 mm²	1.56 mm²
Disc Area	1.93 mm²	1.78 mm²

Fig. 16.4 OCT and color fundus pictures of the right and left optic nerve head in (**a**) a child with subacute LHON presentation: note the small optic disc size, the diffuse RNFL thinning and the temporal optic disc pallor; (**b**) a child with uncategorized early onset before the age of 6: note the medium optic disc size, the temporal RNFL thinning and the nasal RNFL swelling. The OCT software fails to detect the RNFL thinning in the temporal sector due to the floor effect

In the presymptomatic stage, about 4 weeks before the onset of visual loss, topographical analysis of the macular region demonstrated an early involvement of the inner perifoveal ring of the nasal sectors, where the RGC bodies, that contribute to the PMB fibers, are located (Fig. 16.5) [31–33]. In this phase the macular GCL deviation map is more sensitive than the sector analysis provided by OCT to detect initial GCL thinning (Fig. 16.5).

Subsequently, the macular GCL thinning progresses, following a centrifugal and spiral pattern (sequential pattern: inner ring of inferior sector, outer ring of the nasal

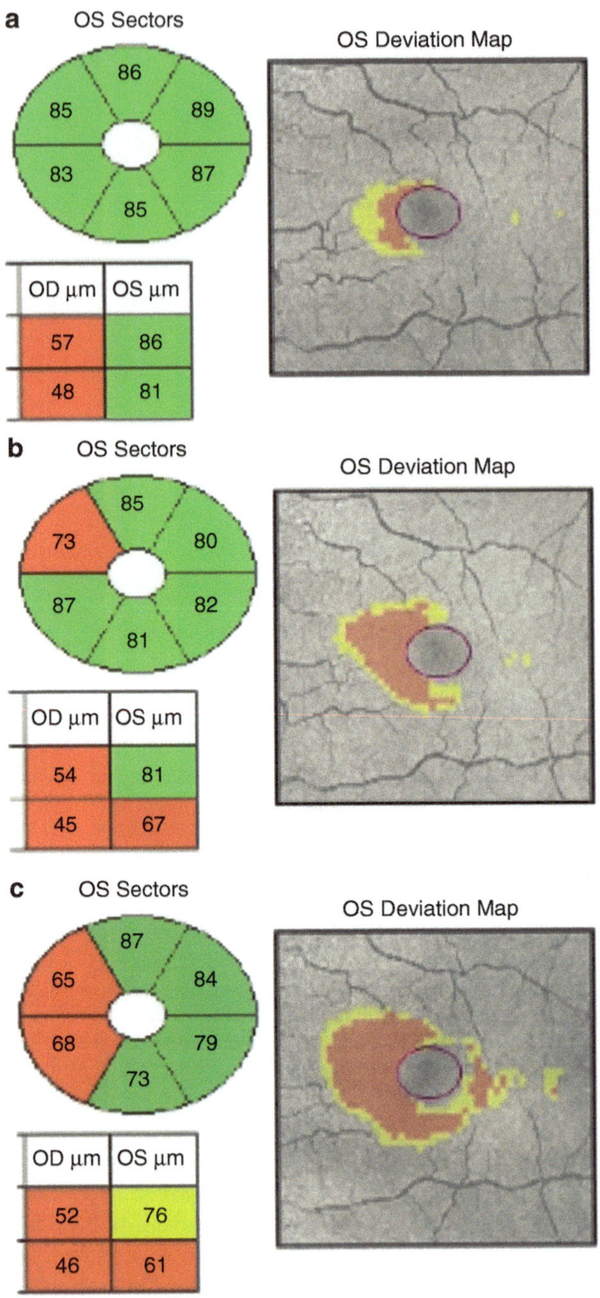

Fig. 16.5 Progressive retinal ganglion cells atrophy in a patient followed from the presymptomatic stage (about 4 weeks before visual loss). Ganglion cell layer sectors analysis and deviation map in pre-symptomatic stage (**a**), at 1 month (**b**), 2 months (**c**) and 5 months (**d**) from disease onset

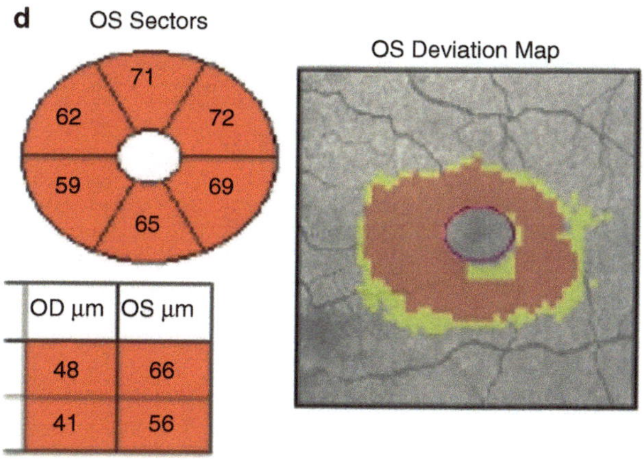

Fig. 16.5 (continued)

sector, inner ring of the temporal and the superior sectors, outer ring of the temporal sector, outer ring of the superior and inferior sectors) [33].

A correlation between GCL thickness and worsening vision was found [30].

16.1.3 Optic Nerve Head Analysis

OCT also enables to investigate the size of the optic nerve head (ONH). Asymptomatic LHON carriers show a larger ONH than symptomatic patients and even healthy controls (Fig. 16.6) [34]. Moreover, the LHON-affected subgroup of patients with visual recovery also had a significantly larger ONH. Therefore, it has been suggested that a larger ONH size, probably associated with less crowding of RGC axons, may represents a favorable prognostic factor, preserving LHON carriers from developing the acute phase of the disease and improving the visual prognosis and in those individuals who develop the optic neuropathy. The role of the ONH size is likely to be related to the mechanical compression of the PMB fibers: the greater space for nerve fibers may reduce the risk of focal compression of swelling axons.

After stratifying LHON affected and carrier patients by mtDNA mutations, 11778/ND4, 3460/ND1 and 3733/ND1 unaffected carriers had larger optic nerve discs than affected patients with the same mutations [26]. 14484/ND6 affected and carrier patients had the same disc size that was larger than the disc size found in patients with the other mutations [34].

Moreover, ONH analysis in subacute childhood LHON patients (classical LHON) showed smaller optic disc areas compared with patients with slowly progressive and subclinical courses of the disease (Fig. 16.4) [27].

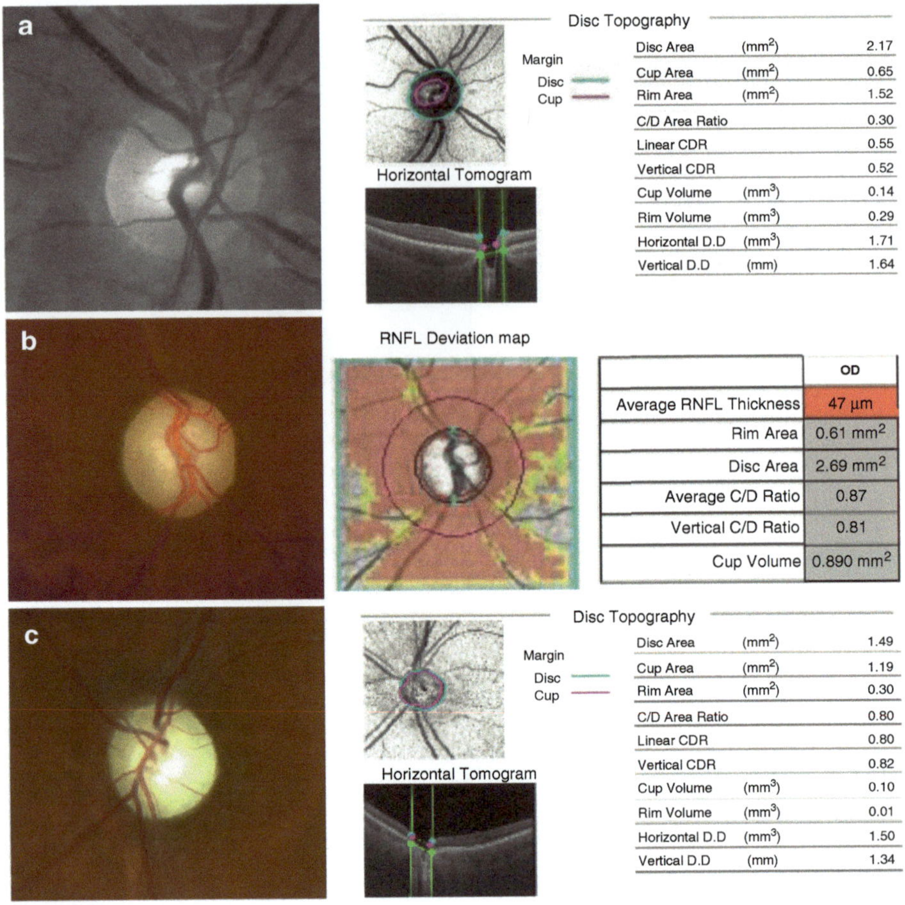

Fig. 16.6 Representative optic nerve head pictures and OCT analysis: (**a**) asymptomatic LHON mutation carrier with large optic disc area; (**b**) chronic LHON patient with large optic disc area and partial visual recovery; (**c**) chronic LHON patient with small optic disc area without visual recovery

16.2 Dominant Optic Atrophy (DOA)

DOA is a similar hereditary degenerative optic neuropathy to LHON, involving preferentially the PMB. However, DOA is due to a mutation in the nuclear genome and is transmitted in a dominant manner. Most cases of DOA have been associated with mutations in the OPA1 gene on the long arm of chromosome 3q28–q29, which encodes a dynamin-related GTPase targeted to mitochondria [35]. Seventy-five percent of DOA patients have a mutation in OPA1 gene; two loci, OPA4 and OPA5, are associated to pure DOA; one locus, OPA2 is associated to xx X-linked form; two loci, OPA6 and OPA7, are related to recessive ceses, two loci, OPA3 and OPA8, are responsable of syndromic recessive or dominant forms [36–38].

DOA patients with OPA1 mutation can be also defined by the mutation type: OPA1 mutation causing haploinsufficiency and OPA1 missense mutation [39].

DOA has a clinical picture more insidious than that of LHON, as it is characterized by very slowly progressive bilateral visual loss starting in childhood and ultimately leading to moderate or severe optic atrophy [40–43]. The disease has incomplete penetrance and variable expression between and within families; it ranges from subclinical manifestations to legal blindness. Twenty percent of DOA patients with OPA1 mutations have a more severe disease with neuromuscular features (DOA plus) [44, 45].

16.2.1 Retinal Nerve Fiber Layer Analysis

OCT analysis of the RNFL in DOA reveals fiber atrophy affecting all quadrants [46–48]. The retinal thinning involves the RNFL and GCL, whereas the photoreceptors are morphologically unaffected (Fig. 16.7).

The RNFL thinning is more pronounced in the temporal and inferior quadrants and less evident in the superior and nasal ones [46–48], confirming the vulnerability of the small fibers of the PMB as a pathognomonic sign of mitochondrial optic neuropathies. Patients with DOA plus disease show a more severe thinning of RNFL in all quadrants compared with simple DOA patients [48].

The progressive fiber loss in affected patients (0.19–0.20 μm/year for the 360° average measurement) is similar to that occurring with age in healthy subjects, where the loss ranges between 0.16 and 0.25 μm/year [49–51]. This observation, in combination to the smaller ONH size of DOA patients (see the next paragraph), suggests that visual loss in DOA patients is related to progressive fiber loss in eyes with already lower congenital or neonatal fiber counts.

The pattern of fiber loss, studied by OCT, in OPA8 patients did not differ from that found in OPA1 patients [52]. A genotype/phenotype correlation, stratifying OCT measurement by OPA1 mutation type, shows that missense mutations had the most severe reductions in both RNFL and macular GCL thickness [31].

16.2.2 Retinal Ganglion Cell Analysis

OCT of DOA patients shows an earlier involvement of the macular RGCs, whose thickness is reduced in all the macular sectors. The thinner sectors were the nasal and inferior ones [31, 53, 54]. As the disease progresses and visual acuity worsens, the macular RGCs measurements correlated with visual acuity better than measures of RNFL thinning (Fig. 16.7) [31, 54]. GCL thickness also declined with age [31].

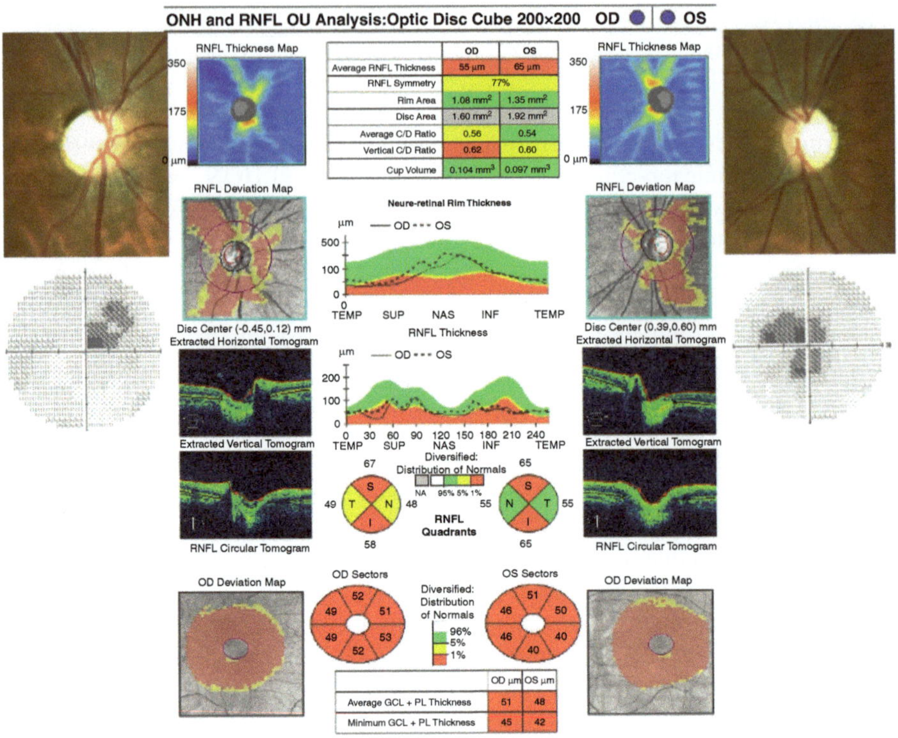

Fig. 16.7 Peripapillary RNFL, macular ganglion cell layer analysis, color fundus image and visual fields in a patient with DOA

16.2.3 Optic Nerve Head Analysis

Patients affected with DOA and carrying OPA1 gene mutations reveal a smaller ONH (both optic disc area and ONH diameters) than controls (Fig. 16.8) [55]. By stratifying these results according to OPA1 mutation, it is possible to identify different degrees of optic disc size, where the mutations range from those associated with a normal optic disc size to those associated with much smaller sizes and more severe clinical features of DOA. The proposed hypothesis is that OPA1 expression regulates apoptosis, thereby playing an important role in the embryonic development of the eye and contributing to the determination of optic disc size and conformation. As stated in the previous paragraph, a constitutive low content of fibers in the optic nerve and the age-related RNFL loss may explain the progressive visual loss in

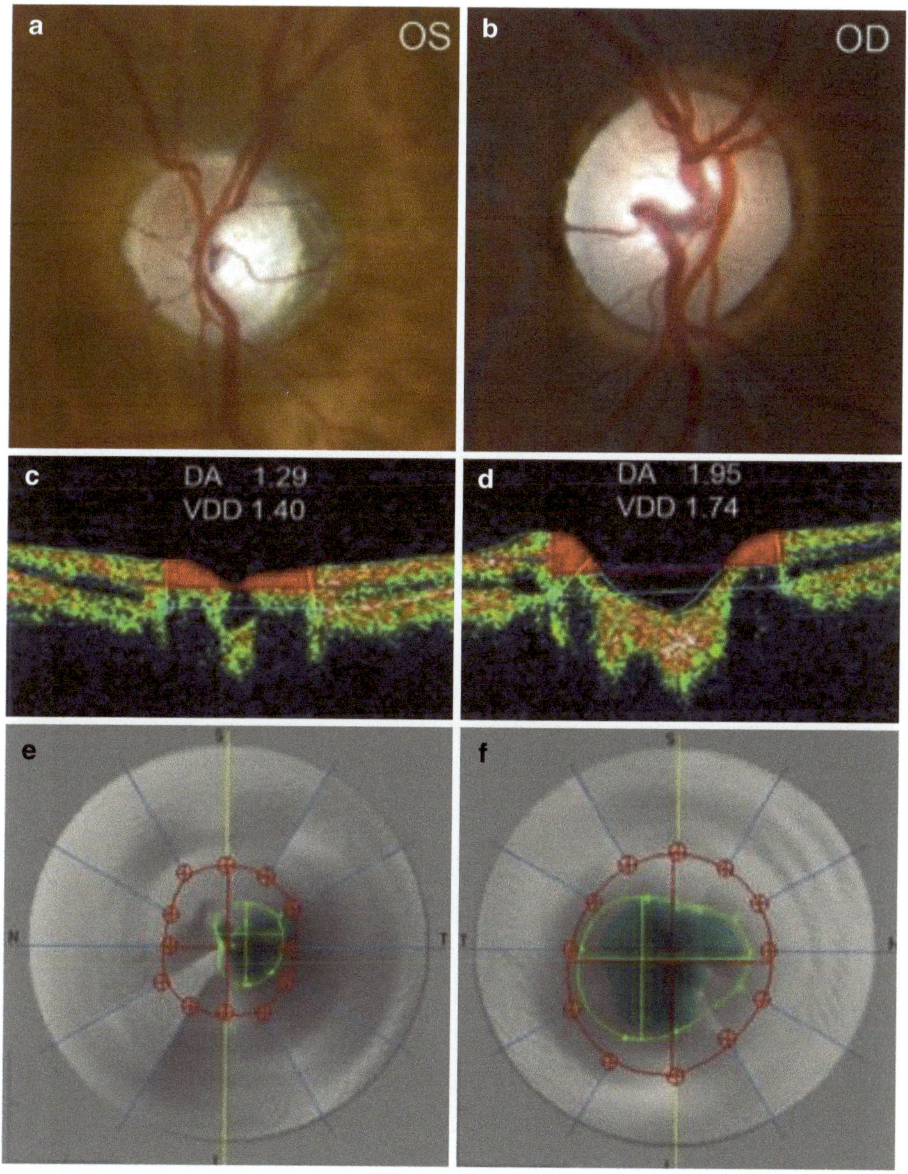

Fig. 16.8 Representative optic nerve head color pictures and OCT analysis of a DOA patient with a small optic disc (**a**, **c**, **e**), and a DOA patient with normal optic disc size (**b**, **d**, **f**). *DA* optic disc area, *VDD* vertical disc diameter (Reproduced with permission from: Gelfand et al. [60])

DOA. DOA patients with the lowest visual acuity have a smaller disc area, measured by OCT, compared to controls [56].

OCT analysis showed that DOA patients who do not recover vision on Idebenone therapy, have thinner RNFL and smaller ONH than patients with visual recovery [55]. This result add further evidence for the prognostic value of OCT in therapeutic protocols.

16.3 Other OCT Macular Findings

OCT analysis of the macular region shows, in addition, that a minority (about 6%) of LHON and DOA patients have microcystic changes in the inner nuclear layer (Fig. 16.9) [57, 58]. Microcystic macular edema (MME) is present in the absence of any leakage at the fluorescein angiography. MME has also been described in inflammatory optic neuritis in MS and NMO [59–64], compressive optic neuropathy [65] and in glaucoma [66].

MME could be related to focal retinal schisis induced by vitreous traction in association with RNFL atrophy [57], or to retrograde transinaptic degeneration in the visual pathways [65, 67], Muller cells dysfunction [68] or inflammation [59].

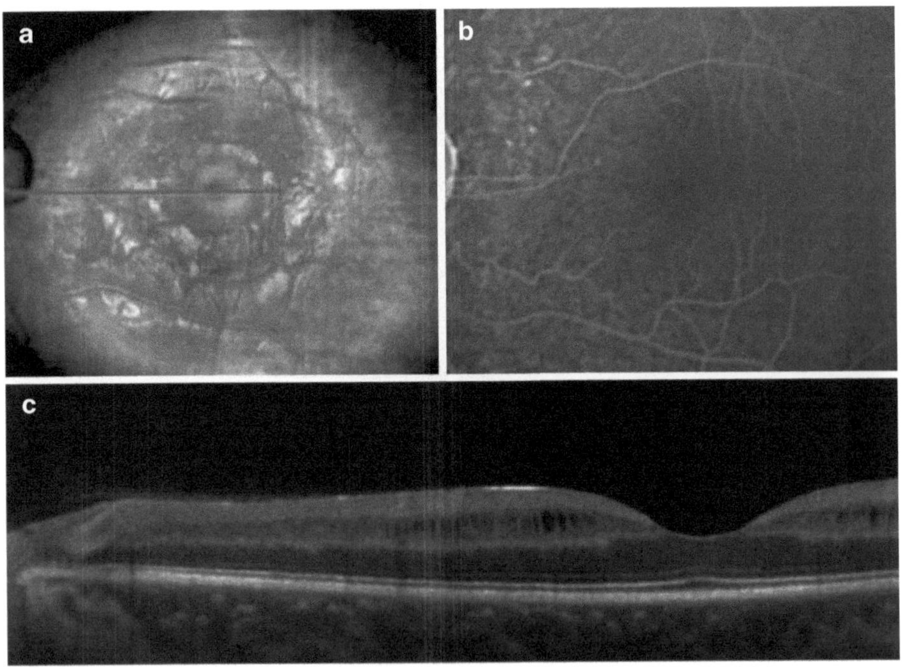

Fig. 16.9 Microcystic macular edema in a patient with LHON. (**a**) Red free fundus picture, (**b**) fluorescein angiography and (**c**) corresponding HD-OCT line of the macula

16.4 OCT and Vascular Supply Analysis

Advances in OCT allowed the study of the choroidal thickness, using enhanced depth imaging (EDI) technique or the swept source OCT (SS-OCT). Moreover, the vascular supply of the optic nerve head, the macula and the choriocapillary is displayable using optical coherence tomography angiography (OCT-A).

Those exams were performed in hereditary optic neuropathies and could elucidate the role of the vasculature in the disease process.

Changes of the choroidal thickness have been documented in LHON patients during disease conversion. Specifically, both macular and peripapillary choroidal thickness increase in the subacute stage and then decrease in the chronic stage, following the same trend of peripapillar RNFL (increased thickness, followed by thinning), but RNFL changes preceded those affecting the choroid [69]. The evidence that increased thickness of axons precedes the increase of choroidal thickness suggests that the first event leads to the other one. The choroidal thickening seen during the LHON subacute stage may be due to a compensatory response to hypoxia and increase oxygen demand. In the chronic stage the choroid was thicker in LHON than in DOA (whereas the RNFL thickness followed an opposite trend being thinner in LHON as compared to DOA) [69].

In LHON, peripapillary teleangectatic blood vessels have been documented in the subacute stage [70–73]. Subsequently, a progressive peripapillary vascular reduction has been detected starting from the temporal and inferior sectors as the disease progresses [74], then spreading to all the other peripapillary vessels in the chronic phase (Fig. 16.10) [74, 75]. Studying the vascular network separately from

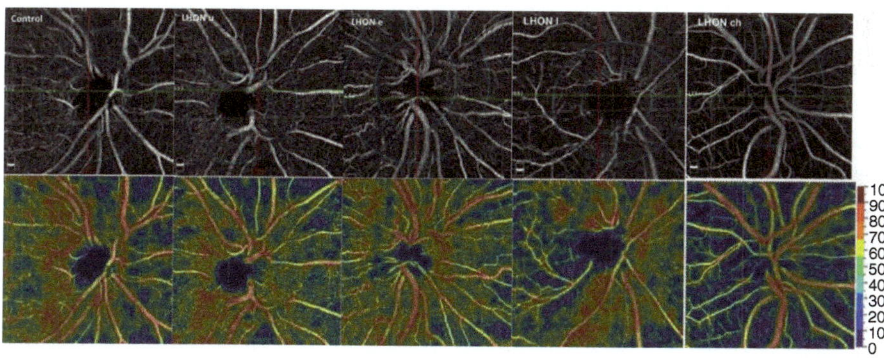

Fig. 16.10 Example of OCT-A in the different stages. Example of vascular visualization of Radial Peripapillary Capillaries (RPC, top images) layer and density maps (bottom images) in 5 groups (control; LHON u: unaffected carrier; LHON e: early subacute stage; LHON l: late subacute stage; LHON ch: chronic stage). Note the progressive vessel density reduction as the disease advances, starting from the temporal sector (Reproduced with the permission from: Balducci et al. [74])

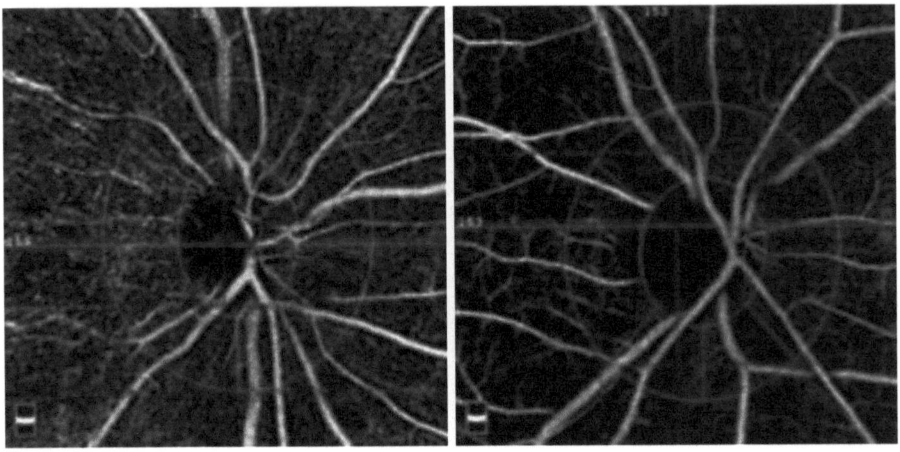

Fig. 16.11 OCT-A of the right optic nerves in a control (left) and Dominant optic atrophy patient (right). Note the diffuse vessel density reduction in DOA patient (Reproduced with the permission from: Balducci et al. [77])

fibers revealed that microvascular changes in the temporal sector preceded the changes of RNFL and mirrored the GCL changes [74]. A recent study [76] found a reduction of the vessel density in the parafoveal region in LHON, mainly confined to the nasal and inferior sectors, corresponding to the PMB. Moreover, an association between the visual loss and the superficial capillary plexus flow impairment was detected [76].

In DOA a reduction of optic nerve head and peripapillary vessel density has been detected (Fig. 16.11) [77].

16.5 Conclusions

Over the last decade, OCT helped us in the diagnosis and follow-up of optic neuropathies. Moreover, the additional informations achieved by OCT and OCT-A about the pathophysiology of LHON and DOA have improved our knowledge on the disease conversion and progression. In the next step, OCT and OCT-A will be able to indicate the timing and the prognosis of future therapeutic approaches.

References

1. Yu-Wai-Man P, Griffiths PG, Chinnery PF. Mitochondrial optic neuropathies disease mechanisms and therapeutic strategies. Prog Retin Eye Res. 2011;30:81–114.
2. Newman NJ. Hereditary optic neuropathies. In: Miller NR, Newman NJ, editors. Walsh and Hoyt's clinical neuro-ophthalmology. 5th ed. Baltimore: Williams & Wilkins; 1998. p. 742–53.
3. Carelli V. Leber's hereditary optic neuropathy. In: Schapira AHV, DiMauro S, editors. Mitochondrial disorders in neurology, Blue books of practical neurology, vol. 26. 2nd ed. Boston: Butterworth-Heinemann; 2002. p. 115–42.

4. Carelli V, Giordano C, d'Amati G. Pathogenic expression of homoplasmic mtDNA mutations needs a complex nuclear-mitochondrial interaction. Trends Genet. 2003;19:257–62.
5. Howell N, Mackey DA. Low-penetrance branches in matrilinear pedigrees with Leber hereditary optic neuropathy. Am J Hum Genet. 1998;63:1220–4.
6. Sadun AA, Kashima Y, Wurdeman AE, et al. Morphological findings in the visual system in a case of Leber's hereditary optic neuropathy. Clin Neurosci. 1994;2:165–72.
7. Kerrison JB, Howell N, Miller NR, et al. Leber hereditary optic neuropathy. Electron microscopy and molecular genetic analysis of a case. Ophthalmology. 1995;102:1509–16.
8. Sadun AA, Win PH, Ross-Cisneros FN, et al. Leber's hereditary optic neuropathy differentially affects smaller axons in the optic nerve. Trans Am Ophthalmol Soc. 2000;98:223–32.
9. Pan BX, Ross-Cisneros FN, Carelli V, Rue KS, Salomao SR, Moraes-Filho MN, Moraes MN, Berezovsky A, Belfort R Jr, Sadun AA. Mathematically modeling the involvement of axons in Leber's hereditary optic neuropathy. Invest Ophthalmol Vis Sci. 2012;53:7608–17.
10. Carelli V, Carbonelli M, de Coo IF, Kawasaki A, Klopstock T, Lagrèze WA, La Morgia C, Newman NJ, Orssaud C, Pott JWR, Sadun AA, van Everdingen J, Vignal-Clermont C, Votruba M, Yu-Wai-Man P, Barboni P. International consensus statement on the clinical and therapeutic management of Leber hereditary optic neuropathy. J Neuroophthalmol. 2017;37:371–81.
11. Nikoskelainen E, Hoyt WF, Nummelin K. Ophthalmoscopic findings in Leber's hereditary optic neuropathy. I. Fundus findings in asymptomatic family members. Arch Ophthalmol. 1982;100:1597–602.
12. Nikoskelainen E, Hoyt WF, Nummelin K. Ophthalmoscopic findings in Leber's hereditary optic neuropathy. II. The fundus findings in affected family members. Arch Ophthalmol. 1983;101:1059–68.
13. Smith JL, Hoyt WF, Susac JO. Ocular fundus in acute Leber optic neuropathy. Arch Ophthalmol. 1973;90:349–54.
14. Riordan-Eva P, Sanders D, Govan GG, et al. The clinical features of Leber's hereditary optic neuropathy defined by the presence of a pathogenic mitochondrial DNA mutation. Brain. 1995;118:319–37.
15. Nikoskelainen EK, Huoponen K, Juvonen V, et al. Ophthalmologic findings in Leber hereditary optic neuropathy, with special reference to mtDNA mutations. Ophthalmology. 1996;103:504–14.
16. Savini G, Barboni P, Valentino ML, Montagna P, Cortelli P, De Negri AM, Sadun F, Bianchi S, Longanesi L, Zanini M, Carelli V. Retinal nerve fiber layer evaluation by optical coherence tomography in unaffected carriers with Leber's hereditary optic neuropathy mutations. Ophthalmology. 2005;112:127–31.
17. Barboni P, Savini G, Valentino ML, Montagna P, Cortelli P, De Negri AM, et al. Retinal nerve fiber layer evaluation by optical coherence tomography in Leber's hereditary optic neuropathy. Ophthalmology. 2005;112:120–6.
18. Hedges TR, Gobuty M, Manfready RA, Erlich-Malona N, Monaco C, Mendoza-Santiesteban CE. The optical coherence tomographic profile of Leber hereditary optic neuropathy. Neuroophthalmology. 2016;40:107–12.
19. Carelli V, Ross-Cisneros FN, Sadun AA. Mitochondrial dysfunction as a cause of optic neuropathies. Prog Retin Eye Res. 2004;23:53–89.
20. Barboni P, Savini G, Feuer WJ, Budenz DL, Carbonelli M, Chicani F, Ramos CD, Salomao SR, De Negri A, Parisi V, Carelli V, Sadun AA. Retinal nerve fiber layer thickness variability in Leber hereditary optic neuropathy carriers. Eur J Ophthalmol. 2012;4(22):985–91.
21. Barboni P, Carbonelli M, Savini G, et al. Natural history of Leber's hereditary optic neuropathy: longitudinal analysis of the retinal nerve fiber layer by optical coherence tomography. Ophthalmology. 2010;117:623–7.
22. Zhang Y, Huang H, Wei S, Qiu H, Gong Y, Li H, Dai Y, Jiang Z, Liu Z. Characterization of retinal nerve fiber layer thickness changes associated with Leber's hereditary optic neuropathy by optical coherence tomography. Exp Ther Med. 2014;7:483–7.

23. Teng D, Peng CX, Qian HY, Li L, Wang W, Wang JQ, Chen B, Zhou HF, Wei SH. Structural impairment patterns in peripapillary retinal fiber layer and retinal ganglion cell layer in mitochondrial optic neuropathies. Int J Ophthalmol. 2018;11:1643–8.
24. Seo JH, Hwang JM, Park SS. Comparison of retinal nerve fibre layers between 11778 and 14484 mutations in Leber's hereditary optic neuropathy. Eye. 2010;24:107–11.
25. Caporali L, Ghelli AM, Iommarini L, Maresca A, Valentino ML, La Morgia C, Liguori R, Zanna C, Barboni P, De Nardo V, Martinuzzi A, Rizzo G, Tonon C, Lodi R, Calvaruso MA, Cappelletti M, Porcelli AM, Achilli A, Pala M, Torroni A, Carelli V. Cybrid studies establish the causal link between the mtDNA m.3890G>A/MT-ND1 mutation and optic atrophy with bilateral brainstem lesions. Biochim Biophys Acta. 2013;1832:445–52.
26. Yum HR, Chae H, Shin SY, Kim Y, Kim M, Park SH. Pathogenic mitochondrial DNA mutations and associated clinical features in Korean patients with Leber's hereditary optic neuropathy. Invest Ophthalmol Vis Sci. 2014;55:8095–101.
27. Barboni P, Savini G, Valentino ML, La Morgia C, Bellusci C, De Negri AM, Sadun F, Carta A, Carbonelli M, Sadun AA, Carelli V. Leber's hereditary optic neuropathy with childhood onset. Invest Ophthalmol Vis Sci. 2006;47:5303–9.
28. Akiyama H, Kashima T, Li D, Shimoda Y, Mukai R, Kishi S. Retinal ganglion cell analysis in Leber's hereditary optic neuropathy. Ophthalmology. 2013;120:1943–4.e5.
29. Mizoguchi A, Hashimoto Y, Shinmei Y, Nozaki M, Ishijima K, Tagawa Y, et al. Macular thickness changes in a patient with Leber's hereditary optic neuropathy. BMC Ophthalmol. 2015;15:27.
30. Moster SJ, Moster ML, Scannell Bryan M, Sergott RC. Retinal ganglion cell and inner plexiform layer loss correlate with visual acuity loss in LHON: a longitudinal, segmentation OCT analysis. Invest Ophthalmol Vis Sci. 2016;57:3872–83.
31. Barboni P, Savini G, Cascavilla M, CAporali L, Milesi J, Borrelli E, et al. Early macular retinal ganglion cell loss in dominant optic atrophy: genotype-phenotype correlation. Am J Ophthalmol. 2014;158:628–36.
32. Zhang Y, Huang H, Wei S, Gong Y, Li H, Dai Y, Zhao S, Wang Y, Yan H. Characterization of macular thickness changes in Leber's hereditary optic neuropathy by optical coherence tomography. BMC Ophthalmol. 2014;14:105.
33. Balducci N, Savini G, Cascavilla ML, La Morgia C, Triolo G, Giglio R, Carbonelli M, Parisi V, Sadun AA, Bandello F, Carelli V, Barboni P. Macular nerve fibre and ganglion cell layer changes in acute Leber's hereditary optic neuropathy. Br J Ophthalmol. 2016;100:1232–7.
34. Ramos CV, Bellusci C, Savini G, et al. Association of optic disc size with development and prognosis of Leber's hereditary optic neuropathy. Invest Ophthalmol Vis Sci. 2009;50:1666–74.
35. Alexander C, Votruba M, Pesch UE, et al. OPA1, encoding a dynamin-related GTPase, is mutated in autosomal dominant optic atrophy linked to chromosome 3q28. Nat Genet. 2000;26:211–5.
36. Ferre M, Amati-Bonneau P, Tourmen Y, Malthièry Y, Reynier P. eOPA1: an online database for OPA1 mutations. Hum Mutat. 2005;25:423–8. PubMed: 15832306.
37. Ferre M, Bonneau D, Milea D, Chevrollier A, Verny C, Dullfus H, et al. Molecular screening of 980 cases of suspected hereditary optic neuropathy with a report on 77 novel OPA1 mutations. Hum Mutat. 2009;30:E692–705.
38. Yu-Wai-Man P, Shankar SP, Biousse V, Miller NR, Bean LJ, Coffee B, et al. Genetic screening for OPA1 and OPA3 mutations in patients with suspected inherited optic neuropathies. Ophthalmology. 2010;118:558–63.
39. Amati-Bonneau P, Valentino ML, Reynier P, Gallardo ME, Bornstein B, Boissière A, et al. OPA1 mutations induce mitochondrial DNA instability and optic atrophy "plus" phenotypes. Brain. 2008;131:338–51.
40. Kjer P. Infantile optic atrophy with dominant mode of inheritance: a clinical and genetic study of 19 Danish families. Acta Ophthalmol Suppl. 1959;164(suppl):1–147.
41. Newman NJ. Hereditary optic neuropathies. In: Miller NR, Newman NJ, editors; Biousse V, Kerrison JB, assoc. editors. Walsh and Hoyt's clinical neuro-ophthalmology, 6th ed., vol. 1. Philadelphia: Lippincott Williams & Wilkins; 2005. p. 465–501.

42. Cohn AC, Toomes C, Hewitt AW, Kearns LS, Inglehearn CF, Craig JE, et al. The natural history of OPA1-related autosomal dominant optic atrophy. Br J Ophthalmol. 2008;92:1333–6.
43. Yu-Wai-Man P, Griffiths PG, Burke A, Sellar PW, Clarke MP, Gnanaraj L, et al. The prevalence and natural history of dominant optic atrophy due to OPA1 mutations. Ophthalmology. 2010;117:1538–46.
44. Amati-Bonneau P, Guichet A, Olichon A, Chevrollier A, Viala F, Miot S, Ayuso C, et al. OPA1 R445H mutation in optic atrophy associated with sensorineural deafness. Ann Neurol. 2005;58:958–63.
45. Hudson G, Amati-Bonneau P, Blakely EL, Stewart JD, He L, Schaefer AM, et al. Mutation of OPA1 causes dominant optic atrophy with external ophthalmoplegia, ataxia, deafness and multiple mitochondrial DNA deletions: a novel disorder of mtDNA maintenance. Brain. 2008;131:329–37.
46. Milea D, Sander B, Wegener M, et al. Axonal loss occurs early in dominant optic atrophy. Acta Ophthalmol. 2010;88:342–6.
47. Barboni P, Savini G, Parisi V, et al. Retinal nerve Fiber layer thickness in dominant optic atrophy measurements by optical coherence tomography and correlation with age. Ophthalmology. 2011;118:2076–80.
48. Yu-Wai-Man P, Bailie M, Atawan A, Chinnery PF, Griffiths PG. Pattern of retinal ganglion cell loss in dominant optic atrophy due to OPA1 mutations. Eye. 2011;25:596–602.
49. Parikh RS, Parikh SR, Sekhar GC, et al. Normal age-related decay of retinal nerve fiber layer thickness. Ophthalmology. 2007;114:921–6.
50. Sung KR, Wollstein G, Bilonick RA, et al. Effects of age on optical coherence tomography measurements of healthy retinal nerve fiber layer, macula and optic nerve head. Ophthalmology. 2009;116:1119–24.
51. Budenz DL, Anderson DR, Varma R, et al. Determinants of normal retinal nerve fiber layer thickness measured by Stratus OCT. Ophthalmology. 2007;114:1046–52.
52. Carelli V, Schimpf S, Fuhrmann N, Valentino ML, Zanna C, Iommarini L, Papke M, Schaich S, Tippmann S, Baumann B, Barboni P, Longanesi L, Rugolo M, Ghelli A, Alavi MV, Youle RJ, Bucchi L, Carroccia R, Giannoccaro MP, Tonon C, Lodi R, Cenacchi G, Montagna P, Liguori R, Wissinger B. A clinically complex form of dominant optic atrophy (OPA8) maps on chromosome 16. Hum Mol Genet. 2011;20:1893–905.
53. Ito Y, Nakamura M, Yamakoshi T, Lin J, Yatsuya H, Terasaki H. Reduction of inner retinal thickness in patients with autosomal dominant optic atrophy associated with OPA1 mutations. Invest Ophthalmol Vis Sci. 2007;48:4079–86.
54. Rönnbäck C, Milea D, Larsen M. Imaging of the macula indicates early completion of structural deficit in autosomal-dominant optic atrophy. Ophthalmology. 2013;120:2672–7.
55. Barboni P, Valentino ML, La Morgia C, Carbonelli M, Savini G, De Negri A, Simonelli F, Sadun F, Caporali L, Maresca A, Liguori R, Baruzzi A, Zeviani M, Carelli V. Idebenone treatment in patients with OPA1-mutant dominant optic atrophy. Brain. 2013;136(Pt2):e231.
56. Barboni P, Carbonelli M, Savini G, Foscarini B, Parisi V, Valentino ML, Carta A, De Negri AM, Sadun F, Zeviani M, Sadun AA, Schimpf S, Wissinger B, Carelli V. OPA1 mutations associated with dominant optic atrophy influence optic nerve head size. Ophthalmology. 2010;117:1547–53.
57. Barboni P, Carelli V, Savini G, Carbonelli M, La Morgia C, Sadun AA. Microcystic macular degeneration from optic neuropathy: not inflammatory, not trans-synaptic degeneration. Brain. 2013;136(Pt 7):e239.
58. Carbonelli M, La Morgia C, Savini G, Cascavilla ML, Borrelli E, Chicani F, do V F Ramos C, Salomao SR, Parisi V, Sebag J, Bandello F, Sadun AA, Carelli V, Barboni P. Macular microcysts in mitochondrial optic neuropathies: prevalence and retinal layer thickness measurements. PLoS One. 2015;10:e0127906.
59. Gelfand JM, Nolan R, Schwatz DM, Graves J, Green AJ. Microcystic macular oedema in multiple sclerosis is associated with disease severity. Brain. 2012;135:1786–93.

60. Gelfand JM, Cree BA, Nolan R, Arnow S, Green AJ. Microcystic inner nuclear layer abnormalities and neuromyelitis optica. JAMA Neurol. 2013;70:629–33.
61. Saidha S, Sotirchos ES, Ibrahim MA, Crainiceanu CM, Gelfand JM, Sepah YJ, et al. Microcystic macular oedema, thickness of the inner nuclear layer of the retina, and disease characteristics in multiple sclerosis: a retrospective study. Lancet Neurol. 2012;11:963–72. Erratum in: Lancet Neurol. 2012;11:1021.
62. Schneider E, Zimmermann H, Oberwahrenbrock T, Kaufhold F, Kadas EM, Petzold A, et al. Optical coherence tomography reveals distinct patterns of retinal damage in neuromyelitis optica and multiple sclerosis. PLoS One. 2013;8:e66151.
63. Balk L, Killestein J, Polman C, Uitdehaag BM, Petzold A. Microcystic macular oedema confirmed, but not specific for MS. Brain. 2012;135:e226. Author reply e227.
64. Kaufhold F, Zimmermann H, Schneider E, Ruprecht K, Paul F, Oberwahrenbrock T, et al. Optic neuritis is associated with inner nuclear layer thickening and microcystic macula edema independently of multiple sclerosis. PLoS One. 2013;8:e71145.
65. Abegg M, Zinkernagel M, Wolf S. Microcystic macular degeneration from optic neuropathy. Brain. 2012;135:e225.
66. Wolff B, Basdekidou C, Vasseur V, Mauget-Faysse M, Sahel JA, Vignal C. Retinal inner nuclear layer microcystic changes in optic nerve atrophy: a novel spectral-domain OCT finding. Retina. 2013;33:2133–8.
67. Jindahra P, Petrie A, Plant GT. The time course of retrograde trans-synaptic degeneration following occipital lobe damage in humans. Brain. 2012;135:534–41.
68. Bhargava P, Calabresi PA. The expanding spectrum of aetiologies causing retinal microcystic macular change. Brain. 2013;136:3212–4.
69. Borrelli E, Triolo G, Cascavilla ML, La Morgia C, Rizzo G, Savini G, Balducci N, Nucci P, Giglio R, Darvizeh F, Parisi V, Bandello F, Sadun AA, Carelli V, Barboni P. Changes in choroidal thickness follow the RNFL changes in Leber's hereditary optic neuropathy. Sci Rep. 2016;6:37332.
70. Ghasemi Falavarjani K, Tian JJ, Akil H, Garcia GA, Sadda SR, Sadun AA. Swept-source optical coherence tomography angiography of the optic disk in optic neuropathy. Retina. 2016;36:S168–77.
71. De Rojas JO, Rasool N, Chen RW, Horowitz J, Odel JG. Optical coherence tomography angiography in Leber hereditary optic neuropathy. Neurology. 2016;87:2065–6.
72. Takayama K, Ito Y, Kaneko H, Kataoka K, Ra E, Terasaki H. Optical coherence tomography angiography in Leber hereditary optic neuropathy. Acta Ophthalmol. 2017;95:e344–5.
73. Akil H, Ghasemi Falavarjani K, Sadda SS, Sadun AA. Optical coherence tomography angiography of the optic disc; an overview. J Ophthalmic Vis Res. 2017;12:98–105.
74. Balducci N, Cascavilla ML, Ciardella A, La Morgia C, Triolo G, Parisi V, Bandello F, Sadun AA, Carelli V, Barboni P. Peripapillary vessel density changes in Leber's hereditary optic neuropathy: a new biomarker. Clin Exp Ophthalmol. 2018; https://doi.org/10.1111/ceo.13326. Epub ahead of print.
75. Kousal B, Kolarova H, Meliska M, Bydzovsky J, Diblik P, Kulhanek J, Votruba M, Honzik T, Liskova P. Peripapillary microcirculation in Leber hereditaryoptic neuropathy. Acta Ophthalmol. 2018. Epub ahead of print.
76. Borrelli E, Balasubruman S, Triolo G, Barboni P, Sadda SS, Sadun AA. Topographic macular microvascular changes and correlation with visual loss in chronic Leber hereditary optic neuropathy. Am J Ophthalmol. 2018;192:217–28.
77. Balducci N, Ciardella A, Gattegna R, Zhou Q, Cascavilla ML, La Morgia C, Savini G, Parisi V, Bandello F, Carelli V, Barboni P. Optical coherence tomography angiography of the peripapillary retina and optic nerve head in dominant optic atrophy. Mitochondrion. 2017;36:60–5.

Trans Neuronal Retrograde Degeneration to OCT in Central Nervous System Diseases

17

Bernardo F. Sánchez-Dalmau, Anna Camós-Carreras, Ruben Torres-Torres, Johannes Keller, Laura Sanchez-Vela, Elena H. Martínez-Lapiscina, and Pablo Villoslada

17.1 Introduction

The anterior visual pathway is composed of axons from retinal ganglion cells, which form the optic nerve, optic chiasm, and optic tract, and synapse in the lateral geniculate nucleus (LGN). The posterior visual pathway is composed of axons from the LGN that form the optic radiations (OR) and project into the visual cortex.

About 90% of retinal axons synapse in the LGN, and travel with the optic radiations to the occipital cortex. The remain 10% project into the pretectal region of the midbrain.

Damage from the posterior to anterior visual pathway requires its transmission through the synapses in the LGN by a process called retrograde trans-synaptic degeneration or trans-neuronal degeneration (Fig. 17.1).

Trans-synaptic retrograde degeneration (TRD) in humans is well known and has been demonstrated from the early twentieth century [1], but clinical evidence of TRD was controversial for many years. In 1982, Beatty et al. [2] reported histological evidence in a case 40 years after occipital lobectomy.

B. F. Sánchez-Dalmau (✉) · A. Camós-Carreras · R. Torres-Torres · J. Keller
Neuroophthalmology Unit, Ophthalmology Department, Hospital Clínic, Barcelona, Spain

Visual Pathway Lab, Neuroimmunology Group, IDIBAPS, Hospital Clínic, Barcelona, Spain
e-mail: acamos@clinic.cat

L. Sanchez-Vela · E. H. Martínez-Lapiscina · P. Villoslada
Visual Pathway Lab, Neuroimmunology Group, IDIBAPS, Hospital Clínic, Barcelona, Spain
e-mail: md072887@uic.es; hernandez@clinic.ub.es; pvillosl@clinic.cat

A. Grzybowski, P. Barboni (eds.), *OCT and Imaging in Central Nervous System Diseases*, https://doi.org/10.1007/978-3-030-26269-3_17

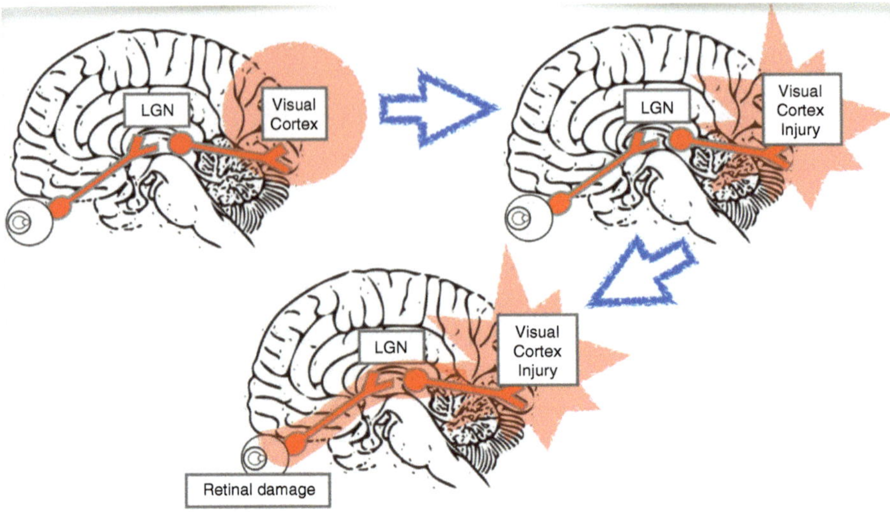

Fig. 17.1 The visual pathway as a model to study trans-synaptic neuronal degeneration

The reasons for this controversy were mainly three:

(a) The presence of retinal degeneration no related with the brain injury
(b) The possibility of direct damage to the optic tracts in patients with occipitotemporal lesions and
(c) The lack of good retinal neurohistology in humans.

The indirect analysis with different techniques like pattern electroretinogram [3–6], fundus photography and ophthalmic examination [7] were used but the results were contradictory.

In this condition, the advent of the Optical Coherence Tomography (OCT) and their subsequent use in neuro-ophthalmology allowed the first reliable and reproducible analysis of the retinal anatomy in humans. Since that moment it was possible to understand the trans-synaptic retrograde degeneration following damage of the central nervous system (CNS) pathways.

Levin suggested in 2005 that retrograde trans-synaptic degeneration of neurons of retinal ganglion cells and their axons in the optic nerve and the optic tract occurred only following prenatal (not post-natal) acquired damage to the posterior visual pathway [8].

More recent studies demonstrated thinning of the retinal nerve fiber layer (RNFL) [9], or in the ganglion cell layer [10], using OCT or thinning of the optic tract using MRI [11, 12] in acquired damage.

The use of OCT to evaluate trans-synaptic retrograde degeneration has been described on different clinical settings such as congenital/long standing homonymous hemianopia, acquired homonymous hemianopia and neurodegenerative diseases like multiple sclerosis or Alzheimer's disease.

17.2 Trans-Synaptic Retrograde Degeneration in Congenital/Long-Standing Homonymous Hemianopia

The first description of using OCT for trans-synaptic retrograde degenerating retinal nerve fiber layer thinning was reported by Cowey [13]. One year later another group, published a report with two female patients with no visual symptoms and homonymous hemianopia secondary to an old occipital infarction showing a RNFL thinning in nasal and temporal regions compatible with the visual field deficit [14].

These results were subsequently confirmed by the same group with a higher number of patients (seven cases) [9]. In both studies there was a strong correlation between the size of brain lesion, visual fields and thinning of the retinal nerve fiber layer, but it was not possible to determine an appropriate temporal sequence between the occipital damage and thinning of the RNFL due to the lack of the exact timing of occipital damage and no follow-up of patients in these series.

17.3 Trans-Synaptic Retrograde Degeneration by OCT in Acquired Homonymous Hemianopia

Jindahra et al. described by first time retinal nerve fiber layer thinning in a series of 19 cases with acquired homonymous hemianopia in 2009 [9]. The observed thinning had the same characteristics and magnitude as previously described in patients with congenital defects.

In 2012, 15 patients with homonymous hemianopia or smaller homonymous visual field defects with occipital cerebral infarction were studied by OCT after the onset of stroke and follow-up in the next years. All patients with homonymous hemianopia showed a retinal nerve fiber layer thinning with a decreasing trend during the period of measurement [15], maximal in the first year after the occipital injury, followed by a much slower rate the following years.

Similar results were observed in another study comparing 46 patients with occipital infarction and 46 healthy controls [16]. The RNFL thickness was reduced significantly as early as 3.6 months in the superior, inferior, and nasal quadrants in the contralateral eyes and in the superior, inferior, and temporal quadrants in the ipsilateral eyes.

The change from the time-domain optical coherence tomography (TD-OCT) to the spectral-domain OCT (SD-OCT) and the development of better segmentation software allowed the measurement of all the retinal layers. Evaluating ganglion cell layer appeared more effective and reliable than the nerve fiber layer of the retina in the quantification of trans-synaptic degeneration. We can quantify only each of the inner layer (RNFL, ganglion cells or inner plexiform), although there is a tendency to group them into two forms, GCcomplex (GCC) including the 3 layers described, or including only the ganglion cell (GCL) and inner plexiform (IPL) layers, forming the GCIP.

Yamashita et al. used this technology in three patients with unilateral posterior cerebral artery (PCA) infarction, all of these patients showed a GCC thinning in the hemiretinae corresponding to the affected hemifields without fundoscopic evidence of optic atrophy [17]. This study showed that RTD of GCL likely begins much earlier.

A study of Keller et al. [18] showed macular GCL atrophy in patients that have suffered a retrogeniculate lesion with at least 1-year evolution. Therefore, the finding of sector macular GCL atrophy proves RTD of neurons in the visual pathway in cases without other ophthalmic or neurological disease. The functional correlation between sector thinning of the GCL and the sensitivity loss of the visual field in the corresponding field indicates that this may occur in lesions regardless their size as shown by Jindahra el al. in quadrantanopic cases [15]. However, we found a significantly stronger correlation between the VF defect and the thickness of GCL rather than that of the peripapillar RNFL. This is probably due to the fact that at the macula, the bodies of the neurons are more numerous and topographically organised to correspond to the VF. In contrast, the anatomical distribution of fibres in the peripapillar RNFL is more complex, making a correlation with the visual field more difficult to establish.

Mitchell et al. [19] found RTD in GCL 15 of 22 patients with homonymous visual field loss due to varying etiologies, but in some cases didn't showed RNFL thinning, and confirm that the RTD again must begin earlier than 1 year. It's remarkable that the RTD clearly didn't occurred in some cases with quadrantanopia with a follow up over 10 years or more.

In other study Shin et al. [20] showed in 22 cases with a significant thinning of GCL, the thinning of RFNL was only observed in 75% of the cases. Moreover, Herro and Lam [21] reported a series of 9 patients with GCL thinning without RNFL loss.

An important element is the presence or absence of blood vessels or other structures that may interfere with the OCT image acquisition. The higher resolution of spectral-domain OCT also allows studying the segmentation of the retina in layers in more detail [17]. It is noteworthy that cases with macular sparing hemi- and quadrantanopia also showed macular GCL atrophy away from the fovea, perhaps explained due to the representation of 15–20° of visual field in the area scanned by the OCT instrument used and the absence of ganglion cells on the fovea.

Similar findings can be observed in patients with homonymous visual field defects after epilepsy surgery (Fig. 17.2).

OCT-Angiography is a new non invasive technique used to study the blood flow in the retinal vessels. There are no published data.

Muñoz-Negrete et al. reported in the 2018 meeting of the American Academy of Ophthalmology a significant decrease of peripapillary and macular vascular density in patients with homonymous visual field defect and retrograde trans-synaptic degeneration and correlation with RNFL and GCC thinning [22].

Our personal data confirm similar results. This technique is improving day by day and new methods of quantification are appearing. New results will be described in the next future.

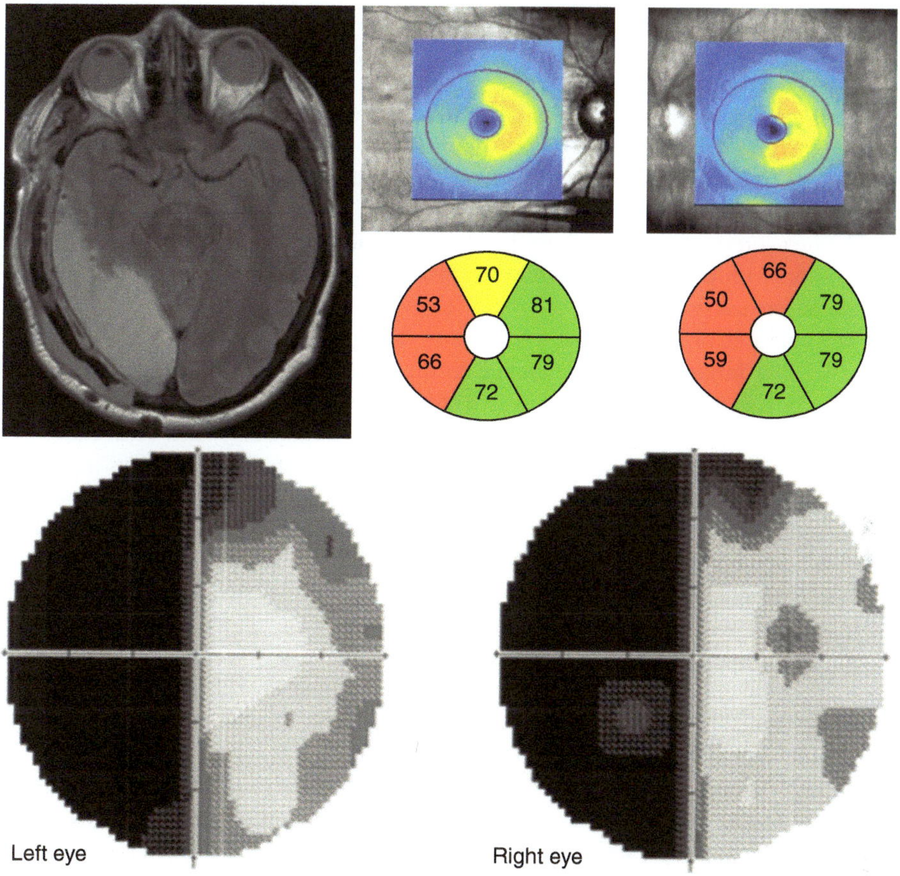

Fig. 17.2 Sectorial ganglion cells layer thinning secondary to an epilepsy surgery, 6 months after surgery. Visual field shows a complete left homonymous hemianopia

17.4 Trans-Synaptic Axonal Degeneration by OCT in Multiple Sclerosis

There is evidence of postmortem atrophy of retinal layers after long-standing disease [23], but due to the multiple CNS lesions that may be developed in patients with multiple sclerosis to establish the presence of trans-synaptic degeneration is difficult.

Because patients with multiple sclerosis lesions can have both the anterior visual pathway and the posterior visual pathway can exist anterograde trans-synaptic degeneration in patients with a history of optic neuritis, and moreover, trans-synaptic retrograde degeneration in patients with lesions of the posterior visual pathway.

This is important, to assess retrograde trans-synaptic degeneration patients who have had previous optic neuritis should be differentiated and excluded from the analysis because trans-synaptic RGC degeneration could be masked by the pronounced loss caused by damage to the anterior visual pathway in multiple sclerosis optic neuritis (MSON). Previous optic neuritis may generate residual impairment of RNFL and CGL distorting the quantification of trans-synaptic degeneration on the anterior visual pathway [24].

The measurement of damage to the anterior visual pathway by OCT [25] and his association with other variables have improved the understanding of neurodegenerative processes in MS.

Gabilondo et al. [26], using a cohort of 100 patients with multiple sclerosis, evaluated the influence of the damage to the posterior visual pathway on retinal atrophy by linear regression analysis. Retinal atrophy was used as the dependent variable, and measures of posterior visual pathway damage and other relevant clinical measures (sex, age at study inclusion, and EDSS score) were used as independent variables. Their regression model indicated that a decrease of 1cm^3 in visual cortex volume predicts a reduction of 0.6 um in retinal nerve fiber layer thickness independent of other variables.

Balk et al. [27] analyzed OCT from 230 patients with MS with and without optic Neuritis (ON) and its relation with occipital volume. They showed that there was a significant amount of atrophy of the inner, but not the outer layers of retina, specifically in the macular RNFL and GCC. The inner nuclear layer and the outer retinal layers of the macular area showed the largest relative thickness in MS with ON, compared with MS without ON or healthy eyes.

Based on these results the authors suggested that in the inner nuclear layer (INL) existed a neural plasticity due to the interaction between bipolar, amacrinal and horizontal cells that blocked the posterior trans-synaptic degeneration, allowing the affectation of ganglion cells only.

Klistorner et al. [28] reported the effects of posterior visual pathway pathology on the retina in MS patients, finding an association between MRI measures of optic radiation integrity and retinal integrity measured by temporal quadrant RNFL thickness using OCT. This finding also supports the occurrence of trans-synaptic degeneration in MS, in this case in a retrograde direction. The authors evaluated the posterior pathways with two methods—lesion analysis and diffusion tensor imaging—with each yielding similar results, increasing confidence in the results and exposing both lesional and non lesional pathology [29]. In this cohort, with optic neuritis–affected eyes specifically excluded, posterior visual pathway pathology accounted for as much as 35–40% of the atrophy of the RNFL. There was also an association between posterior visual pathway integrity and low-contrast letter acuity.

Petracca and colleagues analyzed GCL-IPL and total macular volume as well as RNFL and compared them to various measurements of cortical involvement using MRI in a cohort of 25 patients with primary progressive multiple sclerosis who had not had optic neuritis [30]. They founded that RNFL thickness correlated with thalamic and cortical volume confirming the RTD.

Al-Louzi et al., reported a series of six cases with homonymous, hemi-macular ganglion cell plus inner plexiform (GCIP) thickness reduction in MS lesions of the thalamus (2 cases) and occipital (4 cases) with homonymous hemianopia [31].

Future treatment trials are needed to anticipate that predefined analysis for patients without multiple sclerosis optic neuritis (MSON) are likely to be of stronger statistical power than for patients with previous neuritis, and that alternative measures of disability that better reflect generalized neurological function, including cognition, might need to be used for indirect assessment of diffuse axonal loss in the CNS.

17.5 Trans-Synaptic Axonal Degeneration by OCT in Alzheimer's Disease

Visual impairment is often one of the earliest complaints in patients with Alzheimer's Disease (AD) [32]. Several researchers attribute this impairment to damage in primary the visual cortex with degeneration of cortical areas and secondarily, retrograde loss of nerve fibers in the retina and optic nerve. However, it has been reported the presence of beta-amyloid and tau deposits in the retina [33], its presence in the retinal ganglion cells and internal plexiform layer induce neuroinflammation that could cause retinal degeneration [34]. Accordingly the visual damage is determined by direct toxicity of beta-amyloid and its derivatives in the retina and the retrograde degeneration of retinal nerve fibers.

Thinning of the retinal nerve fiber layer and ganglion cells layer has been described in patients with AD and mild cognitive impairment [35–38] and has good correlation with the Mini Mental State Examination (MMSE) and the disease stage.

It has been postulated that the retinal nerve fiber layer thinning may be the earliest sign of AD even before the hippocampal region damage that affects memory [39].

Larrosa et al. [40] proposed a linear discriminant function (LDF) based on OCT and designed for AD diagnosis. According to their results the most reliable tool for diagnosing Alzheimer's disease was the Spectralis® LDF with an area under the ROC curves of 0.967, sensitivity of 94.3 and specificity of 88.3%.

Lad et al., showed areas of thickening and thinning in NFL and GCIPL in MCI and AD patients, suggesting dynamic changes in the evolution of the disease [41].

A recent systematic review and meta-analysis of 30 studies including 1257 patients, confirmed the associations between retinal measurements of SD OCT and AD, highlighting the potential usefulness of SD-OCT measurements as biomarkers of AD [42].

Despite these promising preliminary studies, it remains to be determined whether the Alzheimer disease affects the retina directly, secondarily by trans-synaptic degeneration, or both.

17.6 Trans-Synaptic Axonal Degeneration in Parkinson

An study revealed RNFL thinning in patients with PD and visual hallucinations as compared to PD patients without hallucinations and controls. With the assumption that patients with PD and hallucinations have dysfunction of the primary visual cortex or visual association cortex, the authors concluded that the RNFL thinning might be the product of retrograde transsynaptic degeneration [43]. In other way, PD can affect directly retinal cells, generating anterograde transsynaptic degeneration in the optic tracts and optic radiations [44].

17.7 Summary

The visual pathway is made up of 4-neuron chain that transfer visual information from the retina to the primary visual cortex. Acute or chronic damage on the posterior visual pathway induce a trans-neuronal retrograde degeneration.

Measuring the degeneration of the anterior visual pathway was difficult before the OCT imaging technology. With this technology the trans-neuronal retrograde degeneration has been well described in several CNS diseases like multiple sclerosis, stroke, Parkinson disease, homonymous hemianopia and Alzheimer's disease.

The OCT allows to measure reliably and noninvasively the macular RNFL and GCC, and these measurements have a high correlation with the CNS lesions and the function of the visual system [45, 46].

OCT helps in evaluation of the magnitude and timing of damage, supporting our understanding the pathophysiology of the diseases and can be used as a reliable biomarker of axonal loss in neurological diseases.

References

1. Campbell AW. Histological studies on the localization of cerebral function. Cambridge: Cambridge University Press; 1905. p. 52–64.
2. Beatty RM, Sadun AA, Smith LEH, Vonsattel JP, Richardson EP. Direct demonstration of transsynaptic degeneration in the human visual system: a comparison of retrograde and anterograde changes. J Neurol Neurosurg Psychiatry. 1982;45:143–6.
3. Stoerig P, Zrenner E. A pattern ERG study of transneuronal retrograde degeneration in the human retina after a post-geniculate lesion. In: Kulikowski JJ, Dickinson CL, Murray JJ, editors. Seeing contour and colour. Oxford: Pergamon Press; 1993. p. 553–556.
4. Porrello G, Falsini B. Retinal ganglion cell dysfunction in humans following post-geniculate lesions: specific spatio–temporal losses revealed by pattern ERG. Vis Res. 1999;39:1739–48.
5. Azzopardi P, King SM, Cowey A. Pattern electroretinograms after cerebral hemispherectomy. Brain. 2001;124:1228–40.
6. Skrandies W, Leipert KP. Visual field defects are not accompanied by electrophysiological evidence of transsynaptic retrograde degeneration. Clin Vis Sci. 1988;3:45–57.
7. Hoyt WF, Kommerell G. Der fundus oculi bei homonymer hemianopie. Klin Mbl Augenhlk. 1973;162:456.

8. Levin LA. Topical diagnosis of chiasmal and retrochiasmal disorders. In: Miller NR, Newman NJ, editors. Walsh and Hoyt's clinical neuro-ophthalmology, 6th ed. Baltimore: Lippincott, Williams & Wilkins; 2005; p. 517.
9. Jindahra P, Petrie A, Plant GT. Retrograde trans-synaptic retinal ganglion cell loss identified by optical coherence tomography. Brain. 2009;132:628–34.
10. Meier PG, Maeder P, Kardon RH, Borruat FX. Homonymous ganglion cell layer thinning after isolated occipital lesion: macular OCT demonstrates transsynaptic retrograde retinal degeneration. J Neuroophthalmol. 2015;35:112–6.
11. Bridge H, Jindahra P, Barbur J, Plant GT. Imaging reveals optic tract degeneration in hemianopia. Invest Ophthalmol Vis Sci. 2011;52:382–8.
12. Millington RS, Yasuda CL, Jindahra P, Jenkinson M, Barbur JL, Kennard C, Cendes F, Plant GT, Bridge H. Quantifying the pattern of optic tract degeneration in human hemianopia. J Neurol Neurosurg Psychiatry. 2014;85:379–86.
13. Cowey A. Fact and artefact and myth about blindsight. Q J Exp Psychol. 2004;57A:577–609.
14. Mehta JS, Plant GT. Optical coherence tomography (OCT) findings in congenital/long-standing homonymous hemianopia. Am J Ophthalmol. 2005;140:727–9.
15. Jindahra P, Petrie A, Plant GT. The time course of retrograde trans-synaptic degeneration following occipital lobe damage in humans. Brain. 2012;135:534–41.
16. Park HYL, Park YG, Cho AH, Park CK. Transneuronal retrograde degeneration of the retinal ganglion cells in patients with cerebral infarction. Ophthalmology. 2013;120:1292–9.
17. Yamashita T, Miki A, Iguchi Y, Kimura K, Maeda F, Kiryu J. Reduced retinal ganglion cell complex thickness in patients with posterior cerebral artery infarction detected using spectral-domain optical coherence tomography. Jpn J Ophthalmol. 2012;56:502–10.
18. Keller J, Sánchez-Dalmau BF, Villoslada P. Lesions in the posterior visual pathway promote trans-synaptic degeneration of retinal ganglion cells. PLoS One. 2014;9:e97444.
19. Mitchell JR, Oliveira C, Tsiouris AJ, Dinkin MJ. Corresponding ganglion cell atrophy in patients with postgeniculate homonymous visual field loss. J Neuroophthalmol. 2015;35:353–9.
20. Shin HY, Park HY, Choi JA, Park CK. Macular ganglion cell-inner plexiform layer thinning in patients with visual field defect that respects the vertical meridian. Graefes Arch Clin Exp Ophthalmol. 2014;252(9):1501–7.
21. Herro AM, Lam BL. Retrograde degeneration of retinal ganglion cells in homonymous hemianopsia. Clin Ophthalmol. 2015;11:1057–64.
22. Muñoz Negrete FJ, Rebolleda G, Jaumandreu L, Sánchez Gutierrez V, De Juan V. Peripapillary and macular vessel density assessed with OCT-A in unilateral retrogeniculate visual pathway lesions. In: Oral communication, American Academy of Ophthalmology 2018 meeting, Chicago.
23. Green AJ, McQuaid S, Hauser SL, et al. Ocular pathology in multiple sclerosis: retinal atrophy and inflammation irrespective of disease duration. Brain. 2010;133:1591–601.
24. Balk LJ, Twisk JWR, Steenwijk MD, Daams M, Tewarie P, Killestein J, et al. A dam for retrograde axonal degeneration in multiple sclerosis? J Neurol Neurosurg Psychiatry. 2014;85:782–9.
25. Galetta KM, Calabresi PA, Frohman EM, Balcer LJ. Optical coherence tomography (OCT): imaging the visual pathway as a model for neurodegeneration. Neurotherapeutics. 2011;8:117–32.
26. Gabilondo I, Martínez-Lapiscina EH, Martínez-Heras E, Fraga-Pumar E, Llufriu S, Ortiz S, et al. Trans-synaptic axonal degeneration in the visual pathway in multiple sclerosis. Ann Neurol. 2014;75:98–107.
27. Balk LJ, Steenwijk MD, Tewarie P, Daams M, Killestein J, Wattjes MP, Vrenken H, Barkhof F, Polman CH, Petzold A. Bidirectional trans-synaptic axonal degeneration in the visual pathway in multiple sclerosis. J Neurol Neurosurg Psychiatry. 2014;85:782–9.
28. Klistorner A, Sriram P, Vootakuru N, Wang C, Barnett MH, et al. Axonal loss of retinal neurons in multiple sclerosis associated with optic radiation lesions. Neurology. 2014;82:2165–72.

29. Sriram P, Wang C, Yiannikas C, Garrick R, Barnett M, Parratt J, Graham SL, Arvind H, Klistorner A. Relationship between optical coherence tomography and electrophysiology of the visual pathway in non-optic neuritis eyes of multiple sclerosis patients. PLoS One. 2014;9:e102546.
30. Petracca M, Cordano C, Cellerino M, Button J, Krieger S, Vancea R, Ghassemi R, Farrell C, Miller A, Calabresi PA, Lublin F, Inglese M. Retinal degeneration in primary progressive multiple sclerosis: a role for cortical lesions? Mult Scler. 2017;23:43–50.
31. Al-Louzi O, Button J, Newsome SD, Calabresi PA, Saidha S. Retrograde trans-synaptic visual pathway degeneration in multiple sclerosis: a case series. Mult Scler. 2017;23:1035–9.
32. Berisha F, Feke GT, Trempe CL, McMeel JW, Schepens CL. Retinal abnormalities in early Alzheimer's disease. Invest Ophthalmol Vis Sci. 2007;48:2285–9.
33. Koronyo Y, Salumbides BC, Black KL, Koronyo-Hamaoui M. Alzheimer's disease in the retina: imaging retinal Aß plaques for early diagnosis and therapy assessment. Neurodegener Dis. 2012;10(1–4):285–93.
34. Garcia-Martin ES, Rojas B, Ramirez AI, de Hoz R, Salazar JJ, Yubero R, Gil P, Triviño A, Ramirez JM. Macular thickness as a potential biomarker of mild Alzheimer's disease. Ophthalmology. 2014;121:1149–51.
35. Iseri PK, Altinaş O, Tokay T, Yüksel N. Relationship between cognitive impairment and retinal morphological and visual functional abnormalities in Alzheimer disease. J Neuroophthalmol. 2006;26:18–24.
36. Kesler A, Vakhapova V, Korczyn AD, Naftaliev E, Neudorfer M. Retinal thickness in patients with mild cognitive impairment and Alzheimer's disease. Clin Neurol Neurosurg. 2011;113:523–6.
37. Kirbas S, Turkyilmaz K, Anlar O, Tufekci A, Durmus M. Retinal nerve fiber layer thickness in patients with Alzheimer disease. J Neuroophthalmol. 2013;33:58–61.
38. Marziani E, Pomati S, Ramolfo P, Cigada M, Giani A, Mariani C, et al. Evaluation of retinal nerve fiber layer and ganglion cell layer thickness in Alzheimer's disease using spectral-domain optical coherence tomography. Invest Ophthalmol Vis Sci. 2013;54:5953–8.
39. He X-F, Liu Y-T, Peng C, Zhang F, Zhuang S, Zhang J-S. Optical coherence tomography assessed retinal nerve fiber layer thickness in patients with Alzheimer's disease: a meta-analysis. Int J Ophthalmol. 2012;5:401–5.
40. Larrosa JM, Garcia-Martin E, Bambo MP, Pinilla J, Polo V, Otin S, et al. Potential new diagnostic tool for Alzheimer's disease using a linear discriminant function for Fourier domain optical coherence tomography. Invest Ophthalmol Vis Sci. 2014;55:3043–51.
41. Lad EM, Mukherjee D, Stinnett SS, Cousins SW, Potter GG, Burke JR, et al. Evaluation of inner retinal layers as biomarkers in mild cognitive impairment to moderate Alzheimer's disease. PLoS One. 2018;13(2):e0192646.
42. Chan VTT, Sun Z, Tang S, Chen, LJ, Wong, A, Tham CC, Wong TJ, Chen C, Kamran Ikram M, Whitson HE, Lad EM, Mok VCT, Cheung CY. Spectral-domain OCT measurements in Alzheimer's disease. A systematic review and meta-analysis. Ophthalmology. 2019;126(4):497–510.
43. Lee JY, Kim JM, Ahn J, Kim HJ, Jeon BS, Kim TW. Retinal nerve fiber layer thickness and visual hallucinations in Parkinson's disease. Mov Disord. 2014;29(1):61–7.
44. Bodis-Wollner I, Kozlowski PB, Glazman S, Miri S. α-Synuclein in the inner retina in Parkinson disease. Ann Neurol. 2014;75:964–6.
45. Moon H, Yoon JY, Lim HT, Sung KR. Ganglion cell and inner plexiform layer thickness determined by spectral domain optical coherence tomography in patients with brain lesions. Br J Ophthalmol. 2015;99(3):329–35.
46. Dinkin M. Trans-synaptic retrograde degeneration in the human visual system: slow, silent, and real. Curr Neurol Neurosci Rep. 2017;17:16.

OCT in Toxic and Nutritional Optic Neuropathies

18

Andrzej Grzybowski, Iwona Obuchowska, and Carl Arndt

18.1 OCT and Toxic Optic Neuropathies

The anterior visual pathways are susceptible to damage from numerous toxic agents [1]. Toxic optic neuropathies can classically be caused by ingestion of numerous substances, including alcohol (methanol, ethylene glycol), antitubercular drugs (ethambutol, isoniazid), antibiotics (linezolid, sulphonamides, chloramphenicol), antimalarials (chloroquine, quinine), anti-cancer drugs (vincristine, methotrexate), antiarrhythmic (digitalis, amiodarone). Although this list of potentially toxic agents for the optic nerves is constantly increasing, due to the current exponential development of new therapies, only few drugs exhibit a firm evidence of causal relationship.

Toxic optic neuropathies, which are clinically often undistinguishable from nutritional optic neuropathies, typically present as painless, progressive, symmetric and bilateral visual impairment due to central or centrocecal scotoma, dyschromatopsia often being the initial symptom. The site of the primary injury can be very variable, including the retina, retinal ganglion cells, intraocular nerve fibre axons, or chiasm. The majority of clinical findings are caused by selective damage to the papillomacular bundle, which fibres are most susceptible due to their long unmyelinated part in the retina and their relatively small calibre. Preferential involvement of the papillomacular bundle is a common feature to many acquired and genetic optic neuropathies. On the cellular level they also share the similar pathophysiology

A. Grzybowski (✉)
University of Warmia and Mazury, Olsztyn, Poland

Institute for Research in Ophthalmology, Poznań, Poland

I. Obuchowska
Department of Ophthalmology, Medical University of Białystok, Białystok, Poland

C. Arndt
Department of Ophthalmology, CHU Reims, Reims, France

A. Grzybowski, P. Barboni (eds.), *OCT and Imaging in Central Nervous System Diseases*, https://doi.org/10.1007/978-3-030-26269-3_18

mechanism based on disruption of oxidative phosphorylation in mitochondria, esp. in retinal ganglion cells, and this is the reason to name them mitochondrial optic neuropathies. Drugs shown to cause mitochondrial optic neuropathy by blocking oxidative phosphorylation include ethambutol, chloramphenicol, linezolid, erythromycin, streptomycin, and antiretroviral drugs [2].

Other drugs provoking optic neuropathy, less strongly related to mitochondrial dysfunction include amiodarone, infliximab, quinine, dapsone, pheniprazine, suramin, and isoniazid [2].

It was suggested that since axonal transport is highly energy dependent and mitochondria need to be transported from the neuron body to the distal synaptic terminals, retinal ganglion cells (RGC) with their long axons are particularly vulnerable [2]. In early drug toxicity mitochondria accumulate within RGC axons, and this is detectable as axonal swelling by OCT [3]. In subacute and chronic stages of mitochondrial optic neuropathies OCT demonstrates RNFL thinning of the papillomacular bundle, esp. in the inferotemporal sector. In the later stages, OCT reveals thinning of RNFL in all layers [2]. Early diagnosis is crucial for intervention, i.e. discontinuation of the drug, which may allow clinical recovery. However, early clinical diagnosis may be difficult, due to the normal ophthalmoscopic appearance of the optic disc pallor. Only at later stages is optic disc pallor or atrophy is clinically visible. For this reason, optical coherence tomography (OCT), has been initially considered as a potential method for early diagnosis and possibly monitoring drug toxicity affecting the retina, the retinal ganglion cells complex or the retinal nerve fiber layer (RNFL). Indeed, beyond its extensive use in glaucoma [4], OCT is now commonly used for the evaluation of various optic neuropathies including optic neuritis, ischemic optic neuropathies, papilledema, traumatic optic neuropathy [5–7]. However, interestingly, the number of OCT studies dedicated to toxic optic neuropathies remains relatively small and no OCT guidelines exist to monitor optic nerve drug toxicities.

18.1.1 Ethambutol

Ethambutol hydrochloride is a bacteriostatic antitubercular agent and probably the most common therapy implicated in toxic optic neuropathy. Ethambutol and its metabolite ethylenediaminodibutyric acid chelates several metal-containing enzyme systems like copper and zinc in the nucleic acid structures of mycobacteria leading to decreased levels of metalloproteins [8, 9]. Similar disruption is seen within the cytochromes of the human mitochondria, leading to apoptosis of retinal ganglion cells [8, 9] and subsequent optic neuropathy [10]. Early animal experiments have also demonstrated ethambutol toxicity affecting the retinal ganglion cells, the optic nerve, chiasm and optic tracts [11, 12].

Ethambutol induced optic neuropathy, which may become clinically patent at any time from 2 to 12 months after the initial treatment, is often reversible, if the condition is early recognized, However, permanent damage may occur at toxic or even standard doses (15–25 mg/kg/day), especially in debilitated patients, i.e. with associated renal failure. The ethambutol induced optic neuropathy has a predilection for the papillo-macular bundle of the retinal nerve fibre layer. Therefore, ophthalmoscopic changes of the optic nerve head are often subtle at the early stages, making OCT a good candidate for early ethambutol optic nerve toxicity detection.

The most common OCT finding in advanced optic nerve ethambutol toxicity is thinning of the retinal nerve fibre layer, especially in the infero-temporal quadrant, corresponding to the papillo-macular bundle [9, 12, 13]. Patients with thinner temporal quadrants display lower visual acuity and significantly reduced colour vision. These OCT findings may also correspond well with the visual field defects on Humphrey visual field analysis. Limited case series have suggested that at early stages, the ethambutol induced optic neuropathy might be associated with increased RNFL thickness [14]. In addition, after cessation of ethambutol, reversible RNFL changes, detectable by OCT may occur [14]. Apart from RML, significant decreases in retinal have been observed at various levels including ganglion cell layer and inner plexiform layer [15, 16].

The up-to-date study, included a group of 21 patients (42 eyes) treated with ethambutol for 2–12 months, showed that early ethambutol-induced optic neuropathy was associated with edema and thickening of peripapillary retinal nerve fiber layer (pRNFL) which persisted for up to 3 months after the onset of symptoms [17]. Also, an initial decrease in the ganglion cell layer plus inner plexus layer (GCIPL) was observed, more remarkable in inner locations (inner ring) than in outer locations. On follow-up OCT, conducted after 6 months, mean thickness of the pRNFL at the temporal, nasal and inferior locations, mean thickness of the inner GCIPL at the temporal, nasal and inferior locations, and mean thickness of the outer GCIPL at the superior and inferior locations were significantly lower than during the baseline examination. The relative decrease in the thickness of the analyzed layers between the first and the second OCT turned out to be markedly more evident for pRNFL than for GCIPL.

The analysis of correlation between the GCIPL thickness and vision recovery after the withdrawal of ethambutol demonstrated a significant positive association between the thickness of the temporal inner GCIPL and the degree of visual acuity improvement within 12 months of the agent discontinuation. A 10-μm loss in the inner GCIPL thickness turned out to be associated with a 0.5 decrease in the amount of logMAR visual acuity recovery at 12 months. No similar relationships were observed at 1, 3 and 6 months after the ethambutol withdrawal, except the temporal inner GCIPL, the thickness of which showed a significant correlation with visual recovery [17]. Taken altogether, these findings imply that temporal GCIPL may serve as an anatomic marker to predict visual acuity improvement both in early-phase neuropathy and at later period, i.e. 12 months after cessation of ethambutol.

Furthermore, the results of this study suggest that the toxic effect of ethambutol is not limited only to the papillomacular bundle, as the damage was observed in both nasal and temporal GCIPL.

An OCT study of patients who received ethambutol at a dose of 15–19 mg/kg/day for approximately 5 months demonstrated that the treatment contributed to an increase in RNFL thickness. The thickness of RNFL returned to its baseline level within 12 months of ethambutol discontinuation. This implies that OCT may be a useful test for early detection of subclinical ethambutol-induced optic neuropathy [18].

Another OCT study of two patients with ethambutol-induced optic neuropathy (developed within 8 and 12 months of the treatment) demonstrated a significant decrease in retinal thickness (especially at the inner ring) when combined RNFL, GCL and IPL map was subjected to the analysis. However, when only the thickness of RNFL was considered, no abnormalities were found in 1 out of the 2 patients. These results suggest that ethambutol may affect both RNFL and retinal GCL [19].

The OCT analysis of pre- and post-treatment RNFL thickness of 38 patients with ethambutol-induced optic neuropathy, who received combined therapy with Boqihuoxue Formula + Methycobal, demonstrated increase of this parameter in all quadrants, especially in the lower and temporal quadrant. These findings imply that OCT may be a useful instrument for the monitoring of treatment effects, and perhaps also recovery after ethambutol discontinuation [20].

In summary, OCT is a potentially interesting tool to assess the degree of optic nerve damage in the ethambutol induced optic neuropathy, especially in the early stages of the condition, when the optic disc has a normal ophthalmoscopic appearance. However, large studies are missing to confirm these preliminary findings, especially regarding early localized temporal RNFL thickening, as an early sign of the disease. Therefore, OCT is not recommended as the sole method for monitoring potential ethambutol optic nerve toxicity.

18.1.2 Methanol

Methanol is a common cause of toxic optic neuropathy especially in the developing world. It is also the most dreaded cause, due to its systemic consequences, potentially leading to metabolic acidosis, visual loss, coma and death. These adverse effects are due to indirect toxicity related to formic acid, catabolised from methyl alcohol via formaldehyde by the enzyme alcohol dehydrogenase in the liver and red blood cells.

The changes in the optic nerves are mostly due to cytotoxic oedema within the retina and the optic nerve, occurring during the first 48 h after methanol ingestion. The retinal ganglion cells and the retrolaminar myelin sheath are also affected due to degeneration of optic nerve axons. Several animal studies also supported these findings by identifying demyelination of optic nerve sheath [21]. The treatment of methanol intoxication is based on ethanol, B-group vitamins, and systemic steroids; however, the prognosis is usually poor and the final visual acuity is counting fingers or worse [22]. It was shown that fomepizole is safe and effective in the treatment of methanol poisoning [23], but high costs limits its availability. The visual improvement after treatment of 2 patients with a combination of intravenous erythropoietin, systemic corticosteroids, vitamins, and folic acid was reported [24]. OCT has been used for exploring macula and peripapillary retina in methanol-induced retinal toxicity, showing peripapillary nerve fibre swelling and accumulation of intraretinal fluid in the acute phase, with subsequent thinning in the chronic phase (Fig. 18.1).

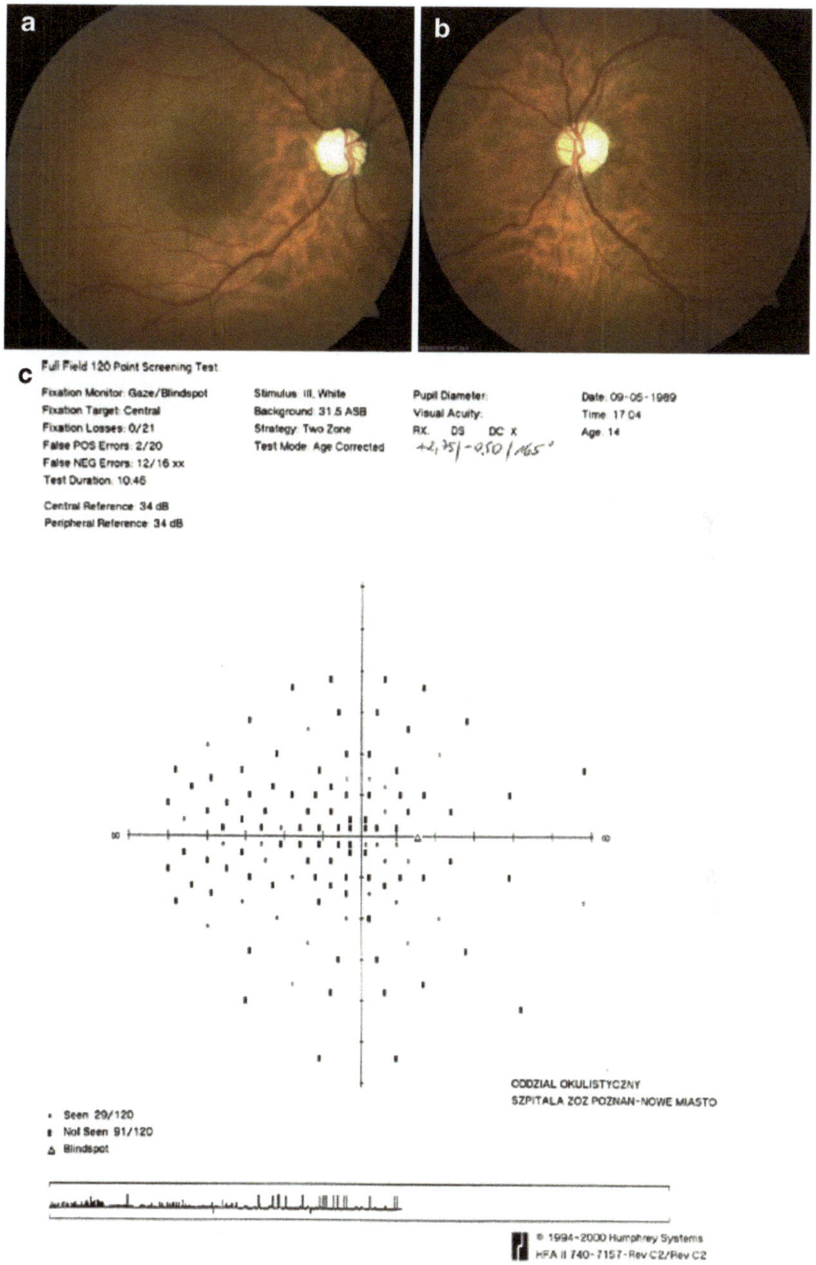

Fig. 18.1 Case report of Methanol Optic Neuropathy. A 40 year old patient with no light perception in both eyes and dilated non-responsive pupils transferred from Toxicology Department after accidental methanol intoxication. After 1-month follow up patient presented improvement of VA in both eyes (counting fingers in right eye and 0.16 in left eye) and kept stable. After 3 months optic nerve atrophy was clearly recognized with pale optic discs in fundoscopy (**a**, **b**), centrocecal scotoma in both eyes (**c**, **d**), decrease in RNFL thickness in both eyes (**e**), and decreased volume of ganglion cells in both eyes (**f**, **g**)

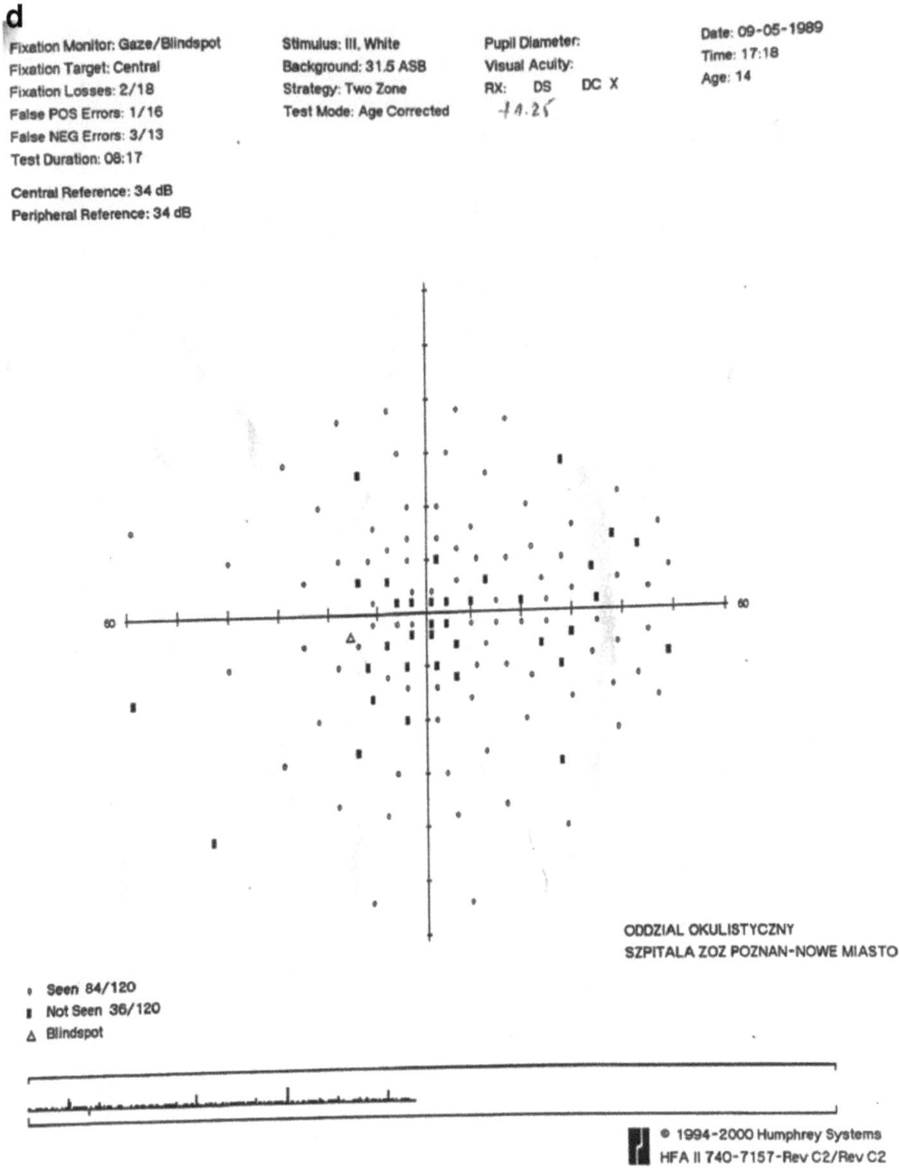

Fig. 18.1 (continued)

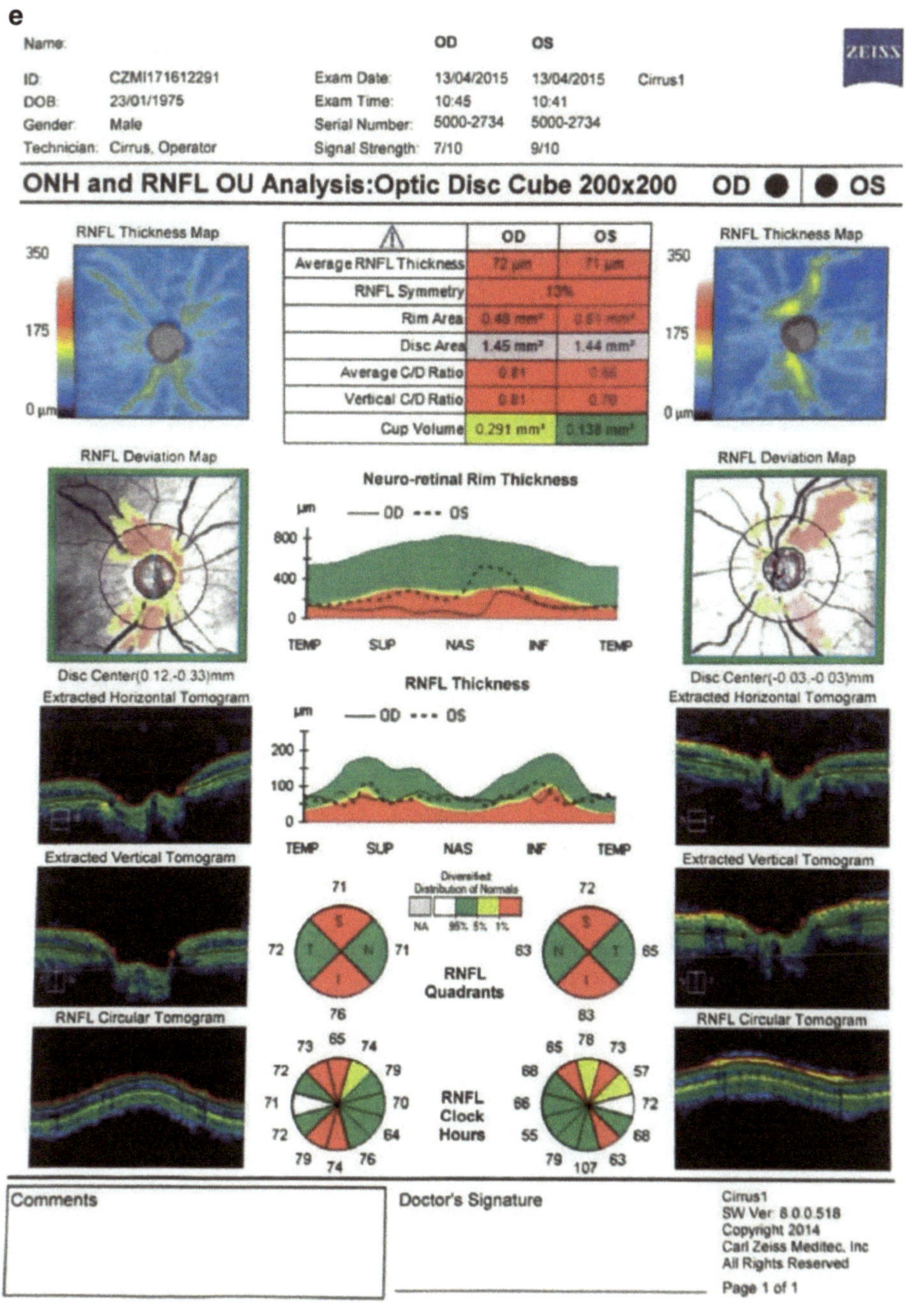

Fig. 18.1 (continued)

f

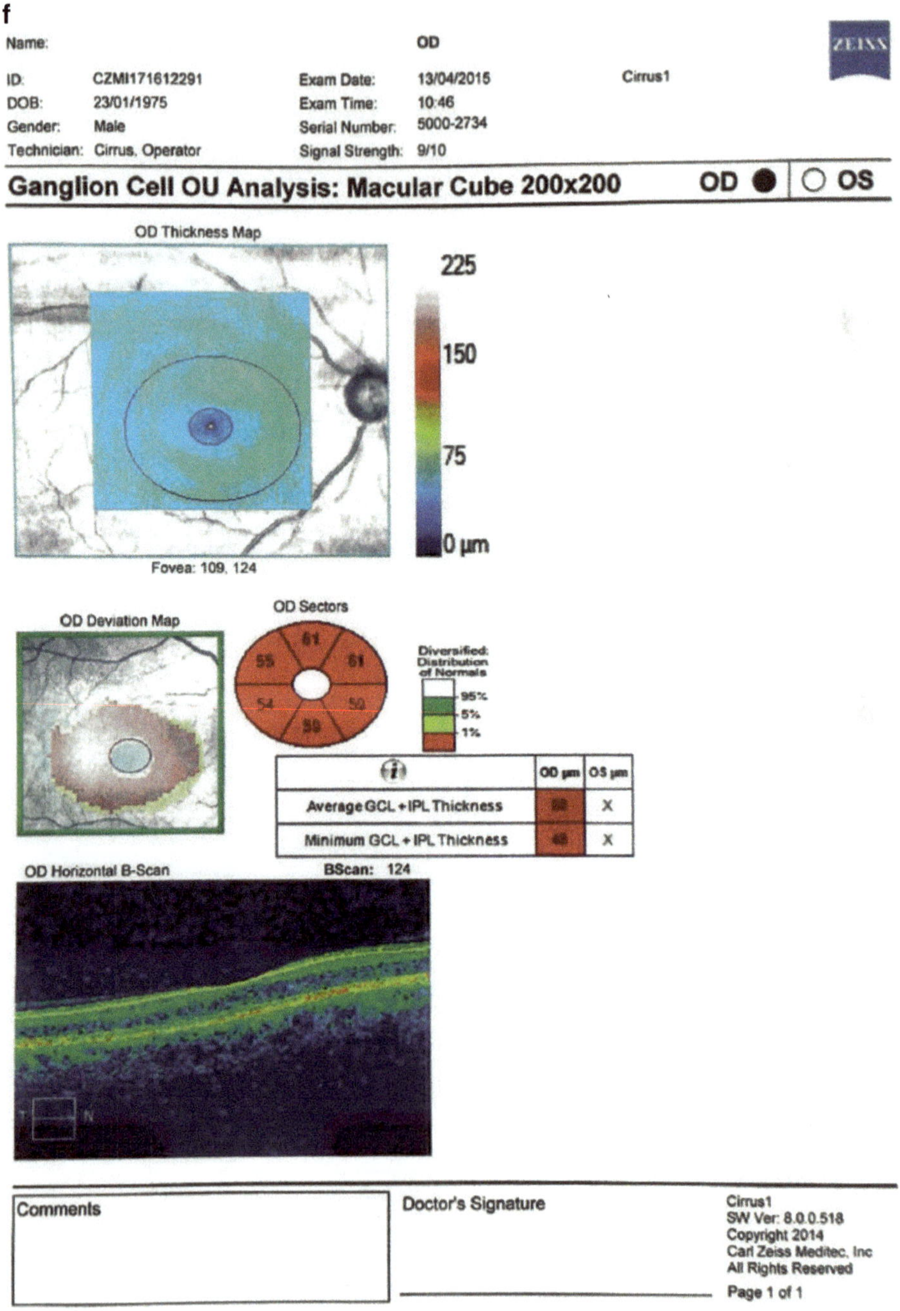

Fig. 18.1 (continued)

g

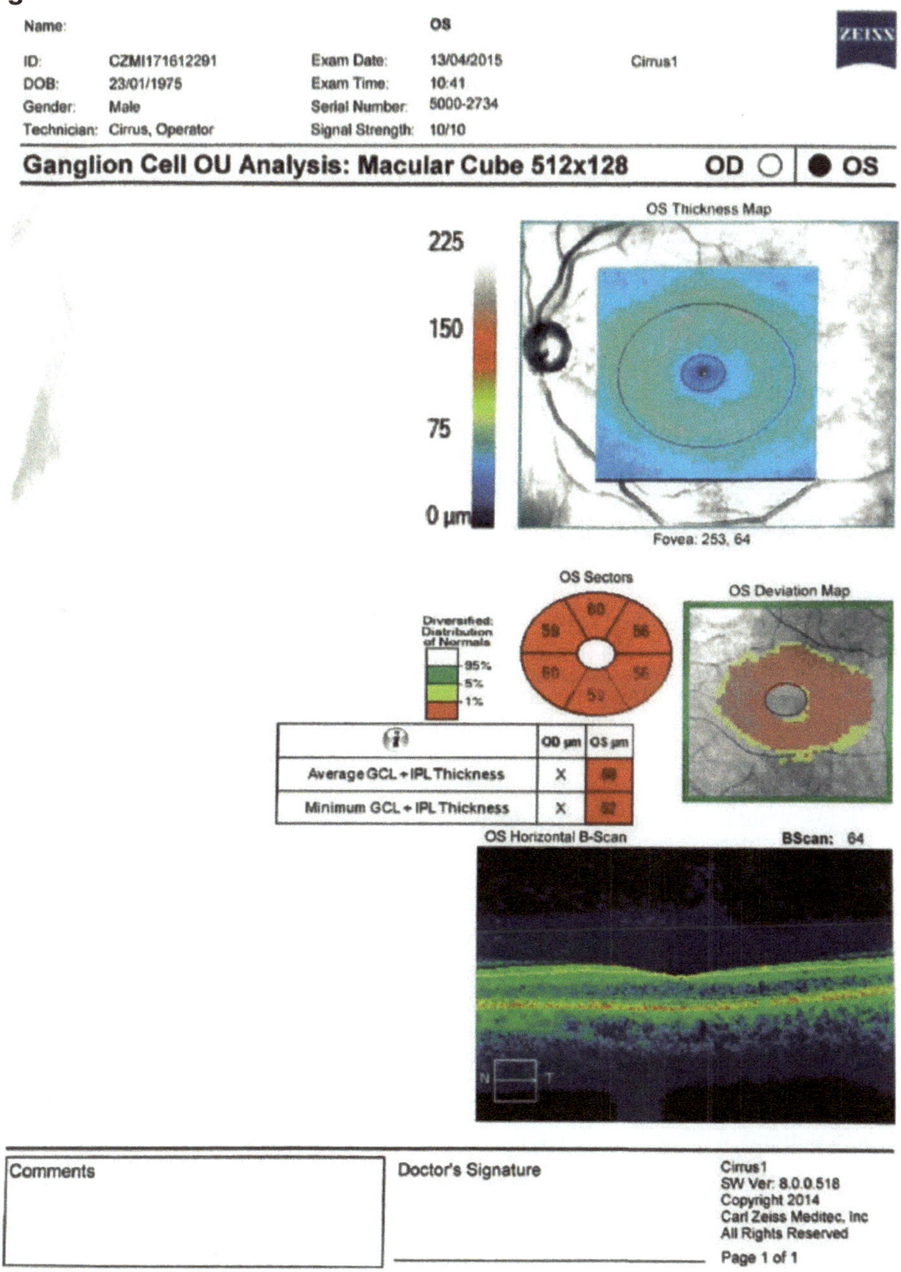

Fig. 18.1 (continued)

Therefore, OCT could he a useful tool in this setting, for evaluation of the severity of retinal edema and the temporal changes in the retinal profile [25].

18.1.2.1 Methanol Toxicity in a 19-Year-Old Female Student: A Case Report

Examination of the patient's right eye revealed inferonasal colobomatous defect of the iris, inferonasal chorioretinal coloboma and tilting and mild peripapillary atrophy of the optic nerve. In the left eye, trace segmental pallor of the temporal optic nerve head was observed during the examination conducted 4 weeks after the methanol ingestion. OCT conducted 4 weeks after the methanol intoxication revealed right ocular changes that corresponded to the coloboma. Neither thinning nor thickening of the RNFL were found in the left eye, other than a mild thinning in the nasal macula. OCT of the macula conducted 8 months after the acute intoxication with methanol revealed multiple retinal microcysts in nasal segments of both eyes. The microcysts appeared highly uniform and localized to the inner nuclear layer. OCT scan of the RNFL was normal, but bilateral wedge-shaped segmental defects of the papillomacular bundles were found during the assessment of ganglion cell layer [26].

The microcysts found on OCT in patients with methanol intoxication are characteristic and unlikely to be confused with those observed in cystoid macular edema. They are highly uniform, small, have characteristic shape and are located in the inner nuclear layer. The microcysts are found in both eyes, occur symmetrically and are not accompanied by macular thickening. In contrast, the cysts observed in cystoid macular edema are larger, more irregular and can also be found in the outer plexiform layer. The lesions are either unilateral or bilateral, asymmetrical.

Several mechanisms of microcyst formation have been proposed thus far, including trans-synaptic retrograde degeneration, glial cell activation and mitochondrial dysfunction. Fluorescein angiography suggests that the lesions have nonvascular etiology. Presence of microcysts in the inner nuclear layer might correspond to retinal ganglion cell loss, and represent a damage to small caliber axons rich in mitochondria in the papillomacular bundle [26].

The OCT study of patients with methanol-induced optic neuropathy demonstrated significant decrease of global RNFL thickness during the following years. The most remarkable loss was detectable in the temporal segments. The highest rate of thickness was seen in the most severely poisoned patients [27]. Therefore, OCT could be a potentially interesting tool to assess the degree of chronic retinal axonal loss in patients with acute methanol-induced optic neuropathy.

18.1.3 Tobacco

The toxic optic neuropathy caused by tobacco seems to be mysterious entity since all confirmed cases were reported many years ago, in the era before OCT and genetic studies. It was shown that at least part of this disorder in fact was Leber's

Hereditary Optic Neuropathy (LHON) [28–30]. It was proposed that smoking, especially in genetically susceptible individuals might affect sulphur metabolism, leading to chronic cyanide intoxication [31, 32]. The disorder was characterized by slowly progressive papillomacular bundle damage, centrocecal scotoma and visual loss. The appearance of the optic nerve is usually normal at the initial stages, with occasional peripapillary dilated vessels and haemorrhages, while pallor ensues only in the later stages [32]. Since the clinical picture of TON is similar to other optic neuropathies, the diagnosis of TON is by exclusion only of other toxic, nutritional and hereditary optic neuropathies. A few new articles [33–35] claimed that they presented patients with tobacco optic neuropathy, but they were undermined as they did not convincingly proofed the diagnosis [36–40].

18.1.4 Amiodarone

Amiodarone is a very efficient antiarrhythmic agent primarily used to treat atrial or ventricular tachyarrhythmias and fibrillation. The clinical presentation of amiodarone induced optic neuropathy may be sometimes indistinguishable from that of non-arteritic anterior ischaemic optic neuropathy (NAION) [41]. Amiodarone induced optic neuropathy has typically an insidious onset with a milder degree of visual loss, a longer duration of disc edema, and is more commonly bilateral than typical NAION, though there can be a considerable overlapping between these two conditions. Furthermore, disc edema and optic neuropathy may continue to progress even after cessation of the drug [41]. The mechanism of amiodarone-induced optic neuropathy is possibly due to the accumulation of cytoplasmic lamellar inclusions in the lysosomes due to binding of amiodarone with phospholipids. These complexes are not degraded by phospholipase enzymes leading to deposition of amiodarone deposits in the optic nerve as well as in other ocular tissues, including cornea and lens.

OCT has shown that in amiodarone-related optic neuropathy, there is transient RNFL thickening, during the initial months of therapy, followed by subsequent axonal loss and optic nerve atrophy [42]. OCT has been proposed as follow-up method for documenting edema or RNFL thinning in this setting.

18.1.5 Linezolid

Linezolid is a widely used broad-spectrum antibiotic. OCT studies demonstrated that patients with the signs of linezolid-induced optic neuropathy presented with microcystic spaces in the retinal nerve fiber layer and at the border of the RNFL and the retinal ganglion cell layer. The microcystic spaces in the RNFL resolved within 6 weeks of linezolid discontinuation. The degree of changes documented on OCT was shown to be proportional to deterioration of visual acuity [43, 44].

18.1.6 Chemotherapy

There is a published case report of neuropathy induced by intravenous chemotherapy (cytarabine and daunorubicin) in a patient with acute myeloid leukemia. OCT, conducted 6 weeks after the onset of symptoms, demonstrated thinning of the retinal nerve fiber layer in both eyes. Moreover, thinning and alteration of the foveal contour were observed in both eyes on OCT of the macula. The progression of changes documented on OCT was no longer observed when the patient was switched to another chemotherapy regimen [45].

18.2 OCT and Nutritional Optic Neuropathies

Nutritional optic neuropathy is more common among alcohol abusers and those who are undernourished [46]. Isolated nutritional optic neuropathies are rare, they are more frequent in regions of famine, where they may be epidemic. Nutritional optic neuropathies may be associated with various causes, including unbalanced diet, bariatric surgery, hunger strike, anorexia nervosa, absorption deficiency of vitamin B [47].

As in toxic neuropathies, the anterior visual pathways are susceptible to nutritional deficiency associating papillomacular bundle damage, central or cecocentral scotoma and reduction of color vision. The primary lesion is not necessarily localized into the optic nerve itself; it may be located at various levels, such as the retinal ganglion cells, nerve fiber layers, chiasm, or the optic tracts [48].

The exact mechanism by which nutritional deficits damage the optic nerve remains largely unknown. Specific deficiencies of vitamin B-12 (cyanocobalamin), thiamine (vitamin B-1) [49], other vitamins (riboflavin, niacin, and pyridoxine), folic acid, copper [50, 51] and other proteins with sulfur-containing amino acids have been associated with optic neuropathies [52]. It has been postulated that these deficiencies affect mitochondrial oxidative phosphorylation, and therefore nutritional optic neuropathies may be part of the acquired mitochondrial optic neuropathies spectrum [53]. The visual prognosis depends on multiple factors, including the cause and the duration of symptoms. At advanced stages of the condition, associated with optic atrophy, recovery is less likely to occur than at early stages [50]. Nutritional optic neuropathies are very rare in children.

Nutritional and toxic optic neuropathies have similar clinical presentations, i.e. bilateral, painless visual loss associated with colour vision disturbances and central scotoma. When an optic neuropathy is suspected, a thorough history should cover diet, drug/toxin exposure, social history (including alcohol consumption) and the professional environment. Treatment of any chronic disease such as pernicious anemia should be elucidated. Sensory symptoms and gait disturbance may be associated, due to either peripheral neuropathy or cerebellar dysfunction. A family history should be taken, to identify environmental factors or predisposition for hereditary optic neuropathies.

Clinically, patients with nutritional optic neuropathies complain of gradual blurring of vision, at far and near. Often, the slow progression of the symptoms delays diagnosis and treatment. Rarely, the visual symptoms may be asymmetric, but almost never strictly unilateral. Dyschromatopsia can be the initial symptom in nutritional optic neuropathies. In case of orbital pain, pain on ocular movement, unilateral vision loss, other diagnoses should be considered.

In nutritional optic neuropathies, visual acuity may vary from minimal reduction of vision to no light perception (NLP). However, most patients have 20/200 vision or better. Both pupils are sluggish to light, and there is no relative afferent pupillary defect due to the bilateral involvement, The optic disc may be normal or slightly hyperemic (Fig. 18.2) in the early stages, with small peripapillary hemorrhages.

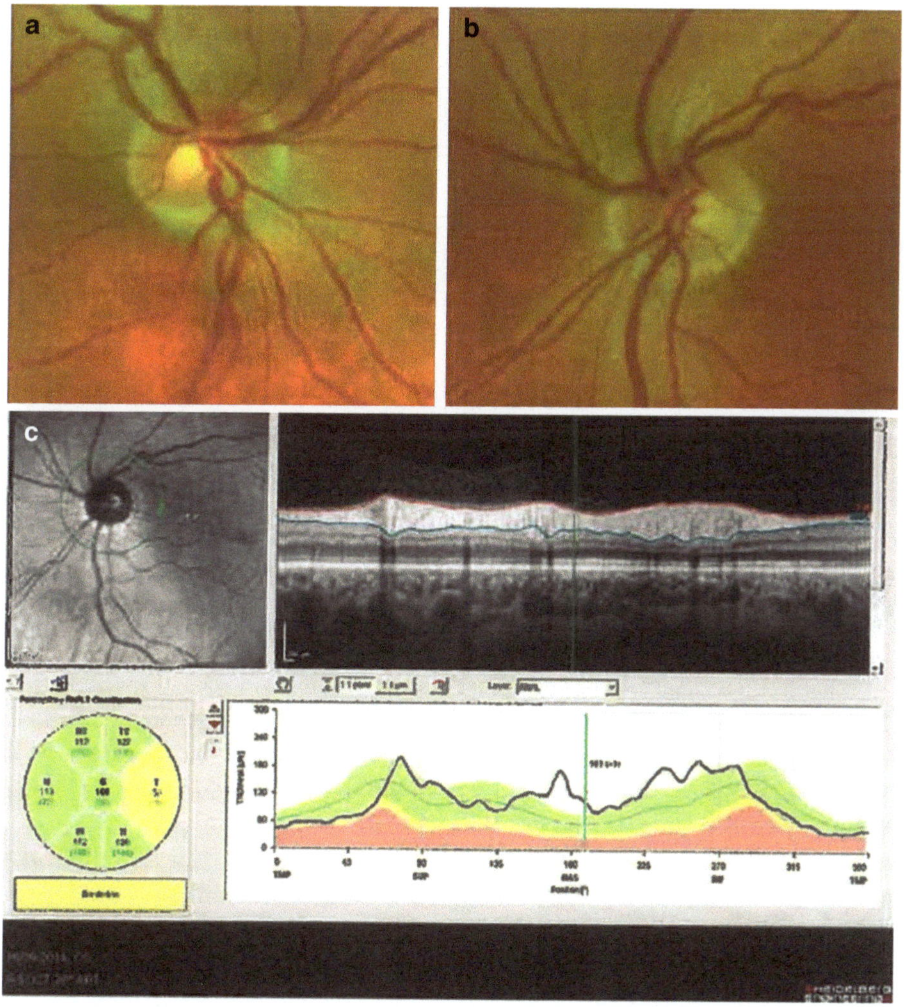

Fig. 18.2 Nutritional optic neuropathy, associated with reduced serum thiamine (Vitamin B 1), in a 30-year-old male patient presenting with blurred vision, painful dysesthesia in both legs and gait instability. Visual acuity was 20/200 in both eyes. Bilateral temporal pallor of the optic discs (**a**, **b**) and moderate reduction of the temporal retinal nerve fibre layer, visible on OCT (**c**, **d**). Vision recovered after intramuscular vitamin Bl administration

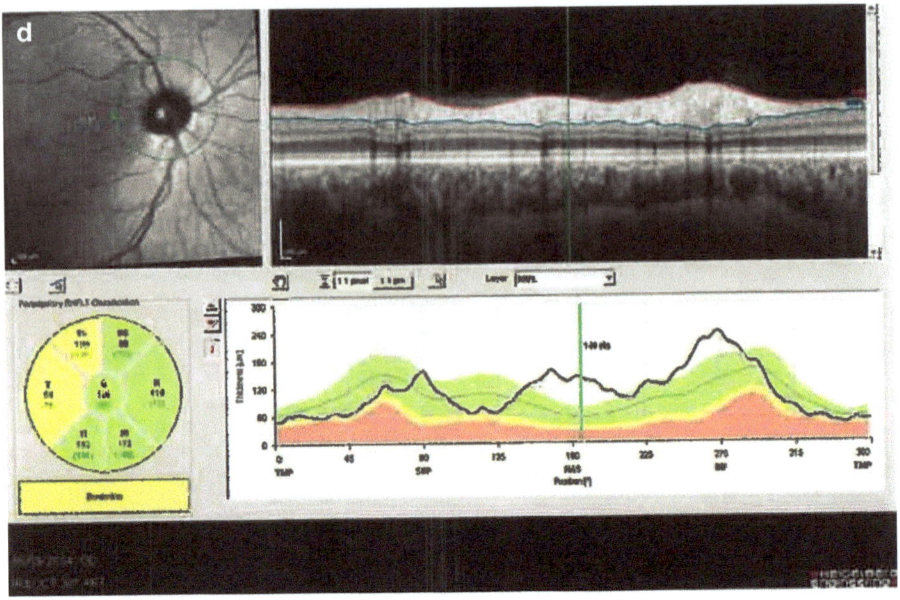

Fig. 18.2 (continued)

After several weeks to months, a papillomacular bundle dropout and temporal disc pallor may occur, followed by optic atrophy (Fig. 18.2). Isolated, purely nutritional optic neuropathies have been rarely explored with OCT, which might be able to closely monitor subtle RNFL changes, i.e. thickening at initial stages, followed at later stages by RML thinning, predominantly encountered in the temporal sector [51] (Figs. 18.3 and 18.4).

A recent OCT study conducted in chronic alcohol and tobacco users demonstrated substantial thinning of the RNFL in all quadrants except the nasal quadrant. The severity of axonal loss in ganglion cells was shown to be proportional to the degree of nicotine dependence. In the case of alcohol abuse, however, the relationship was not as straightforward [54]. These findings suggest that OCT may be a useful screening instrument to predict visual morbidities in persons with nutritional optic neuropathies.

18.2.1 Copper Deficiency

Copper deficiency is an extremely rare finding in patients after bariatric surgeries. According to one published case report, a woman subjected to Roux-en-Y bypass surgery and partial gastrectomy, approximately 3 years after the procedure showed the signs of progressive binocular loss of visual acuity and disorders of color vision with central visual field scotoma in both eyes. OCT conducted 2 months after the

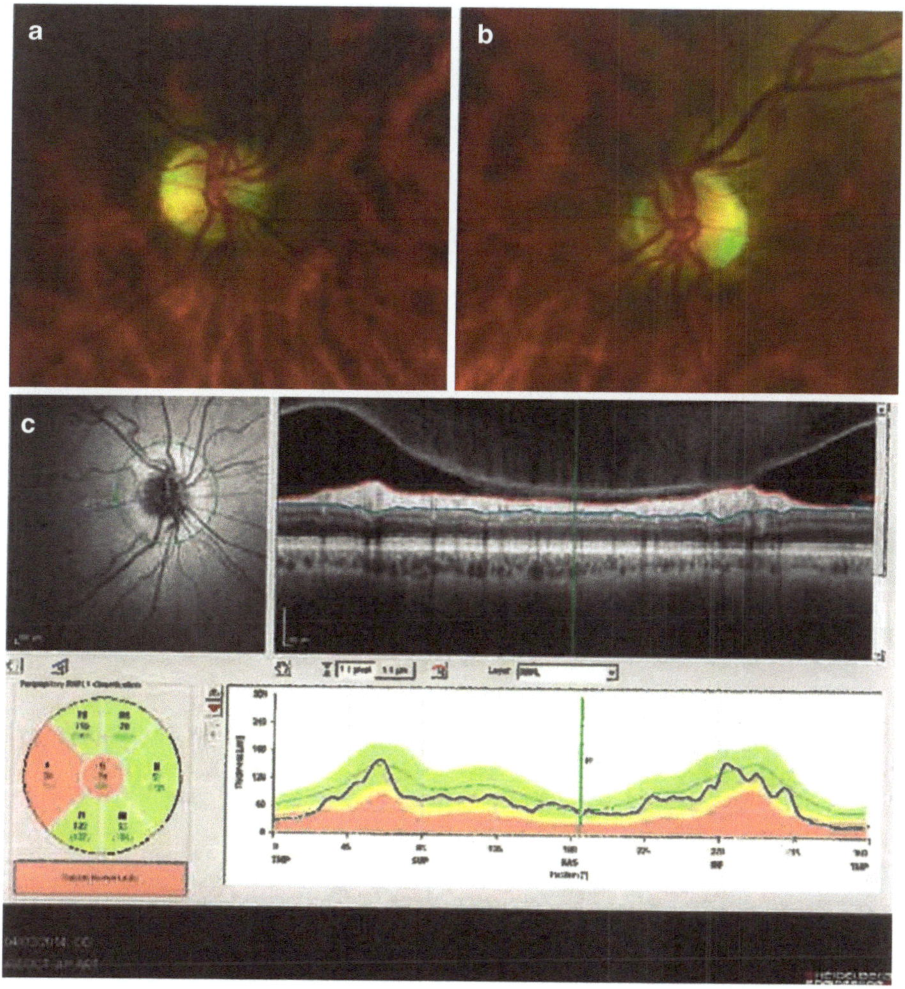

Fig. 18.3 A 60-ycar-old patient presented with bilateral visual loss ongoing for 6 months, (visual acuity was 20/200 in the right eye and 20/400 in the left eye), temporal disc pallor (**a**, **b**) and severe weight loss. There was no history of smoking or alcohol abuse. Decreased RNFL thickness was selectively located in the temporal area (**c**, **d**). Bilateral centrocaecal scotomas were encountered on Goldmann perimetry in both eyes (**e**, **f**). A megaloblastic anemia and folate deficiency was found on the blood test. Eventually a glucagonoma was discovered on abdominal MRI. Malabsorption responsible for malnutrition and particularly for folate deficiency was the suspected mechanism, After successful surgery and folate supplementation, visual acuity improved to 20/30 in the right eye and 20/80 in the left eye

onset of the symptoms revealed binocular thinning of the retinal ganglion cell-inner plexiform layer in the macula. However, the average peripapillary retinal nerve fiber layer thickness was normal. The authors of the report did not provide an explanation for such result of the OCT [55].

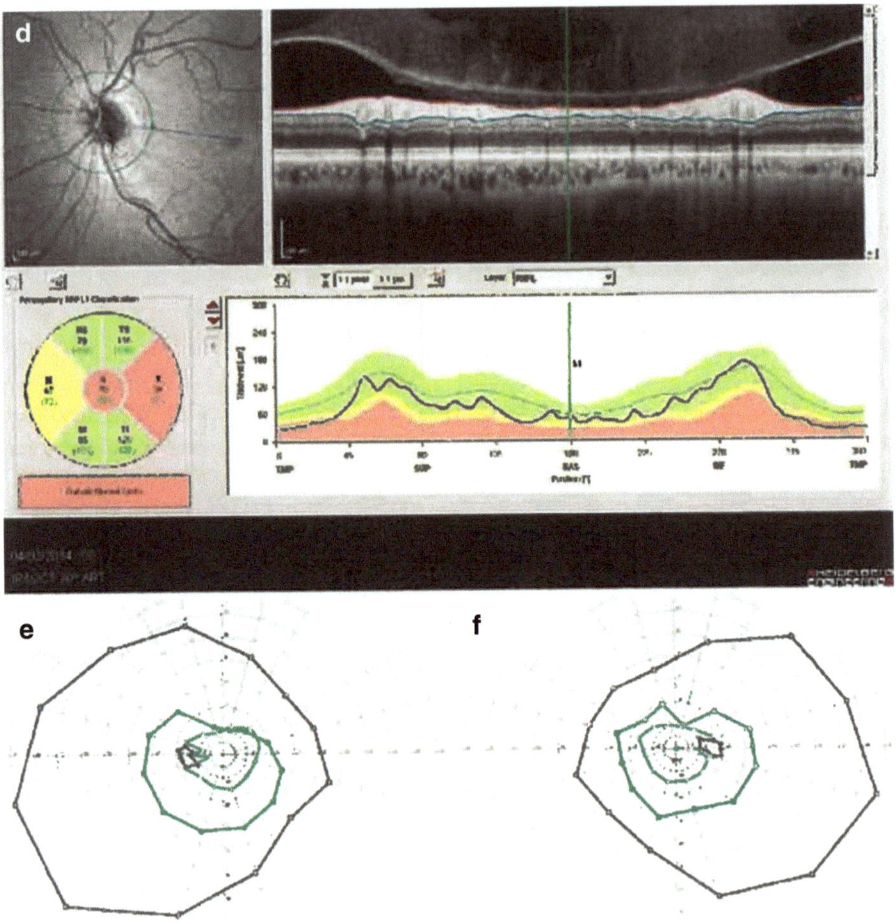

Fig. 18.3 (continued)

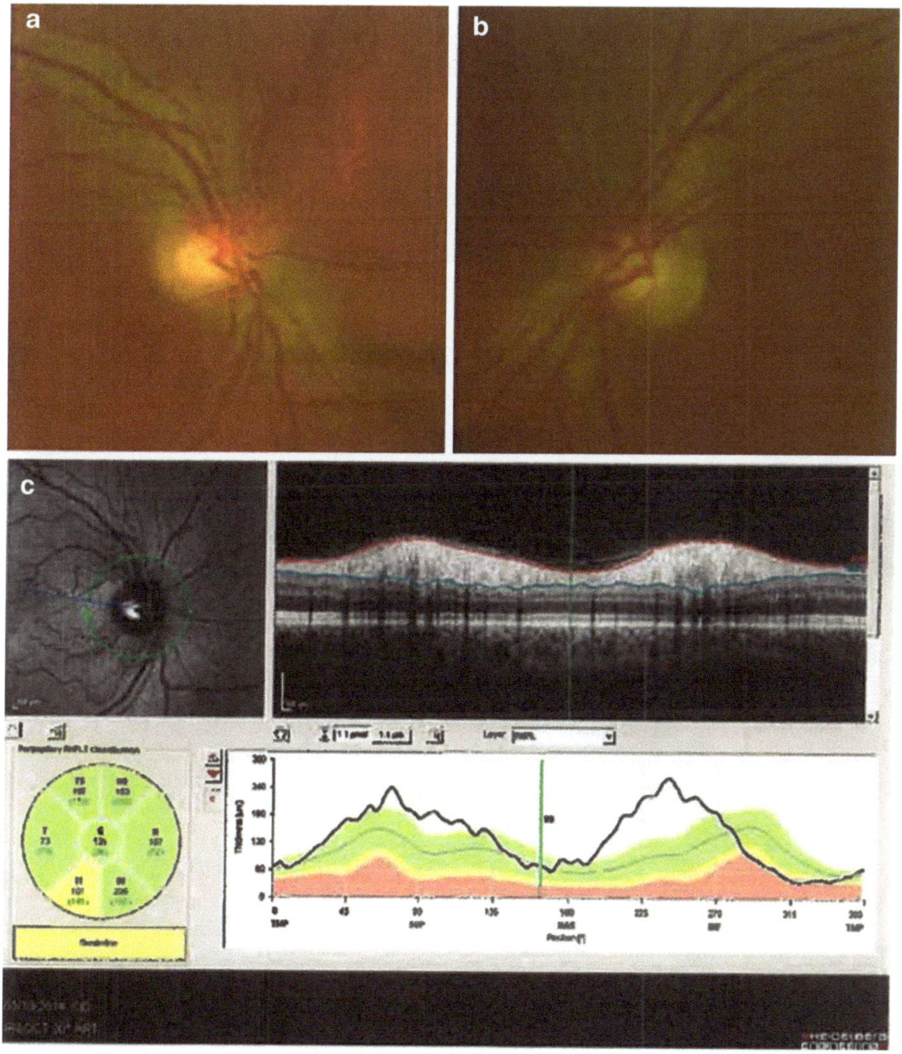

Fig. 18.4 A 40-year-old female patient presented with isolated severe visual loss and a history of mental anorexia in her teens. She stated being well aware of her irregular and unbalanced food intake. Visual acuity was 20/200 in both eyes. The optic disc are slightly hyperaemic with telangiectasia in the peripapillar retina (**a**, **b**). RNFL thickness was at higher normal limit in both eyes (**c**, **d**). The ganglion cell layer was normal in both eyes (**e**, **f**). Leber's hereditary optic neuropathy was ruled out, and the work-up disclosed low vitamin pp and carnitine levels. Six months after supplementation, visual acuity dramatically improved to 20/30 in the right eye and 20/40 in the left eye, although bilateral optic disc pallor had developed and temporal RNFL loss (**g**, **h**) and central ganglion cell loss in both eyes had occurred (**i**, **j**)

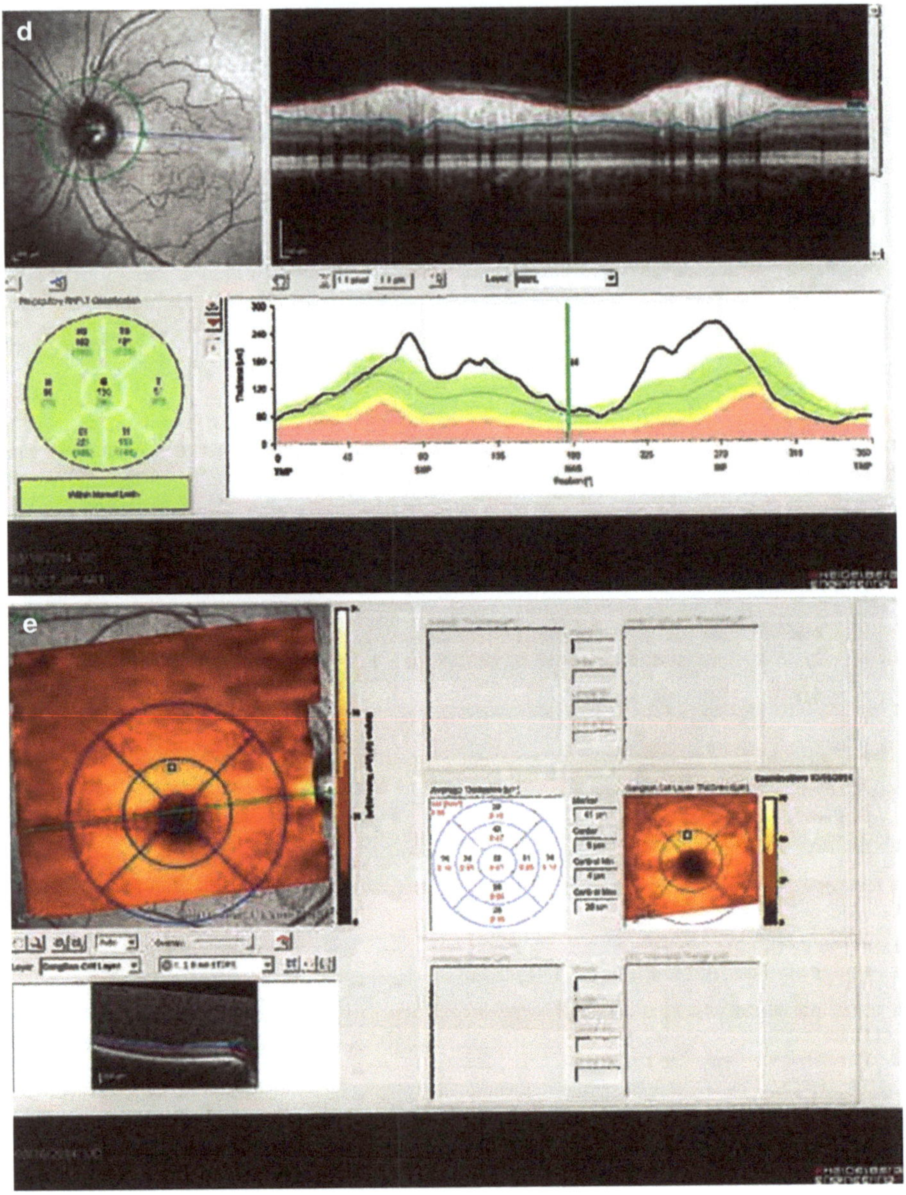

Fig. 18.4 (continued)

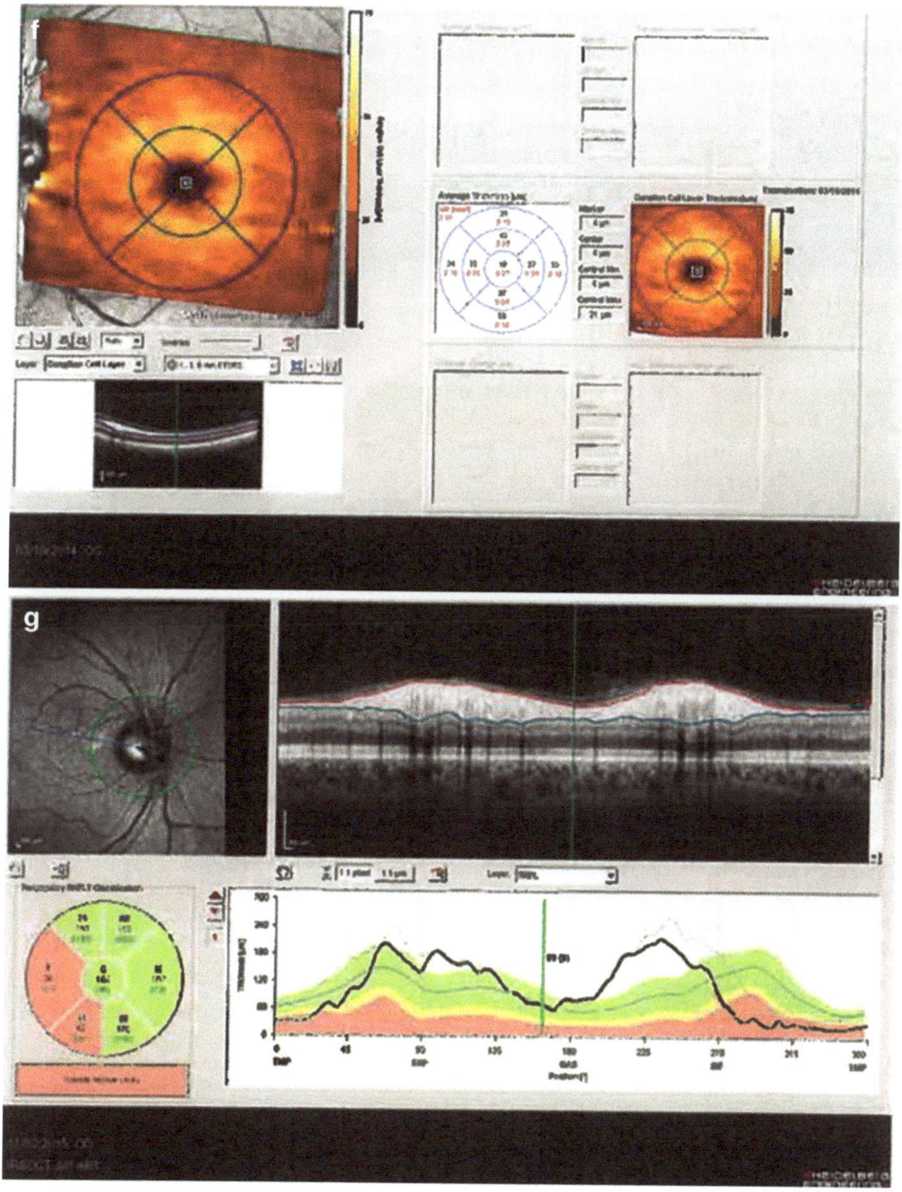

Fig. 18.4 (continued)

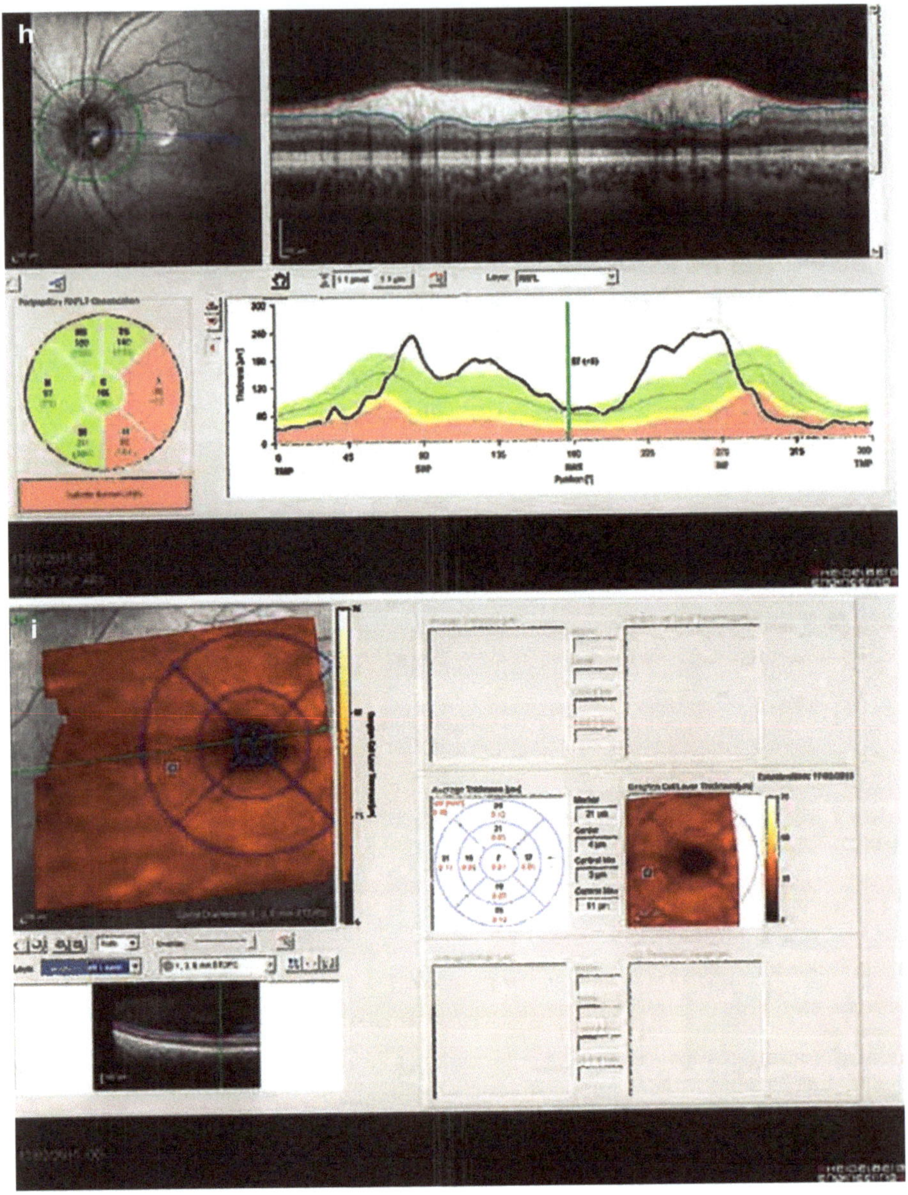

Fig. 18.4 (continued)

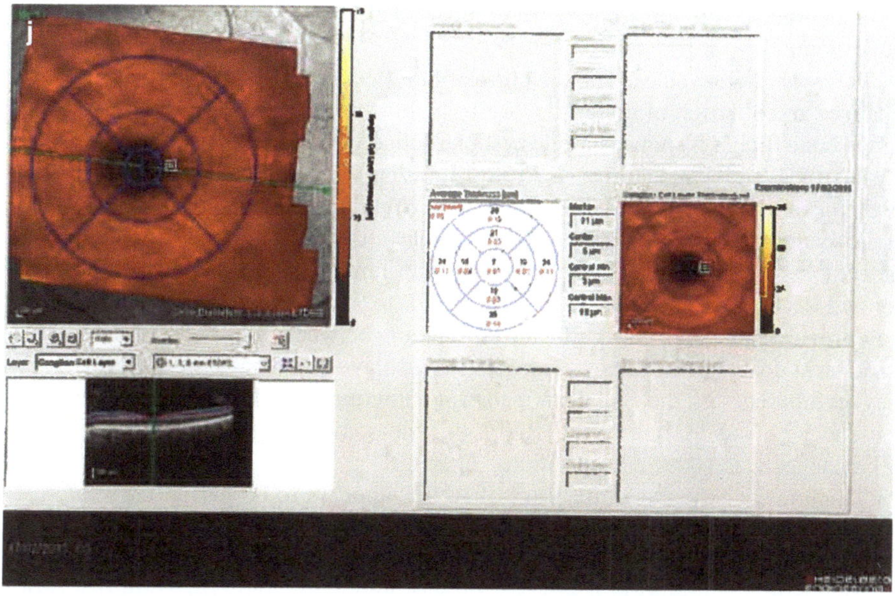

Fig. 18.4 (continued)

18.3 OCT and Antiepileptic Drug Toxic Maculopathy

Vigabatrin (Sabril) is a second-line anti-epileptic drug prescribed in partial epilepsy, with or without secondary generalization (mainly after failure of other drugs). As a first-line/monotherapy, Vigabatrin is licensed only for the treatment of infantile spasms (West's syndrome). Vigabatrin acts as a selective irreversible inhibitor of GABA-transaminase. Treatment therefore causes an increase in the concentration of GABA (gamma aminobutyric acid), the major inhibitory neurotransmitter in the brain but also in the retina. Maximal efficacy in adults is usually seen in the 2–3 g/day range. The recommended maintenance dose in children is 50–100 mg/kg/day.

During its clinical development, vigabatrin has rarely been associated with symptomatic visual field constriction and retinal disorders. In 1997, 3 cases of severe, symptomatic, persistent visual field constriction attributed to vigabatrin (VAVFC) were described by Eke [56].

Vigabatrin toxicity is typically associated with bilateral, concentric, predominantly nasal constriction of visual fields. However, patients with perimetric loss due to vigabatrin exhibit normal visual acuity and are unaware of the visual field constriction unless it extends into the central field [57]. The prevalence of VAVFC varies widely between studies, but is generally estimated to be 30–40% [58, 59].

The precise site of toxicity is controversial, but retina is involved in this condition.

Previous studies have shown correlations between the severity of the ERG changes and duration of therapy, as well as with severity of VAVFC. The amplitude of the cone flicker response has the best predictive value for VAVFC, with a sensitivity of 100% and a specificity of 75% [59]. Therefore, ERG screening is currently used for toxicity detection in patients unable to perform perimetry.

Although visual field (VF) loss may occur in this setting despite any clinically detectable retinal changes, patients on Vigabatrin may exhibit optic nerve head pallor and RNFL thinning (Fig. 18.5) [60]. RNFL loss displayed on time domain OCT has previously shown a significant correlation between VAVFC and cumulative vigabatrin doses [61]. Patients with VAVFC displayed a reduced mean RNFL thickness compared with those under Vigabatrin but without field loss. Since none of the patients with VAVFC had normal RNFL thickness, the OCT sensitivity for detecting VF changes was 100% and specificity 70% [60].

Thickness of the nasal quadrant of RNFL appears to be particularly interesting in predicting vigabatrin associated visual filed constriction, with comparable results in terms of sensitivity (67–100%) and specificity (66–73%) [61, 62]. On the opposite, the temporal RNFL sector was not significantly different from control patients with epilepsy (not treated with gabaergic medications) and healthy volunteers [61, 62].

Thus, time domain and spectral domain optical coherence tomography seem to be reliable, in terms of sensitivity, for detecting RNFL thinning associated with vigabatrin-related visual field loss. It appears that both time domain and spectral domain OCT screening for vigabatrin treated patients may accurately monitor those at risk for VAVFC, especially when they are unable to perform perimetry.

In conclusion, OCT may be useful for quantifying the RNFL and retinal ganglion cells complex parameters in toxic and nutritional optic neuropathies [63]. Several studies have suggested that at early stages, localized, subtle RNFL thickening may be detected with OCT, prior to ophthalmoscopically visible changes. In the long term, localized, followed by diffuse RNFL thinning may occur, witnessing global axonal death.

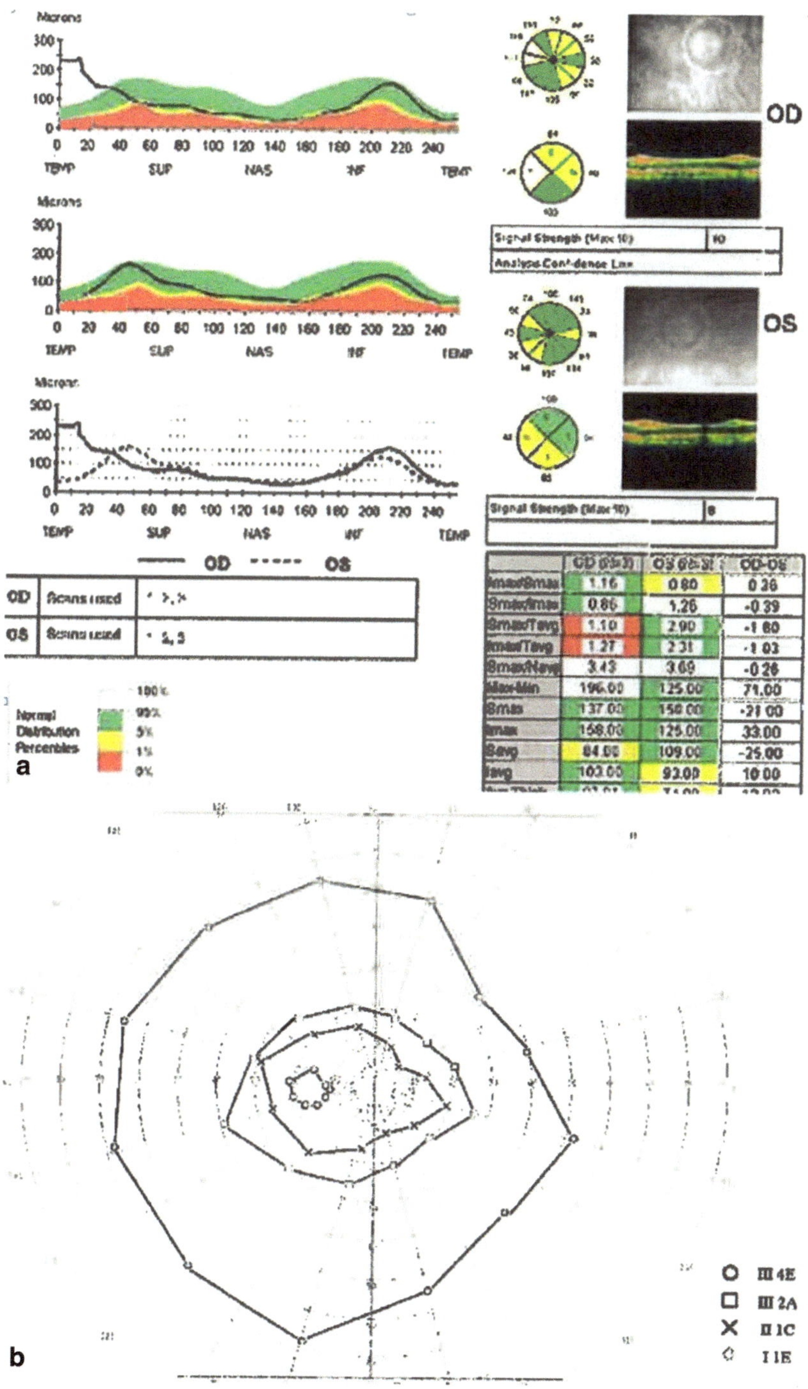

Fig. 18.5 Reduced nasal thickness on time domain OCT (**a**) in a patient treated with vigabatrin and presenting with vigabatrin associated visual field constriction in the nasal hemifield of the left eye (**b**)

References

1. Grzybowski A, Zulsdorff M, Wilhelm H, Tonagel F. Toxic optic neuropathies: an updated review. Acta Ophthalmol. 2015;93:402–10. https://doi.org/10.1111/aos.12515.
2. Wang MY, Sadun AA. Drug-related mitochondrial optic neuropathies. J Neuroophthalmol. 2013;33:172–8.
3. Zoumalan CI, Agarwal M, Sadun AA. Optical coherence tomography can measure axonal loss in patients with ethambutol-induced optic neuropathy. Graefes Arch Clin Exp Ophthalmol. 2005;243:410–6.
4. Sihota R, Sony P, Gupta V, et al. Diagnostic capability of optical coherence tomography in evaluating the degree of glaucomatous retinal nerve fiber damage. Invest Ophthalmol Vis Sci. 2006;47:2006–10.
5. Rebolleda G, Noval S, Contreras I, et al. Optic disc cupping after optic neuritis evaluated with optic coherence tomography. Eye (Lond). 2008;23:890–4.
6. Medeiros FA, Moura FC, Vessani RM, Susanna R. Axonal loss after traumatic optic neuropathy documented by optical coherence tomography. Am J Ophthalmol. 2003;135:406–8.
7. Fisher JB, Jacobs DA, Markowitz CF, et al. Relation of visual function to retinal nerve fiber layer thickness in multiple sclerosis. Ophthalmology. 2006;113:324–32.
8. Kozak SF, Inderlied CB, Hsu HY, et al. The role of copper on ethambutol's antimicrobial action and implications for ethambutol-induced optic neuropathy. Mycobacteriology. 1998;30:83–7.
9. Masvidal D, Parrish RK II, Lam BL. Structural-functional dissociation in presumed ethambutol optic neuropathy. J Neuroophthalmol. 2010;30:305–10.
10. Sadun AA, Wang MY. Ethambutol optic neuropathy: how we can prevent 100,000 new cases of blindness each year. J Neuroophthalmol. 2008;28:265–8.
11. Sivakumaran P, Harrisson AC, Marschner J. Ocular toxicity from ethambutol: a review of four cases and recommended precautions. N Z Med J. 1998;13:428–30.
12. Kinoshita J, Iwata N, Maejima T, Kimotsuki T, Yasuda M. Retinal function and morphology in monkeys with ethambutol-induced optic neuropathy. Invest Ophthalmol Vis Sci. 2012;53:7052–62.
13. Chai SJ, Foroozan R. Decreased retinal nerve fibre layer thickness detected by optical coherence tomography in patients with ethambutol-induced optic neuropathy. Br J Ophthalmol. 2007;91:895–7.
14. Kim U, Hwang JM. Early stage ethambutol optic neuropathy: retinal nerve fiber layer and optical coherence tomography. Eur J Ophthalmol. 2009;19:466–9.
15. Han J, Byun MK, Lee J, Han SY, Lee JB, Han SH. Longitudinal analysis of retinal nerve fiber layer and ganglion cell-inner plexiform layer thickness in ethambutol-induced optic neuropathy. Graefes Arch Clin Exp Ophthalmol. 2015;253:2293–9.
16. Vieira LM, Silva NF, et al. Retinal ganglion cell layer analysis by optical coherence tomography in toxic and nutritional optic neuropathy. J Neuroophthalmol. 2015;35(3):242–5.
17. Lee JY, Choi JH, Park KA, Oh SY. Ganglion cell layer and inner plexiform layer as predictors of vision recovery in ethambutol-induced optic neuropathy: a longitudinal OCT analysis. Invest Ophthalmol Vis Sci. 2018;59:2104–9.
18. Kim KL, Park SP. Visual function test for early detection of ethambutol induced ocular toxicity at the subclinical level. Cutan Ocul Toxicol. 2016;35:228–32.
19. Makino S. Utility of optical coherence tomography in the evaluation of patients with ethambutol-induced optic neuropathy. Int J Ophthalmol Vis Sci. 2014;12(1).
20. Junli X, Qi D, Shuangqing W, Wenyan S, Shanping Z, Liangyu Z. Treatment of ethambutol-induced optic neuropathy by buqihuoxue formula combined with methycobal. Int J Clin Exp Med. 2017;10:7100–15.
21. Fanta H, Mayer-Obcrditsch L. Ein Bcitrag zur Pathologie im Schncrven bci Methylalkoholvergiftung (Tierversuche). Klin Monatsbl Augenheilkd. 1953;122:288–394.
22. Sanaei-zadeh H, Zamani N, Shadnia SH. Outcomes of visual disturbances after methanol poisoning. Clin Toxicol (Phila). 2011;49:102–7.

23. Brent J, McMartin K, Phillips S, Aaron C, Kulig K. Fomepizole for the treatment of methanol poisoning. N Engl J Med. 2001;344:424–9.
24. Pakravan M, Sanjari N. Erythropoietin treatment for methanol optic neuropathy. J Neuroophthalmol. 2012;32:325–8.
25. Fujihara M, Kikuchi M, Kurimoto Y. Methanol-induced retinal toxicity patient examined by optical coherence tomography. Jpn J Ophthalmol. 2006;50:239–41.
26. Klein KA, Warren AK, Baumal CR, Hedges TR III. Optical coherence tomography findings in methanol toxicity. Int J Retina Vitreous. 2017;3:36.
27. Nurieva O, Diblik P, Kuthan P, Sklenka P, Meliska M, Bydzovsky J, Heissigerova J, Urban P, Kotikova K, Navratil T, Komarc M, Seidl Z, Vaneckova M, Pelclova D, Zakharov S. Progressive chronic retinal axonal loss following acute methanol-induced optic neuropathy: four-year prospective cohort study. Am J Ophthalmol. 2018;191:100–15.
28. Cullom ME, Heher KL, Miller NR, Savino PJ, Johns DR. Leber's hereditary optic neuropathy masquerading as tobacco-alcohol amblyopia. Arch Ophthalmol. 1993;111:1482–5.
29. Mackey D, Howell N. Tobacco amblyopia. Am J Ophthalmol. 1994;117:817–9.
30. Johns DR, Heher KL, Miller NR, Smith KH. Leber's hereditary optic neuropathy. Clinical manifestations of the 14484 mutation. Arch Ophthalmol. 1993;111:495–8.
31. Freeman AG. Optic neuropathy and chronic cyanide intoxication: a review. J R Soc Med. 1988;81:103–6.
32. Grzybowski A, Holder GE. Tobacco optic neuropathy (TON) - the historical and present concept of the disease. Acta Ophthalmol. 2011;89:495–9.
33. Behbehani R, Sergott RC, Savino PJ. Tobacco-alcohol amblyopia: a maculopathy? Br J Ophthalmol. 2005;89:1543–4.
34. Kee C, Hwang J-M. Optical coherence tomography in a patient with tobacco-alcohol amblyopia. Eye (Lond). 2008;22:469–70.
35. Moura FC, Monteiro ML. Evaluation of retinal nerve fiber layer thickness measurements using optical coherence tomography in patients with tobacco-alcohol-induced toxic optic neuropathy. Indian J Ophthalmol. 2010;58:143–6.
36. Grzybowski A. Tobacco amblyopia: does it really exist? Eye (Lond). 2007;21:1448–9.
37. Grzybowski A, Pieniazek M. Tobacco-alcohol amblyopia: nonexistent entity. Ind Psychiatry J. 2012;21:79.
38. Grzybowski A, Pieniążek M. Tobacco-alcohol amblyopia does not exist. Acta Ophthalmol. 2014;92:e77–8.
39. Grzybowski A. Mitochondrial optic neuropathies: additional facts and concepts. Clin Exp Ophthalmol. 2013; https://doi.org/10.1111/ceo.
40. Grzybowski A, Pieniazek M. Tobacco-alcohol amblyopia—nonexistent entity cannot be diagnosed. J Neurol Sci. 2013;332:156.
41. Macaluso DC, Shults WT, Fraunfelder FT. Features of amiodarone-induced optic neuropathy. Am J Ophthalmol. 1999;127:610–2.
42. Martínez-López-Portillo A, Martínez-Gamero BO, Mohamed-Noriega J, Cavazos-Adame H, Mohamed-Hamsho J. Behaviour of disc oedema during and after amiodarone optic neuropathy: case report. J Clin Diagn Res. 2014;8:VD04–5.
43. Pilania RK, Arora A, Agarwal A, Jindal AK, Aggarwal K, Krishnan G, Suri D, Gupta A, Singh S, Gupta V. Linezolid-induced mitochondrial toxicity presenting as retinal nerve fiber layer microcysts and optic and peripheral neuropathy in a patient with chronic granulomatous disease. Retin Cases Brief Rep. 2018;25 https://doi.org/10.1097/ICB.0000000000000777.
44. Ishii N, Kinouchi R, Inoue M, Yoshida A. Linezolid-induced optic neuropathy with a rare pathological change in the inner retina. Int Ophthalmol. 2016;36:761–6.
45. David JM, Anupriya A, Sheeja SJ. Presumed chemotherapy-induced optic neuropathy and maculopathy: a case report. Open Ophthalmol J. 2017;11:298–304.
46. Orssaud C, Roche O, Dufier JL. Nutritional optic neuropathies. J Neurol Sci. 2007;262:158–64.
47. Sawicka-Pierko A, Obuchowska I, Hady RH, Mariak Z, Dadan J. Nutritional optic neuropathy following bariatric surgery. Wideochir Inne Tech Maloinwazyjne. 2014;9(4):662–6.

48. Becker M, Masterson K, Delavelle J, Viallon M, Vargas ML, Becker CD. Imaging of the optic nerve. Eur J Radiol. 2010;74:299–313.
49. Gratton SM, Lam BL. Visual loss and optic nerve head swelling in thiamine deficiency without prolonged dietary deficiency. Clin Ophthalmol. 2014;8:1021–4.
50. Pineles SL. Combined optic neuropathy and myelopathy secondary to copper deficiency. Surv Ophthalmol. 2010;55:386–92.
51. Naismith RT, Shepherd JB, Weihl CC, Tutlam NT, Cross AH. Acute and bilateral blindness due to optic neuropathy associated with copper deficiency. Arch Neurol. 2009;66:1025–7.
52. Spinazzi M, De Lazzari F, Tavolato B, Angelini C, Manara R, Armani M. Myelo-opticoneuropathy in copper deficiency occurring after partial gastrectomy: do small bowel bacterial overgrowth syndrome and occult zinc ingestion tip the balance? J Neurol. 2007;254:1012–7.
53. Woon C, Tang RA, Pardo G. Nutrition and optic nerve disease. Semin Ophthalmol. 1995;10:195–202.
54. Ahuja S, Kumar PS, Kumar VP, Kattimani S, Akkilagunta S. Effect of chronic alcohol and tobacco use on retinal nerve fiber layer thickness: a case-control study. BMJ Open Ophthalmol. 2016;1:e000003. https://doi.org/10.1136/bmjophth-2016-000003.
55. Rapoprt Y, Lavin PJM. Nutritional optic neuropathy caused by copper deficiency after bariatric surgery. J Neuroophthalmol. 2016;36:178–81.
56. Eke T, Talbot JF, Lawden MC. Severe persistent visual field constriction associated with vigabatrin. BMJ. 1997;314:180–1.
57. Daneshvar H, Racette L, Coupland SG, Kertes PJ, Guberman A, Zackon D. Symptomatic and asymptomatic visual loss in patients taking vigabatrin. Ophthalmology. 1999;106:1792–8.
58. Lawden MC, Eke T, Degg C, Harding GF, Wild JM. Visual field defects associated with vigabatrin therapy. J Neurol Neurosurg Psychiatry. 1999;67:716–22.
59. Miller NR, Johnson MA, Paul SR, Girkin CA, Perry JD, Endres M, et al. Visual dysfunction in patients receiving vigabatrin: clinical and electrophysiologic findings. Neurology. 1999;53:2082–7.
60. Wild JM, Ahn HS, Baulac M, Bursztyn J, Chiron C, Gandolfo E, et al. Vigabatrin and epilepsy: lessons learned. Epilepsia. 2007;48:1318–27.
61. Versino M, Veggiotti P. Reversibility of vigabratin-induced visual-field defect. Lancet. 1999;354:486.
62. Frisen L, Malmgrcn K. Characterization of vigabatrin-associated optic atrophy. Acta Ophthalmol Scand. 2003;81:466–73.
63. Iorga RE, Moraru A, Ozturk MR, Costin D. The role of optical coherence tomography in optic neuropathies. Rom J Ophthalmol. 2018;62:3–14.

Animal Models in Neuro Ophthalmology 19

Eduardo M. Normando and M. Francesca Cordeiro

19.1 Animal Models of Demyelinating Conditions

Demyelinating conditions such as multiple sclerosis (MS) are a major cause of disability and appropriate neuroprotective strategies have not been successfully developed yet [1]. MS can affect the visual system and therefore the eye can be used as a surrogate in assessing both the natural history of the disease and possible neuroprotective treatments. Although MS is a human specific condition, animal models of similar diseases have been developed such as Experimental autoimmune encephalomyelitis (EAE), viral induced models (mainly mediated by Theiler's Murine Encephalomyelitis Virus), and toxicity-induced models such as the cuprizone model and lysolecithin-induced focal demyelination [2] (Table 19.1).

19.1.1 Experimental Autoimmune Encephalomyelitis (EAE)

EAE is an animal model of neuro-inflammation and is the most commonly used model of MS [3]. It is based on both antigen-antibody and cell-mediated response. It can be induced in several animal species (rat, mouse, rabbit, guinea pig and monkey) by spinal cord homogenate inoculation or by injection of different emulsified proteins or peptides in the animal CNS. The proteins/peptides commonly used to induce EAE are myelin constituent peptides such as myelin basic

E. M. Normando · M. F. Cordeiro (✉)
Imperial College Ophthalmology Research Group (ICORG), Department of Surgery and Cancer, Imperial College London, London, UK

Western Eye Hospital, Imperial College Healthcare NHS Trust, London, UK

Glaucoma and Retinal Neurodegeneration Research, Visual Neuroscience, UCL Institute of Ophthalmology, London, UK
e-mail: m.cordeiro@imperial.ac.uk

A. Grzybowski, P. Barboni (eds.), *OCT and Imaging in Central Nervous System Diseases*, https://doi.org/10.1007/978-3-030-26269-3_19

Table 19.1 Animal models in neuro ophthalmology

Disease	Animal model	Method	Benefits	Limitations	References
MS	EAE (rat, mouse, monkey) Cuprizone, lysolecithin (mouse)	Induced	Similar variation in natural history Simplicity; rapid	Limited brain involvement Reversible	[2–9]
AD	PS-1 and/or PS-2 APP transgenic mutation mouse P301L tau mutation mouse 5xFAD mouse 3xTg-AD mouse	Genetic	Progressive development of senile plaques Robust model of NFT pathology Rapid deposition of large amounts of Aß Follows natural history of AD	Difficult connection between injuries and increased deposition of Aß oligomers 1st generation model No NFT formation	[10–15]
ION	Rat, primate	Rose Bengal injection	Resembles human AION pathology	Does not reflect pathogenesis of -ION	[16]
LHON	CBA/J mice Mice, Rats Mice	Rotenone-induced Mitochondrial ND4 mutation Mitochondrial ND6 mutation	Quick and simple, reproduce the pathophysiologic phenotype–reduced RGC layer thickness, increased apoptosis, decreased retinal metabolic capacity, increased superoxide reproduction of LHON phenotype Clinical, biochemical and anatomical hallmarks of human LHON when induced in animal at 14 and 24 months	The causal role of toxins in human LHON has not been demonstrated The mutation can be fatal (ND4 mutation), technically demanding	[17–19]
NOM	EAE 'passive transfer' mouse Mice	Passive transfer of IgG Injection of IgG	Very similar pathology to human NMO Similar pathology with myelin involvement also	No injury to myelin Dependent on co-injection of human complement	[20]
	"2D2" EAE mouse	Genetic	Similar clinical picture to human NMO	No histological changes in keeping with NMO	[21]

protein (MBP), myelin proteolipid protein (PLP), and myelin oligodendrocyte glycoprotein (MOG). EAE is primarily mediated by specific T cells (CD4+), which migrate to the CNS and cause the autoimmune inflammatory response. The natural history of EAE can be variable, in a similar fashion as in human MS, and it is both species and agent dependent [22]. Hallmark signs include weight loss, ataxia, spastic/flaccid paralysis, and incontinence. The lesions in the EAE model are characterized mainly by spinal inflammation and demyelination, while in human MS, lesions are more commonly seen in the brain [23]. Literature reviews have shown that in recent decades several possible MS therapeutic strategies were successfully tested in animal models of EAE and that it was possible to control the disease in these immune-induced models [4, 5, 24]. However, these successes in animal studies did not translate into a success when it came to human clinical trials [25].

The infection of the central nervous system with the Theiler's virus induces an immune-mediated demyelinating disease and provides an important model for the study of MS [26]. The demyelinating disease induced by Theiler's Murine Encephalomyelitis Virus (TMEV) is similar to chronic-progressive MS and is characterized by demyelination of the CNS mediated by a Th1 response with manifestation of spastic paralysis of the lower limbs. In particular, in the mouse model of TMEV, the damage to myelin is closely dependent on the CD8 mediated antiviral action, demonstrating how brain inflammation could result in demyelination and axonal damage [6, 7, 27, 28].

Alterations in the optic nerve and retina have been described in EAE where optical coherence tomography (OCT) detected GCC changes which may be similar to what is observed in MS [7]. EAE not only promotes apoptosis in the retina, but also causes glial response [8, 9] (Fig. 19.1).

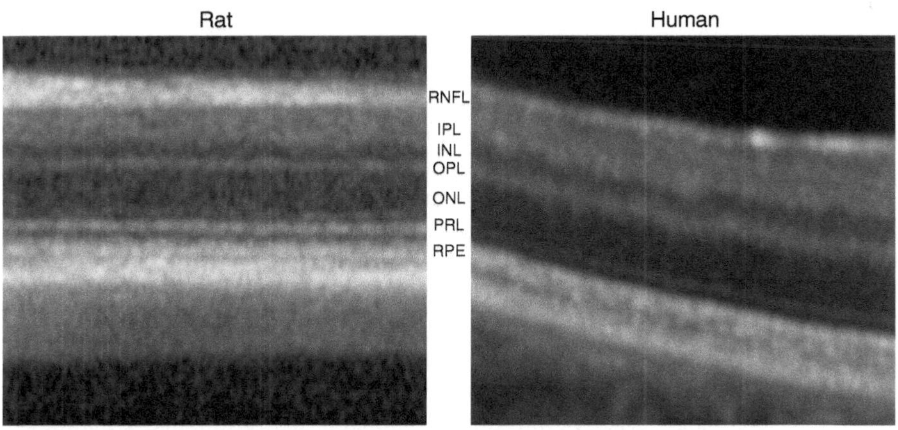

Fig. 19.1 OCT differences between rat retina and human retina. *RNFL* retinal nerve fibre layer, *IPL* inner plexiform layer, *INL* inner nuclear layer, *OPL* outer plexiform layer, *ONL* outer nuclear layer, *PRL* photoreceptor layer, *RPE* retinal pigmented epithelium

19.1.2 Toxic Models of Demyelinating Conditions

Toxic models of demyelination have also been developed. Cuprizone, a copper chelating agent is able to induce rapid oligodendrocyte apoptosis with subsequent demyelination. The most important advantage of the cuprizone model is its simplicity. Mice, orally exposed to cuprizone express a rapid onset of MS like symptoms including ataxia and spastic paralysis. Histological features of this model are oligodendrocyte apoptosis, microglial infiltration, disruption of myelin sheets and macrophage activation which are in keeping with Human MS. Cuprizone impairs visual function, as demonstrated by multifocal electroretinography [29]. However, this is a reversible model; when cuprizone is eliminated from the mouse diet, remyelinization occurs followed by complete restitutio-ad-integrum [8, 20, 30, 31].

Lysolecithin, an activator of phospholipase A2, is also able to induce demyelination when injected into the spinal cord of experimental animals. It generates rapid demyelination due to activation of lymphocytes B and T followed by macrophage infiltration with subsequent disruption of myelin sheets. Like the cuprizone model, after Lysolecithin injection, remyelinization occurs in 6–8 weeks. Hence, this model is also not entirely representative of human MS [21, 32].

In conclusion, none of the currently available animal models of MS can replicate in-toto the human disease and further research is needed in the field.

19.1.3 Animal Models of Neuromyelitis Optica

Neuromyelitis Optica (NMO) is a neuroinflammatory disorder that preferentially targets the optic nerves and spinal cord, causing recurrent and simultaneous inflammation and demyelination of these structures, leading to blindness and paralysis [33]. Once thought to be a subtype of MS, the discovery that NMO is associated with the NMO-IgG biomarker, an antibody which targets the aquaporin-4 (AQP4) water channel on the end feet of astrocytes, has seen it recognised as a spectrum of disorders distinct from MS [34]. Classical presentation is with an episode of optic neuritis causing a loss of vision, or visual field defects and dyschomatopsia occurring in isolation; accompanied by acute spinal cord dysfunction such as paraparesis or quadriparesis with sensory signs, or loss of bladder control.

There is circumstantial evidence from studies which suggests that NMO-IgG is pathogenic in humans, with the presence of the antibodies in patients with transverse myelitis or optic neuritis conferring a strong likelihood that these patients with develop NMO in the future compared to patients who test negative for the antibodies [35]. One animal model of NMO involves passive transfer of NMO-IgG via intraperitoneal injection into the EAE rat model. The IgG appears to exacerbate inflammation and modulate the immune response in the context of this model resulting in complement activation, immunoglobulin deposition, and granulocyte influx in perivascular areas of the spinal cord [36]. These changes represent very similar pathology to that seen in human NMO lesions, however the major limitation in this model is the lack of injury to the myelin. Another model of NMO involves direct injection of NMO-IgG into the brain of mice. Lesion development was dependent on the co-injection of human complement, resulting in similar pathological changes to those seen in human NMO lesions, and in contrast to the rat NMO models also demonstrated damage to the myelin [37]. A genetic animal model of NMO which does not involve IgG has also been developed. The "2D2" EAE model was developed in which mice born with T cells directed against myelin oligodendrocyte glycoprotein (MOG35–55) were crossed with mice that have a transgenic B cell receptor to MOG. The resultant progeny spontaneously developed a clinical picture involving optic neuritis and severe inflammatory spinal cord lesions, with sparing of the brain, as seen in human NMO patients [38]. In this model the drawback was that histological changes such as complement deposition and granulocyte recruitment were not seen. As yet no single animal model has recreated all of the clinical and pathological features of NMO, but a combination of active immunization, passive transfer, and genetic models is helping to elucidate individual pathological events in NMO.

Retinal involvement is a feature of NMO, however, effective animal models of optic neuritis in NMO (NMO-ON) are lacking. Asavapanumas et al. have generated a mouse model of NMO-ON by continuous infusion near the optic chiasm of NMO-IgG [16], Zeka et al. have shown Aquaporin 4-specific T cells and NMO-IgG cause primary retinal damage in a mouse model of NMO [39].

19.2 Animal Models of Ischemic Optic Neuropathy

Ischemic optic neuropathy (ION) is caused by an ischaemia of the optic nerve head and is the most frequent cause of sudden visual loss in patients older than 50 years. ION is characterized by a severe reduction in visual acuity associated with visual field defect, oedema of the optic nerve head and disc haemorrhages. Ischemic optic neuropathy is differentiated into two different clinical forms: non-arteritic (NAION), which is caused by an infarct of the short posterior ciliary arteries associated with anatomical risk factors such as small optic disc; and the arteritic form (AION), which is part of a generalized disease (e.g. giant cells arteritis), caused by an inflammatory reaction. The ischaemic outcome of either event will result in nerve fibre atrophy and often gives rise to a pale optic disc on clinical examination [40, 41].

The major problem regarding animal models of ION lies in the anatomical differences between the optic nerve head (ONH) in human and small animals. The ONH in rodents lacks a lamina cribrosa, and the connective tissue surrounding the axon bundles has different collagen components and hysteresis compared to what is found in humans [42]. The vascular structure of the rodent ONH is also different. While rats have a vascular ring around the ONH which is somewhat similar to primates, mice often lack this anatomical feature [43]. Therefore, this intrinsic inter-species variability translates into completely different manifestations of an ischaemic event. Furthermore, the number of axons which constitute the optic nerve is different between species. Human and non-human primates have 1–1.2 million axons, rats 100,000 and mice 50,000 [44–46]. Again, this crucial anatomical difference results in contrasting manifestations of ONH ischaemia.

The most diffuse model of ION is found in an induced model where a dye (Rose Bengal—RB) is injected intravenously and then locally activated by a focal laser beam (532 nμ) projected onto the ONH of the animal [17]. The activation of the RB provokes reactive oxygen species formation which subsequently triggers platelet activation and capillary endothelial disruption [18]. Repeatability, which was the major problem of this model, has been overcome recently by the introduction of custom made rodent contact lenses which enables constant and reproducible insults [19]. The generated damage has similar features to human ION, however the ischaemia resolves rapidly and the disc oedema disappears after a maximum of 5 days post insult. However, Retinal Ganglion Cell (RGCs) apoptosis occurs and reduction in retinal fibres is clearly visible 1 month after laser exposure using both direct visualization and computerised techniques. The hallmark of the disease, RGC apoptosis is also clearly assessable histologically, alongside structural changes to vessels, ONH oligodendrocytes apoptosis and ONH fibrosis [47, 48]. The same method generates similar results when applied to mice and non-human primates, making this technique a very easy model of ION [49, 50] (Table 19.1). Recent studies have shown that overexpression of Dedicator of cytokinesis 3 (Dock3), which is part of the guanine nucleotide exchange factors family, protects myelin in the corpus callosum in a rodent model of ION [51].

19.3 Animal Models of Leber Hereditary Optic Neuropathy

Leber's hereditary optic neuropathy (LHON) is a rare disorder caused by mitochondrial DNA point mutations in genes coding for specific protein subunits of the respiratory chain complex I (G3460A, T14484C, G11778A) [52, 53]; it is characterized by severe, painless acute unilateral visual loss which becomes bilateral within days or weeks. LHON predominantly affects young men (20 years) and, less frequently, women. However, a small number of paediatric and elderly cases have been reported [54]. The classic manifestation of LHON consists of rapid, painless loss of central vision in one eye, accompanied by dyschromatopsia, followed by the involvement of the fellow eye within days or weeks. The evolution of the visual field defect is generally represented by progressive enlargement of the blind spot with rapid progress towards the central vision. Diagnosis of LHON should be always considered in young male patients with bilateral optic neuritis, regardless of their age [54].

Genetic studies of LHON began over two decades ago, however the pathogenic mechanisms that produce the specific RGCs degeneration are still not fully understood and aetiological therapeutic strategies are still under development. This is due largely to the lack of a good animal models of LHON. The first animal model was generated by intravitreal administration of rotenone, a mitochondrial complex I inhibitor, directly into the mouse eye where histological analysis showed a significant decrease of RGC layer thickness 1 day after injection of rotenone [55]. Another experimental mouse model consists of an intravitreal injection of a genetically-engineered ribozyme. This procedure is responsible for a specific degradation of nuclear mRNA which results in the onset of an optic neuropathy with reduced superoxide dismutase activity and similar histological features observed in patients with LHON [56]. Another model of rodent LHON can be generated by injecting rotenone microspheres directly into the rat's superior colliculus [57]. These animal models showed most common signs of LHON: visual loss within 2 weeks of injection, absence of early RGCs loss with subsequent apoptosis. Intravitreal injections of yeast NADH dehydrogenase (Ndi1) in these models produces restoration of normal vision, which has opened a window of opportunity for novel therapeutic strategies [57]. Genetic models of LHON are also available [10]. A mouse with a G14600A mutation has been developed which results in mouse optic atrophy with synaptosomes and increased ROS production [58].

19.4 Animal Models of Alzheimer's Disease

Alzheimer's disease (AD), the most common cause of dementia, is characterized by the insidious onset of a progressive decline in cognitive function due to the loss of neurons in the brain [59]. The pathology underlying the degeneration of neurons in AD brain is the formation of extracellular senile plaques via amyloid-beta (Aß) deposition and intracellular neurofibrillary tangles (NFTs) via hyperphosphorylation of tau protein [60]. Although much progress has been made in our understanding of AD, early and more accurate diagnosis is currently unavailable, and a definitive diagnosis of AD can still only be made by neuropathology after the patient has died [61]. This prevents effective treatment in the early stages of the disease. Perhaps the main problem in the early diagnosis of AD is the inability to directly visualize changes in the brain.

However, increasing evidence has shown that the retina is also affected in AD, along with the changes in the brain [62, 63]. More significantly, the hallmarks of Alzheimer's in the brain have also been identified in the retina in both animal models and human subjects.

Recent studies have demonstrated that RGCs, the RNFL and inner plexiform of the transgenic mice exhibit a significant rise in the immunoreactivity of Aβ and APP when compared to wild-type mice, with the changes being age-dependent [11, 64, 65]. Histological studies in transgenic AD mouse models have demonstrated the present of Aß in the retina. Using a single transgenic Tg2576 mouse model which contains the APP double Swedish mutation, Liu et al. have shown increased Aß immunoreaction occurring predominantly in the retinal ganglion cell layer and the outer retina [12]. Retinal Aß deposition along with increased APP has also been found in double transgenic mouse models expressing APP and presenilin (PS) mutations; a finding which increased with age [13, 64, 65]. Using a triple transgenic AD mouse model that harbours three mutations of APP, tau and PS, a recent study has also demonstrated increased Aß deposition and tau hyperphosphorylation in the RGC layer compared to age-matched controls. A particularly exciting finding is that retinal Aß plaques in AD mice can be stained with curcumin and imaged *in-vivo*;

and more significantly, that the retinal plaques occurred prior to the development of plaques in the brain [66]. This is hugely relevant as it suggests that retinal changes could potentially be used to make an early diagnosis of AD. Similar to the findings in mice, APP immunoreaction has also been demonstrated in human retina, being prominent in RGCs and the RNFL, and again found in increased abundance with age [14]. In AD patients, Aß specific plaques have been identified in the retina and increased with the severity of the disease by histological analysis of post-mortem eyes [66].

The clinical endpoint for AD pathology is neuronal loss and tissue atrophy in the brain, in which both apoptosis and necrosis play a crucial role [67].

19.4.1 PS-1 and/or PS-2 APP Transgenic Mutation

Copies of human APP and PS1-2, which are implicated in familial AD have been used to create models of transgenic AD mice [68]. Transgenic models generated APP mutation with deposition of amyloid peptide, which is similar but not identical to the one found in human senile plaques, and commonly associated with amyloid angiopathy. Deposit of amyloid peptide are observed with associated dystrophic alterations in axons and dendrites. These models have often been used to understand the natural history of senile plaques [15], to study the plaque removing action of microglia [69], and to study protein interactions [70]. The double APP+ PS1 mutant transgenic models, show a progressive and rapid development of senile plaques at 3 months of age with maximum expression at 12 months [71].

Since the development of this model, several questions have been raised regarding the mechanism of neuronal loss, the accumulation of Aß in the cell body, inflammation, and gliosis. This model has also been used to determine the involvement of oxidative stress in AD [72, 73]. The biggest drawback of this model is the difficulty to draw a connection between symptoms, injuries and increased deposition of Aß oligomers [74]. Another problem of this mouse model is that neurofibrillary tangles (NFTs) are present only in mouse lines that overexpress mutated tau protein [74, 75].

19.4.2 Transgenic Tauopathies

Tauopathies are a group of degenerative diseases characterized histologically by the presence of filamentous inclusions in neurons (neurofibrillary pathology) and occasionally in the glial cells. These filaments are composed of hyperphosphorylated forms of tau protein which together generates NFT. The discovery of the tau gene mutation on chromosome 17 in frontotemporal dementia has facilitated the development of tau-transgenic mice [76–78].

There has been significant progress in the development of models of this group of diseases. In particular mice expressing P301L tau mutation demonstrated that it is possible to generate robust animal models of neurofibrillary pathology [79] which can be assessed in vivo. However, this transgenic model only represents a first generation of mice which are affected by human tauopathies [80].

19.4.3 5 Mutations Model

This model, developed by Oakley et al. is based on 5 mutations that occur in APP and presenilins (PS-1 and PS-2) which lead to an increased production of Aß-42. This model is known as 5xFAD, which represent the five mutations that occur in familial AD. In this model there is a rapid production of Aß-42 that leads to the formation of senile plaques similar to those found in patients with AD [81]. Aß deposits begin at 2 months of age in the neuronal soma and dendrites especially in deep cortical layers, well before the formation of senile plaques.

In this model synaptic dysfunction occurs with aging, showing a marked decrease in synaptophysin, syntaxin and PDS95 and loss of pyramidal cortical neurons [81] with marked memory loss [81, 82]. Moreover it has been reported that this transgenic mouse has behavioural and motor deficiencies [83]. Furthermore, recent studies have shown that 5xFAD mice have early inner retina impairment which precedes neuronal loss in other parts of their brain [84].

This may be a useful model for studying the processes related to the formation of senile plaques, synaptic loss and cognitive decline. This model has the advantage that it produces a large amount of Aß deposition in a short period of time. However, this model does not produce the same NFTs that are characteristic of AD in humans.

19.4.4 Triple-Transgenic Model

In 2003 a triple-transgenic model was described for the first time in which both senile plaques and NFT called 3xTg-AD were present [85].

This mouse expresses extracellular Aß deposits prior to the formation of NFT. This phenotype is in keeping with the natural history of the AD in humans where there is progressive loss of synaptic plasticity followed by extracellular deposits of Aß and the deposition of NFTs, associated with Aß immunoreactivity [86, 87]. Therefore, it is considered that this particular type of transgenic mouse is useful for studying the impact of Aß and tau protein accumulation on synaptic plasticity. Moreover, this model presents with behavioural and cognitive deficits that increase with aging. These characteristics are similar to what happens in humans with AD [88]. Since the creation of the 3xTg-AD mouse, a variety of research projects have been initiated which seek to elucidate our understanding of AD.

It has been demonstrated that the accumulation of Aß which triggers tau deposition occurs before it is undergoes hyperphosphorylation [89, 90]. In 2005, a study showing that chronic nicotine administration exacerbates tauopathy in this model was published [91, 92]. The relationship between Aß, tau and synaptic dysfunction was also assessed [85]. Likewise the ratio of Aß deposition and cognitive deficits was also demonstrated [93]. The 3xTg-AD model has been correlated with glial activation and Aß deposition [94], and has also been used to study the inflammation in specific areas of the CNS in order to evaluate potential inflammatory markers of AD [94]. Furthermore, recent studies have shown accumulation of Tau proteins in the retina in this model which promotes anterograde axonal transport impairment [95]. In a paper published in 2005, primary cultures of 3xTgAD were used to study calcium release induced by caffeine [96]. The triple-transgenic mouse has proven to be a useful model for studying the development of AD, its neurobiochemical, neuropathological and neuropharmacological characteristics. Studies with this model outnumber those made with other types of models. However, there will always be controversy about the extent to which animal models are representative of the disease in humans.

Although an age-dependent increase of the level of RGC apoptosis has been documented histologically in the double AD (APP/PS1) mouse [11, 64], this has not yet been confirmed in real time. Using the triple transgenic mouse model of AD (3xTgAD), it has been attempted to assess both apoptosis and necrosis simultaneously *in-vivo*. Both RGC apoptosis and necrosis are present in the retina of AD mice, and quantitative analysis revealed that the majority of apoptotic RGCs are in their early phase of apoptosis rather than in the late phase or necrosis, compared with age matched controls. This would suggest that early phase apoptosis of RGCs may be characteristic in 3xTgAD mice, and they could be reversed or rescued in this early stage of degeneration.

Increased evidence shows that oxidative stress is heavily implicated in AD pathology, along with increased Aß accumulation and deposition in the brain [97]. As Aß accumulation in the retina has been demonstrated in this AD model [98, 99].

Thus, the novel approach of *in-vivo* retinal imaging not only provides a means to detect RGC death which could reflect the changes in the brain, but also enables differentiation of apoptosing and necrosing processes simultaneously in the same living eye over time.

19.5 Animal Models of Parkinson's Disease

Although the use of L-DOPA has revolutionized the treatment of PD, this is only a symptomatic treatment, which cannot arrest or delay the degeneration of dopaminergic neurons. The most significant obstacle to the development of new neuroprotective drugs is the lack of knowledge of the specific molecular events that lead to neurodegeneration in PD [100].

The development of animal models represents a valuable tool for testing therapeutic strategies.

In PD, studies in a wide range of invertebrates have shown that AS is normally present in retinal cells [101]. Moreover the genetic expression of AS mRNA and protein is distributed across the different retinal layers [102]. Compared to AD there are fewer animal studies that focus on retinal changes in PD with more emphasis on understanding the molecular mechanisms involved in dopaminergic neuronal death in the brain. The rodent and non-human primates models of the PD retina can be broadly categorised into neuropharamacological agents targeting catecholaminergic neurons (neurotoxins) and those based on genetic manipulations relevant to PD or sometimes used in combination [103]. To date, the agents used to induce degeneration of cells producing dopamine include MPTP (1-Methyl-4-phenyl-1,2,3,6-tetrahydropyridine) [104], and pesticides such as rotenone [105].

The treatment of animals with neurotoxins such as rotenone, paraquat, 6-OHDA, MPTP and -synuclein, provide important models for the study of the causes and the molecular mechanisms involved in the death of dopaminergic neurons in PD. Although these toxins induce CNS neurodegeneration, each one produces different clinical and neuropathological effects. Each neurotoxic model of PD has its own advantages and disadvantages and currently no one model is capable of representing all aspects of PD. For this reason, the choice of toxins used to induce a PD model is related to the type of study to be undertaken [106]. A summary of models is presented in the table below (Table 19.2).

19.5.1 Paraquat (1,1′-Dimethyl-4,4′-Bipyridinium Dichloride)

When administered systemically in rodents, paraquat can induce reduced motor activity, a dose dependent loss of dopaminergic neurons in the SN, and a reduction of dopaminergic fibres in the striatum [107]. Rats treated with paraquat are reported to also express pathological levels of α-syn in the SN [108]. However, a limitation of this model is that paraquat also induces severe lung, liver, and kidney toxicity causing a high mortality rate in treated animals [109].

19.5.2 6-OHDA (6-Hydroxyl Dopamine or 2, 4, 5-Trihydroxy Phenethylamine)

6-OHDA does not easily cross the Blood Brain Barrier (BBB) and therefore cannot reach toxic concentrations in the CNS following a systemic administration. However, systemic administration of 6-OHDA causes damage to the peripheral nervous system [131]. Due to its inability to cross the BBB, direct administration of 6-OHDA in different brain area has been achieved using stereotactic methods to better model PD [106]. Used firstly on rats, the direct administration of 6-OHDA has subsequently been characterised in mice and monkeys [110–114]. The most common method to induce a lesion in the nigrostriatal pathway is the unilateral administration of 6-OHDA in the forebrain bundle (which includes the nigrostriatal tract) or in the striatum [132], however, a bilateral lesion with 6-OHDA is fatal. After direct administration of 6-OHDA, apoptosis of dopaminergic neurons is reported to occur within 24 h [133]. The maximum reduction in the levels of striatal DA occurs between 3 and 4 days after lesion onset, when the residual striatal

Table 19.2 Comparing the common animal models of PD

Model	Administration route	Type of damage	Histological findings	Symptoms	Disadvantages	References
Paraquat	Systemic	Loss of striatal dopaminergic fibres	α-syn inclusions	Reduced motor activity	Active on other neurotransmitter	[107–109]
6-OHDA	Local, stereotaxic	Loss of striatal dopaminergic neurons	Absence of α-syn inclusions	Rotational behaviours	Intracranial injections are fatal	[110–114]
MPTP	Systemic, subcutaneous, intravenous, intraperitoneal or intramuscular	Selective loss of Da neurons, reduced DA fibers	Absence of α-syn inclusions	Reduced motor activity	Acute model, does not progress	[115–118]
α-synuclein	Viral vectors, transgenic model	Selective degeneration of dopaminergic neurons	Overexpression of α-syn	Heavily reduced motor activity	Scarce evidence of neuronal death	[119–122]
Rotenone	Systemic, subcutaneous, intravenous, intraperitoneal or intramuscular	Loss of striatal dopaminergic neurons	α-syn inclusions, reduced tyrosine hydroxylase levels, nigrostriatal microglial activation	Reduced motor activity, altered posture, sleep and gastrointestinal alteration	Time consuming, high rate of mortality	[123–127]
LRRK-2	Transgenic	Minor loss of striatal dopaminergic neurons	Presence of Lewy bodies	Reduced motor activity	Absence of α-syn inclusions, poorly reproducible	[128–130]

DA neuron population is reduced to less than 20% of age matched controls [134]. Therefore, this is a rapid model but very invasive. The presence of Lewy's Bodies (LB) has not yet been documented in this model.

19.5.3 MPTP (1-Methyl-4-Phenyl-1,2,3,6-Tetrahydropyridine)

Neuropathological data, derived mainly from experiments on non-human primates, has demonstrated that administration of MPTP causes damage to the nigrostriatal dopaminergic pathway similar to that found in PD [115]. The most reliable and reproducible disease model is induced through systemic administration of MPTP via intranasal [135], subcutaneous [136], intravenous [137], intra-peritoneal [138] or intramuscular [139] injection. As in human PD, a large loss of dopaminergic neurons in the CNS and ventral tegmental area is reported in this model [116, 117]. However, MPTP induced models of PD do not present with LBs [118].

19.5.4 α-Synuclein

Chronologically, the most recent model of PD, this model is based on the genetic link between Parkinson's disease and neuropathological effect of α-synuclein (α-syn) [119]. There are two types of α-syn animal models, either transgenic or non-transgenic. Transgenic model organisms in Drosophila and mice have been developed which over-express both the human wild-type α-syn and the mutated (A3OP and A53T) forms [140]. In models of Drosophila a significant loss of DA neurons is reported, while murine models do not demonstrate significant anomalies in dopaminergic neurons [120]. Non-transgenic models are based instead on the insertion of α-syn encoding genes into the SNPC using viral vectors [121, 122]. The mutation of α-syn in this way is reported to cause the selective degeneration of dopaminergic neurons in the rat SNPC, with the formation of cytoplasmic structures containing a-syn which are very similar to LBs [141].

19.5.5 Rotenone ((2R, 6aS, 12aS)-1, 2, 6, 6a, 12, 12a-Hexahydro-2-Isopropenyl-8, 9-Dimethoxy Chromeno [3, 4-b] Furo (2, 3-H) Chromen-6-One)

Among the various models of PD, the rotenone model has recently drawn particular attention because it reproduces most of the motor defect symptoms and the histopathological features of PD [142, 143].

This insecticide found in the roots of leguminous plants, interacts specifically with the mitochondrial respiratory chain complex [144]. Rotenone acts by blocking the mitochondrial electron transport form complex I to CoenzymeQ10 leading to energy starvation and cellular death.

Rotenone may have initially been used by Indians as a poison when hunting for fish [145]. Today it is commonly used as a pesticide due to its high biodegradability, degrading within days. It is highly lipophilic so it quickly passes through the cell membrane, the blood brain barrier and accumulates in subcellular organelles such as mitochondria [146]. Both pulsatile [147] and chronic [123] administration of rotenone *in-vivo* and *in-vitro* models induces degeneration of nigrostriatal neurons, with formation of cytoplasmic inclusions similar to Lewy bodies, oxidative damage and parkinsonian bradykinesia and rigidity.

The mechanism by which complex I dysfunction induces neurotoxicity is still not known. The most common pathway seems to involve increased levels of oxidative stress [148], resulting in reduced levels of glutathione and oxidative modification of DNA, lipids, proteins and antioxidants such as α-tocopherol [149, 150]. Inhibition of Complex I was also demonstrated to increase levels of H_2O_2 and inhibition of Reactive Oxygen Species (ROS) [151]. It is believed that increased levels of ROS are mediated by microglia, which are also activated by the rotenone [152]. This massive oxidative stress produces alterations in mitochondrial function and activation of the apoptosing cascade [151]. The resulting decrease in intracellular levels of ATP causes the opening of Na^+K^+-ATP channels [153]. It has been shown that the hyperpolarization induced by the application of rotenone on dopamine cells of the CNS is mediated by the opening of these channels. In addition, the dopaminergic cells that contain the SUR-1 subunit of the Na^+ K^+-ATP channels are more sensitive to metabolic changes induced by the toxin [154].

The selectivity of rotenone on the dopaminergic system has been explained on the basis of the cytotoxic effect mediated by the same endogenous mechanism [155]. It has been shown that rotenone induced blockade of mitochondrial complex I occurs in all cells indiscriminately [156], but this inhibition does not induce cell death in non-dopaminergic cells. The association between ROS—dopamine in dopaminergic cells could be the basis of the initial apoptotic process [157].

Biehlmaier et al. have demonstrated that rotenone-treated rats show a depletion of DA in the striatum and substantia nigra (SN), in association to a significant reduction in retinal dopaminergic amacrine cells, similar to that found in PD patients [107, 158].

In 2000, it was first reported that chronic systemic rotenone exposure in rats produced phenotypical features of PD. Rotenone is reported to exert highly selective toxicity on DA neurons both *in-vitro* [159, 160] and *in-vivo* [123, 161, 162].

The mechanisms of action of rotenone are various [163]; rotenone is reported to inhibit mitochondrial complex 1, impeding the oxidation of NADH to NAD^+ so causing a reduction in cellular respiration [163]. The consequence of complex 1 inhibition is a cascade of events which leads to elevated oxidative stress [164] and ultimately apoptosis [165].

In-vivo models have been obtained through different routes of rotenone administration; Oral administration (via food), is reported to cause only mild neurotoxicity [124]. Stereotactic administration of rotenone in the medial forebrain bundle is reported to cause depletion of striatal DA neurons [166]. Systemic administration, including intravenous (i.v.), subcutaneous (s.c.), or intraperitoneal (I.P.), has been found to induce the formation of α-syn cytoplasmatic particles, in the substantia nigra of treated rats in a similar manner to the typical LBs found in PD [123, 167]. Systemic administration of rotenone is also reported to promote the production of pro inflammatory factors and microglial activation triggering further oxidative insult to DA neurons [168, 169].

Rotenone administration also causes symptomatic changes in rodents including motor rigidity, behavioural alterations, catalepsy, sleep and gastrointestinal alterations. L-DOPA therapy is able to reverse temporarily the motor deficits reported in these models [170, 171]. Furthermore, systemic rotenone administration, frequently causes neurotoxicity and mortality in a dose-dependent manner.

Systemic rotenone administration has been reported, through its ability to penetrate all cells, to act also on non-dopaminergic neurons such as Retinal Ganglion Cells (RGCs) [172]. Additional supporting evidence for the use of rotenone as a PD model can be found in epidemiological studies which demonstrated a correlation between PD and rotenone exposure in humans [173, 174].

19.5.6 LRRK2 Model (Table 19.3)

Leucine Rich Repeat Kinase (LRRK2) is a gene responsible for coding an enzyme called dardarin which has kinase activities and is responsible for signal transmission, protein-protein interaction, and amino acid phosphorylation [185]. Mutation of the *lrrk2* gene has been implicated in the pathogenesis of familial PD [128].

Table 19.3 Mutation involved in genetic PD

	Locus	Gene	Transmission	Number of family	Reference
PARK 1	4q21-23	α-synuclein	AD	18	[175]
PARK 2	6q25-27	Parkin	AR	Many	[176]
PARK 3	2p13	–	AD	6	[177]
PARK 4	4q21-23	α-synuclein	AD	Many	[178]
PARK 5	4p14	Ubiquitin	AD	1	[179]
PARK 6	1p35-36	Pink-1	AR	Sporadic cases	[180]
PARK 7	1p36	DJ-1	AR	2	[181]
PARK 8	12p11-q13	Dardarin (LRKK2)	AD	Many + sporadic cases	[182, 183]
PARK 9	1p36	–	AR	Kulford-Rakeb Syndrome	[184]

lrrk2 was associated with the locus Park8 (Parkinson family of type 8) for the first time in 2002, in a large Japanese family that presented parkinsonian symptoms with autosomal dominant inheritance, but without the appearance of Lewy bodies [129]. Since 2004, mutations in *lrrk2*-linked to PD have been found in many families, which also included cases with the presence of LBs [128]. The relationship between PD and *lrrk2* was later confirmed by gene sequencing which has revealed numerous pathogenic amino acid substitutions [186]. The *lrrk2* mutation Gly2019Ser is the most frequent replacement in the Caucasian population, which is statistically present in 0.5–2% of cases of sporadic and 5% of MP in familial Parkinsonism [187]. The probability that a heterozygote manifests symptoms below the age of 50 is less than 20%, but this increases with age to more than 80% after 75 years [130]. Biopsies of the substantia nigra of patients with PD caused by expression of mutated LRRK2 show the presence of Lewy bodies [188, 189]. La Morgia and colleagues have shown also retinal modifications in patients affected by the mutation of *lrrk2* [190] and reported the same RNFL thinning that occurs in patients with sporadic PD [191]. Retinal modifications have also been shown in a LRRK2 transgenic Drosophila melanogaster model [192]. Using this model, Hindle et al. demonstrated a loss of visual response and concomitant photoreceptor degeneration.

19.6 Conclusion

Accessibility and cost efficiency combined with the great accessibility of the eye make animal models a precious tool for studying the natural history of neuro-ophthalmological diseases suggesting these models could provide a source of novel biomarkers for the early diagnosis and follow up of neurodegenerative diseases. Nevertheless, due to anatomical and physiological differences, the validity of animal models is closely related to the level of similarity with the human pathology. Therefore prudence should be always applied in choosing the appropriate model for each individual neuro-ophthalmological condition.

References

1. Sormani MP, Bruzzi P. Can we measure long-term treatment effects in multiple sclerosis? Nat Rev Neurol. 2015;11:176–82.
2. Gold R, Hartung HP, Toyka KV. Animal models for autoimmune demyelinating disorders of the nervous system. Mol Med Today. 2000;6(2):88–91.
3. Hoglund RA, Maghazachi AA. Multiple sclerosis and the role of immune cells. World J Exp Med. 2014;4(3):27–37.
4. Vesterinen HM, Sena ES, ffrench-Constant C, Williams A, Chandran S, Macleod MR. Improving the translational hit of experimental treatments in multiple sclerosis. Mult Scler. 2010;16(9):1044–55.
5. Pryce G, O'Neill JK, Croxford JL, Amor S, Hankey DJ, East E, et al. Autoimmune tolerance eliminates relapses but fails to halt progression in a model of multiple sclerosis. J Neuroimmunol. 2005;165(1–2):41–52.

6. Mecha M, Carrillo-Salinas FJ, Mestre L, Feliu A, Guaza C. Viral models of multiple sclerosis: neurodegeneration and demyelination in mice infected with Theiler's virus. Prog Neurobiol. 2013;101–102:46–64.
7. Manogaran P, Walker-Egger C, Samardzija M, Waschkies C, Grimm C, Rudin M, et al. Exploring experimental autoimmune optic neuritis using multimodal imaging. NeuroImage. 2018;175:327–39.
8. Maganti RJ, Hronowski XL, Dunstan RW, Wipke BT, Zhang X, Jandreski L, et al. Defining changes in the spatial distribution and composition of brain lipids in the shiverer and cuprizone mouse models of myelin disease. J Histochem Cytochem. 2019;67:203–19.
9. Horstmann L, Schmid H, Heinen AP, Kurschus FC, Dick HB, Joachim SC. Inflammatory demyelination induces glia alterations and ganglion cell loss in the retina of an experimental autoimmune encephalomyelitis model. J Neuroinflammation. 2013;10:120.
10. Ratican SE, Osborne A, Martin KR. Progress in gene therapy to prevent retinal ganglion cell loss in Glaucoma and Leber's hereditary optic neuropathy. Neural Plast. 2018;2018:7108948.
11. Shimazawa M, Inokuchi Y, Okuno T, Nakajima Y, Sakaguchi G, Kato A, et al. Reduced retinal function in amyloid precursor protein-over-expressing transgenic mice via attenuating glutamate-N-methyl-d-aspartate receptor signaling. J Neurochem. 2008;107(1):279–90.
12. Liu B, Rasool S, Yang Z, Glabe CG, Schreiber SS, Ge J, et al. Amyloid-peptide vaccinations reduce {beta}-amyloid plaques but exacerbate vascular deposition and inflammation in the retina of Alzheimer's transgenic mice. Am J Pathol. 2009;175(5):2099–110.
13. Dutescu RM, Li QX, Crowston J, Masters CL, Baird PN, Culvenor JG. Amyloid precursor protein processing and retinal pathology in mouse models of Alzheimer's disease. Graefe's Arch Clin Exp Ophthalmol. 2009;247(9):1213–21.
14. Loffler KU, Edward DP, Tso MO. Immunoreactivity against tau, amyloid precursor protein, and beta-amyloid in the human retina. Invest Ophthalmol Vis Sci. 1995;36(1):24–31.
15. Park JH, Widi GA, Gimbel DA, Harel NY, Lee DH, Strittmatter SM. Subcutaneous Nogo receptor removes brain amyloid-beta and improves spatial memory in Alzheimer's transgenic mice. J Neurosci. 2006;26(51):13279–86.
16. Asavapanumas N, Ratelade J, Papadopoulos MC, Bennett JL, Levin MH, Verkman AS. Experimental mouse model of optic neuritis with inflammatory demyelination produced by passive transfer of neuromyelitis optica-immunoglobulin G. J Neuroinflammation. 2014;11:16.
17. Zhao BQ, Suzuki Y, Kondo K, Kawano K, Ikeda Y, Umemura K. A novel MCA occlusion model of photothrombotic ischemia with cyclic flow reductions: development of cerebral hemorrhage induced by heparin. Brain Res Brain Res Protoc. 2002;9(2):85–92.
18. Mosinger JL, Olney JW. Photothrombosis-induced ischemic neuronal degeneration in the rat retina. Exp Neurol. 1989;105(1):110–3.
19. Bernstein SL, Johnson MA, Miller NR. Nonarteritic anterior ischemic optic neuropathy (NAION) and its experimental models. Prog Retin Eye Res. 2011;30(3):167–87.
20. Praet J, Guglielmetti C, Berneman Z, Van der Linden A, Ponsaerts P. Cellular and molecular neuropathology of the cuprizone mouse model: clinical relevance for multiple sclerosis. Neurosci Biobehav Rev. 2014;47C:485–505.
21. van der Star BJ, Vogel DY, Kipp M, Puentes F, Baker D, Amor S. In vitro and in vivo models of multiple sclerosis. CNS Neurol Disord Drug Targets. 2012;11(5):570–88.
22. Kuerten S, Lehmann PV. The immune pathogenesis of experimental autoimmune encephalomyelitis: lessons learned for multiple sclerosis? J Interf Cytokine Res. 2011;31(12):907–16.
23. Handel AE, Lincoln MR, Ramagopalan SV. Of mice and men: experimental autoimmune encephalitis and multiple sclerosis. Eur J Clin Investig. 2011;41(11):1254–8.
24. Gogoleva VS, Atretkhany KN, Drutskaya MS, Mufazalov IA, Kruglov AA, Nedospasov SA. Cytokines as mediators of neuroinflammation in experimental autoimmune encephalomyelitis. Biochemistry (Mosc). 2018;83(9):1089–103.
25. Friese MA, Montalban X, Willcox N, Bell JI, Martin R, Fugger L. The value of animal models for drug development in multiple sclerosis. Brain J Neurol. 2006;129(Pt 8):1940–52.

26. Takizawa S, Kaneyama T, Tsugane S, Takeichi N, Yanagisawa S, Ichikawa M, et al. Role of the Programmed Death-1 (PD-1) pathway in regulation of Theiler's murine encephalomyelitis virus-induced demyelinating disease. J Neuroimmunol. 2014;274(1–2):78–85.
27. Martinez NE, Karlsson F, Sato F, Kawai E, Omura S, Minagar A, et al. Protective and detrimental roles for regulatory T cells in a viral model for multiple sclerosis. Brain Pathol. 2014;24(5):436–51.
28. Zhang J, Lipton HL, Perelson AS, Dahari H. Modeling the acute and chronic phases of Theiler murine encephalomyelitis virus infection. J Virol. 2013;87(7):4052–9.
29. Namekata K, Kimura A, Harada C, Yoshida H, Matsumoto Y, Harada T. Dock3 protects myelin in the cuprizone model for demyelination. Cell Death Dis. 2014;5:e1395.
30. Sachs HH, Bercury KK, Popescu DC, Narayanan SP, Macklin WB. A new model of cuprizone-mediated demyelination/remyelination. ASN Neuro. 2014;6(5).
31. Praet J, Guglielmetti C, Berneman Z, Van der Linden A, Ponsaerts P. Cellular and molecular neuropathology of the cuprizone mouse model: clinical relevance for multiple sclerosis. Neurosci Biobehav Rev. 2014;47:485–505.
32. Nastasijevic B, Wright BR, Smestad J, Warrington AE, Rodriguez M, Maher LJ 3rd. Remyelination induced by a DNA aptamer in a mouse model of multiple sclerosis. PLoS One. 2012;7(6):e39595.
33. Huang TL, Lin KH, Wang JK, Tsai RK. Treatment strategies for neuromyelitis optica. Ci Ji Yi Xue Za Zhi. 2018;30(4):204–8.
34. Jones MV, Collongues N, de Seze J, Kinoshita M, Nakatsuji Y, Levy M. Review of animal models of neuromyelitis optica. Mult Scler Relat Disord. 2012;1(4):174–9.
35. Frohman EM, Kerr D. Is neuromyelitis optica distinct from multiple sclerosis?: something for "lumpers" and "splitters". Arch Neurol. 2007;64(6):903–5.
36. Kinoshita M, Nakatsuji Y, Kimura T, Moriya M, Takata K, Okuno T, et al. Neuromyelitis optica: passive transfer to rats by human immunoglobulin. Biochem Biophys Res Commun. 2009;386(4):623–7.
37. Saadoun S, Waters P, Bell BA, Vincent A, Verkman AS, Papadopoulos MC. Intra-cerebral injection of neuromyelitis optica immunoglobulin G and human complement produces neuromyelitis optica lesions in mice. Brain J Neurol. 2010;133(Pt 2):349–61.
38. Bettelli E, Baeten D, Jager A, Sobel RA, Kuchroo VK. Myelin oligodendrocyte glycoprotein-specific T and B cells cooperate to induce a Devic-like disease in mice. J Clin Invest. 2006;116(9):2393–402.
39. Zeka B, Hastermann M, Kaufmann N, Schanda K, Pende M, Misu T, et al. Aquaporin 4-specific T cells and NMO-IgG cause primary retinal damage in experimental NMO/SD. Acta Neuropathol Commun. 2016;4(1):82.
40. Arnold AC, Hepler RS. Natural history of nonarteritic anterior ischemic optic neuropathy. J Neuroophthalmol. 1994;14(2):66–9.
41. Arnold AC. Pathogenesis of nonarteritic anterior ischemic optic neuropathy. J Neuroophthalmol. 2003;23(2):157–63.
42. Albrecht MC. Comparative anatomy of the optic nerve head and inner retina in non-primate animal models used for glaucoma research. Open Ophthalmol J. 2008;2:94–101.
43. Bernstein SL, Guo Y, Kelman SE, Flower RW, Johnson MA. Functional and cellular responses in a novel rodent model of anterior ischemic optic neuropathy. Invest Ophthalmol Vis Sci. 2003;44(10):4153–62.
44. Williams RW, Strom RC, Rice DS, Goldowitz D. Genetic and environmental control of variation in retinal ganglion cell number in mice. J Neurosci. 1996;16(22):7193–205.
45. Perry VH, Henderson Z, Linden R. Postnatal changes in retinal ganglion cell and optic axon populations in the pigmented rat. J Comp Neurol. 1983;219(3):356–68.
46. Morrison JC, Cork LC, Dunkelberger GR, Brown A, Quigley HA. Aging changes of the rhesus monkey optic nerve. Invest Ophthalmol Vis Sci. 1990;31(8):1623–7.
47. Goldenberg-Cohen N, Guo Y, Margolis F, Cohen Y, Miller NR, Bernstein SL. Oligodendrocyte dysfunction after induction of experimental anterior optic nerve ischemia. Invest Ophthalmol Vis Sci. 2005;46(8):2716–25.

48. Khalilpour S, Latifi S, Behnammanesh G, Majid A, Majid ASA, Tamayol A. Ischemic optic neuropathy as a model of neurodegenerative disorder: a review of pathogenic mechanism of axonal degeneration and the role of neuroprotection. J Neurol Sci. 2017;375:430–41.
49. Feng G, Mellor RH, Bernstein M, Keller-Peck C, Nguyen QT, Wallace M, et al. Imaging neuronal subsets in transgenic mice expressing multiple spectral variants of GFP. Neuron. 2000;28(1):41–51.
50. Chen CS, Johnson MA, Flower RA, Slater BJ, Miller NR, Bernstein SL. A primate model of nonarteritic anterior ischemic optic neuropathy. Invest Ophthalmol Vis Sci. 2008;49(7):2985–92.
51. Kokona D, Haner NU, Ebneter A, Zinkernagel MS. Imaging of macrophage dynamics with optical coherence tomography in anterior ischemic optic neuropathy. Exp Eye Res. 2017;154:159–67.
52. Ziccardi L, Sadun F, De Negri AM, Barboni P, Savini G, Borrelli E, et al. Retinal function and neural conduction along the visual pathways in affected and unaffected carriers with Leber's hereditary optic neuropathy. Invest Ophthalmol Vis Sci. 2013;54(10):6893–901.
53. Rasool N, Lessell S, Cestari DM. Leber hereditary optic neuropathy: bringing the lab to the clinic. Semin Ophthalmol. 2016;31(1–2):107–16.
54. La Morgia C, Carbonelli M, Barboni P, Sadun AA, Carelli V. Medical management of hereditary optic neuropathies. Front Neurol. 2014;5:141.
55. Zhang X, Jones D, Gonzalez-Lima F. Mouse model of optic neuropathy caused by mitochondrial complex I dysfunction. Neurosci Lett. 2002;326(2):97–100.
56. Qi X, Lewin AS, Hauswirth WW, Guy J. Suppression of complex I gene expression induces optic neuropathy. Ann Neurol. 2003;53(2):198–205.
57. Marella M, Seo BB, Thomas BB, Matsuno-Yagi A, Yagi T. Successful amelioration of mitochondrial optic neuropathy using the yeast NDI1 gene in a rat animal model. PLoS One. 2010;5(7):e11472.
58. Lin CS, Sharpley MS, Fan W, Waymire KG, Sadun AA, Carelli V, et al. Mouse mtDNA mutant model of Leber hereditary optic neuropathy. Proc Natl Acad Sci U S A. 2012;109(49):20065–70.
59. Musardo S, Saraceno C, Pelucchi S, Marcello E. Trafficking in neurons: searching for new targets for Alzheimer's disease future therapies. Eur J Pharmacol. 2013;719(1–3):84–106.
60. Nogueras-Ortiz CJ, De Jesus-Cortes HJ, Vaquer-Alicea J, Vega IE. Novel autoimmune response in a tauopathy mouse model. Front Neurosci. 2014;7:277.
61. Ni R, Gillberg PG, Bergfors A, Marutle A, Nordberg A. Amyloid tracers detect multiple binding sites in Alzheimer's disease brain tissue. Brain J Neurol. 2013;136(Pt 7):2217–27.
62. Krantic S, Torriglia A. Retina: source of the earliest biomarkers for Alzheimer's disease? J Alzheimers Dis. 2014;40:237–43.
63. Novak P, Kontsekova E, Zilka N, Novak M. Ten years of tau-targeted immunotherapy: the path walked and the roads ahead. Front Neurosci. 2018;12:798.
64. Ning A, Cui J, To E, Ashe KH, Matsubara J. Amyloid-beta deposits lead to retinal degeneration in a mouse model of Alzheimer disease. Invest Ophthalmol Vis Sci. 2008;49(11):5136–43.
65. Perez SE, Lumayag S, Kovacs B, Mufson EJ, Xu S. Beta-amyloid deposition and functional impairment in the retina of the APPswe/PS1DeltaE9 transgenic mouse model of Alzheimer's disease. Invest Ophthalmol Vis Sci. 2009;50:793–800.
66. Koronyo-Hamaoui M, Koronyo Y, Ljubimov AV, Miller CA, Ko MK, Black KL, et al. Identification of amyloid plaques in retinas from Alzheimer's patients and noninvasive in vivo optical imaging of retinal plaques in a mouse model. NeuroImage. 2011;54(Suppl 1):S204–17.
67. de Lemos ML, de la Torre AV, Petrov D, Brox S, Folch J, Pallas M, et al. Evaluation of hypoxia inducible factor expression in inflammatory and neurodegenerative brain models. Int J Biochem Cell Biol. 2013;45(7):1377–88.
68. Duff K, Eckman C, Zehr C, Yu X, Prada CM, Perez-tur J, et al. Increased amyloid-beta42(43) in brains of mice expressing mutant presenilin 1. Nature. 1996;383(6602):710–3.

69. Simard AR, Soulet D, Gowing G, Julien JP, Rivest S. Bone marrow-derived microglia play a critical role in restricting senile plaque formation in Alzheimer's disease. Neuron. 2006;49(4):489–502.
70. Yao J, Taylor M, Davey F, Ren Y, Aiton J, Coote P, et al. Interaction of amyloid binding alcohol dehydrogenase/Abeta mediates up-regulation of peroxiredoxin II in the brains of Alzheimer's disease patients and a transgenic Alzheimer's disease mouse model. Mol Cell Neurosci. 2007;35(2):377–82.
71. Holcomb L, Gordon MN, McGowan E, Yu X, Benkovic S, Jantzen P, et al. Accelerated Alzheimer-type phenotype in transgenic mice carrying both mutant amyloid precursor protein and presenilin 1 transgenes. Nat Med. 1998;4(1):97–100.
72. Schuessel K, Schafer S, Bayer TA, Czech C, Pradier L, Muller-Spahn F, et al. Impaired Cu/Zn-SOD activity contributes to increased oxidative damage in APP transgenic mice. Neurobiol Dis. 2005;18(1):89–99.
73. Esposito L, Raber J, Kekonius L, Yan F, Yu GQ, Bien-Ly N, et al. Reduction in mitochondrial superoxide dismutase modulates Alzheimer's disease-like pathology and accelerates the onset of behavioral changes in human amyloid precursor protein transgenic mice. J Neurosci. 2006;26(19):5167–79.
74. Duyckaerts C, Potier MC, Delatour B. Alzheimer disease models and human neuropathology: similarities and differences. Acta Neuropathol. 2008;115(1):5–38.
75. Hutton M, Lewis J, Dickson D, Yen SH, McGowan E. Analysis of tauopathies with transgenic mice. Trends Mol Med. 2001;7(10):467–70.
76. Gotz J, Chen F, van Dorpe J, Nitsch RM. Formation of neurofibrillary tangles in P3011 tau transgenic mice induced by Abeta 42 fibrils. Science. 2001;293(5534):1491–5.
77. Higuchi M, Ishihara T, Zhang B, Hong M, Andreadis A, Trojanowski J, et al. Transgenic mouse model of tauopathies with glial pathology and nervous system degeneration. Neuron. 2002;35(3):433–46.
78. Lewis J, McGowan E, Rockwood J, Melrose H, Nacharaju P, Van Slegtenhorst M, et al. Neurofibrillary tangles, amyotrophy and progressive motor disturbance in mice expressing mutant (P301L) tau protein. Nat Genet. 2000;25(4):402–5.
79. Terwel D, Lasrado R, Snauwaert J, Vandeweert E, Van Haesendonck C, Borghgraef P, et al. Changed conformation of mutant Tau-P301L underlies the moribund tauopathy, absent in progressive, nonlethal axonopathy of Tau-4R/2N transgenic mice. J Biol Chem. 2005;280(5):3963–73.
80. Gotz J, Deters N, Doldissen A, Bokhari L, Ke Y, Wiesner A, et al. A decade of tau transgenic animal models and beyond. Brain Pathol. 2007;17(1):91–103.
81. Oakley H, Cole SL, Logan S, Maus E, Shao P, Craft J, et al. Intraneuronal beta-amyloid aggregates, neurodegeneration, and neuron loss in transgenic mice with five familial Alzheimer's disease mutations: potential factors in amyloid plaque formation. J Neurosci. 2006;26(40):10129–40.
82. Ohno M, Cole SL, Yasvoina M, Zhao J, Citron M, Berry R, et al. BACE1 gene deletion prevents neuron loss and memory deficits in 5XFAD APP/PS1 transgenic mice. Neurobiol Dis. 2007;26(1):134–45.
83. Jawhar S, Trawicka A, Jenneckens C, Bayer TA, Wirths O. Motor deficits, neuron loss, and reduced anxiety coinciding with axonal degeneration and intraneuronal Abeta aggregation in the 5XFAD mouse model of Alzheimer's disease. Neurobiol Aging. 2012;33(1):196 e29–40.
84. Criscuolo C, Cerri E, Fabiani C, Capsoni S, Cattaneo A, Domenici L. The retina as a window to early dysfunctions of Alzheimer's disease following studies with a 5xFAD mouse model. Neurobiol Aging. 2018;67:181–8.
85. LaFerla FM, Oddo S. Alzheimer's disease: Abeta, tau and synaptic dysfunction. Trends Mol Med. 2005;11(4):170–6.
86. Oddo S, Caccamo A, Shepherd JD, Murphy MP, Golde TE, Kayed R, et al. Triple-transgenic model of Alzheimer's disease with plaques and tangles: intracellular Abeta and synaptic dysfunction. Neuron. 2003;39(3):409–21.

87. Oddo S, Caccamo A, Kitazawa M, Tseng BP, LaFerla FM. Amyloid deposition precedes tangle formation in a triple transgenic model of Alzheimer's disease. Neurobiol Aging. 2003;24(8):1063–70.
88. Gimenez-Llort L, Blazquez G, Canete T, Johansson B, Oddo S, Tobena A, et al. Modeling behavioral and neuronal symptoms of Alzheimer's disease in mice: a role for intraneuronal amyloid. Neurosci Biobehav Rev. 2007;31(1):125–47.
89. Rissman RA, Poon WW, Blurton-Jones M, Oddo S, Torp R, Vitek MP, et al. Caspase-cleavage of tau is an early event in Alzheimer disease tangle pathology. J Clin Invest. 2004;114(1):121–30.
90. Oddo S, Billings L, Kesslak JP, Cribbs DH, LaFerla FM. Abeta immunotherapy leads to clearance of early, but not late, hyperphosphorylated tau aggregates via the proteasome. Neuron. 2004;43(3):321–32.
91. Oddo S, Caccamo A, Green KN, Liang K, Tran L, Chen Y, et al. Chronic nicotine administration exacerbates tau pathology in a transgenic model of Alzheimer's disease. Proc Natl Acad Sci U S A. 2005;102(8):3046–51.
92. Smith IF, Green KN, LaFerla FM. Calcium dysregulation in Alzheimer's disease: recent advances gained from genetically modified animals. Cell Calcium. 2005;38(3–4):427–37.
93. Billings LM, Oddo S, Green KN, McGaugh JL, LaFerla FM. Intraneuronal Abeta causes the onset of early Alzheimer's disease-related cognitive deficits in transgenic mice. Neuron. 2005;45(5):675–88.
94. Janelsins MC, Mastrangelo MA, Oddo S, LaFerla FM, Federoff HJ, Bowers WJ. Early correlation of microglial activation with enhanced tumor necrosis factor-alpha and monocyte chemoattractant protein-1 expression specifically within the entorhinal cortex of triple transgenic Alzheimer's disease mice. J Neuroinflammation. 2005;2:23.
95. Chiasseu M, Alarcon-Martinez L, Belforte N, Quintero H, Dotigny F, Destroismaisons L, et al. Tau accumulation in the retina promotes early neuronal dysfunction and precedes brain pathology in a mouse model of Alzheimer's disease. Mol Neurodegener. 2017;12(1):58.
96. Smith IF, Hitt B, Green KN, Oddo S, LaFerla FM. Enhanced caffeine-induced Ca2+ release in the 3xTg-AD mouse model of Alzheimer's disease. J Neurochem. 2005;94(6):1711–8.
97. Lee CW, Shih YH, Kuo YM. Cerebrovascular pathology and amyloid plaque formation in Alzheimer's disease. Curr Alzheimer Res. 2014;11(1):4–10.
98. Alexandrov PN, Pogue A, Bhattacharjee S, Lukiw WJ. Retinal amyloid peptides and complement factor H in transgenic models of Alzheimer's disease. Neuroreport. 2011;22(12):623–7.
99. Savini G, Barboni P, Carbonelli M, Hoffer KJ. Comparison of methods to measure corneal power for intraocular lens power calculation using a rotating Scheimpflug camera. J Cataract Refract Surg. 2013;39(4):598–604.
100. Worth PF. How to treat Parkinson's disease in 2013. Clin Med. 2013;13(1):93–6.
101. Martínez-Navarrete GC, Martín-Nieto J, Esteve-Rudd J, Angulo A, Cuenca N. Alpha synuclein gene expression profile in the retina of vertebrates. Mol Vis. 2007;13:949–61.
102. Brancato R, Pece A, Carassa R. Central retinal artery occlusion after local anesthesia for blepharoplasty. Graefes Arch Clin Exp Ophthalmol. 1991;229(6):593–4.
103. Gubellini P, Kachidian P. Animal models of Parkinson's disease: an updated overview. Rev Neurol. 2015;171:750–61.
104. Nicklas WJ, Vyas I, Heikkila RE. Inhibition of NADH-linked oxidation in brain mitochondria by 1-methyl-4-phenyl-pyridine, a metabolite of the neurotoxin, 1-methyl-4-phenyl-1,2,5,6-tetrahydropyridine. Life Sci. 1985;36(26):2503–8.
105. McNaught KS, Perl DP, Brownell AL, Olanow CW. Systemic exposure to proteasome inhibitors causes a progressive model of Parkinson's disease. Ann Neurol. 2004;56(1):149–62.
106. Bove J, Prou D, Perier C, Przedborski S. Toxin-induced models of Parkinson's disease. NeuroRx. 2005;2(3):484–94.
107. Blesa J, Phani S, Jackson-Lewis V, Przedborski S. Classic and new animal models of Parkinson's disease. J Biomed Biotechnol. 2012;2012:845618.

108. Manning-Bog AB, McCormack AL, Li J, Uversky VN, Fink AL, Di Monte DA. The herbicide paraquat causes up-regulation and aggregation of alpha-synuclein in mice: paraquat and alpha-synuclein. J Biol Chem. 2002;277(3):1641–4.
109. Freire C, Koifman S. Pesticide exposure and Parkinson's disease: epidemiological evidence of association. Neurotoxicology. 2012;33(5):947–71.
110. Annett LE, Torres EM, Clarke DJ, Ishida Y, Barker RA, Ridley RM, et al. Survival of nigral grafts within the striatum of marmosets with 6-OHDA lesions depends critically on donor embryo age. Cell Transplant. 1997;6(6):557–69.
111. Crofts HS, Dalley JW, Collins P, Van Denderen JC, Everitt BJ, Robbins TW, et al. Differential effects of 6-OHDA lesions of the frontal cortex and caudate nucleus on the ability to acquire an attentional set. Cereb Cortex. 2001;11(11):1015–26.
112. He Y, Appel S, Le W. Minocycline inhibits microglial activation and protects nigral cells after 6-hydroxydopamine injection into mouse striatum. Brain Res. 2001;909(1–2):187–93.
113. Ma KH, Huang WS, Chen CH, Lin SZ, Wey SP, Ting G, et al. Dual SPECT of dopamine system using [99mTc]TRODAT-1 and [123I]IBZM in normal and 6-OHDA-lesioned formosan rock monkeys. Nucl Med Biol. 2002;29(5):561–7.
114. Lundblad M, Picconi B, Lindgren H, Cenci MA. A model of L-DOPA-induced dyskinesia in 6-hydroxydopamine lesioned mice: relation to motor and cellular parameters of nigrostriatal function. Neurobiol Dis. 2004;16(1):110–23.
115. Allen JM, Cross AJ, Crow TJ, Javoy-Agid F, Agid Y, Bloom SR. Dissociation of neuropeptide Y and somatostatin in Parkinson's disease. Brain Res. 1985;337(1):197–200.
116. Seniuk NA, Tatton WG, Greenwood CE. Dose-dependent destruction of the coeruleus-cortical and nigral-striatal projections by MPTP. Brain Res. 1990;527(1):7–20.
117. Sirinathsinghji DJ, Kupsch A, Mayer E, Zivin M, Pufal D, Oertel WH. Cellular localization of tyrosine hydroxylase mRNA and cholecystokinin mRNA-containing cells in the ventral mesencephalon of the common marmoset: effects of 1-methyl-4-phenyl-1,2,3,6-tetrahydropyridine. Brain Res Mol Brain Res. 1992;12(1–3):267–74.
118. Ovadia A, Zhang Z, Gash DM. Increased susceptibility to MPTP toxicity in middle-aged rhesus monkeys. Neurobiol Aging. 1995;16(6):931–7.
119. Blandini F, Armentero MT. Animal models of Parkinson's disease. FEBS J. 2012;279(7):1156–66.
120. Corti O, Lesage S, Brice A. What genetics tells us about the causes and mechanisms of Parkinson's disease. Physiol Rev. 2011;91(4):1161–218.
121. Lindgren HS, Lelos MJ, Dunnett SB. Do alpha-synuclein vector injections provide a better model of Parkinson's disease than the classic 6-hydroxydopamine model? Exp Neurol. 2012;237(1):36–42.
122. Recchia A, Debetto P, Negro A, Guidolin D, Skaper SD, Giusti P. Alpha-synuclein and Parkinson's disease. FASEB J. 2004;18(6):617–26.
123. Betarbet R, Sherer TB, MacKenzie G, Garcia-Osuna M, Panov AV, Greenamyre JT. Chronic systemic pesticide exposure reproduces features of Parkinson's disease. Nat Neurosci. 2000;3(12):1301–6.
124. Marking LL. Oral toxicity of rotenone to mammals, Investigations in fish control. Washington: U.S. Fish and Wildlife Service; 1988.
125. Mastroberardino PG, Hoffman EK, Horowitz MP, Betarbet R, Taylor G, Cheng D, et al. A novel transferrin/TfR2-mediated mitochondrial iron transport system is disrupted in Parkinson's disease. Neurobiol Dis. 2009;34(3):417–31.
126. Lapointe N, St-Hilaire M, Martinoli MG, Blanchet J, Gould P, Rouillard C, et al. Rotenone induces non-specific central nervous system and systemic toxicity. FASEB J. 2004;18(6):717–9.
127. Drolet RE, Cannon JR, Montero L, Greenamyre JT. Chronic rotenone exposure reproduces Parkinson's disease gastrointestinal neuropathology. Neurobiol Dis. 2009;36(1):96–102.
128. Houlden H, Singleton AB. The genetics and neuropathology of Parkinson's disease. Acta Neuropathol. 2012;124(3):325–38.

129. Gasser T. Molecular genetic findings in LRRK2 American, Canadian and German families. J Neural Transm Suppl. 2006;70:231–4.
130. Farrer MJ. Genetics of Parkinson disease: paradigm shifts and future prospects. Nat Rev Genet. 2006;7(4):306–18.
131. Zheng LF, Wang ZY, Li XF, Song J, Hong F, Lian H, et al. Reduced expression of choline acetyltransferase in vagal motoneurons and gastric motor dysfunction in a 6-OHDA rat model of Parkinson's disease. Brain Res. 2011;1420:59–67.
132. Javoy F, Sotelo C, Herbet A, Agid Y. Specificity of dopaminergic neuronal degeneration induced by intracerebral injection of 6-hydroxydopamine in the nigrostriatal dopamine system. Brain Res. 1976;102(2):201–15.
133. Jeon BS, Jackson-Lewis V, Burke RE. 6-Hydroxydopamine lesion of the rat substantia nigra: time course and morphology of cell death. Neurodegeneration. 1995;4(2):131–7.
134. Faull RL, Laverty R. Changes in dopamine levels in the corpus striatum following lesions in the substantia nigra. Exp Neurol. 1969;23(3):332–40.
135. Lao CL, Kuo YH, Hsieh YT, Chen JC. Intranasal and subcutaneous administration of dopamine D3 receptor agonists functionally restores nigrostriatal dopamine in MPTP-treated mice. Neurotox Res. 2013;24(4):523–31.
136. Kim JI, Yang EJ, Lee MS, Kim YS, Huh Y, Cho IH, et al. Bee venom reduces neuroinflammation in the MPTP-induced model of Parkinson's disease. Int J Neurosci. 2011;121(4):209–17.
137. Liu K, Shi N, Sun Y, Zhang T, Sun X. Therapeutic effects of rapamycin on MPTP-induced parkinsonism in mice. Neurochem Res. 2013;38(1):201–7.
138. Yabuki Y, Ohizumi Y, Yokosuka A, Mimaki Y, Fukunaga K. Nobiletin treatment improves motor and cognitive deficits seen in MPTP-induced Parkinson model mice. Neuroscience. 2013;259C:126–41.
139. Masilamoni GJ, Bogenpohl JW, Alagille D, Delevich K, Tamagnan G, Votaw JR, et al. Metabotropic glutamate receptor 5 antagonist protects dopaminergic and noradrenergic neurons from degeneration in MPTP-treated monkeys. Brain. 2011;134(Pt 7):2057–73.
140. Xun Z, Sowell RA, Kaufman TC, Clemmer DE. Quantitative proteomics of a presymptomatic A53T alpha-synuclein drosophila model of Parkinson disease. Mol Cell Proteomics. 2008;7(7):1191–203.
141. Recchia A, Rota D, Debetto P, Peroni D, Guidolin D, Negro A, et al. Generation of a alpha-synuclein-based rat model of Parkinson's disease. Neurobiol Dis. 2008;30(1):8–18.
142. Betarbet R, Sherer TB, Greenamyre JT. Animal models of Parkinson's disease. BioEssays. 2002;24(4):308–18.
143. Schober A. Classic toxin-induced animal models of Parkinson's disease: 6-OHDA and MPTP. Cell Tissue Res. 2004;318(1):215–24.
144. Schuler F, Casida JE. Functional coupling of PSST and ND1 subunits in NADH:ubiquinone oxidoreductase established by photoaffinity labeling. Biochim Biophys Acta. 2001;1506(1):79–87.
145. Prance G. The poisons and narcotics of the Amazonian Indians. J R Coll Physicians Lond. 1999;33(4):368–76.
146. Talpade DJ, Greene JG, Higgins DS Jr, Greenamyre JT. In vivo labeling of mitochondrial complex I (NADH:ubiquinone oxidoreductase) in rat brain using [(3)H]dihydrorotenone. J Neurochem. 2000;75(6):2611–21.
147. Alam M, Schmidt WJ. Rotenone destroys dopaminergic neurons and induces parkinsonian symptoms in rats. Behav Brain Res. 2002;136(1):317–24.
148. Sherer TB, Betarbet R, Testa CM, Seo BB, Richardson JR, Kim JH, et al. Mechanism of toxicity in rotenone models of Parkinson's disease. J Neurosci. 2003;23(34):10756–64.
149. Alam ZI, Jenner A, Daniel SE, Lees AJ, Cairns N, Marsden CD, et al. Oxidative DNA damage in the parkinsonian brain: an apparent selective increase in 8-hydroxyguanine levels in substantia nigra. J Neurochem. 1997;69(3):1196–203.
150. Floor E, Wetzel MG. Increased protein oxidation in human substantia nigra pars compacta in comparison with basal ganglia and prefrontal cortex measured with an improved dinitrophenylhydrazine assay. J Neurochem. 1998;70(1):268–75.

151. Tada-Oikawa S, Hiraku Y, Kawanishi M, Kawanishi S. Mechanism for generation of hydrogen peroxide and change of mitochondrial membrane potential during rotenone-induced apoptosis. Life Sci. 2003;73(25):3277–88.
152. Beal MF. Mitochondria, oxidative damage, and inflammation in Parkinson's disease. Ann N Y Acad Sci. 2003;991:120–31.
153. Aguilar-Bryan L, Clement JP, Gonzalez G, Kunjilwar K, Babenko A, Bryan J. Toward understanding the assembly and structure of KATP channels. Physiol Rev. 1998;78(1):227–45.
154. Liss B, Bruns R, Roeper J. Alternative sulfonylurea receptor expression defines metabolic sensitivity of K-ATP channels in dopaminergic midbrain neurons. EMBO J. 1999;18(4):833–46.
155. Stokes AH, Hastings TG, Vrana KE. Cytotoxic and genotoxic potential of dopamine. J Neurosci Res. 1999;55(6):659–65.
156. Spector S, Sjoerdsma A, Udenfriend S. Blockade of endogenous norepinephrine synthesis by alpha-methyl-tyrosine, an inhibitor of tyrosine hydroxylase. J Pharmacol Exp Ther. 1965;147:86–95.
157. Sakka N, Sawada H, Izumi Y, Kume T, Katsuki H, Kaneko S, et al. Dopamine is involved in selectivity of dopaminergic neuronal death by rotenone. Neuroreport. 2003;14(18):2425–8.
158. Biehlmaier O, Alam M, Schmidt WJ. A rat model of parkinsonism shows depletion of dopamine in the retina. Neurochem Int. 2007;50(1):189–95.
159. Marey-Semper I, Gelman M, Levi-Strauss M. A selective toxicity toward cultured mesencephalic dopaminergic neurons is induced by the synergistic effects of energetic metabolism impairment and NMDA receptor activation. J Neurosci Off J Soc Neurosci. 1995;15(9):5912–8.
160. Huang J, Liu H, Gu W, Yan Z, Xu Z, Yang Y, et al. A delivery strategy for rotenone microspheres in an animal model of Parkinson's disease. Biomaterials. 2006;27(6):937–46.
161. Feng Y, Liang ZH, Wang T, Qiao X, Liu HJ, Sun SG. alpha-Synuclein redistributed and aggregated in rotenone-induced Parkinson's disease rats. Neurosci Bull. 2006;22(5):288–93.
162. Xiong N, Huang J, Zhang Z, Zhang Z, Xiong J, Liu X, et al. Stereotaxical infusion of rotenone: a reliable rodent model for Parkinson's disease. PLoS One. 2009;4(11):e7878.
163. Xiong N, Long X, Xiong J, Jia M, Chen C, Huang J, et al. Mitochondrial complex I inhibitor rotenone-induced toxicity and its potential mechanisms in Parkinson's disease models. Crit Rev Toxicol. 2012;42(7):613–32.
164. Testa CM, Sherer TB, Greenamyre JT. Rotenone induces oxidative stress and dopaminergic neuron damage in organotypic substantia nigra cultures. Brain Res Mol Brain Res. 2005;134(1):109–18.
165. Isenberg JS, Klaunig JE. Role of the mitochondrial membrane permeability transition (MPT) in rotenone-induced apoptosis in liver cells. Toxicol Sci. 2000;53(2):340–51.
166. Heikkila RE, Nicklas WJ, Vyas I, Duvoisin RC. Dopaminergic toxicity of rotenone and the 1-methyl-4-phenylpyridinium ion after their stereotaxic administration to rats: implication for the mechanism of 1-methyl-4-phenyl-1,2,3,6-tetrahydropyridine toxicity. Neurosci Lett. 1985;62(3):389–94.
167. Schmidt WJ, Alam M. Controversies on new animal models of Parkinson's disease pro and con: the rotenone model of Parkinson's disease (PD). J Neural Transm Suppl. 2006;70:273–6.
168. Hu LF, Lu M, Tiong CX, Dawe GS, Hu G, Bian JS. Neuroprotective effects of hydrogen sulfide on Parkinson's disease rat models. Aging Cell. 2010;9(2):135–46.
169. Pan-Montojo F, Anichtchik O, Dening Y, Knels L, Pursche S, Jung R, et al. Progression of Parkinson's disease pathology is reproduced by intragastric administration of rotenone in mice. PLoS One. 2010;5(1):e8762.
170. Alam M, Schmidt WJ. L-DOPA reverses the hypokinetic behaviour and rigidity in rotenone-treated rats. Behav Brain Res. 2004;153(2):439–46.
171. Alam M, Mayerhofer A, Schmidt WJ. The neurobehavioral changes induced by bilateral rotenone lesion in medial forebrain bundle of rats are reversed by L-DOPA. Behav Brain Res. 2004;151(1–2):117–24.

172. Kamalden TA, Ji D, Osborne NN. Rotenone-induced death of RGC-5 cells is caspase independent, involves the JNK and p38 pathways and is attenuated by specific green tea flavonoids. Neurochem Res. 2012;37(5):1091–101.
173. Hancock DB, Martin ER, Mayhew GM, Stajich JM, Jewett R, Stacy MA, et al. Pesticide exposure and risk of Parkinson's disease: a family-based case-control study. BMC Neurol. 2008;8:6.
174. Dhillon AS, Tarbutton GL, Levin JL, Plotkin GM, Lowry LK, Nalbone JT, et al. Pesticide/environmental exposures and Parkinson's disease in East Texas. J Agromedicine. 2008;13(1):37–48.
175. Polymeropoulos MH, Lavedan C, Leroy E, Ide SE, Dehejia A, Dutra A, Pike B, Root H, Rubenstein J, Boyer R, Stenroos ES, Chandrasekharappa S, Athanassiadou A, Papapetropoulos T, Johnson WG, Lazzarini AM, Duvoisin RC, Di Iorio G, Golbe LI, Nussbaum RL. Mutation in the α-synuclein gene identified in families with Parkinson's disease. Science. 1997;276(5321):2045–7.
176. Kitada T, Asakawa S, Hattori N, Matsumine H, Yamamura Y, Minoshima S, Yokochi M, Mizuno Y, Shimizu N. Mutations in the parkin gene cause autosomal recessive juvenile parkinsonism. Nature. 1998;392(6676):605–8.
177. Gasser T, Müller-Myhsok B, Wszolek ZK, Oehlmann R, Calne DB, Bonifati V, Bereznai B, Fabrizio E, Vieregge P, Horstmann RD. A susceptibility locus for Parkinson's disease maps to chromosome 2p13. Nat Genet. 1998;18(3):262–5.
178. Singleton AB, Farrer M, Johnson J, Singleton A, Hague S, Kachergus J, Hulihan M, Peuralinna T, Dutra A, Nussbaum R, Lincoln S, Crawley A, Hanson M, Maraganore D, Adler C, Cookson MR, Muenter M, Baptista M, Miller D, Blancato J, Hardy J, Gwinn-Hardy K. Alpha-synuclein locus triplication causes Parkinson's disease. Science. 2003;302(5646):841.
179. Leroy E, Boyer R, Auburger G, Leube B, Ulm G, Mezey E, Harta G, Brownstein MJ, Jonnalagada S, Chernova T, Dehejia A, Lavedan C, Gasser T, Steinbach PJ, Wilkinson KD, Polymeropoulos MH. The ubiquitin pathway in Parkinson's disease. Nature. 1998;395(6701):451–2.
180. Valente EM, Bentivoglio AR, Dixon PH, Ferraris A, Ialongo T, Frontali M, Albanese A, Wood NW. Localization of a novel locus for autosomal recessive early-onset parkinsonism, PARK6, on human chromosome 1p35-p36. Am J Hum Genet. 2001;68(4):895–900.
181. Bonifati V, Rizzu P, van Baren MJ, Schaap O, Breedveld GJ, Krieger E, Dekker MC, Squitieri F, Ibanez P, Joosse M, van Dongen JW, Vanacore N, van Swieten JC, Brice A, Meco G, van Duijn CM, Oostra BA, Heutink P. Mutations in the DJ-1 gene associated with autosomal recessive early-onset parkinsonism. Science. 2003;299(5604):256–9.
182. Funayama M, Hasegawa K, Kowa H, Saito M, Tsuji S, Obata F. A new locus for Parkinson's disease (PARK8) maps to chromosome 12p11.2-q13.1. Ann Neurol. 2002;51(3):296–301.
183. Bonifati V, Rohé CF, Breedveld GJ, Fabrizio E, De Mari M, Tassorelli C, Tavella A, Marconi R, Nicholl DJ, Chien HF, Fincati E, Abbruzzese G, Marini P, De Gaetano A, Horstink MW, Maat-Kievit JA, Sampaio C, Antonini A, Stocchi F, Montagna P, Toni V, Guidi M, Dalla Libera A, Tinazzi M, De Pandis F, Fabbrini G, Goldwurm S, de Klein A, Barbosa E, Lopiano L, Martignoni E, Lamberti P, Vanacore N, Meco G, Oostra BA, Italian Parkinson Genetics Network. Early-onset parkinsonism associated with PINK1 mutations: frequency, genotypes, and phenotypes. Neurology. 2005;65(1):87–95.
184. Hampshire DJ, Roberts E, Crow Y, Bond J, Mubaidin A, Wriekat AL, Al-Din A, Woods CG. Kufor-Rakeb syndrome, pallido-pyramidal degeneration with supranuclear upgaze paresis and dementia, maps to 1p36. J Med Genet. 2001;38(10):680–2.
185. Chan SL, Angeles DC, Tan EK. Targeting leucine-rich repeat kinase 2 in Parkinson's disease. Expert Opin Ther Targets. 2013;17(12):1471–82.
186. Lesage S, Brice A. Parkinson's disease: from monogenic forms to genetic susceptibility factors. Hum Mol Genet. 2009;18(R1):R48–59.

187. Peeraully T, Tan EK. Genetic variants in sporadic Parkinson's disease: East vs West. Parkinsonism Relat Disord. 2012;18(Suppl 1):S63–5.
188. Mamais A, Raja M, Manzoni C, Dihanich S, Lees A, Moore D, et al. Divergent alpha-synuclein solubility and aggregation properties in G2019S LRRK2 Parkinson's disease brains with Lewy Body pathology compared to idiopathic cases. Neurobiol Dis. 2013;58:183–90.
189. Healy DG, Falchi M, O'Sullivan SS, Bonifati V, Durr A, Bressman S, et al. Phenotype, genotype, and worldwide genetic penetrance of LRRK2-associated Parkinson's disease: a case-control study. Lancet Neurol. 2008;7(7):583–90.
190. La Morgia C, Barboni P, Rizzo G, Carbonelli M, Savini G, Scaglione C, et al. Loss of temporal retinal nerve fibers in Parkinson disease: a mitochondrial pattern? Eur J Neurol. 2013;20(1):198–201.
191. Satue M, Garcia-Martin E, Fuertes I, Otin S, Alarcia R, Herrero R, et al. Use of Fourier-domain OCT to detect retinal nerve fiber layer degeneration in Parkinson's disease patients. Eye. 2013;27(4):507–14.
192. Hindle SJ, Elliott CJ. Spread of neuronal degeneration in a dopaminergic, Lrrk-G2019S model of Parkinson disease. Autophagy. 2013;9(6):936–8.

OCT in Glaucoma

20

Harsha Rao, Kaweh Mansouri, and Robert Weinreb

20.1 Introduction

Glaucoma is a chronic optic neuropathy characterised by progressive loss of retinal ganglion cells (RGCs) [1]. It is the leading cause of irreversible blindness in the world. A recent systematic review and meta-analysis estimated that the number of people aged between 40 and 80 years with glaucoma worldwide was 64.3 million, and that it would increase to 76.0 million in 2020 and 111.8 million in 2040 [2]. Another recent meta-analysis reported that the number of people blind due to glaucoma worldwide was 2.1 million and those visually impaired due to glaucoma was 4.2 million [3]. The meta-analysis also reported that between 1990 and 2010, the number of people blind due to glaucoma increased by 0.8 million or 62% and those visually impaired increased by 2.3 million or 83%, respectively [3]. As the loss of RGCs in glaucoma is irreversible, early detection of the disease is of utmost importance because appropriate treatment can prevent or slow disease progression and therefore, preserve vision.

Glaucoma is characterised by typical optic nerve head (ONH) and retinal nerve fiber layer (RNFL) changes with or without the presence of correlating visual field (VF) loss. Detection of VF loss by means of standard automated perimetry (SAP) has been one of the mainstays in the diagnosis and monitoring of glaucoma. However, the subjective nature of perimetry creates large variability in results, which make it difficult to reliably assess and monitor the disease. Structural

H. Rao
Narayana Nethralaya, Bengaluru, India

K. Mansouri
Glaucoma Center, Montchoisi Clinic, Swiss Vision Network, Lausanne, Switzerland

R. Weinreb (✉)
Shiley Eye Institute, Hamilton Glaucoma Center, and Viterbi Family Department of Ophthalmology, University of California, San Diego, La Jolla, CA, USA
e-mail: rweinreb@ucsd.edu

A. Grzybowski, P. Barboni (eds.), *OCT and Imaging in Central Nervous System Diseases*, https://doi.org/10.1007/978-3-030-26269-3_20

changes in the ONH and RNFL often are visible before the appearance of detectable loss by SAP [4, 5]. The ability to detect structural loss at the level of the ONH and peripapillary RNFL is, therefore, fundamental in the diagnosis and management of glaucoma. Clinical examination of the ONH and RNFL is routinely done on a slit-lamp biomicroscope using a high powered convex lens. Although detecting glaucoma by this method is fairly simple in moderate and severe stages of the disease, identification of subtle ONH and RNFL changes in early glaucoma requires training and experience. Another method of detecting glaucoma is the evaluation of optic disc stereo-photographs. Both these methods, however, are subjective, and the agreement even among experts in detecting glaucomatous changes either clinically or on disc photographs is far from excellent [6, 7]. The other major drawback of these methods is that changes can only be qualitatively assessed but cannot be quantified. These limitations are overcome by optical coherence tomography (OCT) imaging of ONH and RNFL. OCT provides objective assessment of structural changes in glaucoma by reproducibly quantifying the changes in ONH and RNFL.

OCT technology has evolved from time-domain (TD-) to spectral-domain technology (SD-OCT) which is faster and provides greater resolution (axial resolution of 5 μm). As a result of improved resolution, it is now possible to evaluate each layer of the retina separately using SD-OCT. This has led to a renewed interest in evaluating the macular changes in glaucoma [8]. Macula contains approximately 50% of all RGCs. RGC layer in the macula contains seven layers of RGC bodies in contrast to the peripheral retina where the RGC layer is only one cell thick [9]. Therefore, evaluation of macula, especially the inner retinal layers (ganglion cell layer and the inner plexiform layer), along with ONH and RNFL, has gained importance in glaucoma.

Current OCT devices evaluate the ONH, peripapillary RNFL as well as the macula using cube scans for assessing the amount of structural damage in glaucoma. Below is a description of the way ONH, RNFL and macular analysis is performed by different OCT devices.

20.2 ONH Analysis of OCT

Glaucoma is a disease that primarily affects the RGCs and their axons, which travel through the ONH into the optic nerve. Loss of RGCs and their axons, therefore show typical features on the ONH, such as increased cup-to-disc ratio, thinning of the neuroretinal rim (NRR) and NRR notching. Clinical characteristics such as NRR thinning and increased optic disc cupping differentiate glaucoma from other optic neuropathies [10].

ONH analysis with OCT is performed by automated software. Different manufacturers of OCT devices have their own proprietary softwares for ONH analysis, which vary slightly from each other. A brief description of the automated ONH analysis performed in commonly used OCT devices is important to understand the differences between the reported measurements.

The software of one OCT device identifies the termination of Bruch's membrane as the disc margin from the 3-dimensional data set. The software then generates a set of vectors from the disc margin to points on the vitreoretinal interface for each radial direction and calculates a trapezoidal, cross-sectional area associated with each vector. For each point on the disc margin, the vector that produces the minimum cross-sectional area is identified and each of these vectors is geometrically transformed into the plane of the optic disc to provide a 2-D representation of the 3-D data acquired by the imaging software. In this manner, the cup margin is defined by a set of optimal vectors and the neuro-retinal rim area is calculated as a piecewise sum of the corresponding minimum trapezoidal, cross-sectional areas. One of the difficulties in clinical assessment of the ONH is when the viewing angle of the ophthalmologist is not the same as the ONH axis, for example in tilted discs, where the neuro-retinal rim appears foreshortened. The 2-D representation of the ONH provided is as though the viewing angle is parallel to the ONH axis which minimizes the problem of foreshortening (Fig. 20.1) [11].

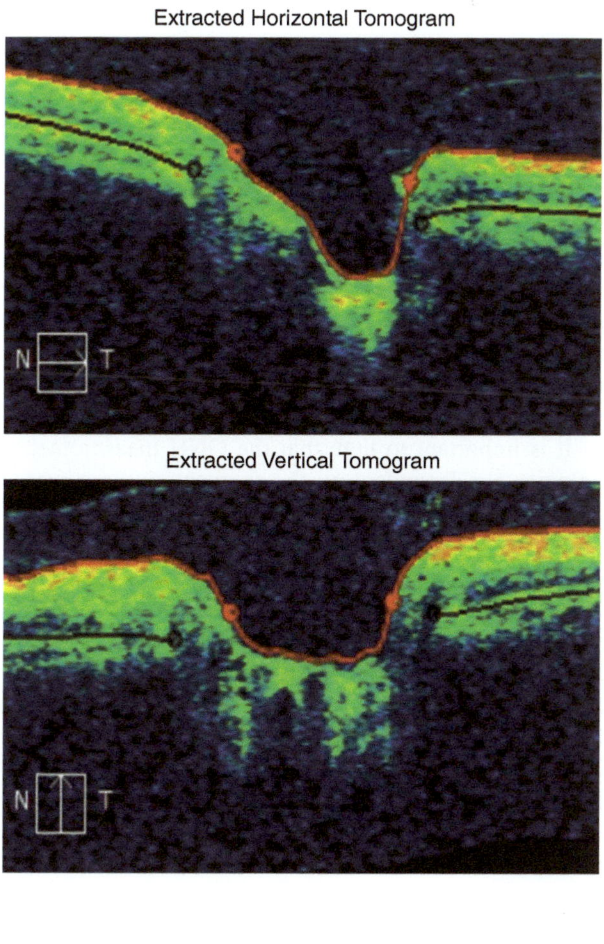

Fig. 20.1 Automated segmentation of the optic nerve head on an OCT device. Open black circles represent the termination of Bruch's membrane and the red circles represent the demarcation between neuroretinal rim and cup

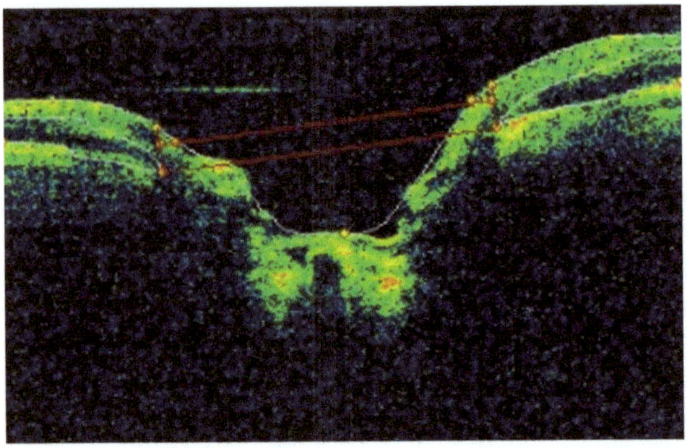

Fig. 20.2 Automated segmentation of the optic nerve head with another OCT software. The lower red straight line represents the line connecting the retinal pigment epithelium (RPE) tips and another red line is drawn 150 μm above and parallel to this plane. The optic nerve head tissue above the upper red line (between the 3 yellow colored circles) is defined as the neuroretinal rim tissue (source: Optovue.com)

The software of another OCT device detects the retinal pigment epithelium (RPE) tips automatically and then delineates the optic disc margin by joining the RPE tips. The optic cup is defined by fitting a plane 150 μm parallel to and above the plane that fit the coordinates of the RPE tips. ONH tissue above the cup line and within the perpendicular lines drawn from the RPE tips to the surface of the retina is considered as the neuroretinal rim (Fig. 20.2).

The software of yet another OCT device identifies the termination of the Bruch's membrane and delineates the Bruch's membrane opening (BMO) which acts as a surrogate for the disc margin. It subsequently calculates a parameter called minimum rim width (MRW) which is the minimum distance between the BMO line and the surface of the rim tissue (Fig. 20.3).

It is important to note that the ONH measurements of different imaging technologies are dependent on the segmentation performed by the propriety software and are not necessarily interchangeable with each other.

20.3 Peripapillary RNFL Analysis of OCT

RNFL contains the axons of the RGCs and the loss of the axons in glaucoma manifests as RNFL thinning and wedge shaped RNFL defects around the ONH (peripapillary region). Like for the ONH, different manufacturers of OCT devices have their own proprietary automated softwares for segmenting the peripapillary RNFL and measuring its thickness. Softwares of most OCT devices measure the RNFL thickness along a circle 3.46/3.45 mm in diameter positioned evenly around the center of the optic disc (Figs. 20.4 and 20.5). Software of another OCT device uses

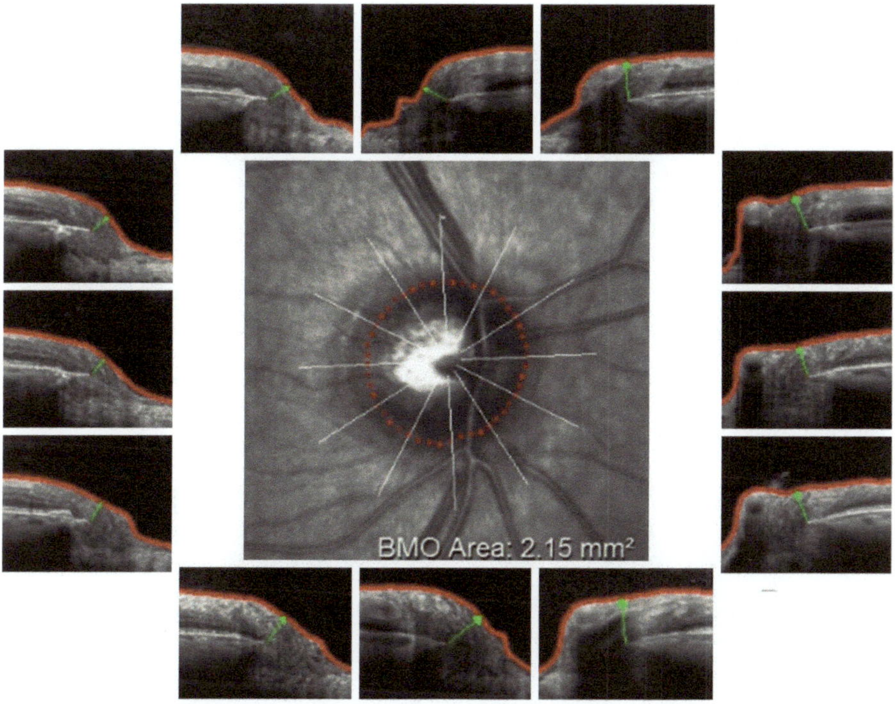

Fig. 20.3 The software of another OCT device identifies the termination of Bruch's membrane (Bruch's membrane opening, BMO) as the disc margin. The green lines represent the minimum rim width (MRW) which is the shortest distance between the BMO and the surface of the rim tissue at various locations

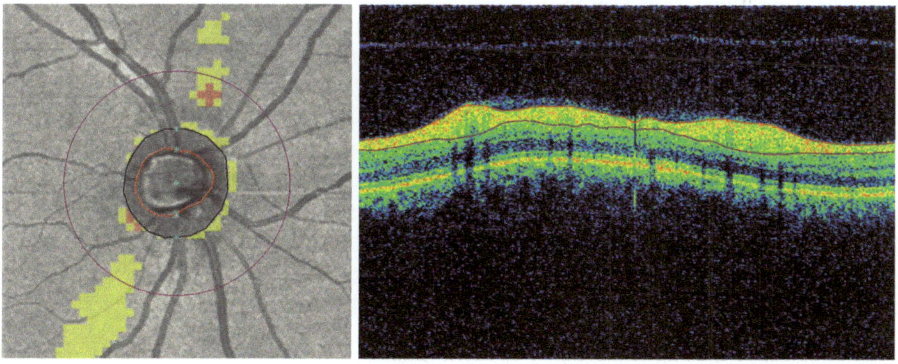

Fig. 20.4 Left image shows the circle scan (in purple color) along which peripapillary retinal nerve fiber layer (RNFL) thickness is measured on an OCT device. Right image shows the segmentation of RNFL; red line marks the internal limiting membrane and purple line marks the lower border of the RNFL

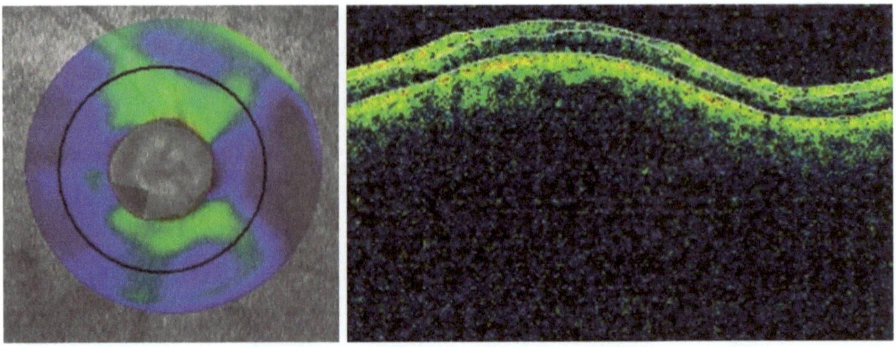

Fig. 20.5 Left image shows the circle scan along which retinal nerve fiber layer (RNFL) thickness is measured on a different OCT device. Right image shows the segmentation of RNFL displayed by the upper two white lines on the B scan image (source: Optovue.com)

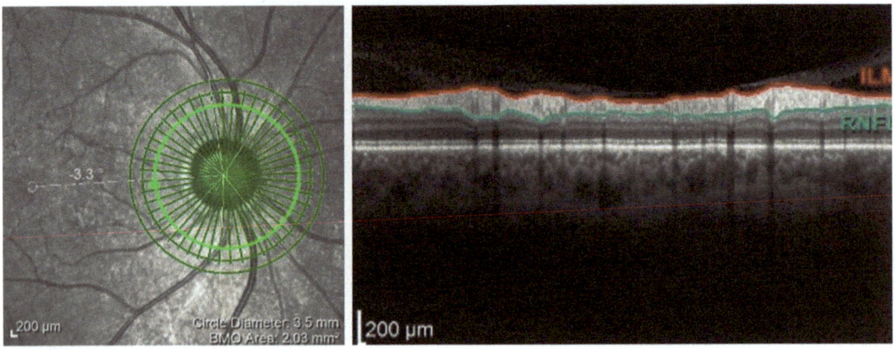

Fig. 20.6 Left image shows the circle scans (green) along which retinal nerve fiber layer (RNFL) thickness is measured on another OCT device. FoDi (fovea to disc) alignment technology (blue line) is used here to overcome the effect of eye rotation and head tilt on RNFL measurements and to match with alignment of the normative database. Right image shows the segmentation of RNFL; red line marks the internal limiting membrane and blue line marks the lower border of the RNFL

Fovea-to-Disc alignment technology that automatically tracks and aligns circle scans of 3.45 mm diameter to overcome measurement errors due to changing head and/or eye position during scanning (Fig. 20.6). This alignment technology improves the reproducibility of RNFL measurements.

Studies have shown that the RNFL thickness values vary between different SD-OCT devices and cannot be used interchangeably [12, 13].

20.4 Macular Analysis of OCT

Macula contains the greatest density of RGCs and therefore, loss of RGCs result in thinning of the inner retinal layers at the macula. Thinning of inner retinal layers at the macula, however, cannot be assessed either clinically using slit-lamp biomicroscope or on fundus photographs. This macular information provided by OCT therefore is unique.

Different manufacturers of OCT devices have different proprietary automated software for segmenting the inner retinal layers and measuring their thicknesses at the macula (which roughly is a region 8° in radius from the center of the fovea). Software of one OCT device measures the GCL and IPL thickness together as ganglion cell-inner plexiform layer (GCIPL) thickness (Fig. 20.7) while another measures the RNFL and GCIPL thickness together as ganglion cell complex (GCC, Fig. 20.8). Another device measures the thicknesses of each retinal layer separately (Fig. 20.9).

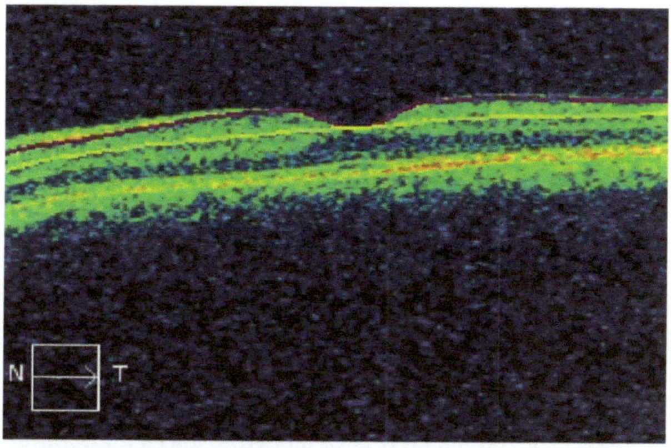

Fig. 20.7 Macular imaging of an OCT device which evaluates ganglion cell layer and inner plexiform layer together as ganglion cell-inner plexiform layer (GCIPL) thickness. Purple and yellow lines demonstrate the segmentation of GCIPL

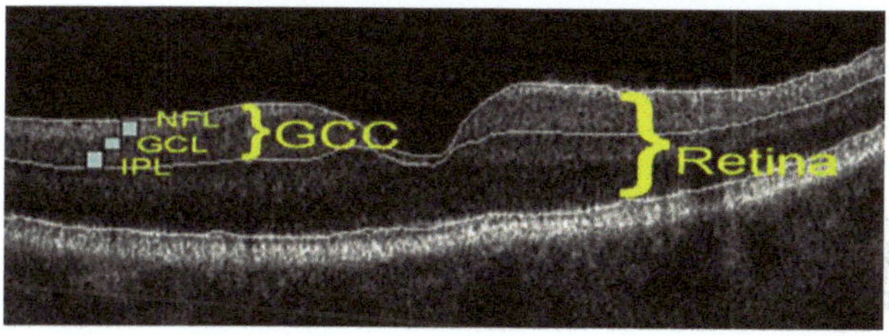

Fig. 20.8 Macular imaging of an OCT device which evaluates retinal nerve fiber layer, ganglion cell layer and inner plexiform layer together as ganglion cell complex (GCC) thickness. The two white lines on the top demonstrate the segmentation of GCC (source: Optovue.com)

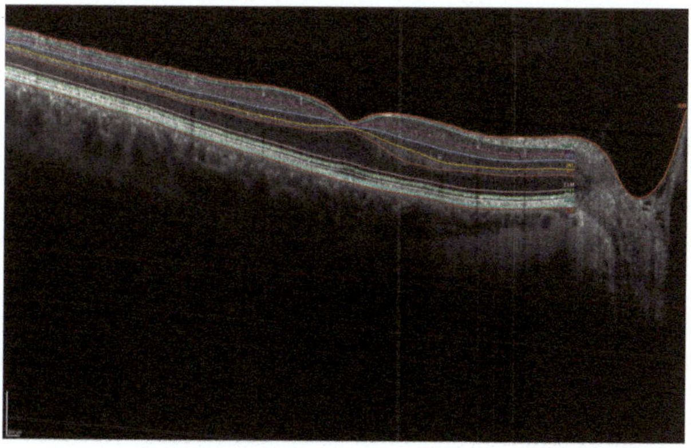

Fig. 20.9 Macular imaging from an OCT device which segments each layer of the retina and measures the thickness of each layer of retina separately (source: Heidelberg Engineering)

20.5 Interpreting the ONH, RNFL and Macular Measurements of OCT in Normal and Glaucoma Eyes

Once the ONH, RNFL and macular scans are acquired and segmentation performed, the software of the OCT calculates certain parameters. All these measurements are then compared with an age-matched reference database within the device to quantify glaucomatous damage and are interpreted either as "within normal limits (color-coded as green)" or "borderline (coded as yellow)" or "outside normal limits (coded as red)". The parameter is coded in green if the subject's measurement falls between the 5th and the 95th percentile values of the reference database ($p > 5\%$). The parameter is flagged in yellow if the measurement falls between the 5th and the 1st percentile values ($p < 5\%$ and $p > 1\%$) and "red" if the measurement falls below the lowest 1 percentile value ($p < 1\%$) of the reference database.

Figure 20.10 shows the ONH and RNFL report of a normal and a glaucomatous eye and Fig. 20.11 shows the macular (GCIPL) analysis report of a normal (Fig. 20.11a) and a glaucoma (Fig. 20.11b) patient from a commercially available OCT device. Figure 20.12 shows the results of ONH, RNFL and macular imaging from another OCT device in a normal subject (Fig. 20.12a) and a glaucoma patient (Fig. 20.12b). Figures 20.13, 20.14 and 20.15 show the ONH, RNFL and macular analysis report respectively of a normal and a glaucomatous patient from yet another OCT device.

Most of these reports show (1) a thickness map: in which RNFL/macular thickness measurements are represented in pseudocolors (hot colors such as red and orange represent thicker, and cool colors such as green and blue represent thinner measurements), (2) deviation and sector/clock-hour maps: in which the RNFL/macular thickness is compared with the reference database and coded either as green, yellow or red as described previously.

RNFL/macular thickness map is reported to be better than the deviation and the clock hour map to detect structural abnormalities in early glaucoma [14, 15]. Deviation and clock hour maps rely on the reference database to classify a measurement as normal, suspect or outside normal limits. The reference database has strict inclusion criteria and because of the wide range of "normal", significant reduction of the structural measurements is required before a measurement is labelled as outside normal limits of the reference database.

20.6 Role of OCT in Diagnosing Glaucoma

Multiple studies have evaluated the ability of OCT in diagnosing glaucoma. A Cochrane review of these studies found the ONH and RNFL measurements to have excellent abilities to diagnose glaucoma [16]. In clinical practice, OCT imaging has been found to be especially useful in eyes with suspicious optic discs and normal VF. Figure 20.16 shows an eye with a glaucomatous optic disc (showing

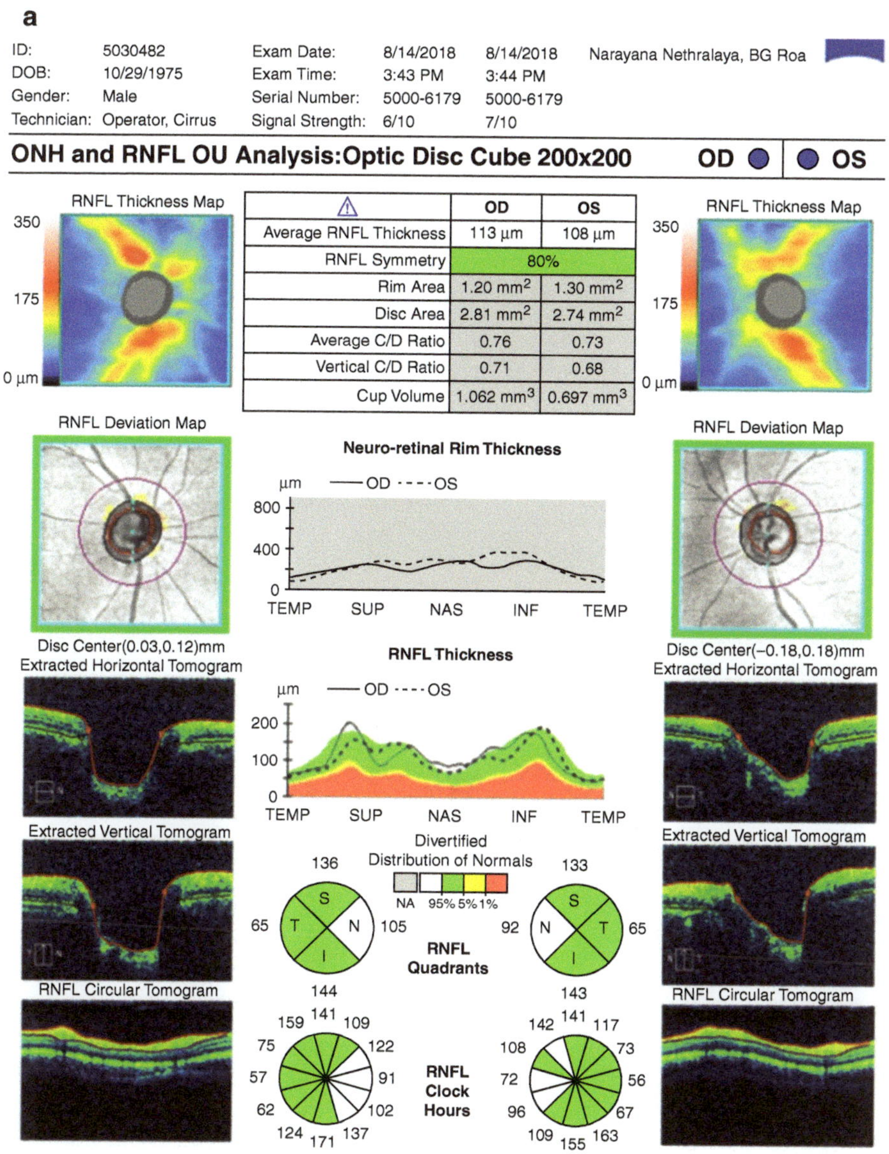

Fig. 20.10 Optic nerve head (ONH) and retinal nerve fiber layer (RNFL) reports of a normal subject (**a**) and a glaucoma patient (**b**). Compared to a normal eye, glaucomatous eye shows cool colors (blues, greens) on the "RNFL thickness map" representing thinning of RNFL (seen in the superior quadrant of the right eye and inferior quadrant of the left eye, **b**), red and yellow regions on the "deviation map" and "quadrant and clock hour maps" corresponding to the regions of RNFL thinning, RNFL and neuroretinal rim thickness falling in the red or yellow shaded region at corresponding locations around the disc on "TSNIT profile map" and reduction in the "summary parameters" in the tables which are color-coded in yellow or red

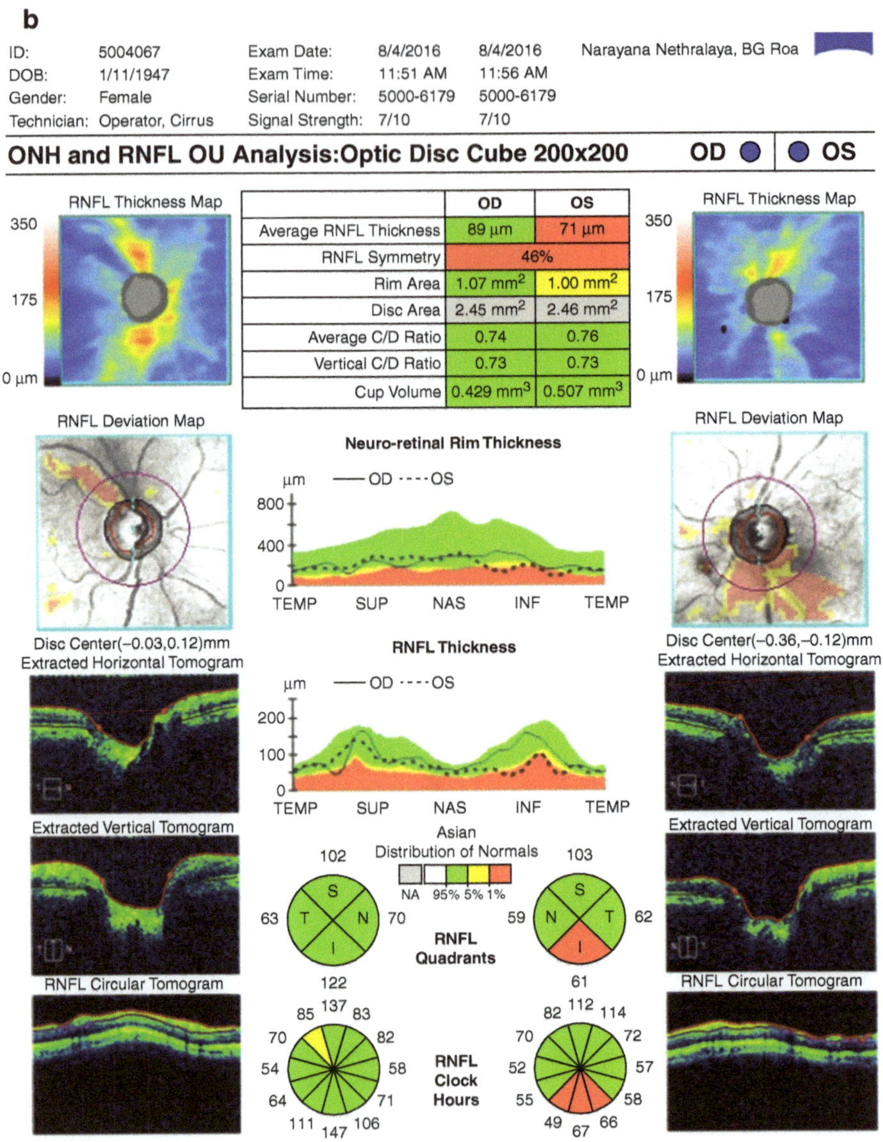

Fig. 20.10 (continued)

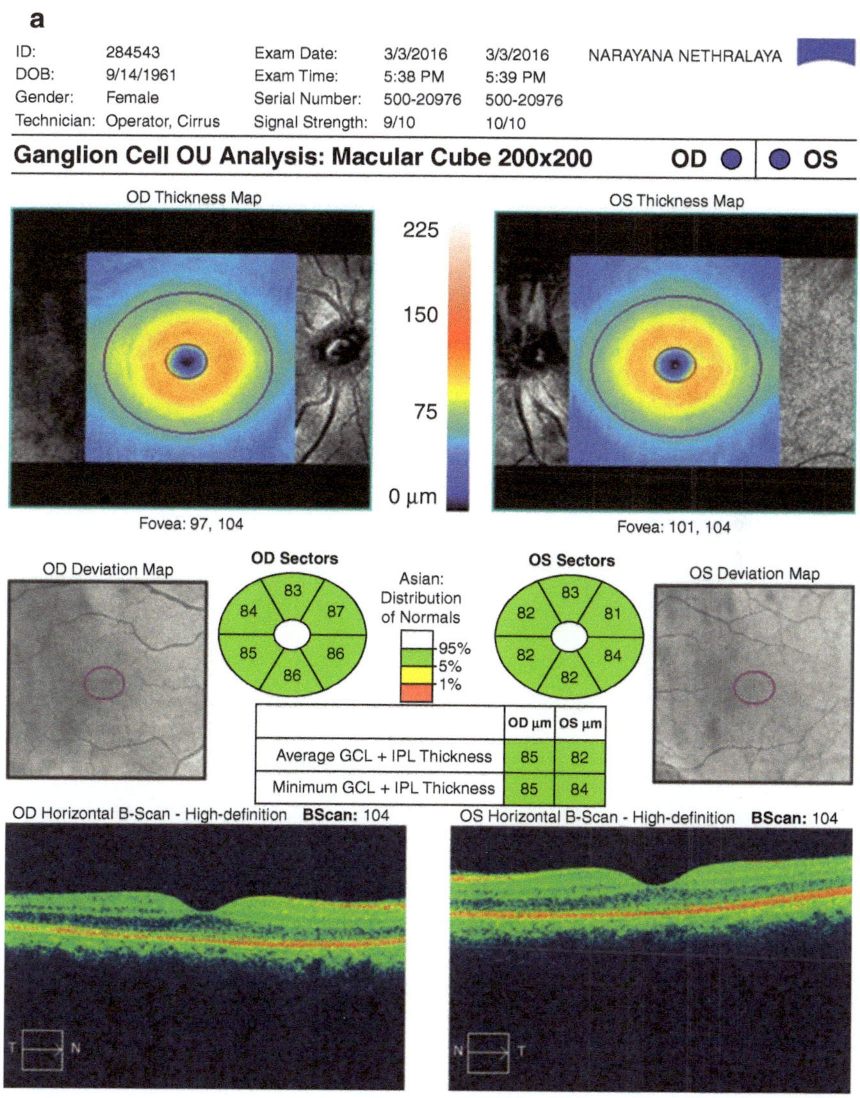

Fig. 20.11 Macular scan of a normal subject (**a**) and a glaucoma patient (**b**) showing the analysis of ganglion cell-inner plexiform layer (GCIPL) thickness. Interpretation of the macular report is similar to that described for the retinal nerve fiber layer (RNFL) report in Fig. 20.10. Figure (**b**) shows normal GCIPL thickness in right eye but superior GCIPL thinning in left eye, which is shown on GCIPL thickness, deviation and sector maps

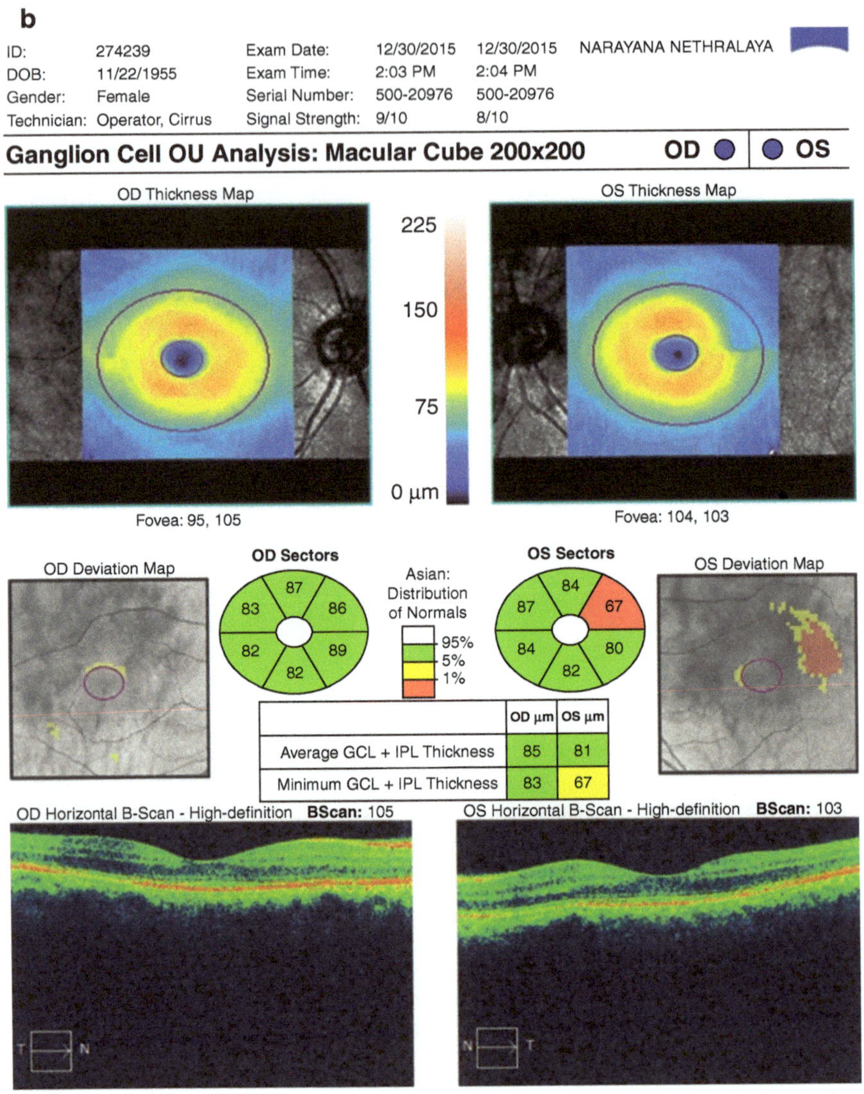

Fig. 20.11 (continued)

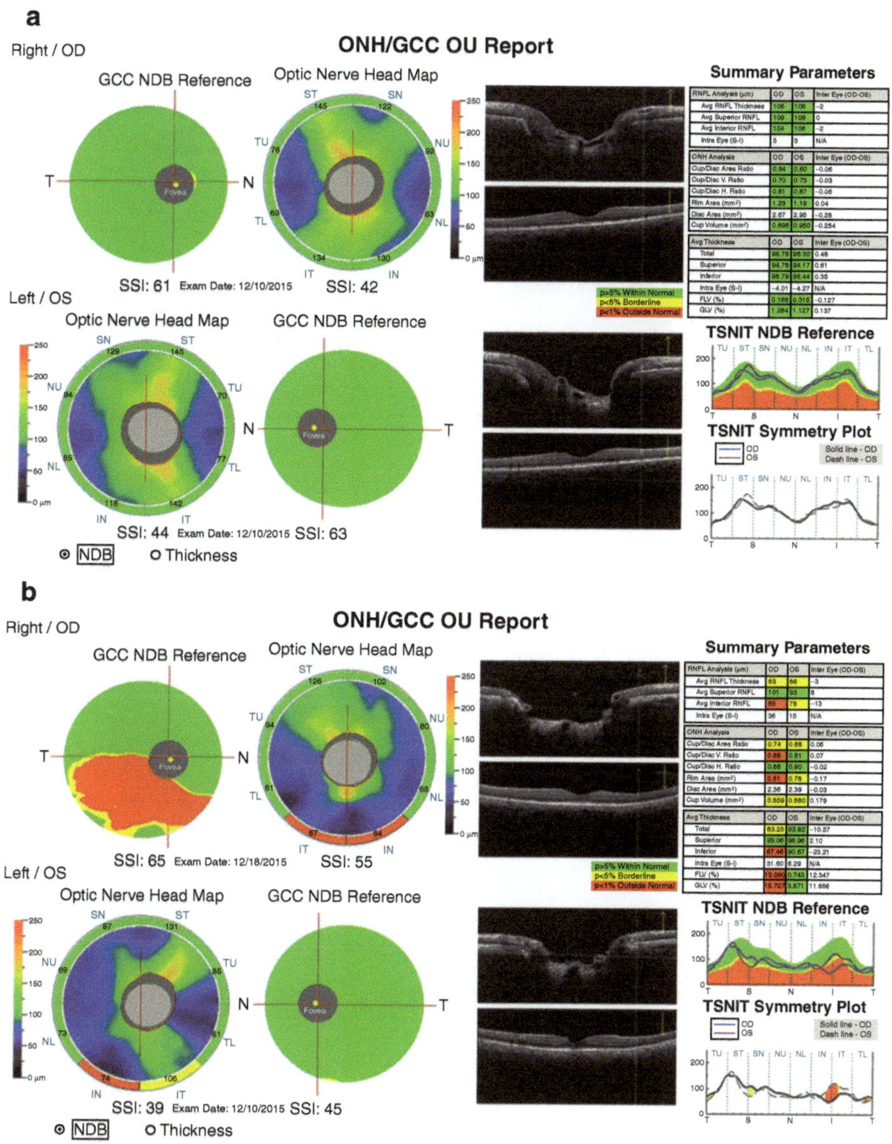

Fig. 20.12 Optic nerve head (ONH), retinal nerve fiber layer (RNFL) and ganglion cell complex (GCC) analysis report of a normal subject (**a**) and a glaucoma patient (**b**) from an OCT device. The interpretation of the report is similar to that described in Fig. 20.10. Figure (**b**) shows RNFL and GCC thinning in the inferior quadrant of right eye. Left eye in (**b**) shows inferior quadrant RNFL thinning without any GCC abnormality

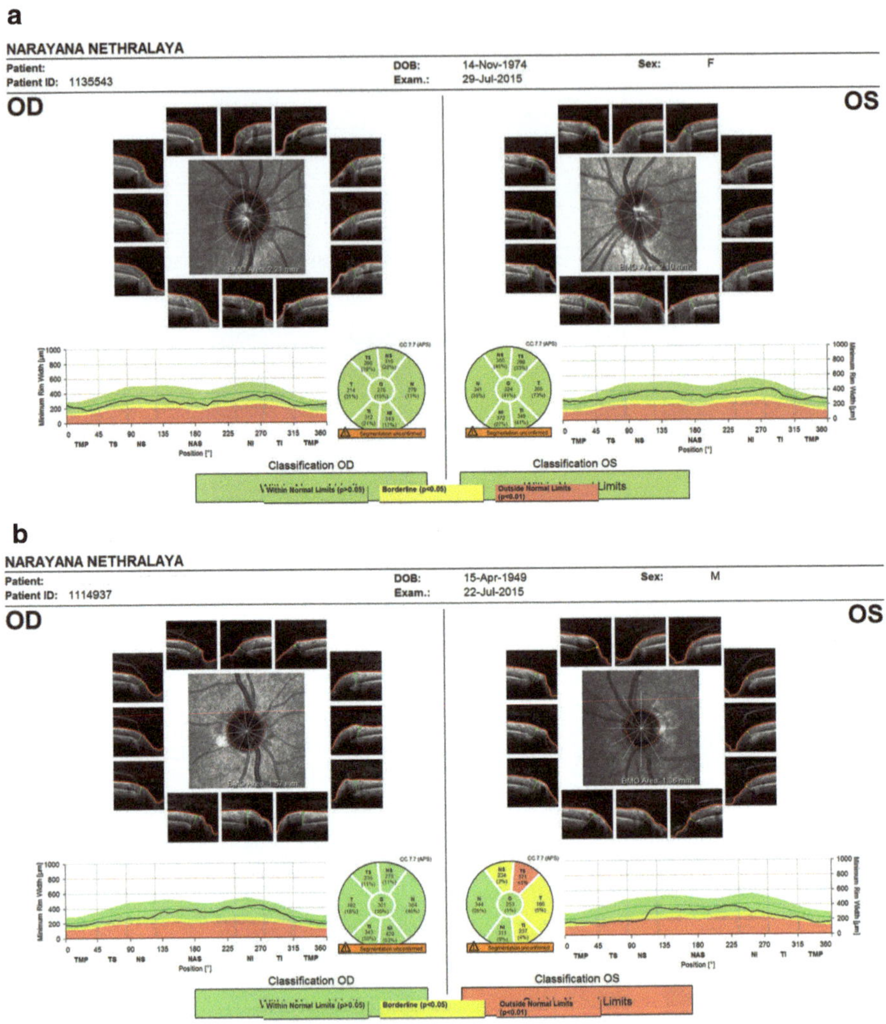

Fig. 20.13 Optic nerve head (ONH) report of a normal subject (**a**) and a glaucoma patient (**b**) from another OCT device showing the minimum rim width (MRW) at different sectors. Compared to the normal MRW measurements in Figure (**a**), Figure (**b**) shows MRW being thinner in the superior, temporal and inferior regions of left eye

a

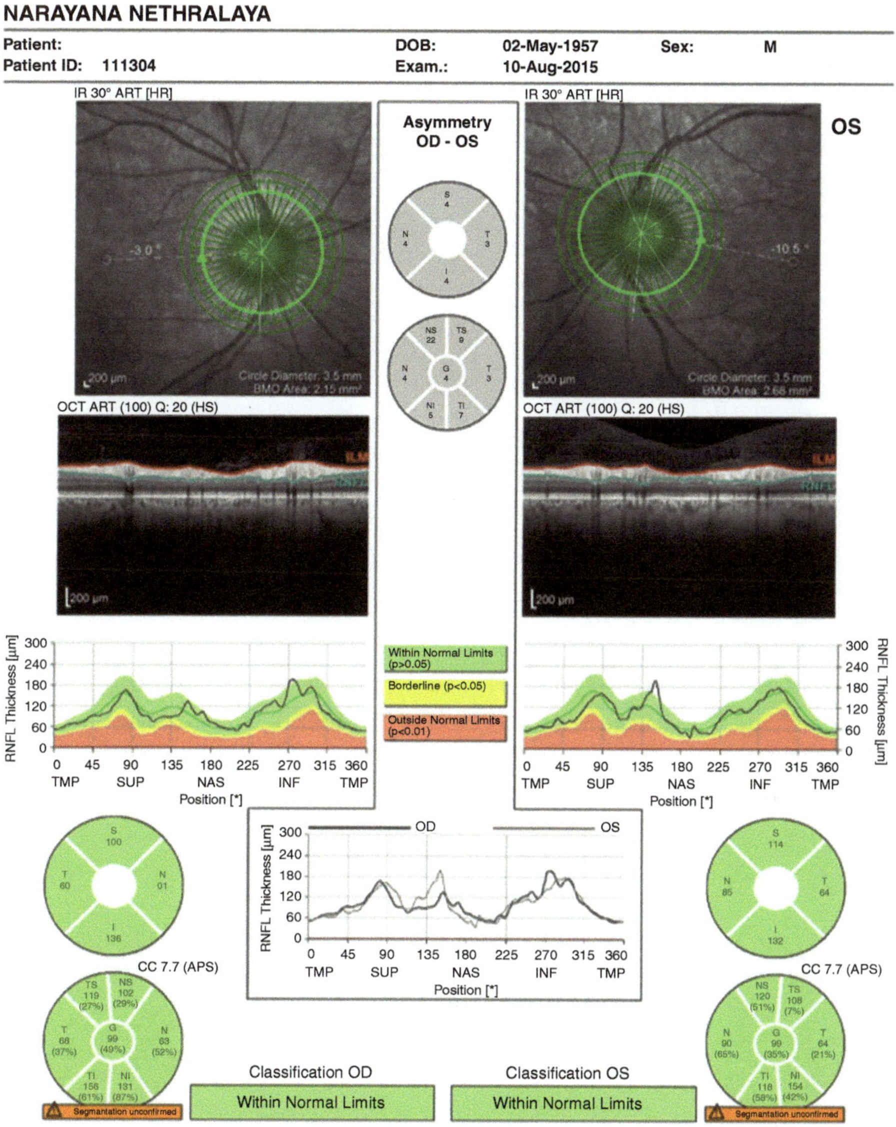

Fig. 20.14 Retinal nerve fiber layer (RNFL) report of a normal subject (**a**) and a glaucoma patient (**b**) from another OCT device. Compared to the RNFL report of the normal subject, glaucoma patient shows inferotemporal RNFL thinning in both eyes

b

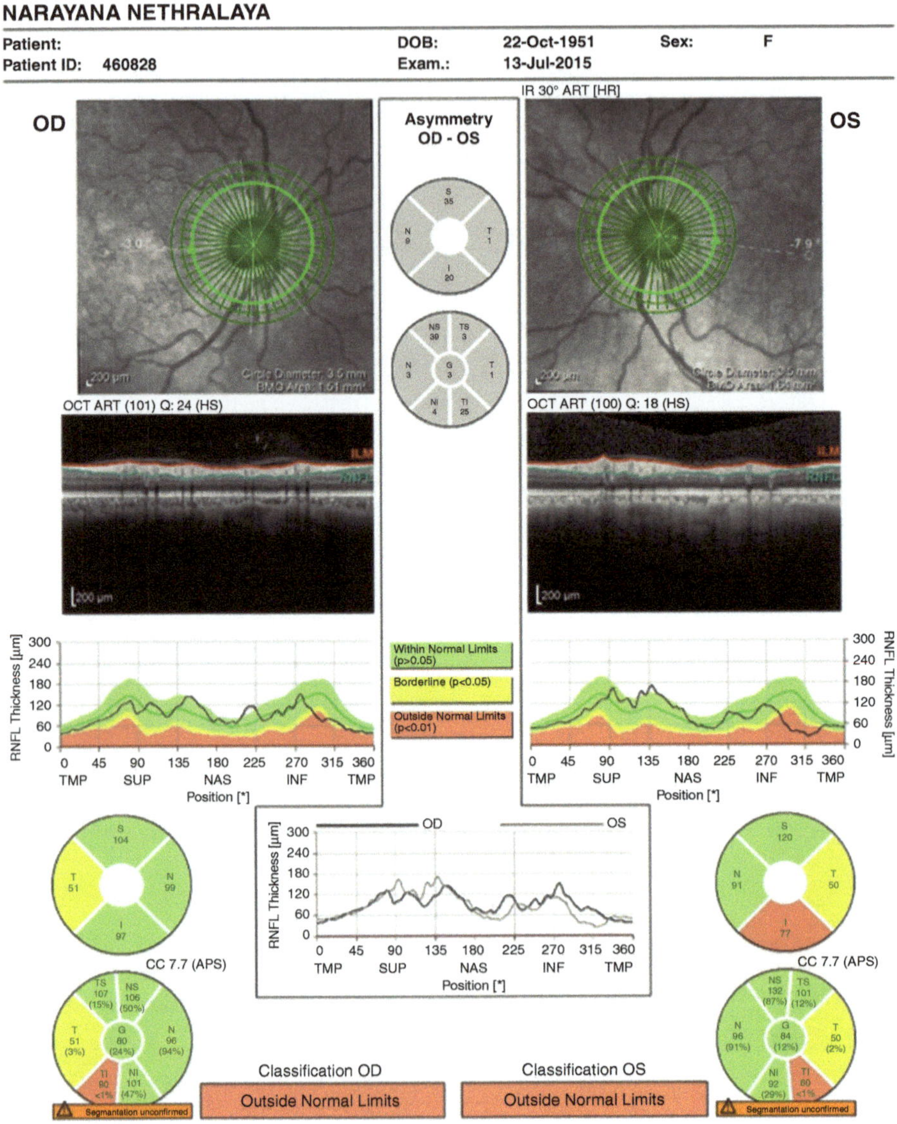

Fig. 20.14 (continued)

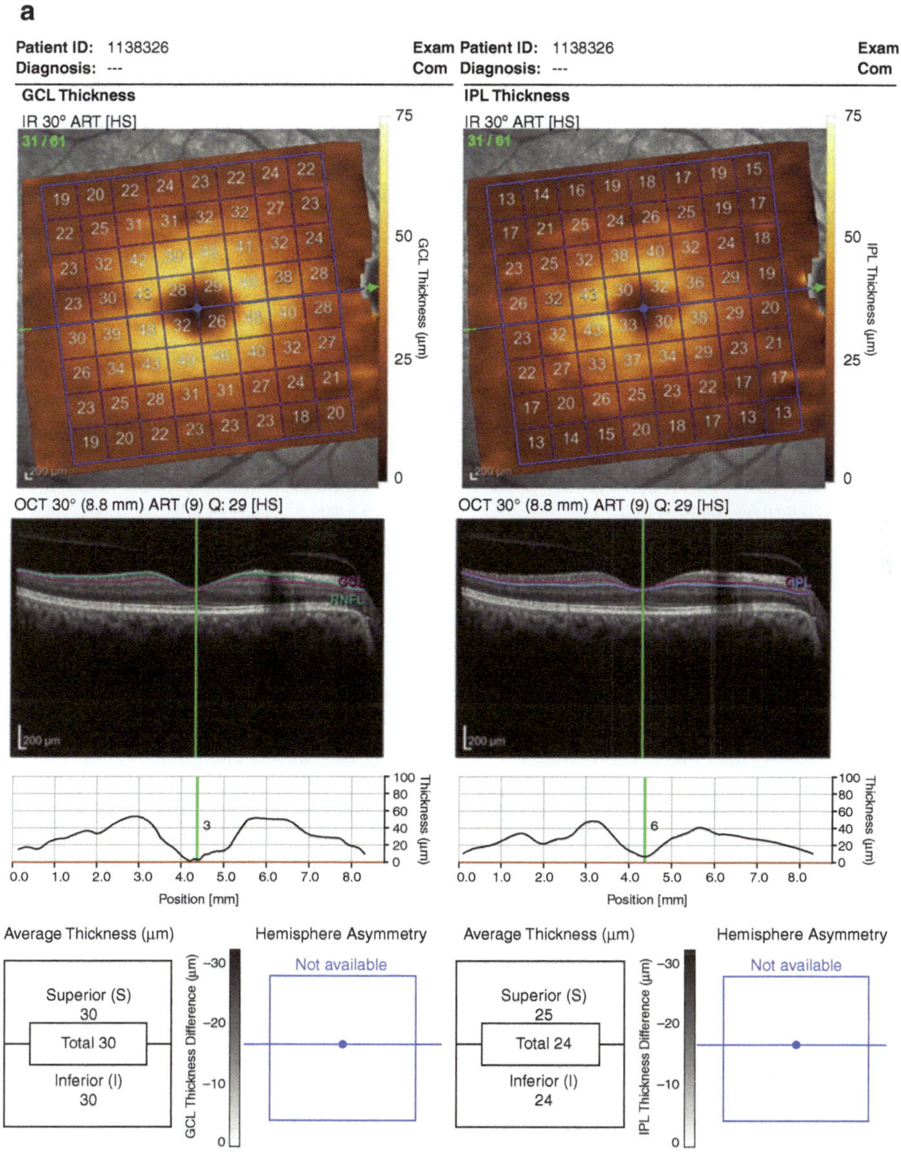

Fig. 20.15 Macular analysis report of a normal (**a**) and a glaucomatous eye (**b**) from another OCT device. Each layer of retina is analysed separately in this device, and ganglion cell layer (GCL) and inner plexiform layer (IPL) analysis is shown here. For each layer, the thickness is assessed at 64 cubes across the entire scan region and overlaid on the thickness map. The comparison between the superior and inferior hemispheres is also provided. Compared to the normal eye, the glaucomatous eye shows thinning of both the GCL and IPL in the inferior hemisphere

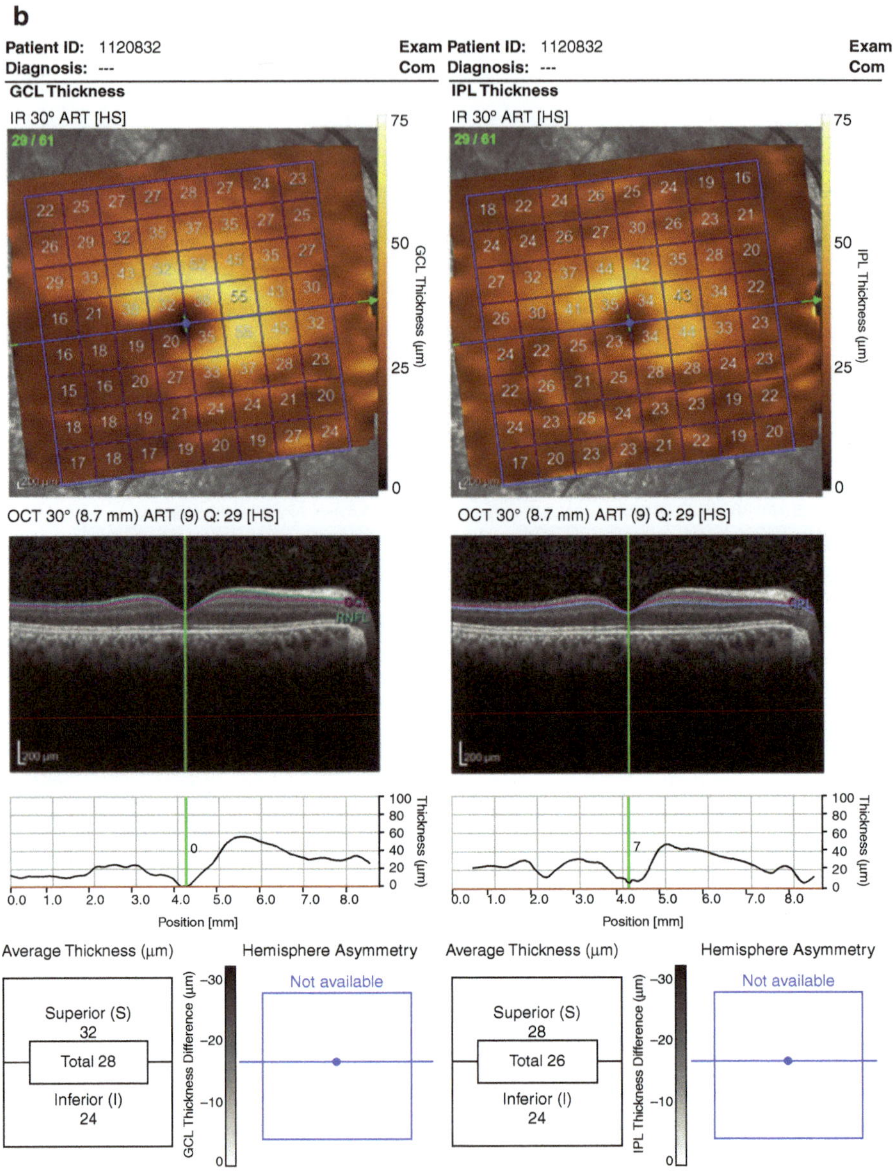

Fig. 20.15 (continued)

neuroretinal rim thinning and the presence of a RNFL defect inferiorly) and normal VF. OCT confirms the presence of RNFL thinning and quantifies it, enabling monitoring over time for progression. A study by Kuang et al. found that OCT was able to detect RNFL thinning 8 years before the development of VF defects [17]. Figure 20.17 shows an eye with a suspicious optic disc and a probable nasal defect on VF. OCT confirms the presence of RNFL thinning inferiorly which aids in the diagnosis and monitoring of this patient.

Structural changes in glaucoma are detectable on the ONH, RNFL and macular scans of OCT; however, it is still not clear which of these parameters detects glaucoma early. A systematic review reported RNFL measurements to be better than the inner retinal measurements at macula for diagnosing glaucoma [18]. However, it is useful to evaluate glaucomatous damage both on the ONH/RNFL and macular OCT scans to better understand the severity and pattern of structural loss.

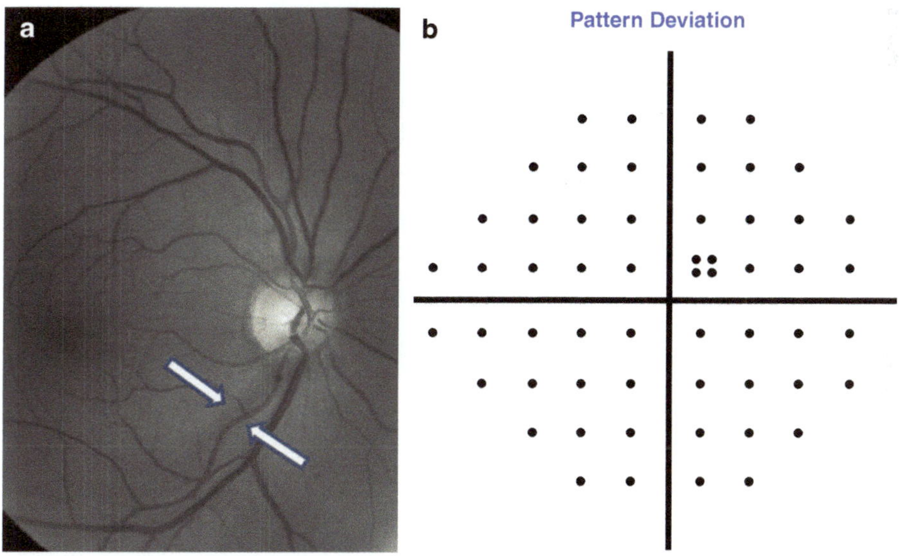

Fig. 20.16 An example of a right eye showing neuroretinal rim thinning and the presence of a retinal nerve fiber layer (RNFL) defect inferiorly on the optic disc photograph (**a**) but normal visual field (**b**). OCT confirms the presence of RNFL thinning on RNFL thickness map, deviation map and clock-hour map (**c**). Reproduced with permission from [102]

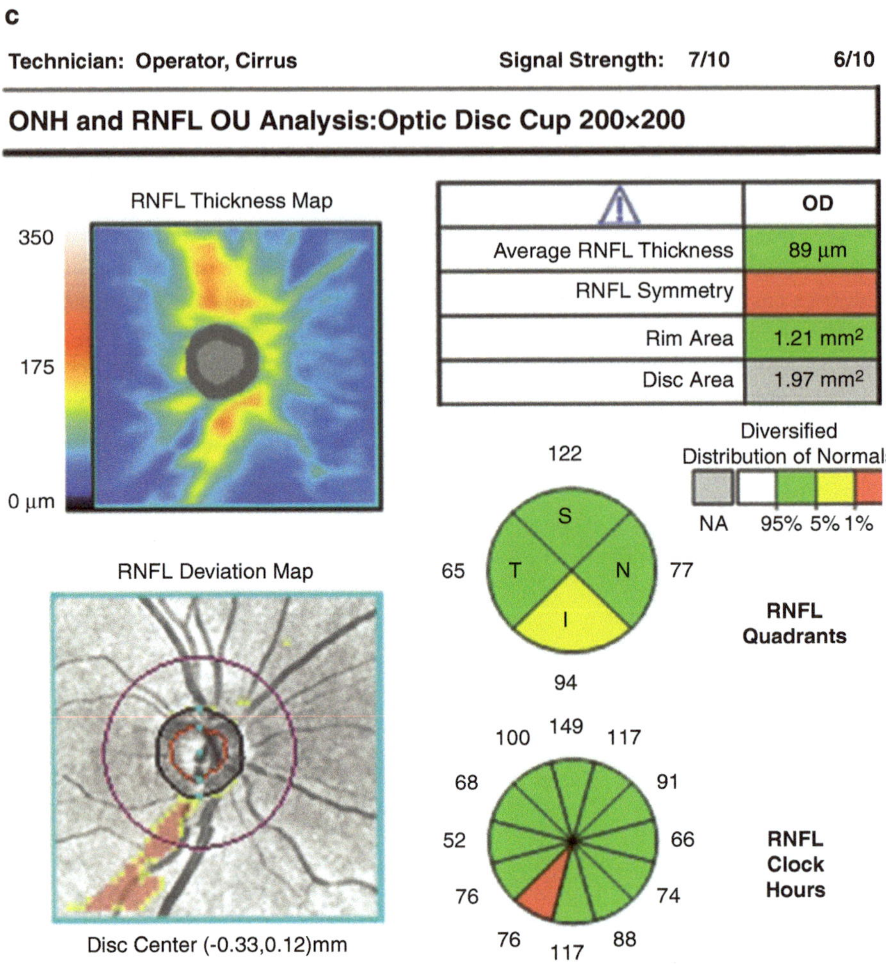

Fig. 20.16 (continued)

20.7 OCT in Monitoring Glaucoma Progression

One of the most challenging aspects in the management of glaucoma is to diagnose progression early and accurately. Like for VF, software to detect progression on OCT also employ trend and event-based analyses. A trend-based analysis estimates the rate of change (slope) of the parameter over time. An event-based analysis determines progression if the amount of change crosses a particular pre-set value (threshold).

Figure 20.18a shows the ONH/RNFL progression report of one OCT device which uses both the trend and the event based progression analyses. The report includes three analyses:

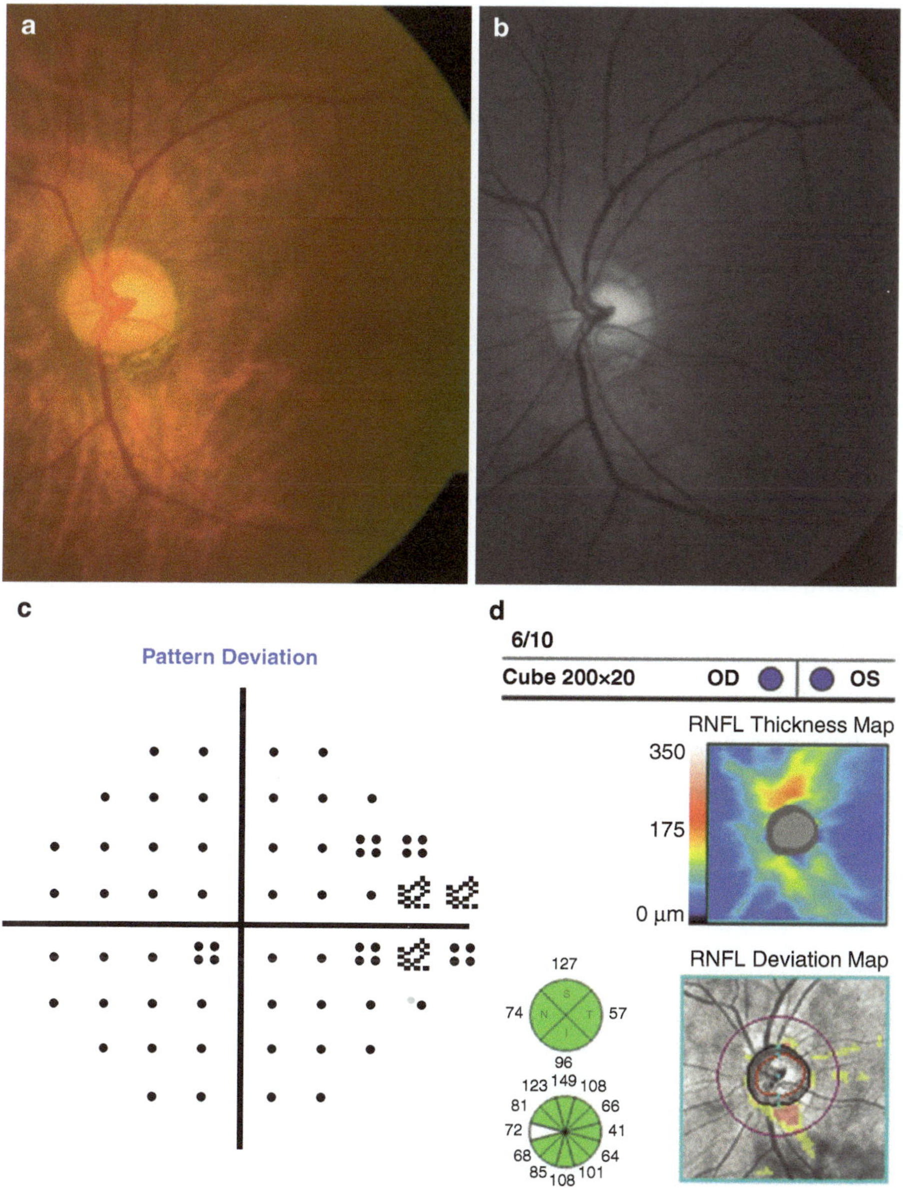

Fig. 20.17 An example of an eye showing suspicious optic disc (**a**), a possible inferotemporal retinal nerve fiber layer (RNFL) defect on red-free photograph (**b**) and a probable nasal defect on visual fields (**c**). OCT confirms the presence of inferotemporal RNFL thinning on the thickness map and deviation map (**d**). It can be noted that the clock-hour and quadrant maps do not show any RNFL abnormality; these maps are known to have a poorer diagnostic ability as compared to the thickness and deviation maps. Reproduced with permission from [102]

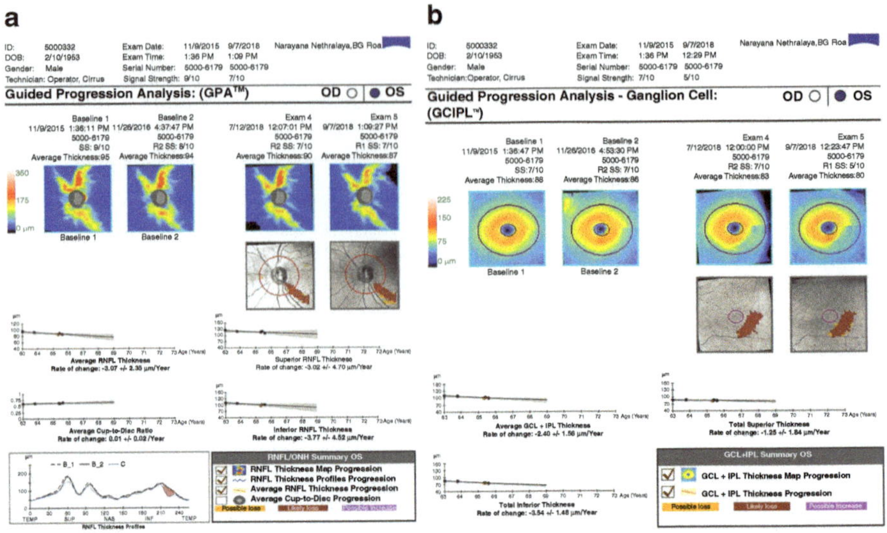

Fig. 20.18 Optic nerve head (ONH)/retinal nerve fiber layer (RNFL) progression analysis of an OCT device (**a**) showing disease progression on both event and trend-based methods. Two good quality baseline exams are required for all analyses and two good quality follow-up exams are required to confirm "likely change" in the ONH and RNFL parameters. The progression report includes "RNFL thickness change map", an event-based analysis, which marks out the RNFL regions which have changed by an amount greater than the test-retest variability, "RNFL thickness graphs", trend-based analyses, which evaluate the rate of change of superior, inferior and average RNFL thickness measurements over time and "RNFL thickness profile analysis", also an event-based analysis, which detects the regions on the RNFL profile graph that have decreased beyond the expected test-retest variability. Macular (GCIPL thickness) analysis (**b**) showing disease progression on both event and trend-based methods. The report of GCIPL progression analysis, similar to the ONH/RNFL report, includes "GCIPL thickness change map", an event-based analysis, and "GCIPL thickness graphs", a trend-based analysis

1. a chronological display of RNFL thickness maps and RNFL thickness change maps
2. average cup to disc ratio (CDR), superior, inferior and average RNFL thickness graphs representing rate of change, and
3. RNFL thickness profiles comparing the current exam to the baseline exams.

Two good quality baseline exams are required for these analyses and two good quality follow-up exams are required to confirm likely change in the ONH and RNFL parameters. Statistically significant changes are summarized with color-codes for possible or likely RNFL thickness loss (or possible RNFL thickness increase).

RNFL thickness map and thickness change map is an event-based analysis, which compares the follow-up exams with the baseline exams and marks out the RNFL regions which have changed by an amount greater than the test-retest variability. When a particular region exceeded the test-retest variability for the first time, it is flagged as a "possible loss" and coded in yellow. When the same region shows a change beyond the test-retest variability in a subsequent exam, it is flagged as a "likely loss" and coded in red. When a particular region shows an increase in RNFL thickness beyond the test-retest variability, it is flagged as a "possible increase" and coded in lavender. In the absence of concurrent retinal pathologies, "possible increase" generally occurs if the baseline exams include poor quality scans with an improvement in scan quality subsequently. RNFL thickness change map is preferred to detect focal changes.

RNFL thickness profile analysis is also an event-based analysis, which compares the RNFL profile of the current examination with that of the baseline exams. It detects the regions on the RNFL profile graph that have decreased beyond the expected test-retest variability. The regions showing the change are flagged as "possible loss", "likely loss" or "possible increase" as mentioned above. RNFL thickness profile analysis, like the RNFL thickness and change map, is preferred to detect focal changes.

Average cup to disc ratio (CDR) and RNFL thickness graphs use a trend-based analysis to evaluate the rate of change of average CDR, superior, inferior and average RNFL thickness measurements over time. Rate of change in these trend-based analyses is estimated using linear regression. The individual data points (from each examination) are highlighted (color-coded) to indicate when the parameter value changed by an amount greater than the test-retest variability. The result shows up as "possible loss" when the rate of loss is statistically significant for only a single visit and is indicated by a yellow symbol. The result shows up as "likely loss" when the rate of loss is statistically significant for two visits in a row and is indicated by a red symbol. Average thickness graphs are preferred to detect diffuse changes unlike the previous two maps. Figure 20.18b shows the macular progression analysis report which is interpreted similar to the RNFL progression report detailed above.

Figure 20.19 shows the progression analysis report from another OCT device which employs a trend-based method to evaluate the rate of change of RNFL and macular (GCC) thickness over time. The rate of change is high-lighted (as

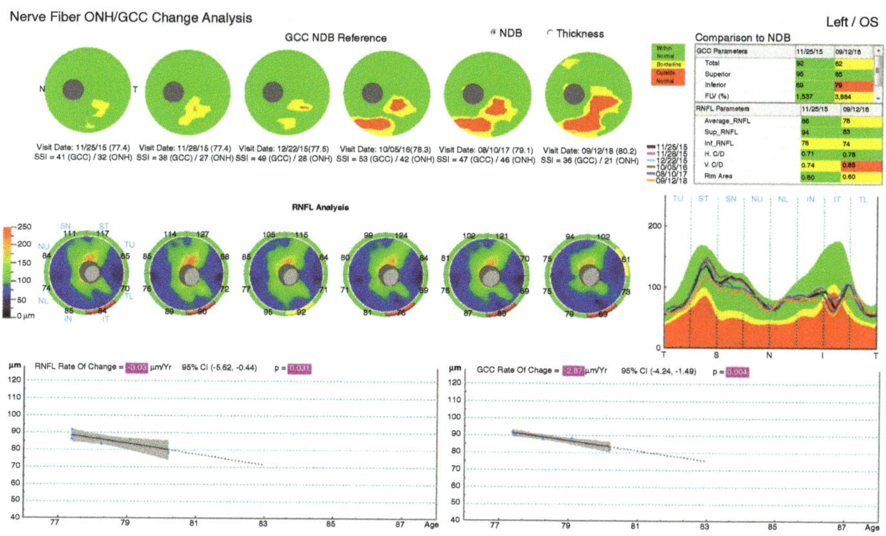

Fig. 20.19 Retinal nerve fiber layer (RNFL) and ganglion cell complex (GCC) thickness progression analysis of an OCT device showing significant deterioration of average RNFL and GCC thickness on the trend-based analysis

represented in the figure) according to the p value of the slope. In the example, both RNFL and GCC thickness are decreasing at a magnitude which is significant.

Figure 20.20 shows the trend-based analysis of the global RNFL thickness (Fig. 20.20a) and the global MRW (Fig. 20.20b) of an OCT device. The analysis shows the magnitude of slope associated with the change in the parameters with time and also the p value associated with the slope.

As demonstrated above, OCT analyses ONH, RNFL and macular parameters for progression; however, it is of interest to evaluate which of these parameters is useful in detecting progression early and at all stages of disease severity. Kim et al. investigated the temporal relationship between GCIPL and corresponding peripapillary RNFL thinning on the OCT deviation maps in 151 patients with early-stage POAG [19]. The scans were performed at baseline and 3 years later. They found that in eyes with early glaucoma, GCIPL change is frequently detected before corresponding peripapillary RNFL change. They concluded that peripapillary RNFL analysis alone likely would overlook macular damage and macular imaging should be included in the imaging algorithm for the serial observation of patients with glaucoma [19]. In another study, Hwang et al. found progression to be more frequent in RNFL than GCIPL thickness [20]. Of the 106 eyes that showed either RNFL and/or GCIPL progression in a cohort of 527 glaucoma eyes, 54 eyes (50.9%) showed progression earlier on RNFL thickness, 13 eyes (12.3%) showed progression earlier on GCIPL thickness, and 39 eyes (36.8%) showed progression both on RNFL and GCIPL thickness simultaneously [20]. Another study by Hou et al. investigated the temporal relationship among progressive macular GCIPL thinning, progressive RNFL thinning, and VF progression in 136 patients (231 eyes) with POAG followed up for ≥5 years [21]. GPA detected progressive GCIPL thinning in 57 eyes (24.7%) and progressive RNFL thinning in 66 eyes (28.6%) with at a specificity of 95.5% and 91.0%, respectively. In their study, eyes with progressive GCIPL thinning had a higher risk for progressive RNFL thinning (hazard ratio, HR = 5.27; 95% CI: 2.89–9.62), and eyes with progressive RNFL thinning also had a higher risk for progressive GCIPL thinning (HR = 2.99; 95% CI: 1.48–6.02). Eyes with progressive GCIPL and RNFL thinning were at a higher risk of VF progression. However, eyes with VF progression were not at risk of progressive RNFL or GCIPL thinning [21]. They concluded that progressive GCIPL thinning and progressive RNFL thinning are mutually predictive, and integrating GCIPL and RNFL measurements is relevant to facilitate early detection of disease deterioration in glaucoma patients [21]. Another recent study demonstrated that the macular and ONH parameters of OCT have the ability to detect progression even in advanced cases of glaucoma where the RNFL thickness had reached a "floor" (explained below) [22]. All the OCT parameters are complementary to each other and analysing all of them increases the sensitivity to detect progression. Therefore, it is preferable to obtain both the RNFL/ONH and macular scans at all follow-up examinations, and to consider the severity of glaucoma before deciding the OCT parameter to be used for detecting structural progression. However, it is to be noted that the use of multiple OCT parameters increases the number of eyes that are falsely labelled as progressing.

The magnitude of decrease in OCT measurements that is clinically significant is also debatable. Studies have reported a change of 4 μm for GCIPL, 5 μm for average RNFL and 7 μm for inferior and superior sector RNFL thickness to be clinically significant [23, 24], and this can be used as a thumb rule to aid decision making.

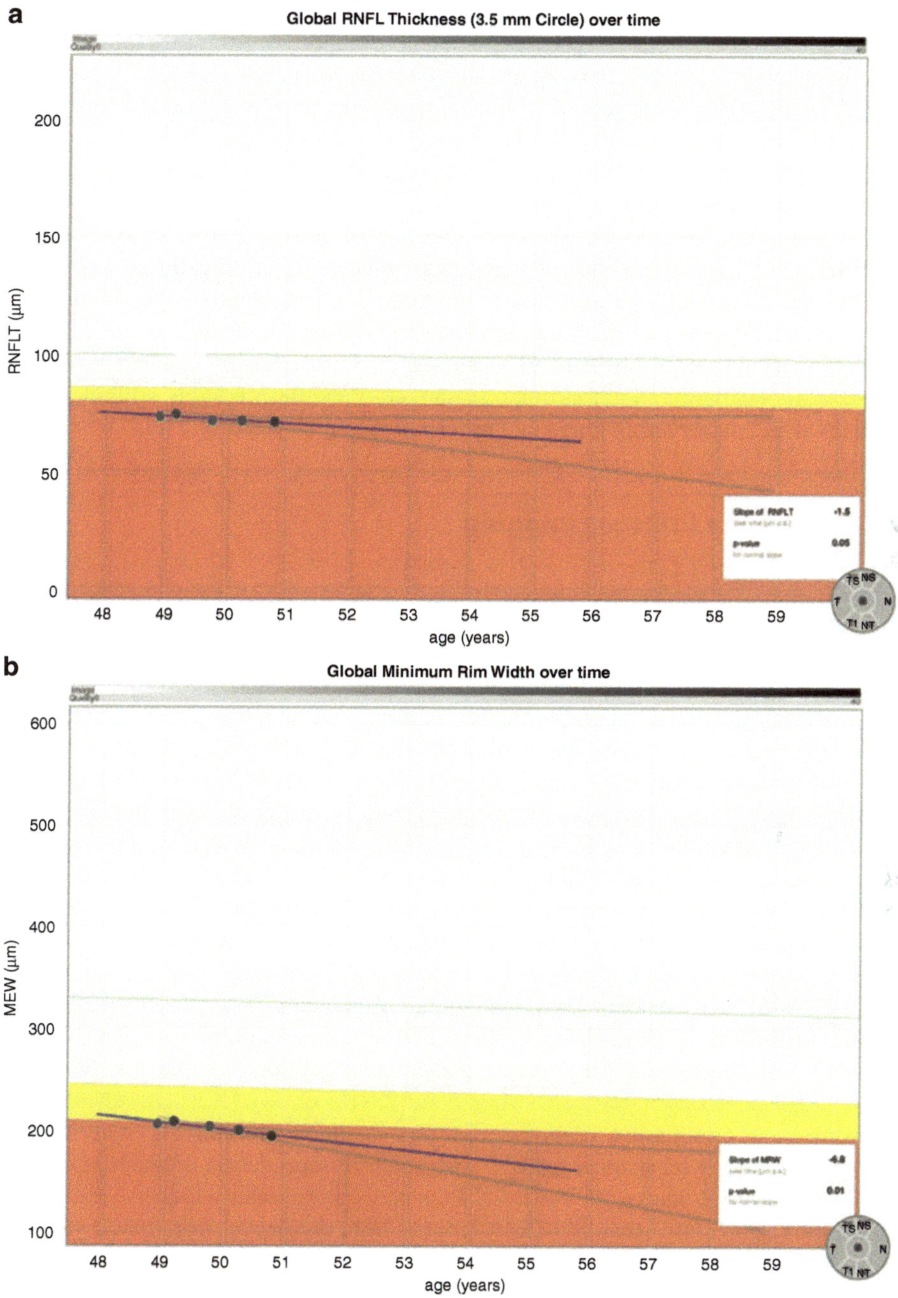

Fig. 20.20 Trend-based progression analysis of global retinal nerve fiber layer (RNFL) thickness (**a**) and minimum rim width (MRW, **b**) of an OCT device (source: Dr. Sebastian Rausch, Heidelberg Engineering)

The relevance of the glaucoma progression on OCT is frequently questioned because it is believed that VF progression is more important from the patients' perspective. However, studies have shown that OCT progression precedes VF progression [25, 26]. Also, faster rate of RNFL loss has been shown to be associated with faster decline in quality of life [27]. OCT therefore offers the possibility of detecting patients at high risk of VF progression, following them up more closely and a possibility of augmenting treatment early.

It is important to note that the OCT progression analysis gives us statistically significant change, but not clinically significant change. Therefore, the results of the OCT progression analysis should not be interpreted independently but in the context of the entire clinical picture. It is important to consider the results of the clinical evaluation (intraocular pressure, disease stage, occurrence of disc hemorrhage, increase in beta peripapillary atrophic region, etc.) and the VF along with the OCT findings while determining glaucoma progression.

20.8 Lamina Cribrosa Imaging

The lamina cribrosa (LC) is a multi-layered sieve-like structure in the sclera where retinal ganglion cell axons exit from the eye. The LC has been known to play a critical role in the pathogenesis of glaucoma [28]. Blockage of axonal transport within the LC has been proposed as a salient pathogenic mechanism for glaucoma. It is assumed that the LC provides mechanical support to the nerve fibers traversing the deeper ocular structures. Deformation of LC presumably from elevated IOP likely hinders axoplasmic flow and thus disrupts transport of trophic factors critical to retinal ganglion cells, thereby causing neuronal death that is characteristic of glaucoma. Furthermore, the LC represents a biomechanical discontinuity in the spherical casing of the eye, so that the globe is more vulnerable to stress loading that may play a role in glaucoma. Understanding such forces that affect the structure of the LC, through both focal and general morphologic changes, would clarify the mechanisms of glaucoma. A detailed study of the LC, however, requires accurate and clear visualization of this structure. Clinical examination of the LC structures cannot be performed routinely with current diagnostic methods.

Advances in OCT technology have enabled in vivo visualization of the LC now [29–31]. The enhanced depth imaging (EDI) technique for example, has provided better image contrast for the deep portion of the ONH [32, 33]. OCT light-attenuation software such as adaptive compensation has further improved LC visibility by effective blood-vessel shadow removal and better differentiation of tissue boundaries [34, 35]. Swept-source OCT (SS-OCT), which incorporates a longer-wavelength (1050 nm) light source than SD-OCT, reduces light dispersion from blood vessels, thereby allowing for high-resolution imaging of the LC [36].

LC findings on OCT are commonly categorized in terms of position (LC depth and LC insertion depth), curvature or shape, and microarchitectural change (LC defect) [37].

LC depth (LCD, Fig. 20.21) is defined as the maximum or mean vertical distance from the anterior LC surface to the reference plane of Bruch's membrane opening (BMO). Multiple studies have demonstrated that the LCD is greater in eyes with glaucoma compared to healthy eyes [38–40]. LCD was also noted to reduce when the IOP in glaucomatous eyes was lowered after the introduction of medical therapy [41], or after glaucoma filtration surgery [42, 43]. In prospective studies, greater LCD was also associated with greater visual field progression [44] and faster rates of retinal nerve fibre layer (RNFL) thinning [45]. However, one of the limitation of calculating LCD is that it requires the use of a reference plane and BMO, which is used as the reference plane commonly, includes choroidal thickness in its measurement. Choroidal thickness varies with age and other non-glaucomatous pathologies and therefore can affect the LCD measurement [46, 47].

Similar to LCD, lamina cribrosa insertion (LCI, Fig. 20.21), the region wherein the vascular perfusion from the capillaries of the short posterior ciliary artery drains to the LC [48], is reported to migrate posteriorly in glaucoma [49]. Determining LCI depth also requires the use of a reference plane.

To overcome the challenges of LCD and LCI depth determination, LC curvature, which does not require the use of a reference plane, has been proposed as an alternative structural parameter that is useful in glaucoma. LC curvature has been evaluated by measuring the difference between the mean LCD and the anterior LCI depth, in both the horizontal and vertical meridians [50]. LC curvature is reported to have a significantly better diagnostic performance than LCD [40].

All the above LC parameters on OCT are based only on the anterior surface of LC and the posterior surface of LC is difficult to image on OCT [51].

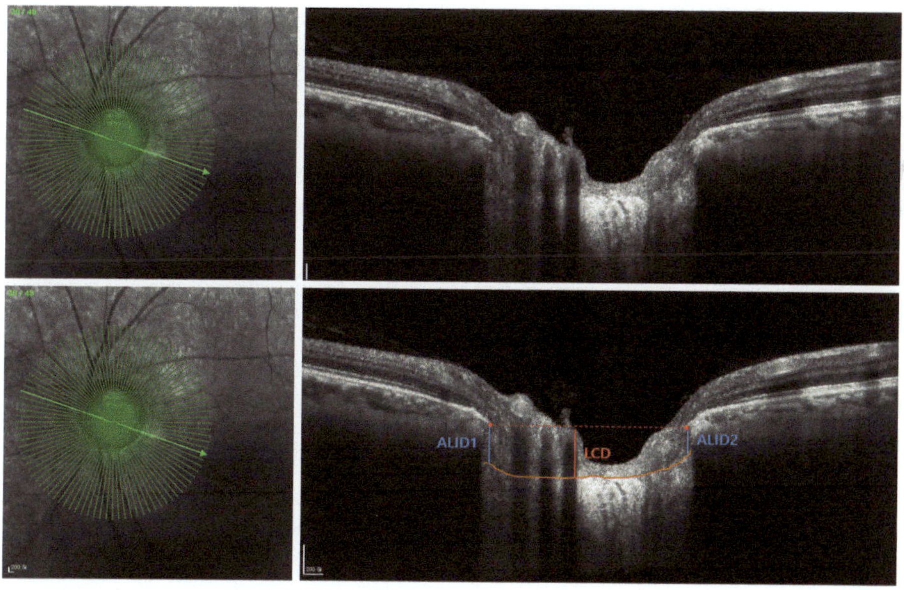

Fig. 20.21 The anterior laminar insertion depth (ALID) is defined as the perpendicular distance between the Bruch's membrane openings (BMO, red dots) and the anterior laminar insertion (ends of the orange line). The lamina cribrosa depth (LCD) is measured as the vertical distance between the BMO reference plane (red dotted line) and the maximally depressed point of the anterior laminar surface (orange line) (Image courtesy: Minh H. Suh, Department of Ophthalmology, Haeundae Paik Hospital, Inje University College of Medicine, Busan, South Korea)

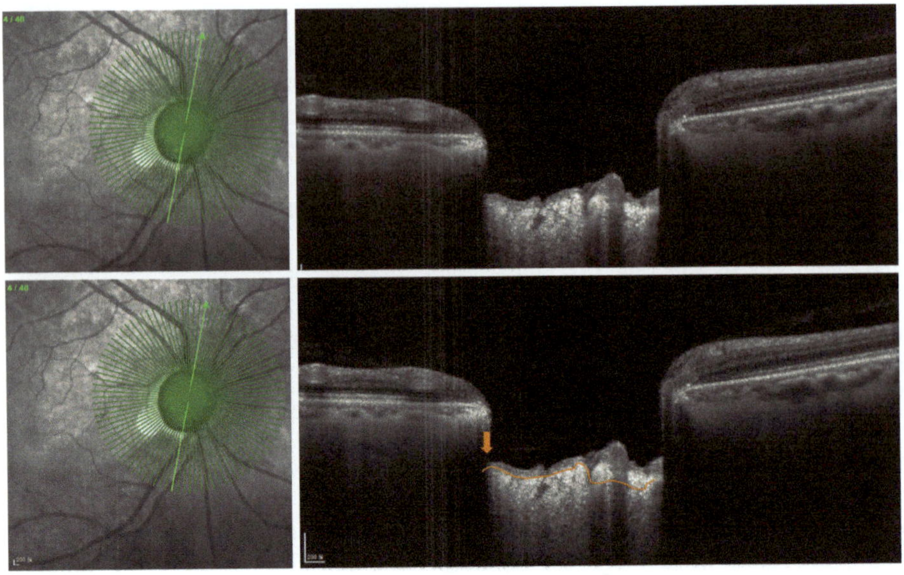

Fig. 20.22 Focal lamina cribrosa defect (FLD) observed in the inferotemporal region of the optic nerve head (Image courtesy: Minh H. Suh, Department of Ophthalmology, Haeundae Paik Hospital, Inje University College of Medicine, Busan, South Korea)

Focal LC defect (FLD) is representative of focal LC-microstructural change. On OCT, it is seen as an anterior laminar surface irregularity manifesting as a laminar hole or disinsertion that violates the normal smooth curvilinear contours of the LC (Fig. 20.22) [52]. FLD presents clinically as an acquired pit of optic nerve, rim thinning or notching, and has shown a spatial correlation with VF defect and localized RNFL defects [53, 54]. FLDs are also associated with presence of disc hemorrhages [55, 56]. Eyes with FLDs showed a faster rate of glaucoma progression [57–60].

20.9 Limitations of OCT

OCT imaging requires clear media for good quality scans. Segmentation algorithms of OCT softwares fail in poor quality scans leading to erroneous measurements. Image quality is known to significantly affect the ability of OCT to detect glaucomatous defects [61, 62].

Using OCT in highly myopic eyes is challenging as a result of poor image quality and comparisons drawn using a dissimilar reference database.

OCT measurements are known to level off in more advanced stages of glaucoma. RNFL thickness, for example, levels off when the corresponding functional loss on automated perimetry reaches a severity of −10 to −15 dB [63]. Further deterioration in the glaucoma severity causes little change in the RNFL thickness, resulting in a floor effect (Fig. 20.23). It has to be noted that the floor may be at different levels for different OCT parameters and GCIPL and ONH measurements may still be able to detect progression in eyes where the RNFL thickness has reached a floor [22].

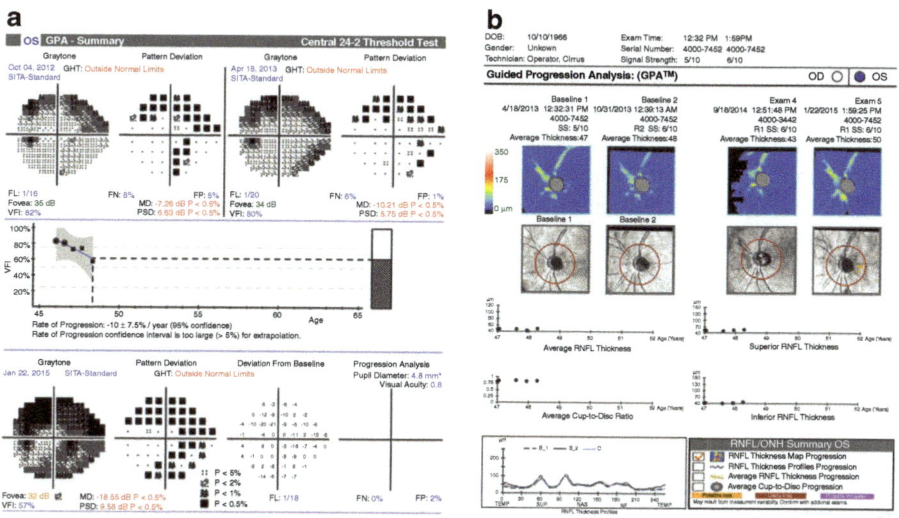

Fig. 20.23 An example of a glaucomatous eye showing obvious progression on visual fields (**a**) but showing no progression on retinal nerve fiber layer (RNFL) analysis of OCT (**b**) due to the 'floor effect'. Reproduced with permission from [102]

Certain clinical findings that are crucial in decision making, like neuroretinal rim pallor and disc hemorrhages, are not picked up by the OCT.

20.10 OCT Angiography

OCT has also been used to non-invasively delineate the vasculature of the retina and ONH. Doppler OCT was one of the earliest techniques developed for vascular imaging. It assessed blood flow by comparing phase differences between adjacent A-scans [64]. Although Doppler OCT was appropriate for large vessels around the disc, it was not sensitive enough to measure accurately the low velocities in small vessels that make up the ONH and retinal microcirculation. The search for a simple, non-invasive, reproducible method of evaluating the ocular blood flow has recently lead to the development of a technique called OCT angiography (OCTA).

OCTA is capable of imaging large vessels as well as microvasculature of the retina and ONH by performing multiple OCT scans of the same region. The variation in OCT signal at each location is then studied. Moving particles, such as red blood cells, result in a high variance of the OCT signal between repeated scans and this is used to identify blood vessels. Several algorithms have been developed to interpret the OCT signals and to delineate the blood vessels. Split spectrum amplitude decorrelation angiography (SSADA; Angiovue, RTVue-XR SD-OCT, Optovue Inc., Fremont, CA) is one such algorithm that uses the variation in the intensity of the OCT signal to identify blood vessels. The fluctuating value of OCT intensities is considered as the decorrelation (D). Thus, pixels in the B-scan frame where blood is flowing have fluctuating intensities and yield high D values (approaching 1).

Pixels in the B-scan frames that contain static tissue yield small D values (approaching 0) [65]. The principles of SSADA have been explained in detail by Jia et al. [66]. The optical microangiography (OMAG), another algorithm that performs OCTA (Angioplex, Cirrus HD-OCT, Carl Zeiss Meditec Inc., Dublin, CA), uses the variation in intensity as well as the phase difference of the OCT signals for vessel delineation. As the time required to obtain the scan with OCTA is close to 3 s, involuntary saccades and changes in fixation during data acquisition can lead to motion artifacts that may confound the interpretation of the final OCT angiogram. Active eye tracking is therefore an essential feature of the OCTA devices.

Retina is segmented into different slabs, such as choriocapillaris, outer and deep retina and superficial retina, and vessels in each of these slabs is presented in 2-dimensional format. Figure 20.24 shows the macular scan of one OCTA device.

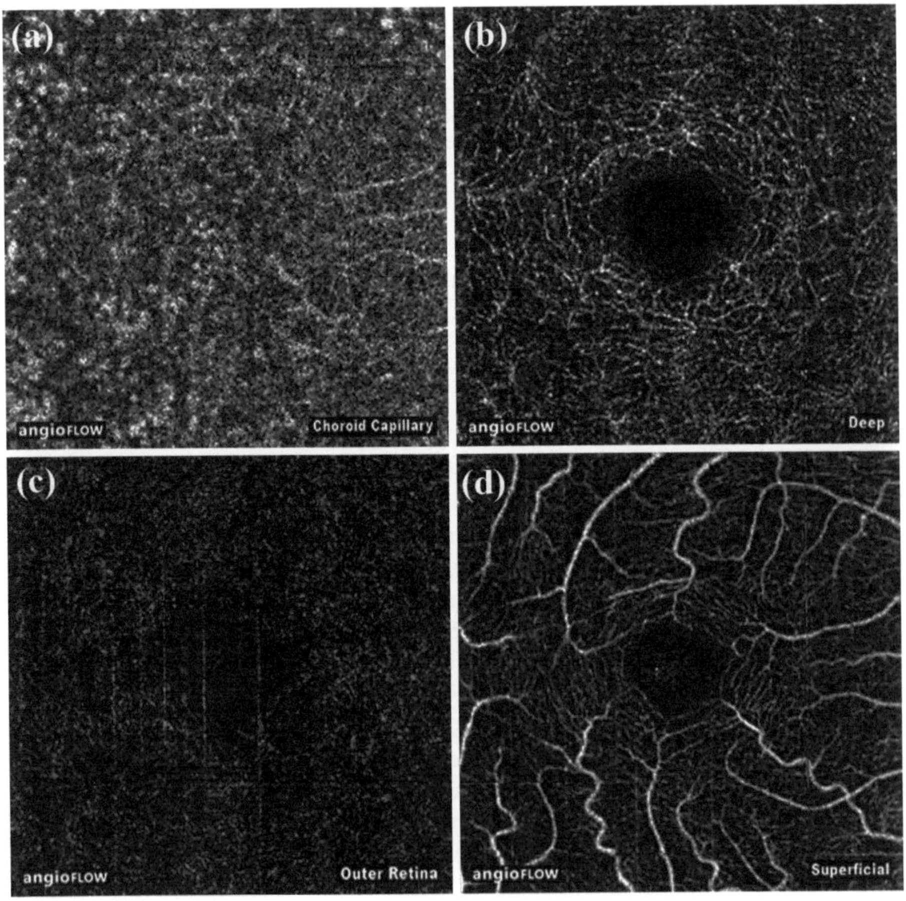

Fig. 20.24 Angiography slabs of the macular scan obtained using spectral domain optical coherence tomography showing the choriocapillaris (**a**), deep retinal (**b**), outer retinal (**c**) and superficial retinal (**d**) slabs

The macular OCTA scan is performed using a volumetric scan covering a 3 × 3 mm area. More recently 6 × 6 mm scans of the macula are also available. The superficial retinal slab extends from 3 μm below the ILM to 15 μm below the inner plexiform layer (IPL). Deep retinal slab extends from 15 μm below IPL to 70 μm below the IPL. Outer retinal slab extends from 70 μm below the IPL to 30 μm below the retinal pigment epithelium (RPE) and choroid capillary slab extends from 30 μm below the RPE to 60 μm below the RPE.

The optic disc OCTA scan is performed using volumetric scans covering an area of 4.5 × 4.5 mm. The optic disc region, similar to the macular region, is divided into several slabs for further analysis. Figure 20.25 shows the optic disc scan of one OCTA device. The most superficial "vitreous" slab is usually used for assessing neovascularization of the disc and is not used in glaucoma. The "nerve head" layer

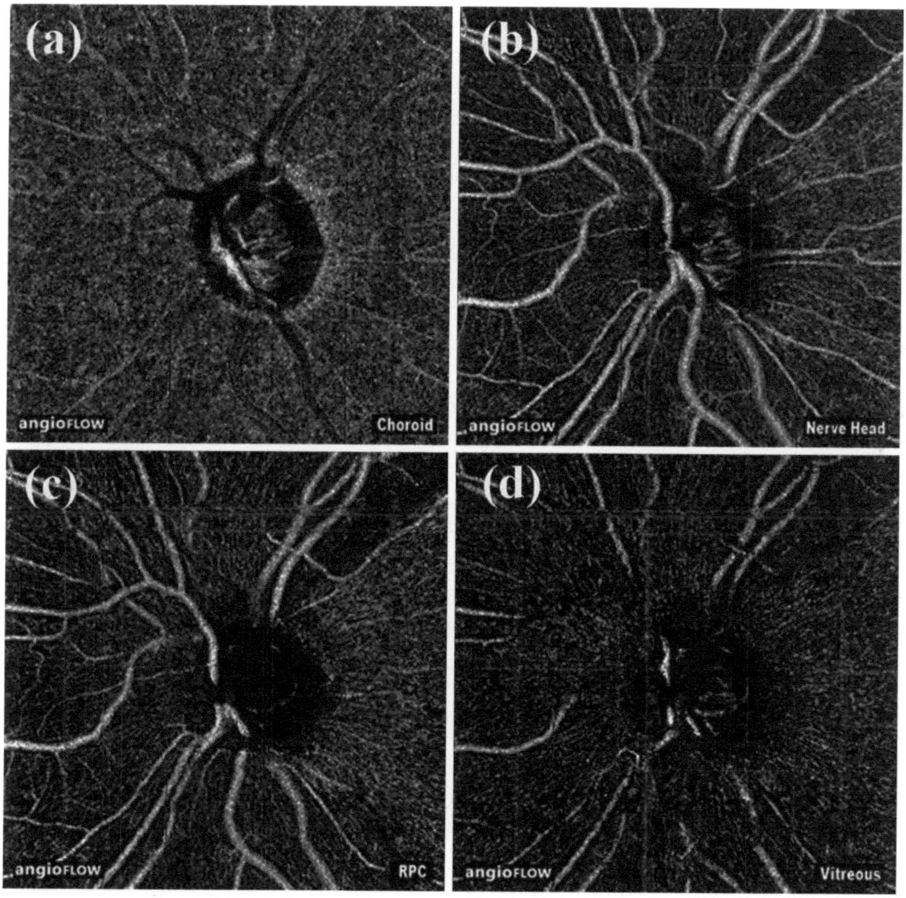

Fig. 20.25 Angiography slabs of the optic nerve head scan obtained using spectral domain optical coherence tomography showing the choroid (**a**), nerve head (**b**), radial peripapillary capillary, RPC (**c**) and vitreous (**d**) slabs

extends from the internal limiting membrane (ILM) to 150 μm posterior and is used for assessing the vasculature within the optic disc. The "radial peripapillary capillary (RPC)" layer extends from the ILM to the posterior boundary of the RNFL and is used for assessing the vascular supply of the RNFL layer of the peripapillary region. And the "choroidal slab" is used to assess the deep retinal and choroidal vasculature.

OCTA quantifies the ocular circulation using two parameters: flow index and vessel density. Flow index is defined as the average decorrelation values in the measured area, and vessel density, which is the most widely used OCTA parameter, is defined as the percentage area occupied by vessels in the measured area [65]. The threshold decorrelation value used to separate blood vessel and static tissue is set at 0.125, which is two standard deviations above the mean decorrelation value in the foveal avascular zone, a region devoid of vessels. Quantification of vessel density can be performed in the nerve head and the RPC slab of the optic disc scan, but not the choroidal slab. After acquiring the optic disc scan, the software automatically fits an ellipse to the optic disc margin. The region within this margin is referred to as the "inside disc" region. The peripapillary region is defined as a 0.75 mm-wide elliptical annulus extending from the optic disc boundary. This region is further divided in 6 sectors based on the Garway-Heath map.

Similarly, vessel densities can also be determined for the superficial vascular plexus of the macula scan. The macular region is divided in the small central foveal area and a 1.5 mm wide parafoveal, circular annulus. This parafoveal region is divided in 2 hemispheres of 180° each (superior and inferior). Additionally, it is also divided into 4 sectors of 90° each (nasal, inferior, superior, and temporal sectors). The current OCTA machines do not contain a normative database for comparison of the patient's vessel densities. Currently these comparisons are made in research studies using control eyes.

20.11 OCTA Report of a Normal Eye

Figure 20.26 shows the peripapillary OCTA report of a normal eye (showing normal optic disc and visual field). The OCTA report shows (Fig. 20.26a) angiography image showing large vessels and a dense network of capillaries in the RPC segment (Fig 20.26b) En face image (Fig. 20.26d, e) B scan showing the segmentation lines (for the RPC segment) along with the blood vessels detected by the SSADA algorithm (Fig. 20.26f) Heat map showing dense network of vessels in the peripapillary region; represented by warm colors such as red and yellow (Fig. 20.26c) Table showing the vessel density in the entire scan region and various sectors.

Figure 20.27 shows a macular OCTA report of a normal eye showing the superficial retinal vessels. Macular scan is performed using a 3 × 3 mm scan. The interpretation of the report is similar to that of the peripapillary report described earlier.

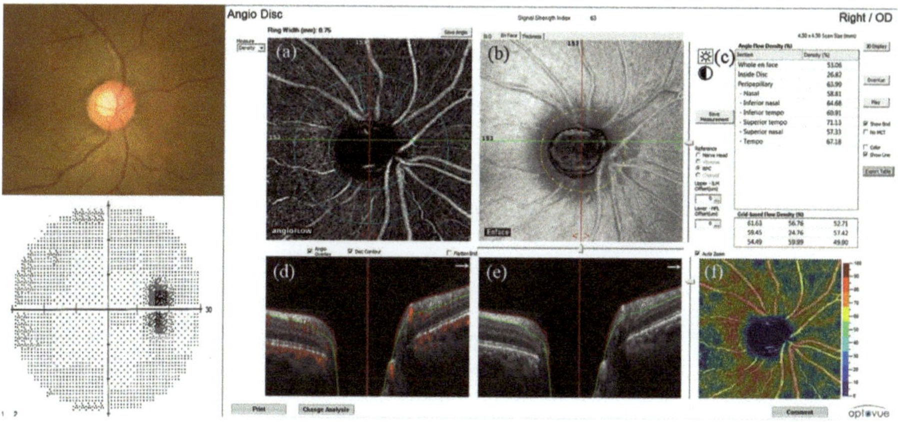

Fig. 20.26 Peripapillary OCTA report of an eye showing normal optic disc (upper left), normal retinal nerve fiber layer on enface image (**b**) and normal visual fields (lower left). The OCTA report shows dense radial peripapillary capillaries on the angiography image (**a**) and heat map (**f**) with vessel densities in different sectors quantified in the table (**c**). Segmentation of the angiography slab on B scan is shown in (**d**) and (**e**). Flow signals on the B scan is shown in (**d**)

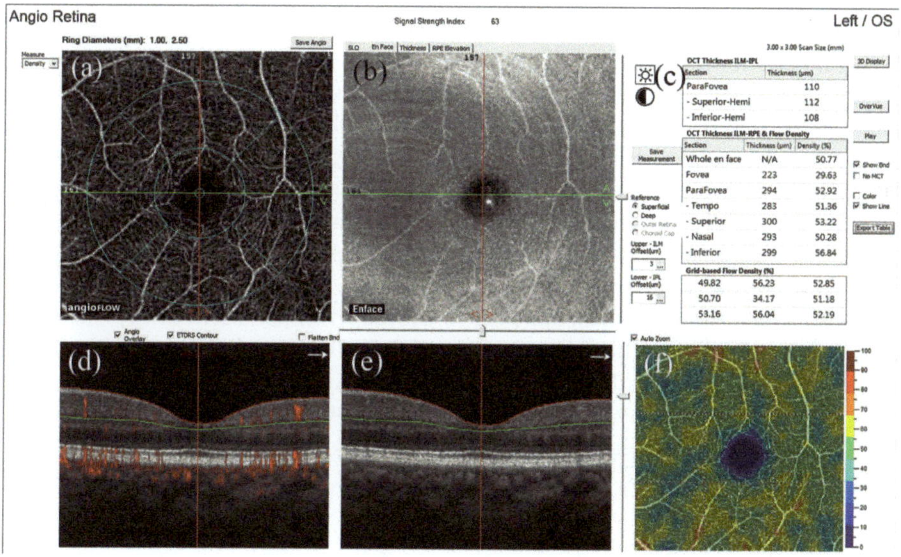

Fig. 20.27 Macular OCTA report showing the superficial retinal vessels of a normal eye. The OCTA report shows dense capillaries on the angiography image (**a**) and heat map (**f**) with vessel densities in different sectors quantified in the table (**c**). Enface image of the macula is shown in (**b**). Segmentation of the angiography slab on B scan is shown in (**d**) and (**e**). Flow signals on the B scan is shown in (**d**)

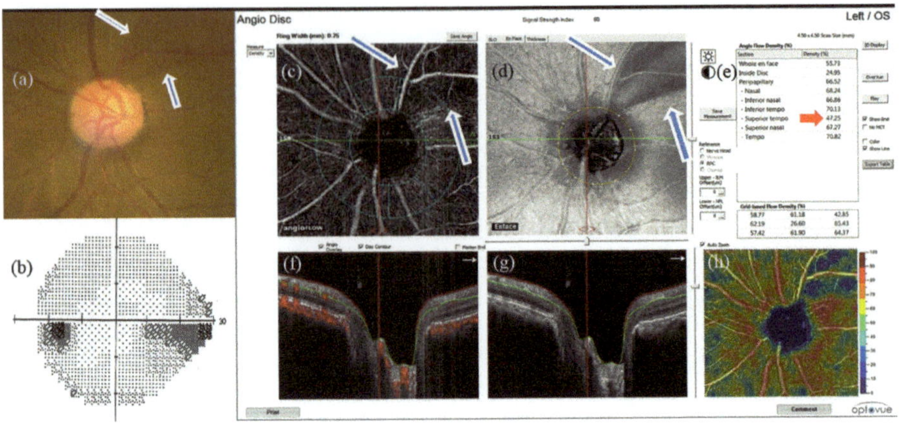

Fig. 20.28 Peripapillary OCTA report of a glaucomatous eyes with mild disease. Optic disc photograph (**a**) shows superior neuroretinal rim notch and superotemporal RNFL defect (indicated by arrows on the disc photograph) with a correlating inferior hemifield defect on the visual fields (**b**). OCTA report shows reduced vessel density in the superotemporal region as indicated by the arrows on the angiography (**c**) and heat map (**h**), along with a decrease in the vessel density in the corresponding region on the table (**e**, red arrow). Enface map (**d**) also shows the RNFL defect. fegmentation of the angiography slab on B scan is shown in (**f**) and (**g**). Flow signals on the B scan is shown in (**f**)

20.12 OCTA Report of a Glaucomatous Eye

Figure 20.28 shows a glaucomatous eye (mild severity of disease) with a superior neuroretinal rim notch and superotemporal RNFL defect (indicated by arrows on the disc photograph) with a correlating inferior hemifield defect on the visual fields. OCTA shows reduced vessel density in the superotemporal region on the angiography and the heat map, along with a decrease in the vessel density in the corresponding sector.

Figure 20.29 shows an eye with advanced glaucoma. OCTA shows gross loss of capillaries on the angiography and heat map, along with a decrease in the vessel densities in all peripapillary sectors in the Table.

Figure 20.30 shows a glaucomatous eye with superior hemifield defect and a corresponding inferior ganglion cell complex (GCC) thinning. OCTA shows reduced superficial retinal vessel density in the inferior macular region noted on the heat map. Figure 20.31 shows the heat map of macular OCTA scan of the same eye performed with 6 × 6 mm scan. Compared to the 3 × 3 mm scan, the vessel dropouts are more obvious on the 6 × 6 mm scan.

20.13 A Quantitative Analysis of OCTA Changes in Different Subtypes of Glaucoma

(i) POAG: All the initial studies with OCTA were performed in eyes with primary open angle glaucoma (POAG) and showed reduced flow index and vessel density inside the ONH and in the peripapillary region of eyes with POAG compared to controls [65, 67–69]. Multiple studies subsequently showed that the OCTA vessel densities measured in the macular regions were also reduced in eyes with glau-

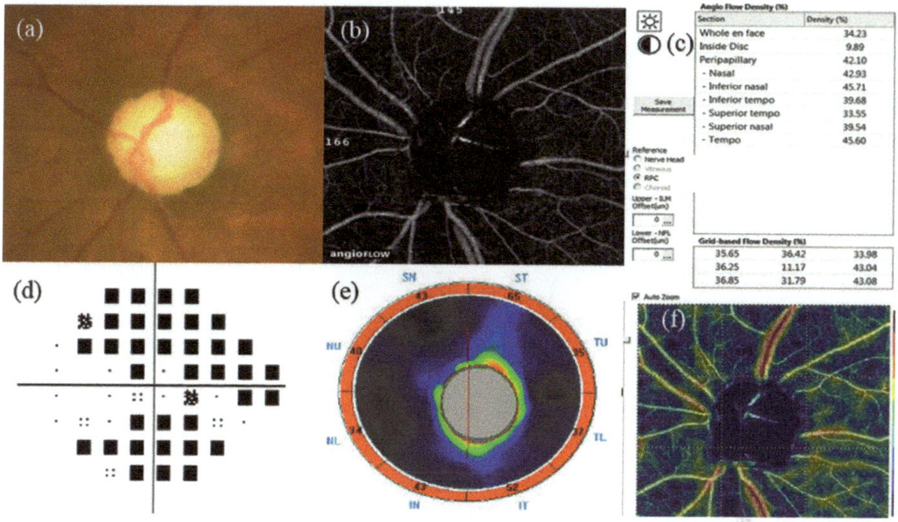

Fig. 20.29 Peripapillary OCTA report of a glaucomatous eyes with advanced disease, which shows advanced disc damage (**a**), bi-arcuate visual field loss (**d**) and diffuse RNFL thinning (**e**). OCTA report shows gross loss of capillaries on the angiography (**b**) and heat map (**f**), along with a decrease in the vessel densities in all peripapillary OCTA sectors in the table (**c**)

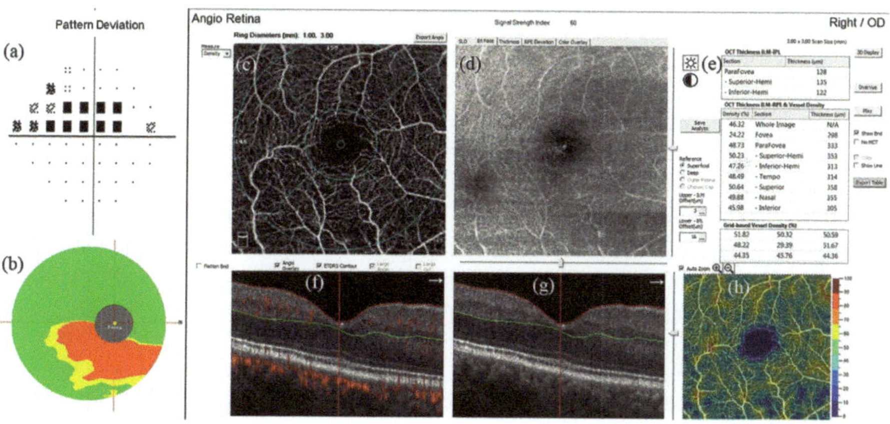

Fig. 20.30 Macular OCTA report of a glaucomatous eye which shows a superior hemifield defect (**a**) and a corresponding inferior ganglion cell complex thinning (**b**). OCTA shows reduced superficial macular vessel density in the inferior region on the angiography map (**c**), better noted on the heat map (**h**) and quantified in the table (**e**). Enface image of the macula is shown in (**d**). Segmentation of the angiography slab on B scan is shown in (**f**) and (**g**). Flow signals on the B scan is shown in (**f**)

coma compared to control eyes [70, 71]. Peripapillary vessel density reduction was found to be significantly greater than that inside the ONH and the macular region in glaucomatous eyes [70]. Vascular theory of glaucoma is considered to be more applicable in eyes developing glaucomatous damage at low/normal IOP. A few studies, therefore, compared the OCTA measurements in POAG eyes

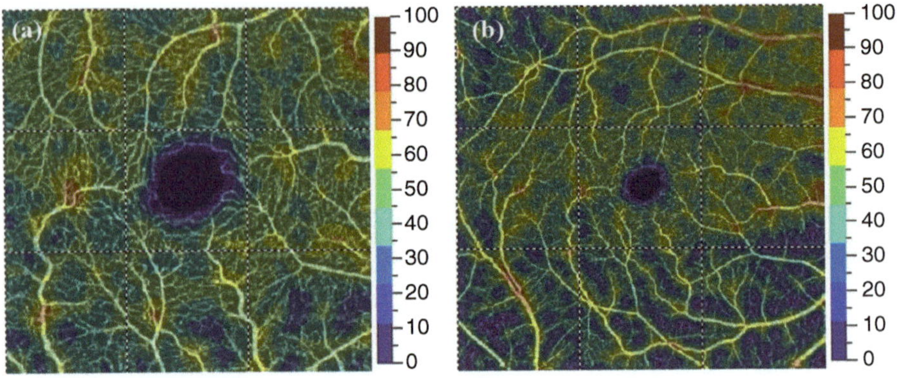

Fig. 20.31 Macular OCTA report of the eye shown in Fig. 20.30 imaged using a 3 × 3 mm (**a**) and a 6 × 6 mm scan (**b**). Compared to the 3 × 3 mm scan, the vessel dropouts are more obvious on the 6 × 6 mm scan

showing damage at low/normal IOP and high IOP. However, no differences in OCTA measurements were seen between these two POAG groups [70, 72].

(ii) Angle closure glaucoma: OCTA measurements in primary angle closure glaucoma (PACG) were found to be similar to that in POAG when the severity of disease was matched for [73]. Like POAG (described below), OCT neuronal (NRR, RNFL and GCC) measurements had a better diagnostic ability compared to OCTA vessel density measurements (inside ONH, in peripapillary and macular regions) in PACG [74]. Moghimi et al. demonestrated that in acute primary angle closure glaucoma, vessel density decreased over 6 weeks after an the attack compared with the contralateral unaffected eyes. In contrast, there was an initial increase in RNFL thickness that was followed by a subsequent decrease [75].

(iii) Pseudoexfoliation glaucoma: A few studies have evaluated the superficial retinal vasculature in the peripapillary region of PXG eyes and have reported that the reduction of vessel densities was greater in PXG compared to POAG eyes of similar disease severity [76, 77].

20.14 OCTA Changes in Perimetrically Intact Regions of Glaucomatous Eyes

It is important to determine the temporal relationship of vessel density reduction on OCTA with respect to RNFL thinning and visual field defects. This would help us develop strategies to detect the disease in the earliest stages. A longitudinal study is required to address this question. However, OCTA is a relatively new technology and there are, currently, no longitudinal studies addressing this question. As an alternate approach, studies have been performed in eyes with established perimetric glaucoma, whose visual field defects are limited to one hemifield; and the vascular changes in regions corresponding to the intact hemifield have been examined. These studies have found reduced peripapillary vessel density and RNFL thickness in the hemiretina corresponding to the perimetrically intact hemifield compared to that of healthy eyes [78–81]. One of these studies also found that the temporal sector of the perimetrically intact hemifield (corresponding to the region of papillomacular bundles) showed reduced vessel density in the presence of normal RNFL thickness [79]. This suggested that there may be regional variations in the alterations of RNFL thickness and vessel density measurements, and OCTA changes may precede RNFL changes in some sectors. In a longitudinal study with 13 months follow up by Shoji et al., eyes with POAG had significantly faster loss of macula vessel density than either glaucoma-suspect or healthy eyes. Serial OCTA measurements also detected glaucomatous change in macula vessel density in eyes without evidence of change in GCC thickness [82].

20.15 Comparing OCTA with OCT Measurements in Diagnosing Glaucoma

A number of studies have compared the diagnostic abilities of OCTA measurements (vessel densities of the inside disc, peripapillary and macular regions) with corresponding OCT measurements (ONH neuroretinal rim area, RNFL and macular thickness) in glaucoma.

A few studies comparing the diagnostic abilities (area under the receiver operating characteristic curves [AUC] and sensitivities at high specificities) of peripapillary vessel densities and RNFL thickness in POAG have found them to similar [68, 69, 73]. Depending on the severity of glaucoma patients included in these studies, the AUCs of both peripapillary vessel density and RNFL thickness have ranged between 0.85 to 0.95. A few other studies have reported a better diagnostic ability of RNFL thickness compared to peripapillary vessel density in POAG [71, 83]. In spite of the AUCs being similar, one study showed that the sensitivity to detect glaucoma in early stages of severity was better with RNFL thickness compared to peripapillary vessel density measurements [71]. Diagnostic abilities of vessel density measurements inside ONH were found to be significantly lesser than that of the OCT measured NRR area [71]. Similar to the peripapillary measurements, diagnostic ability of superficial retinal vessel density at macula was found to be similar to that of macular GCC thickness by one study [84] while the same was found to be inferior to GCC thickness by another study [71]. However, macular vessel densities in all these studies were evaluated on 3 × 3 mm scans, and a subsequent study showed that evaluating the macular vessel densities on 6 × 6 mm scans would be able to better detect glaucomatous changes [85]. It is still not clear if OCTA measured vessel density changes occur before or after OCT measured neuronal (NRR, RNFL and GCC) changes in glaucoma. Longitudinal studies in the future should be able to clarify this.

20.16 OCTA of the Peripapillary Choroid

Peripapillary choroidal circulation is of particular interest in glaucoma as it may be a surrogate marker for the perfusion of the deep ONH structures. Recently, choroidal microvasculature dropout (CMvD, Fig. 20.32), defined as the complete loss of

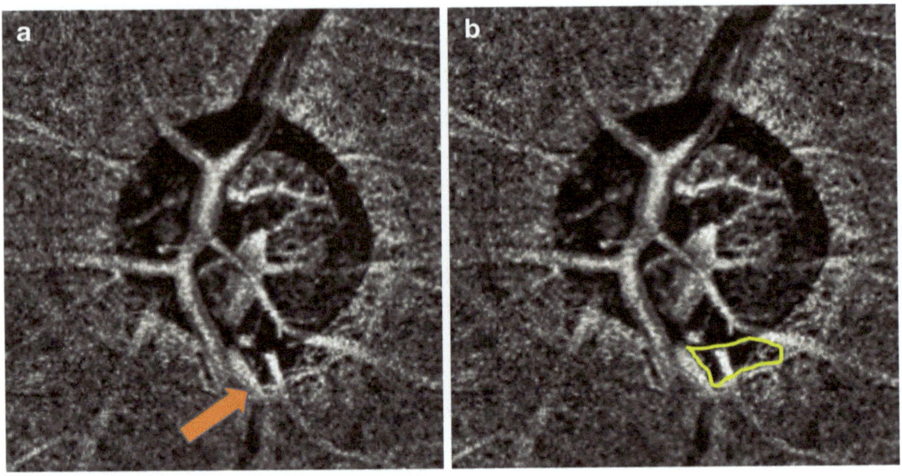

Fig. 20.32 Choroidal OCTA slab of a glaucomatous eye showing the presence of choroidal microvasculature dropout (CMvD) in the inferior region (**a**). Arrow points to the CMvD. Yellow line marks out the boundary of the CMvD (**b**)

choriocapillaris in localized regions of parapapillary atrophy (PPA), has been observed using OCTA in POAG eyes [86, 87]. CMvD has been shown to be a true perfusion defect using indocyanine green angiography [88]. Studies have also reported a topographic association between the location of CMvD and structural defects (RNFL thinning and lamina cribrosa defects) as well as functional defects (visual field loss) in POAG eyes [86, 89–91]. CMvD is a relatively novel finding in glaucoma and the clinical implications of it are not fully known. It has been argued that CMvD is likely to precede glaucomatous ONH damage [92]. A recent study reported an association between CMvD and progressive RNFL thinning in POAG eyes with DH [93]. Longitudinal studies are required to determine the clinical implication of CMvD in glaucoma.

20.17 Factors Affecting OCTA Measurements

Unlike the neuronal elements, vasculature is affected by multiple factors other than glaucoma. A study evaluated the effect of subject-related (age, gender, systemic hypertension and diabetes), eye-related (refractive error, optic disc size) and technology-related (signal strength index, SSI of the scans) determinants on the peripapillary and macular vessel densities in normal eyes [94]. It found that peripapillary vessel densities were higher in females. Peripapillary vessel densities were lower, while the macular vessel density was higher, in subjects with hypertension. Most of the vessel densities were lower in subjects with diabetes. In addition to these factors, SSI of the OCTA scans showed a significant positive association with the vessel densities of all regions. Vessel densities were higher in scans with higher

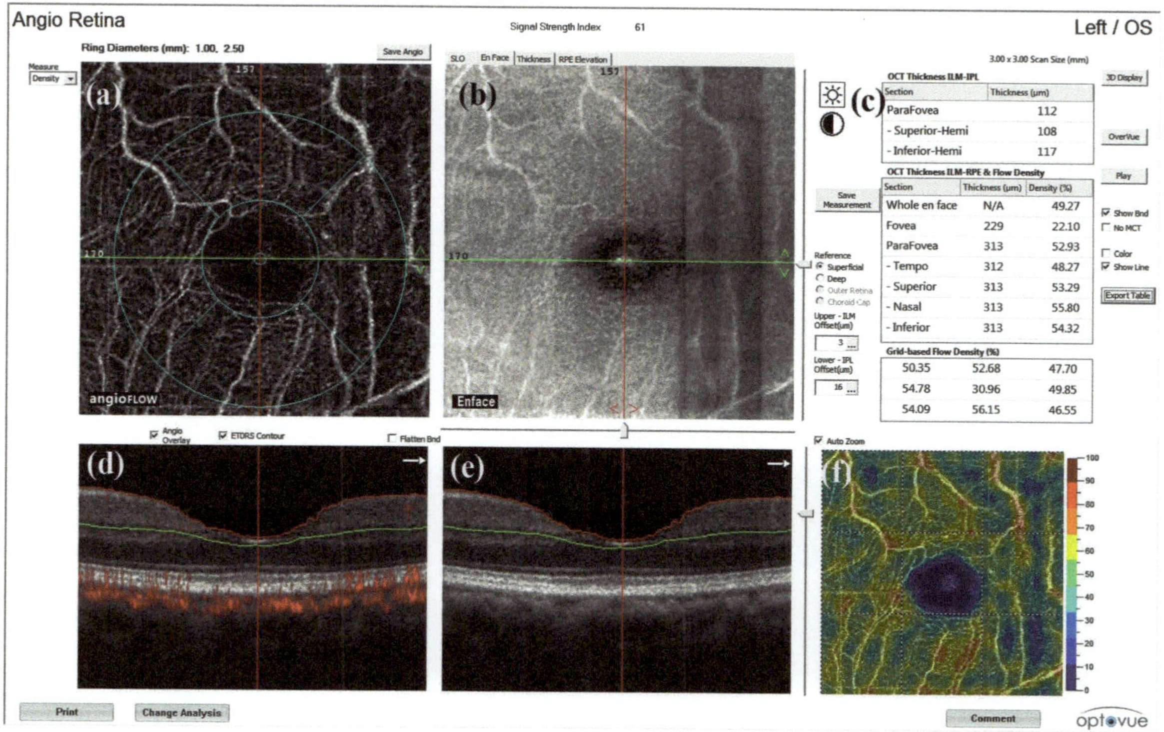

Fig. 20.33 Macular OCTA scan showing two types of artifacts; motion artifacts, recognized as vertical bands temporally on the en face map (**b**) and duplication of vessels, recognized inferiorly and nasally on the angiography map (**a**). These artifacts cause a decrease in vessel density in the temporal sector and increase in vessel density in the nasal and inferior sectors (noted on the heat map [**f**] and table [**c**]). Segmentation of the angiography slab on B scan is shown in (**d**) and (**e**). Flow signals on the B scan is shown in (**d**)

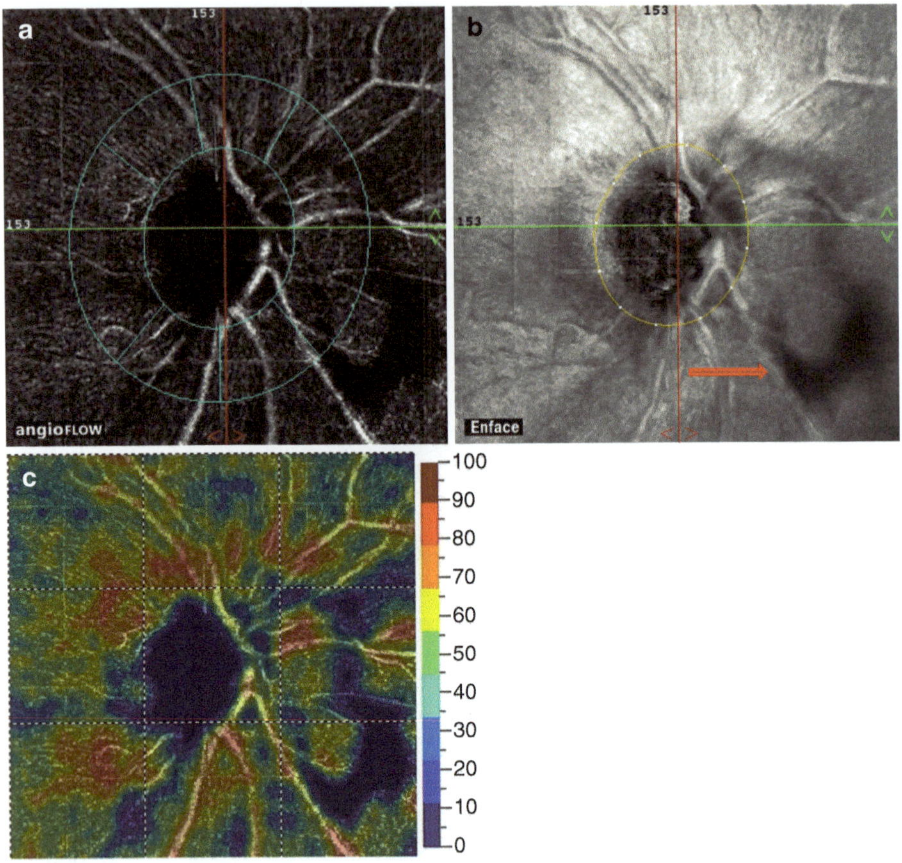

Fig. 20.34 Vitreous opacity (red arrow on en face map [**b**]) casting a shadow, as seen on the angiography map (**a**) and causing a falsely reduced vessel density on the heat map (**c**)

SSI values [94]. These results should be considered while interpreting the vessel densities in glaucoma.

20.18 Limitations and Recent Advances in OCTA

Motion artifacts are common with OCTA imaging due to the prolonged time required to acquire the scans; in spite of methods available to account for the artifacts (Fig. 20.33). This is true even in research settings and multiple studies have also reported high number of poor quality images with OCTA [95–98]. Two significant improvements incorporated recently to overcome the issue of poor quality scans are (1) real time eye tracking technology, for controlling the motion artifacts more effectively [99] and, (2) high-density (HD) scanning mode, for improving the resolution of the scans. A recent study has reported that the number of poor quality scans significantly decreased with the incorporation of these improvements [100].

Media opacities, especially vitreous opacities, can significantly affect the quality of OCTA scans and the quantification of vessel densities (Fig. 20.34).

OCTA technology is able to evaluate the superficial retinal vessels well but not the deeper retinal and choroidal vasculature. This is because the signals from the superficial retinal vessels project on to the deeper layers causing artifacts known as the projection artifacts [66]. Detection of CMvD, for example, is affected by the presence of projection artifacts. Newer methods of projection artifact correction have been tried and the newer generations of OCTA (projection resolved OCTA) are likely to evaluate the deeper retinal and choroidal vasculature better [101].

20.19 Summary

The introduction of OCT, has caused a paradigm shift in glaucoma diagnosis and monitoring. The information derived from OCT complements the information derived from the clinical examination and VF assessment in detecting glaucoma or its progression.

Acknowledgements This work is supported in part by NIH grant R01 EY029058 and, in part, an unrestricted grant from Research to Prevent Blindness (New York, NY).

References

1. Weinreb RN, Aung T, Medeiros FA. The pathophysiology and treatment of glaucoma: a review. JAMA. 2014;311:1901–11.
2. Tham YC, Li X, Wong TY, et al. Global prevalence of glaucoma and projections of glaucoma burden through 2040: a systematic review and meta-analysis. Ophthalmology. 2014;121:2081–90.
3. Bourne RR, Taylor HR, Flaxman SR, et al. Number of people blind or visually impaired by glaucoma worldwide and in world regions 1990-2010: a meta-analysis. PLoS One. 2016;11:e0162229.
4. Quigley HA, Addicks EM. Quantitative studies of retinal nerve fiber layer defects. Arch Ophthalmol. 1982;100:807–14.
5. Harwerth RS, Carter-Dawson L, Smith EL 3rd, et al. Neural losses correlated with visual losses in clinical perimetry. Invest Ophthalmol Vis Sci. 2004;45:3152–60.
6. Abrams LS, Scott IU, Spaeth GL, et al. Agreement among optometrists, ophthalmologists, and residents in evaluating the optic disc for glaucoma. Ophthalmology. 1994;101:1662–7.
7. Jampel HD, Friedman D, Quigley H, et al. Agreement among glaucoma specialists in assessing progressive disc changes from photographs in open-angle glaucoma patients. Am J Ophthalmol. 2009;147:39–44 e1.
8. Zeimer R, Asrani S, Zou S, et al. Quantitative detection of glaucomatous damage at the posterior pole by retinal thickness mapping. A pilot study. Ophthalmology. 1998;105:224–31.
9. Curcio CA, Allen KA. Topography of ganglion cells in human retina. J Comp Neurol. 1990;300:5–25.
10. Burgoyne C. The morphological difference between glaucoma and other optic neuropathies. J Neuroophthalmol. 2015;35(Suppl 1):S8–s21.
11. Mwanza JC, Oakley JD, Budenz DL, Anderson DR. Ability of cirrus HD-OCT optic nerve head parameters to discriminate normal from glaucomatous eyes. Ophthalmology. 2011;118:241–8 e1.

12. Leite MT, Rao HL, Weinreb RN, et al. Agreement among spectral-domain optical coherence tomography instruments for assessing retinal nerve fiber layer thickness. Am J Ophthalmol. 2011;151:85–92 e1.
13. Pierro L, Gagliardi M, Iuliano L, et al. Retinal nerve fiber layer thickness reproducibility using seven different OCT instruments. Invest Ophthalmol Vis Sci. 2012;53:5912–20.
14. Hwang YH, Kim YY, Kim HK, Sohn YH. Ability of cirrus high-definition spectral-domain optical coherence tomography clock-hour, deviation, and thickness maps in detecting photographic retinal nerve fiber layer abnormalities. Ophthalmology. 2013;120:1380–7.
15. Hwang YH, Jeong YC, Kim HK, Sohn YH. Macular ganglion cell analysis for early detection of glaucoma. Ophthalmology. 2014;121:1508–15.
16. Michelessi M, Lucenteforte E, Oddone F, et al. Optic nerve head and fibre layer imaging for diagnosing glaucoma. Cochrane Database Syst Rev. 2015:CD008803.
17. Kuang TM, Zhang C, Zangwill LM, et al. Estimating lead time gained by optical coherence tomography in detecting glaucoma before development of visual field defects. Ophthalmology. 2015;122:2002–9.
18. Oddone F, Lucenteforte E, Michelessi M, et al. Macular versus retinal nerve fiber layer parameters for diagnosing manifest glaucoma: a systematic review of diagnostic accuracy studies. Ophthalmology. 2016;123:939–49.
19. Kim YK, Ha A, Na KI, et al. Temporal relation between macular ganglion cell-inner plexiform layer loss and peripapillary retinal nerve Fiber layer loss in glaucoma. Ophthalmology. 2017;124:1056–64.
20. Hwang YH, Kim Y, Chung JK, Lee KB. Glaucomatous progression in the retinal nerve fibre and retinal ganglion cell-inner plexiform layers determined using optical coherence tomography-guided progression analysis. Clin Exp Optom. 2018;101:666–73.
21. Hou HW, Lin C, Leung CK. Integrating macular ganglion cell inner plexiform layer and parapapillary retinal nerve fiber layer measurements to detect glaucoma progression. Ophthalmology. 2018;125:822–31.
22. Lavinsky F, Wu M, Schuman JS, et al. Can macula and optic nerve head parameters detect glaucoma progression in eyes with advanced circumpapillary retinal nerve fiber layer damage? Ophthalmology. 2018;125:1907–12.
23. Mwanza JC, Chang RT, Budenz DL, et al. Reproducibility of peripapillary retinal nerve fiber layer thickness and optic nerve head parameters measured with cirrus HD-OCT in glaucomatous eyes. Invest Ophthalmol Vis Sci. 2010;51:5724–30.
24. Kim KE, Yoo BW, Jeoung JW, Park KH. Long-term reproducibility of macular ganglion cell analysis in clinically stable glaucoma patients. Invest Ophthalmol Vis Sci. 2015;56:4857–64.
25. Miki A, Medeiros FA, Weinreb RN, et al. Rates of retinal nerve fiber layer thinning in glaucoma suspect eyes. Ophthalmology. 2014;121:1350–8.
26. Yu M, Lin C, Weinreb RN, et al. Risk of visual field progression in glaucoma patients with progressive retinal nerve fiber layer thinning: a 5-year prospective study. Ophthalmology. 2016;123:1201–10.
27. Gracitelli CP, Abe RY, Tatham AJ, et al. Association between progressive retinal nerve fiber layer loss and longitudinal change in quality of life in glaucoma. JAMA Ophthalmol. 2015;133:384–90.
28. Quigley HA, Addicks EM. Regional differences in the structure of the lamina cribrosa and their relation to glaucomatous optic nerve damage. Arch Ophthalmol. 1981;99:137–43.
29. Kagemann L, Ishikawa H, Wollstein G, et al. Ultrahigh-resolution spectral domain optical coherence tomography imaging of the lamina cribrosa. Ophthalmic Surg Lasers Imaging. 2008;39:S126–31.
30. Inoue R, Hangai M, Kotera Y, et al. Three-dimensional high-speed optical coherence tomography imaging of lamina cribrosa in glaucoma. Ophthalmology. 2009;116:214–22.
31. Lee EJ, Kim TW, Weinreb RN, et al. Three-dimensional evaluation of the lamina cribrosa using spectral-domain optical coherence tomography in glaucoma. Invest Ophthalmol Vis Sci. 2012;53:198–204.

32. Lee EJ, Kim TW, Weinreb RN, et al. Visualization of the lamina cribrosa using enhanced depth imaging spectral-domain optical coherence tomography. Am J Ophthalmol. 2011;152:87–95 e1.
33. Park SC, De Moraes CG, Teng CC, et al. Enhanced depth imaging optical coherence tomography of deep optic nerve complex structures in glaucoma. Ophthalmology. 2012;119:3–9.
34. Girard MJ, Strouthidis NG, Ethier CR, Mari JM. Shadow removal and contrast enhancement in optical coherence tomography images of the human optic nerve head. Invest Ophthalmol Vis Sci. 2011;52:7738–48.
35. Mari JM, Strouthidis NG, Park SC, Girard MJ. Enhancement of lamina cribrosa visibility in optical coherence tomography images using adaptive compensation. Invest Ophthalmol Vis Sci. 2013;54:2238–47.
36. Mansouri K, Nuyen B, N Weinreb R. Improved visualization of deep ocular structures in glaucoma using high penetration optical coherence tomography. Expert Rev Med Devices. 2013;10:621–8.
37. Kim YW, Jeoung JW, Kim YK, Park KH. Clinical implications of in vivo lamina cribrosa imaging in glaucoma. J Glaucoma. 2017;26:753–61.
38. Furlanetto RL, Park SC, Damle UJ, et al. Posterior displacement of the lamina cribrosa in glaucoma: in vivo interindividual and intereye comparisons. Invest Ophthalmol Vis Sci. 2013;54:4836–42.
39. Park SC, Brumm J, Furlanetto RL, et al. Lamina cribrosa depth in different stages of glaucoma. Invest Ophthalmol Vis Sci. 2015;56:2059–64.
40. Lee SH, Kim TW, Lee EJ, et al. Diagnostic power of lamina cribrosa depth and curvature in glaucoma. Invest Ophthalmol Vis Sci. 2017;58:755–62.
41. Lee EJ, Kim TW, Weinreb RN, Kim H. Reversal of lamina cribrosa displacement after intraocular pressure reduction in open-angle glaucoma. Ophthalmology. 2013;120:553–9.
42. Reis AS, O'Leary N, Stanfield MJ, et al. Laminar displacement and prelaminar tissue thickness change after glaucoma surgery imaged with optical coherence tomography. Invest Ophthalmol Vis Sci. 2012;53:5819–26.
43. Lee EJ, Kim TW, Weinreb RN. Reversal of lamina cribrosa displacement and thickness after trabeculectomy in glaucoma. Ophthalmology. 2012;119:1359–66.
44. Wu Z, Lin C, Crowther M, et al. Impact of rates of change of lamina cribrosa and optic nerve head surface depths on visual field progression in glaucoma. Invest Ophthalmol Vis Sci. 2017;58:1825–33.
45. Lee EJ, Kim TW, Kim M, Kim H. Influence of lamina cribrosa thickness and depth on the rate of progressive retinal nerve fiber layer thinning. Ophthalmology. 2015;122:721–9.
46. Rhodes LA, Huisingh C, Johnstone J, et al. Variation of laminar depth in normal eyes with age and race. Invest Ophthalmol Vis Sci. 2014;55:8123–33.
47. Johnstone J, Fazio M, Rojananuangnit K, et al. Variation of the axial location of Bruch's membrane opening with age, choroidal thickness, and race. Invest Ophthalmol Vis Sci. 2014;55:2004–9.
48. Hayreh SS. Blood flow in the optic nerve head and factors that may influence it. Prog Retin Eye Res. 2001;20:595–624.
49. Lee KM, Kim TW, Weinreb RN, et al. Anterior lamina cribrosa insertion in primary open-angle glaucoma patients and healthy subjects. PLoS One. 2014;9:e114935.
50. Kim YW, Jeoung JW, Kim DW, et al. Clinical assessment of lamina cribrosa curvature in eyes with primary open-angle glaucoma. PLoS One. 2016;11:e0150260.
51. Girard MJ, Tun TA, Husain R, et al. Lamina cribrosa visibility using optical coherence tomography: comparison of devices and effects of image enhancement techniques. Invest Ophthalmol Vis Sci. 2015;56:865–74.
52. Kiumehr S, Park SC, Syril D, et al. In vivo evaluation of focal lamina cribrosa defects in glaucoma. Arch Ophthalmol. 2012;130:552–9.
53. You JY, Park SC, Su D, et al. Focal lamina cribrosa defects associated with glaucomatous rim thinning and acquired pits. JAMA Ophthalmol. 2013;131:314–20.
54. Tatham AJ, Miki A, Weinreb RN, et al. Defects of the lamina cribrosa in eyes with localized retinal nerve fiber layer loss. Ophthalmology. 2014;121:110–8.

55. Sharpe GP, Danthurebandara VM, Vianna JR, et al. Optic disc hemorrhages and laminar disinsertions in glaucoma. Ophthalmology. 2016;123:1949–56.
56. Kim YK, Park KH. Lamina cribrosa defects in eyes with glaucomatous disc haemorrhage. Acta Ophthalmol. 2016;94:e468–73.
57. Faridi OS, Park SC, Kabadi R, et al. Effect of focal lamina cribrosa defect on glaucomatous visual field progression. Ophthalmology. 2014;121:1524–30.
58. Moghimi S, Zangwill LM, Manalastas PIC, et al. Association between lamina cribrosa defects and progressive retinal nerve fiber layer loss in glaucoma. JAMA Ophthalmol. 2019;137:425–33.
59. Park HL, Lee J, Jung Y, Park CK. Optic disc hemorrhage and lamina cribrosa defects in glaucoma progression. Sci Rep. 2017;7:3489.
60. Park HL, Kim SI, Park CK. Influence of the lamina cribrosa on the rate of global and localized retinal nerve fiber layer thinning in open-angle glaucoma. Medicine (Baltimore). 2017;96:e6295.
61. Rao HL, Addepalli UK, Yadav RK, et al. Effect of scan quality on diagnostic accuracy of spectral-domain optical coherence tomography in glaucoma. Am J Ophthalmol. 2014;157:719–27 e1.
62. Rao HL, Addepalli UK, Yadav RK, et al. Factors affecting the ability of the spectral domain optical coherence tomograph to detect photographic retinal nerve fiber layer defects. PLoS One. 2014;9:e116115.
63. Hood DC, Kardon RH. A framework for comparing structural and functional measures of glaucomatous damage. Prog Retin Eye Res. 2007;26:688–710.
64. Wang Y, Bower BA, Izatt JA, et al. Retinal blood flow measurement by circumpapillary Fourier domain Doppler optical coherence tomography. J Biomed Opt. 2008;13:064003.
65. Jia Y, Morrison JC, Tokayer J, et al. Quantitative OCT angiography of optic nerve head blood flow. Biomed Opt Express. 2012;3:3127–37.
66. Jia Y, Tan O, Tokayer J, et al. Split-spectrum amplitude-decorrelation angiography with optical coherence tomography. Opt Express. 2012;20:4710–25.
67. Jia Y, Wei E, Wang X, et al. Optical coherence tomography angiography of optic disc perfusion in glaucoma. Ophthalmology. 2014;121:1322–32.
68. Liu L, Jia Y, Takusagawa HL, et al. Optical coherence tomography angiography of the peripapillary retina in glaucoma. JAMA Ophthalmol. 2015;133:1045–52.
69. Yarmohammadi A, Zangwill LM, Diniz-Filho A, et al. Optical coherence tomography angiography vessel density in healthy, glaucoma suspect, and glaucoma eyes. Invest Ophthalmol Vis Sci. 2016;57:OCT451–9.
70. Rao HL, Pradhan ZS, Weinreb RN, et al. Regional comparisons of optical coherence tomography angiography vessel density in primary open-angle glaucoma. Am J Ophthalmol. 2016;171:75–83.
71. Rao HL, Pradhan ZS, Weinreb RN, et al. A comparison of the diagnostic ability of vessel density and structural measurements of optical coherence tomography in primary open angle glaucoma. PLoS One. 2017;12:e0173930.
72. Scripsema NK, Garcia PM, Bavier RD, et al. Optical coherence tomography angiography analysis of perfused peripapillary capillaries in primary open-angle glaucoma and normal-tension glaucoma. Invest Ophthalmol Vis Sci. 2016;57:OCT611–OCT20.
73. Rao HL, Kadambi SV, Weinreb RN, et al. Diagnostic ability of peripapillary vessel density measurements of optical coherence tomography angiography in primary open-angle and angle-closure glaucoma. Br J Ophthalmol. 2017;101:1066–70.
74. Rao HL, Pradhan ZS, Weinreb RN, et al. Vessel density and structural measurements of optical coherence tomography in primary angle closure and primary angle closure glaucoma. Am J Ophthalmol. 2017;177:106–15.
75. Moghimi S, SafiZadeh M, Fard MA, et al. Changes in optic nerve head vessel density after acute primary angle closure episode. Invest Ophthalmol Vis Sci. 2019 Feb 1;60(2):552–8.
76. Suwan Y, Geyman LS, Fard MA, et al. Peripapillary perfused capillary density in exfoliation syndrome and exfoliation glaucoma versus POAG and healthy controls: an OCTA study. Asia Pac J Ophthalmol (Phila). 2018;7:84–9.

77. Park JH, Yoo C, Girard MJA, et al. Peripapillary vessel density in glaucomatous eyes: comparison between pseudoexfoliation glaucoma and primary open-angle glaucoma. J Glaucoma. 2018;27:1009–16.
78. Yarmohammadi A, Zangwill LM, Diniz-Filho A, et al. Peripapillary and macular vessel density in patients with glaucoma and single-hemifield visual field defect. Ophthalmology. 2017;124:709–19.
79. Pradhan ZS, Dixit S, Sreenivasaiah S, et al. A sectoral analysis of vessel density measurements in perimetrically intact regions of glaucomatous eyes: an optical coherence tomography angiography study. J Glaucoma. 2018;27:525–31.
80. Pradhan ZS, Puttaiah NK. Optic Nerve Head and Retinal Nerve Fiber Layer Imaging in the Diagnosis and Management of Glaucoma. In: Prajna NV, Editor. Peyman's Principles and Practice of Ophthalmology. New Delhi: Jaypee Brothers Medical Publishers, 2018:1081–93.
81. Chen CL, Bojikian KD, Wen JC, et al. Peripapillary retinal nerve fiber layer vascular microcirculation in eyes with glaucoma and single-hemifield visual field loss. JAMA Ophthalmol. 2017;135:461–8.
82. Shoji T, Zangwill LM, Akagi T, et al. Progressive Macula Vessel Density Loss in Primary Open-Angle Glaucoma: A Longitudinal Study. Am J Ophthalmol 2017;182:107–17.
83. Chihara E, Dimitrova G, Amano H, Chihara T. Discriminatory power of superficial vessel density and prelaminar vascular flow index in eyes with glaucoma and ocular hypertension and normal eyes. Invest Ophthalmol Vis Sci. 2017;58:690–7.
84. Chen HS, Liu CH, Wu WC, et al. Optical coherence tomography angiography of the superficial microvasculature in the macular and peripapillary areas in glaucomatous and healthy eyes. Invest Ophthalmol Vis Sci. 2017;58:3637–45.
85. Takusagawa HL, Liu L, Ma KN, et al. Projection-resolved optical coherence tomography angiography of macular retinal circulation in glaucoma. Ophthalmology. 2017;124:1589–99.
86. Suh MH, Zangwill LM, Manalastas PI, et al. Deep retinal layer microvasculature dropout detected by the optical coherence tomography angiography in glaucoma. Ophthalmology. 2016;123:2509–18.
87. Lee EJ, Kim TW, Lee SH, Kim JA. Underlying microstructure of parapapillary deep-layer capillary dropout identified by optical coherence tomography angiography. Invest Ophthalmol Vis Sci. 2017;58:1621–7.
88. Lee EJ, Lee KM, Lee SH, Kim TW. Parapapillary choroidal microvasculature dropout in glaucoma: a comparison between optical coherence tomography angiography and indocyanine green angiography. Ophthalmology. 2017;124:1209–17.
89. Lee EJ, Lee SH, Kim JA, Kim TW. Parapapillary deep-layer microvasculature dropout in glaucoma: topographic association with glaucomatous damage. Invest Ophthalmol Vis Sci. 2017;58:3004–10.
90. Shin JW, Kwon J, Lee J, Kook MS. Choroidal microvasculature dropout is not associated with myopia, but is associated with glaucoma. J Glaucoma. 2018;27:189–96.
91. Rao HL, Sreenivasaiah S, Riyazuddin M, et al. Choroidal microvascular dropout in primary angle closure glaucoma. Am J Ophthalmol. 2019;199:184–92.
92. Lee EJ, Kim TW, Kim JA, Kim JA. Central visual field damage and parapapillary choroidal microvasculature dropout in primary open-angle glaucoma. Ophthalmology. 2018;125:588–96.
93. Park HL, Kim JW, Park CK. Choroidal microvasculature dropout is associated with progressive retinal nerve Fiber layer thinning in glaucoma with disc hemorrhage. Ophthalmology. 2018;125:1003–13.
94. Rao HL, Pradhan ZS, Weinreb RN, et al. Determinants of peripapillary and macular vessel densities measured by optical coherence tomography angiography in normal eyes. J Glaucoma. 2017;26:491–7.
95. Suh MH, Zangwill LM, Manalastas PI, et al. Optical coherence tomography angiography vessel density in glaucomatous eyes with focal lamina cribrosa defects. Ophthalmology. 2016;123:2309–17.
96. Hollo G. Intrasession and between-visit variability of sector peripapillary angioflow vessel density values measured with the angiovue optical coherence tomograph in different retinal layers in ocular hypertension and glaucoma. PLoS One. 2016;11:e0161631.

97. Spaide RF, Fujimoto JG, Waheed NK. Image artifacts in optical coherence tomography angiography. Retina. 2015;35:2163–80.
98. Venugopal JP, Rao HL, Weinreb RN, et al. Repeatability of vessel density measurements of optical coherence tomography angiography in normal and glaucoma eyes. Br J Ophthalmol. 2018;102:352–7.
99. Camino A, Zhang M, Gao SS, et al. Evaluation of artifact reduction in optical coherence tomography angiography with real-time tracking and motion correction technology. Biomed Opt Express. 2016;7:3905–15.
100. Venugopal JP, Rao HL, Weinreb RN, et al. Repeatability and comparability of peripapillary vessel density measurements of high-density and non-high-density optical coherence tomography angiography scans in normal and glaucoma eyes. Br J Ophthalmol. 2019;103:949–54.
101. Campbell JP, Zhang M, Hwang TS, et al. Detailed vascular anatomy of the human retina by projection-resolved optical coherence tomography angiography. Sci Rep. 2017;7:42201.
102. Rao HL, Pradhan ZS, Puttaiah NK. Optic Nerve Head and Retinal Nerve Fiber Layer Imaging in the Diagnosis and Management of Glaucoma. In: Prajna NV, Editor. Peyman's Principles and Practice of Ophthalmology. New Delhi: Jaypee Brothers Medical Publishers; 2018:1081–93.

OCT in Amblyopia

21

Paolo Nucci, Andrea Lembo, Stefano Lucentini, and Francesco Pichi

Amblyopia is one of the most common cause of monocular visual loss in children and young adults in many countries and can be defined as a disorder characterized by a dysfunction of the processing of visual information [1]. It results from degradation of the retinal image during the period of visual development, which historically has been thought to be the first 6 years of life [2]. Therefore, amblyopia never occurs in isolation; the disease is not the cause, but the effect of another pathological process. Amblyopia can be seen as a result of either disuse, due to the absence of a clear image on the retina (anisometropia or deprivation), or misuse, due to abnormal binocular interaction (strabismus) [3]. In fact, primary types of amblyopia include anisometropia, strabismus, form deprivation and high bilateral refractive errors. In particular, the degradation of the image, and subsequent central suppression that leads to amblyopia results from one of the three causal processes.

In 2003, the American Association for Pediatric Ophthalmology and Strabismus (AAPOS) published a list of risk factors for amblyopia [4]; Arnold et al. [5] attempted to estimate cut-off found by the AAPOS in a meta-analysis. The following results were obtained: approximate prevalence of anisometropia of 1.2%, hyperopia of 6%, astigmatism of 15%, myopia of 0.6%, strabismus of 2.5%, and a visual acuity less than 20/40 of 6%. The mean combined prevalence found was 21% ± 2% compared to a prevalence of amblyopia 20/40 and worse of 2.5%. The estimated prevalence of amblyopia in adults is 2–9% [6], and it still seems to be the leading cause of monocular vision loss in people aged between 20 and 70 years [7]. In light of these data, it is easy to think how important an early diagnosis of amblyopia is.

P. Nucci · A. Lembo (✉) · S. Lucentini
Department of Clinical Sciences and Community Health, Istituto di Ricovero e Cura a Carattere Scientifico (IRCCS) Multimedica, University of Milan, Eye Clinic San Giuseppe Hospital, Milan, Italy
e-mail: paolo.nucci@unimi.it; stefano.lucentini@unimi.it

F. Pichi
Eye Institute, Cleveland Clinic Abu Dhabi, Abu Dhabi, United Arab Emirates

A. Grzybowski, P. Barboni (eds.), *OCT and Imaging in Central Nervous System Diseases*, https://doi.org/10.1007/978-3-030-26269-3_21

The diagnosis of unilateral amblyopia is made when reduced visual acuity is recorded in the presence of an amblyogenic factor, and not explained by another ocular abnormality. Residual visual deficits after correction of any amblyogenic factor (for example by spectacles prescription) are assumed to be due to amblyopia [3]. A widely-accepted definition of amblyopia based on visual acuity is two or more Snellen or logMAR lines difference between eyes in best-corrected visual acuity. A one-line difference is usually a normal result, based on test-retest variability [8]. One important feature of visual acuity testing to diagnose amblyopia is that there is a distribution or range of typical visual acuity in any population. This range changes with age because of neural maturational processes [3].

Although clinical ocular examination is most often normal in amblyopia, microscopic anatomical and structural abnormalities have been found, starting from Hubel and Wiesel's pioneering work [9] in the retina, lateral geniculate bodies, and visual cortex [10–12]. Amblyopia is thought to be related to abnormalities in the visual cortex. However, it is quite controversial whether the choroid and retina are involved in the pathologic changes of amblyopia. With the advent of OCT in ophthalmology, there have been numerous attempts to investigate the structural differences in macular and peripapillary retinal nerve fiber layer (RNFL) in amblyopic patients [13–15]. Despite the use of more and more advanced techniques, conflicting results have often been found. Khan [16] compared the anterior and posterior ocular architecture of amblyopic and normal fellow eyes in 14 patients with *hyperopic anisometropic amblyopia*. Subjects were children between 5 and 10 years of age, with hyperopia >1.5 D and unilateral amblyopia with an interocular difference in spherical equivalent of at least 1D. Patients were examined using two tools: corneal topography to measure anterior and posterior corneal curvature, corneal thickness and volume, anterior chamber volume and depth; and OCT for RNFL, central macular thickness and macular volume measurements. In these children, corneal topography and OCT revealed no differences ($P > 0.05$) in the anterior and posterior architecture between the amblyopic and the fellow eye. Wu et al. [17] examined a larger sample, including 72 children (range 5–16 years) to compare the RNFL and macular thickness in amblyopic eyes with that in fellow eyes. All enrolled children had unilateral hyperopic anisometropic amblyopia and normal vision in the contralateral eye. After a full ophthalmological assessment, OCT scans were performed using a spectral domain OCT (3D-OCT 1000). The foveolar thickness, central macular thickness and four quadrants of the inner and outer macular thickness were measured for each subject. Peripapillary RNFL thickness was measured using the "fast RNFL thickness (3.4mm diameter)" scan protocol, which consisted of six radial line scans. OCT measurements found thicker foveolas and peripapillary RNFL in eyes with hyperopic anisometropic amblyopia compared to the contralateral eyes, but no changes in 1-mm central macular thickness (Fig. 21.1). This difference between foveolar thickness and 1-mm central macular thickness needs further histopathologic investigation. No correlation was found between severity of anisometropia and differences of peripapillary RNFL thickness, or between central macular thickness and foveal thickness in the contralateral eyes, suggesting far more complex

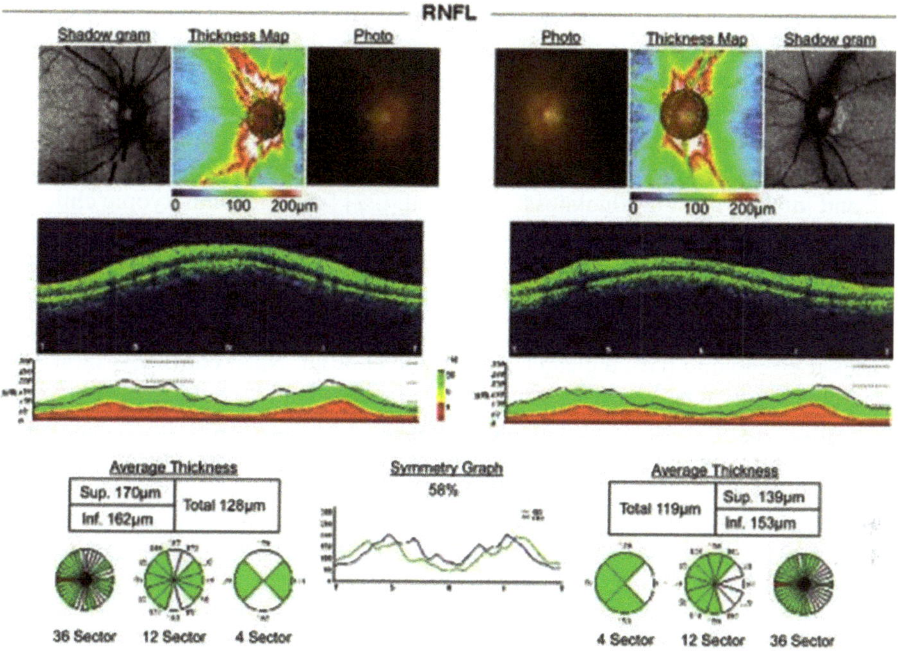

Fig. 21.1 OCT of retinal nerve fiber layer (RNFL) in a patient with hyperopic anisometropic amblyopia (Courtesy of Wu SQ, et al. Macular and peripapillary retinal nerve fiber layer thickness in children with hyperopic anisometropic amblyopia. Int J Ophthalmol. 2013;6(1):85–9)

pathophysiologic mechanisms for anisometropic amblyopia than we currently know. An interesting biological theory regarding differences in RNFL thickness in eyes with and without amblyopia proposes that in humans the total population of cells in the ganglion cell layer is at its highest approximately between 18 and 30 weeks of gestation and declines rapidly thereafter [18]. The number of axons in the human optic nerve decreases too during gestation [19]. Absence of normal visual stimulation may contribute to the reduced apoptosis of retinal ganglion cells in amblyopic eyes, eventually leading to thicker RNFL compared to non-amblyopic eye. Yen et al. [20] mentioned that the physiological postnatal ganglion cell reduction could be inhibited in amblyopia, while Kok et al. [21] concluded that an hypothetical arrest of the normal ganglion cell reduction is expected to lead to an abnormally thick retinal thickness, especially the pericentral retinal thickness. A second hypothesis seems to regard the macula, which becomes thicker rather than thinner in the perifoveal retina in 6-month embryos, manifesting a slight protrusion. Wu et al. [17] found that the foveola was significantly thicker in amblyopic eyes than in the fellow eyes (181.4 ± 14.2 µm *vs* 175.2 ± 13.3 µm, $P < 0.01$). In their studies, blurred vision could lead to insufficient stimulation in the amblyopic eye, affecting the normal maturation of the macula, including movement of Henle's fibers away from the fovea and a decrease in foveal cone diameter, which would result in increased foveolar thickness.

Regarding myopic amblyopia, Pang et al. [22] conducted a study on 31 children with a mean age of 9.56 years and mean spherical equivalent in amblyopic eyes of −10.79 ± 3.40 diopters. Patients were scanned with OCT using the "Fast macular thickness protocol". The following ten parameters were measured for each subject: foveal minimum thickness, average foveal thickness, inner nasal, superior, temporal, and inferior macular thickness, outer nasal, superior, temporal, and inferior macular thickness. Pang et al. [22] found that amblyopic children with unilateral high myopia tend to have a thicker fovea and thinner inner and outer layers in the amblyopic eye compared to the normal fellow eye (Fig. 21.2).

Another important parameter that can be detected at OCT and that can be investigated in amblyopic eyes is the thickness of the choroid. Nowadays, the EDI OCT makes it possible to have a clearer view of the choroid. Nishi et al. [23] showed a different choroidal profile in the amblyopic eyes and found the subfoveal choroid of eyes with hyperopic anisometropic amblyopia significantly thicker than that of the fellow eyes and the age-matched normal eyes (Fig. 21.3). Xu et al. [24] investigated the choroidal thickness (CT) in children with amblyopia through SD-OCT and found that in the subfoveal area, the choroid was thicker in amblyopic eyes than in fellow eyes and control eyes as well. In contrast, Niyaz et al. [25] found that the

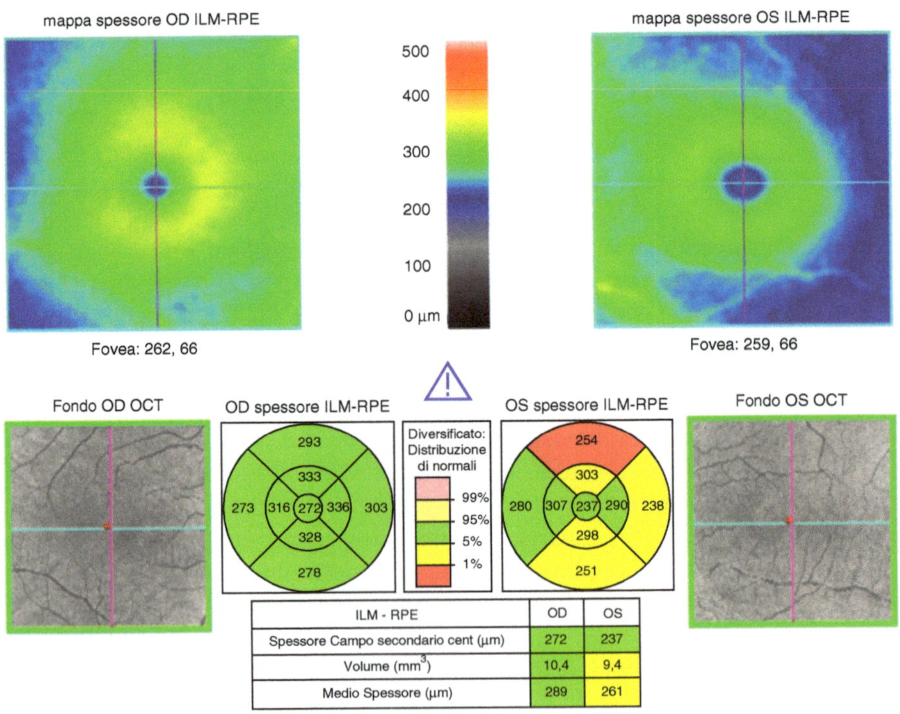

Fig. 21.2 OCT images from an amblyopic subject (OD: amblyopic eye; OS: fellow eye). Refractive error OD: −6.00–1.25 × 165, OS: −1.25 sph (Thanks to F. Bonsignore—University Eye Clinic-Ospedale San Giuseppe, Milan)

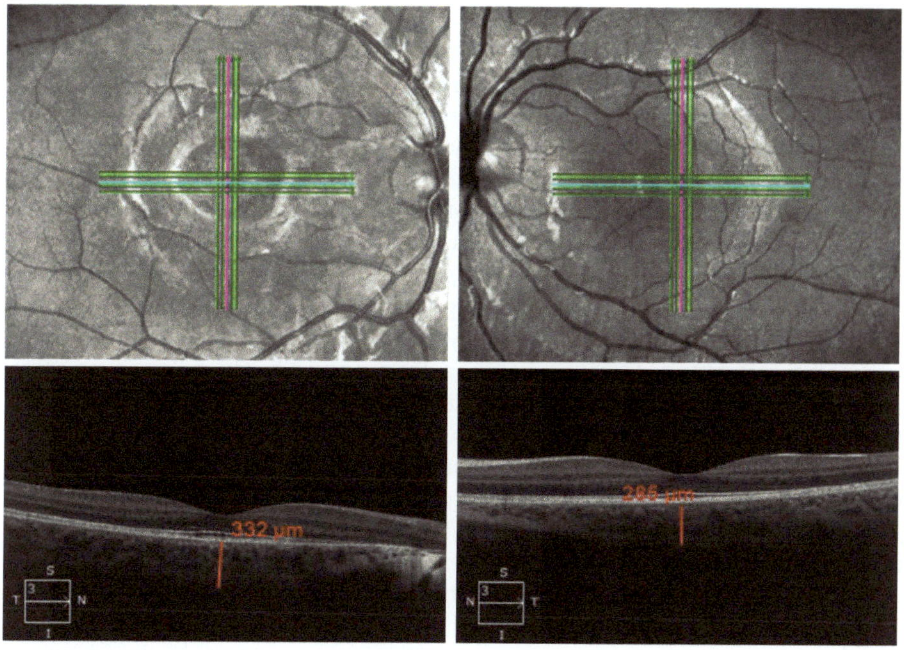

Fig. 21.3 Enhanced depth imaging spectral domain optical coherence tomographic (EDI-SD-OCT) images of an anisohypermetropic amblyopic eye (right) and control eye (left) (Thanks to F. Bonsignore—University Eye Clinic-Ospedale San Giuseppe, Milan)

choroidal thickness was not significantly different between amblyopic and fellow eyes in strabismus 175 patients.

Moreover, Pang et al. [26] showed that the increased central macular thickness of eyes with myopic anisometropic amblyopia tended to decrease to the fellow eye level after amblyopia treatment (refractive correction and patching). These results indicate that anatomic changes may be present in the retinas of amblyopic children with unilateral high myopia and these changes could be partially reversible with proper treatment. Anisometropia as the most frequent cause of amblyopia has been evaluated in numerous studies. However, anisometropia associated with high myopia has often been excluded from these studies. The few studies investigating *anisometropic amblyopia* caused by unilateral high myopia have concluded that this type of amblyopia had poorer treatment outcomes [27]. Underlying structural abnormalities and macular hypoplasia have been proposed as causes for the poor treatment outcomes in myopic anisometropia [28, 29]. Knowledge of the macular structure and associated factors in amblyopia associated with unilateral high myopia will help the understanding of this disease and may assist clinicians in predicting treatment outcomes. Studies that have focused on comparison between *strabismic and anisometropic amblyopia*, have found differences between the two defects. Dickmann et al. [30] conducted a study to determine whether RNFL thickness, macular thickness, and foveal volume in patients with unilateral amblyopia differed between the amblyopic and the fellow eye. Stratus OCT was performed on 80 eyes of 40 patients (mean age, 15.2 years; range, 5–56 years) with unilateral amblyopia divided into 20 strabismic and 20 anisometropic. OCT found that the difference in RNFL thickness between the amblyopic and fellow eyes was no statistically significant ($p > 0.05$) in both groups. Conversely, macular thickness and foveal volume in strabismic amblyopia were 5% lower in the fellow eye than in the amblyopic one. On the other hand, in the anisometropic group there was no significant difference between eyes in either macular thickness or foveal volume. Dickmann et al. [31] found similar results on 15 patients with strabismic anisometropia and 15 patients with anisometric amblyopia. In both groups, mean foveal volume and RNFL thickness did not differ significantly between eyes. Only macular thickness in the strabismic group differed significantly between the amblyopic and fellow eyes. This statistically significant difference, also established in other studies [15, 30], was not present in the refractive amblyopia group: amblyopia of different etiologies could therefore be associated with different changes of the retinal tissues. Thickening of the amblyopic fovea could be related to a developmental arrest, with incomplete formation of the foveal depression, even if it's difficult to determine whether this may be caused by a direct effect of abnormal sensory output or the consequence of primary alteration of visual cortex and the lateral geniculate nucleus (Fig. 21.2). There was also a significant correlation between RNFL thickness and macular sensitivity measured with microperimetry (strabismic group, $r = 0.84$, $P = 0.002$; anisometropic group, $r = 0.66$, $P = 0.02$). Although visual fields generally appear normal, amblyopia can be associated with small central and paracentral scotoma in some amblyopic eyes but do not need further evaluations, especially if the patient is asymptomatic. If a deep focal deficit is found, causes of organic pathologies (for example optic neuropathy) should be investigated. Data from Dickmann et al. [31] study suggest that the anatomical differences of RNFL thickness between the amblyopic and the fellow eye could determine the difference in macular sensitivity between the two eyes. Additional studies with larger, more diverse cohorts are needed to reveal whether these findings can be confirmed. Szigeti et al. [32] used OCT imaging and image segmentation methodology on 38 patients (range 6–67 years) with different types of amblyopia (strabismus without anisometropia, anisometropia without strabismus, strabismus with anisometropia). They detected structural changes in the outer nuclear layer of the fovea, suggesting the possible involvement of photoreceptor. There is ***growing*** evidence showing that photoreceptors may be affected in amblyopia. For example, Enoch [33] using the Stiles-Crawford function suggested that photoreceptor orientation is abnormal in amblyopic eyes, while other Authors did not found indication of retinal dysfunction at the level of the cones in amblyopic eyes [25]. Nishi et al. [23] used SD OCT to analyze the thickness of the outer nuclear layer (ONL), photoreceptor inner segment (IS) layer and outer segment (OS) layer of 21 patients (mean 6.0 ± 2.3 years) with anisohypermetropic amblyopia and 25 age-matched controls (mean 5.6 ± 1.9 years). Additionally, they assessed the effects of optical treatments on the photoreceptor layer. Results showed that the length of the OS was significantly lower in the amblyopic eyes (42.4 ± 4.6 μm, $p = 0.03$) compared to the fellow eyes (48.0 ± 6.6 μm).

One year after the optical treatment, the best-corrected visual acuity (BCVA) improved and the length of the OS was significantly increased ($p = 0.0001$). The change of BCVA was significantly correlated with the change of the length of the OS 1 year after the treatment ($r = 0.52$; $p = 0.0004$). Even if the number of patients is exiguous and children enrolled have only hyperopic anisometropic amblyopia, this study suggest that there are qualitative and quantitative differences in the microstructure of photoreceptors of amblyopic fovea from normal one. Furthermore, optical treatment in anisohypermetropic amblyopia can induce dynamic changes in photoreceptors (increase in the OS length in the amblyopic eyes after the optical treatment, with significant correlation between the increased OS length and better BCVA). Anyway, the relationship between these morpho-structural changes and the amblyopia is still far from being clearly understood. Further studies are warranted to investigate better these changes [34].

As we previously anticipated, various studies in the latest 5 years investigated through OCT the correlation between Choroidal Thickness (CT) changes and amblyopia (both anisometropic and strabismic amblyopia) in children. A Meta-Analysis by Liu et al. [35], which includes 11 clinical trial involving 449 patients, indicated that the amblyopic process may involve the choroid. The results showed that the CT was thicker in the amblyopic eyes than in both the fellow and control eyes from the fovea to the temporal and nasal cavities at different interval (range: 0.5–3 mm) points. Sub-Foveal Choroideal Thickness (SFCT) did not differ between anisometropic and strabismic amblyopia. Congruously with previous study, foveola was thicker in the amblyopic eyes than that in the visually normal control eyes. In this regard, the authors provide a suggestive theory to explain the CT thicker in amblyopic eyes. A thicker retina may require additional blood for nourishment. Therefore, the CT may have to increase to supply additional blood to the retina. Increased choroidal blood flow can cause choroidal thickening. Using split-spectrum amplitude-decorrelation angiography OCT (SSADA-OCT), simply known as OCT-Angiography, Guo et al. [36] discovered that 86.4% of the amblyopic eyes displayed a blurry choroidocapillary network and that 68.2% of the amblyopic eyes had a dark atrophic patch. The authors said that it was possible that the choriocapillary atrophy patch caused a wide range of compensatory dilatation of its surrounding capillaries, and because of this, blurry images occurred. Dilatation of the choroidal vessels may lead to increased CT. All the studies included in the Meta-Analysis by Liu used SD-OCT. This could be a potential bias if we consider that swept source OCT (SS-OCT) is recognized as the latest landmark in choroidal imaging. Up to date, Araki et al. [37] published the only study which investigate the macular retinal and choroidal thickness in amblyopic eyes using SS-OCT. The design of the study is similar to those included in the Meta-Analysis, but the results are quite surprising: although there were significant differences in CT with hyperopic anisometropic amblyopia group (CT significantly greater than that of amblyopic fellow and normal eyes), there was no significant difference in CT for the strabismic amblyopia group respect to amblyopic fellow and normal eyes. The discrepancy in CT between the two types of amblyopia may be due to both differences in ocular size and underlying mechanism.

Aslan Bayhan et al. [38] assessed changes in CT during amblyopia treatment using (SD-OCT). 40 patients (aged 3–9 years) with hyperopic anisometropic amblyopia underwent treatment with refractive correction alone for 16 weeks and if needed, with refractive correction and patching treatment thereafter (6 months). CT was measured at the fovea, and at two different distances (1.5–3.00 mm) temporally and nasally to the fovea in the amblyopic eyes and fellow eyes during treatment and in the control subjects (n = 22). CT at all locations decreased significantly after treatment in the amblyopic eyes. These findings indicate that thicker CT in amblyopic eyes partially regresses after amblyopia treatment.

However, considering these results, further studies are necessary to clear the causal relationship and the mechanisms involved between amblyopia and changes in CT.

Recently, the OCT technology was implemented with the introduction of the Optical Coherence Tomographic Angiography (OCT-A). This new technique provides a non invasive visualization of the microvasculature of the retina, allowing the identification of the superficial retinal capillary plexus (SCP), the deep retinal capillary plexus (DCP), and the choroid. An increasing number of studies have been conducted with the use of OCT-A in the field of retinal pathology. Some pioneering studies have extended OCT-A application even to amblyopic eyes.

Lonngi et al. [39] examined 63 eyes of 59 children (age < 18 years), 13 (21%) were amblyopic (anisometropic and refractive amblyopia) and 50 (79%) were control eyes. The objective of the study was to evaluate SCP and DCP in terms of vessel density, as a percentage, at Macular as well as optic nerve localizations. No abnormality in papillary and peripapillary vessel density was found between the two groups: this result is consistent with the findings of the Pediatric Eye Disease Investigator Group which used OCT and reported no difference in global or quadrantic RNFL thickness compared with the fellow non amblyopic eyes [40]. However OCT-A revealed a significantly lower vessel density of the DCP, with a mean of a 5.7% reduction in the 6 × 6-mm macular scan in children with amblyopia. This reduction was a mean of 1.8% in the SCP.

The same group [41] also investigated choriocapillaris vessel density by OCT-A in a total of 20 eyes of 16 patients with amblyopia and 25 eyes of 25 controls. Mean choriocapillaris vessel density was significantly higher (74.8 ± 5.8) in the amblyopic group than in the control group (71.1 ± 3.6), even after adjusting for age and refractive error (P = 0.012). Also outer parafoveal macular thickness (the inner boundary of the inner nuclear layer to the retinal pigment epithelium outer boundary) was significantly greater in amblyopic eyes than in control eyes, congruously with previous studies [23].

Sobral et al. [42] evaluated the highest number of amblyopic children using OCT-A up to date (July 2018). They enrolled the largest cohort of amblyopic patients compared to the same number of control patients in order to overcome the limitations of sample size in the previous studies investigating the vascularization of amblyopic eyes in children using OCT-A [36, 40]. SCP and DCP were evaluated in terms of both vascular density (anatomical parameter) and flow area (functional parameter). They found a significant decreased macular vascular density of SCP

(53.07 ± 2.55% vs 54.96 ± 3.33% [P = 0.0171]) and macular flow area of SCP (1.45 ± 0.11 mm^2 vs 1.50 ± 0.09 [P = 0.0305]) in the amblyopic eyes compared with the fellow ones. Compared with randomly selected eyes of controls, amblyopic eyes showed a statistically significant decrease in the macular flow area of the SCP (P = 0.005) and of the DCP (P = 0.002), in the macula vascular density of the SCP (P = 0.022) and in the optic disk flow area (P = 0.004) (Fig. 21.4). Data on macular vascular density of the SCP and DCP are similar to the findings of Yilmaz, Lonngi and colleagues [39, 43]. Data on reduced macular and optic disk flow area in the amblyopic eyes represent original findings. However, the clinical significance and utility of these findings are thus far unknown.

It remains to be determined whether the documented microvascularization defect is the cause or a consequence of the amblyopia. The main limitations of these studies with OCT-A on amblyopia include lack of masking of observers and the absence

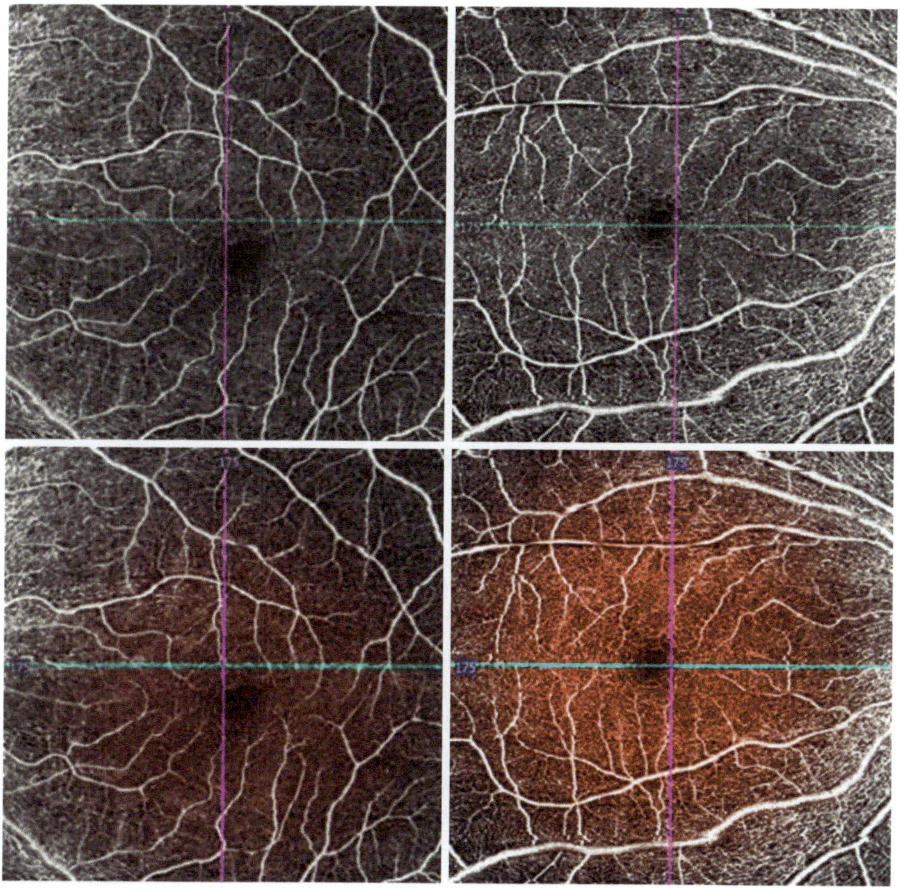

Fig. 21.4 Vessel density of SCP of an amblyopic eye (right) and a control eye (left). Vessel density of SCP is lower in the amblyopic eye (Thanks to F. Bonsignore—University Eye Clinic-Ospedale San Giuseppe, Milan)

of deprivational amblyopia cases in the amblyopia group. Future randomized, masked studies, with larger numbers of subjects will better confirm some of these issues. It would be useful also to obtain follow-up studies after treatment to show if there is any change in these vascular parameters.

As far as *deprivation amblyopia* in congenital cataract patients is concerned, the first study [44] investigating the structural difference of macular and peripapillary RNFL using OCT in this pathology has been conducted on a small sample. In Kim et al. work, 14 unilateral pseudophakic children with deprivational amblyopia and 14 age-matched normal children (mean age, 7.45 ± 2.57 years) were scanned with Cirrus HD-OCT. Macular, RNFL, and ganglion cell-inner plexiform layer thicknesses were measured, and compared between the eyes after correction for axial length-related magnification errors. OCT demonstrated significant increase in nasal RNFL thickness compared to fellow non-amblyopic eyes and age-matched normal eyes. The macular and macular ganglion cell-inner plexiform layer thickness did not show any significant difference. These results are quite contrasting if compared to data emerged from subsequent studies. Bansal et al. [45] compared the retinal nerve fiber layer thickness (RNFLT) and central macular thickness (CMT) in pediatric patients (age group 4–16 years) with unilateral congenital or developmental cataract (n = 15) and bilateral cataract (n = 15), and age-matched controls (n = 15). RNFLT and CMT were measured using SD-OCT in normal controls and 3 months postoperatively in children with unilateral and bilateral cataract. Children with unilateral cataract showed significant thinning of superior, nasal, and temporal RNFL compared to the fellow eyes as well as age-matched normal eyes on OCT. The CMT was inferior in deprivational amblyopic eyes than in age-matched normal eyes, but there was no significant difference compared to the fellow nonamblyopic eyes. In bilateral cataract, RNFLT was significantly thinner in superior and nasal quadrants as compared to age-matched normal eyes. Conversely, Al-Haddad et al. [46] found increased CMT in 14 eyes with deprivational amblyopia from pediatric cataract compared to 20 age-matched control eyes and this was correlated with the severity of amblyopia.

Several older studies reported a decrease in nasal visual fields in children treated for unilateral congenital cataract [47]. Kanamori et al. [48] demonstrated the relationship between visual field sensitivity at each tested location in standard automated perimetry and peripapillary RNFL thickness measured with Stratus OCT; the nasal sectoral RNFL corresponded well with nasal visual field area. Taken together, decreased nasal visual field in previous reports may have been due to increased nasal sectoral peripapillary RNFL thickness, as shown in Enoch study [33].

We can therefore conclude that OCT is certainly a rapid, non-invasive, office-based imaging technique allowing objective quantification of retinal structures with high resolution, including determination of peripapillary RNFL thickness, macular thickness and choroidal thickness (CT) so that it can be successfully applied also in young children. The recent introduction of OCT-A represent a new fascinating method to evaluate the retinal microvasculature in a non invasive way. Its application in amblyopia field is giving new interesting results regarding anatomical and functional changes of retinal vascular plexus which occurs in amblyopic eyes. These data have to be considered preliminary, but this new technology will improve, for sure, our knowledge on amblyopia mechanisms and related retinal changes. Nevertheless, evidence for direct retinal changes in eyes with amblyopia has been controversial: the results of these studies are equivocal with regard to whether macular, peripapillary RNFL and choroidal thicknesses differ in amblyopic eyes and between amblyopia subgroups (anisometropic, strabismic, deprivational). Moreover, the majority of the studies have been limited to strabismic or anisometropic amblyopia, and analyzed the fellow non amblyopic eyes as control [44]. Further randomized, masked studies with larger sample are required, especially as regards myopic anisometropic and deprivational amblyopia.

References

1. McKee SP, Levi DM, Movshon JA. The pattern of visual deficits in amblyopia. J Vis. 2003;3(5):380–405.
2. Crawford ML, Harwerth RS, Smith EL, von Noorden GK. Keeping an eye on the brain: the role of visual experience in monkeys and children. J Gen Psychol. 1993;120(1):7–19.
3. Holmes JM, Clarke MP. Amblyopia. Lancet. 2006;367(9519):1343–51.
4. Donahue SP, Arnold RW, Ruben JB. Preschool vision screening: what should we be detecting and how should we report it? Uniform guidelines for reporting results of preschool vision screening studies. J AAPOS. 2003;7(5):314–6.
5. Arnold RW. Amblyopia risk factor prevalence. J Pediatr Ophthalmol Strabismus. 2013;50(4):213–7.
6. Attebo K, Mitchell P, Cumming R, Smith W, Jolly N, Sparkes R. Prevalence and causes of amblyopia in an adult population. Ophthalmology. 1998;105(1):154–9.
7. National Eye Institute Office of Biometry and Epidemiology. Report on the National Eye Institute's Visual Acuity Impairment Survey Pilot Study. Washington: US Department of Health and Human Services; 1984.
8. Holmes JM, Beck RW, Repka MX, Leske DA, Kraker RT, Blair RC, et al. The amblyopia treatment study visual acuity testing protocol. Arch Ophthalmol. 2001;119(9):1345–53.
9. Wiesel TN, Hubel DH. Single-cell responses in striate cortex of kittens deprived of vision in one eye. J Neurophysiol. 1963;26:1003–17.
10. Williams C, Papakostopoulos D. Electro-oculographic abnormalities in amblyopia. Br J Ophthalmol. 1995;79(3):218–24.
11. Von Noorden GK, Crawford ML. The lateral geniculate nucleus in human strabismic amblyopia. Invest Ophthalmol Vis Sci. 1992;33(9):2729–32.
12. Horton JC, Hocking DR. Timing of the critical period for plasticity of ocular dominance columns in macaque striate cortex. J Neurosci. 1997;17(10):3684–709.
13. Dickmann A, Petroni S, Perrotta V, Parrilla R, Aliberti S, Salerni A, et al. Measurement of retinal nerve fiber layer thickness, macular thickness, and foveal volume in amblyopic eyes using spectral-domain optical coherence tomography. J AAPOS. 2012;16(1):86–8.
14. Repka MX, Kraker RT, Tamkins SM, Suh DW, Sala NA, Beck RW. Retinal nerve fiber layer thickness in amblyopic eyes. Am J Ophthalmol. 2009;148(1):143–7.
15. Huynh SC, Samarawickrama C, Wang XY, Rochtchina E, Wong TY, Gole GA, et al. Macular and nerve fiber layer thickness in amblyopia: the Sydney Childhood Eye Study. Ophthalmology. 2009;116(9):1604–9.
16. Khan AO. A comparison between the amblyopic eye and normal fellow eye ocular architecture in children with hyperopic anisometropic amblyopia. J AAPOS. 2013;17(1):115–6.
17. Wu SQ, Zhu LW, Xu QB, Xu JL, Zhang Y. Macular and peripapillary retinal nerve fiber layer thickness in children with hyperopic anisometropic amblyopia. Int J Ophthalmol. 2013;6(1):85–9.

18. Provis JM, van Driel D, Billson FA, Russell P. Development of the human retina: patterns of cell distribution and redistribution in the ganglion cell layer. J Comp Neurol. 1985;233(4):429–51.
19. Provis JM, van Driel D, Billson FA, Russell P. Human fetal optic nerve: overproduction and elimination of retinal axons during development. J Comp Neurol. 1985;238(1):92–100.
20. Yen MY, Cheng CY, Wang AG. Retinal nerve fiber layer thickness in unilateral amblyopia. Invest Ophthalmol Vis Sci. 2004;45(7):2224–30.
21. Kok PH, de Kinkelder R, Braaksma-Besselink YC, Kalkman J, Prick LJ, Sminia ML, et al. Anomalous relation between axial length and retinal thickness in amblyopic children. J AAPOS. 2013;17(6):598–602.
22. Pang Y, Goodfellow GW, Allison C, Block S, Frantz KA. A prospective study of macular thickness in amblyopic children with unilateral high myopia. Invest Ophthalmol Vis Sci. 2011;52(5):2444–9.
23. Nishi T, Ueda T, Hasegawa T, Miyata K, Ogata N. Choroidal thickness in children with hyperopic anisometropic amblyopia. Br J Ophthalmol. 2014;98(2):228–32.
24. Xu J, Zheng J, Yu S, Sun Z, Zheng W, Qu P, Chen Y, Chen W, Yu X. Macular choroidal thickness in unilateral amblyopic children. Invest Ophthalmol Vis Sci. 2014;55(11):7361–8.
25. Niyaz L, Yücel OE, Arıtürk N, Terzi O. Choroidal thickness in strabismus and amblyopia cases. Strabismus. 2017;25(2):56–9.
26. Pang Y, Frantz KA, Block S, Goodfellow GW, Allison C. Effect of amblyopia treatment on macular thickness in eyes with myopic anisometropic amblyopia. Invest Ophthalmol Vis Sci. 2015;56(4):2677–83.
27. Kutschke PJ, Scott WE, Keech RV. Anisometropic amblyopia. Ophthalmology. 1991; 98(2):258–63.
28. Nucci P, Drack AV. Refractive surgery for unilateral high myopia in children. J AAPOS. 2001;5(6):348–51.
29. Saw SM, Gazzard G, Shih-Yen EC, Chua WH. Myopia and associated pathological complications. Ophthalmic Physiol Opt. 2005;25(5):381–91.
30. Dickmann A, Petroni S, Salerni A, Dell'Omo R, Balestrazzi E. Unilateral amblyopia: an optical coherence tomography study. J AAPOS. 2009;13(2):148–50.
31. Dickmann A, Petroni S, Perrotta V, Salerni A, Parrilla R, Aliberti S, et al. A morpho-functional study of amblyopic eyes with the use of optical coherence tomography and microperimetry. J AAPOS. 2011;15(4):338–41.
32. Szigeti A, Tátrai E, Szamosi A, Vargha P, Nagy ZZ, Németh J, et al. A morphological study of retinal changes in unilateral amblyopia using optical coherence tomography image segmentation. PLoS One. 2014;9(2):e88363.
33. Enoch JM. Receptor amblyopia. Am J Ophthalmol. 1959;48(3, Part 2):262–74.
34. Delint PJ, Weissenbruch C, Berendschot TT, Norren DV. Photoreceptor function in unilateral amblyopia. Vis Res. 1998;38(4):613–7.
35. Liu Y, Dong Y, Zhao K. A meta-analysis of choroidal thickness changes in unilateral amblyopia. J Ophthalmol. 2017;2017:2915261.
36. Guo L, Tao J, Xia F, Yang Z, Ma X, Hua R. In vivo optical imaging of amblyopia: digital subtraction autofluorescence and split-spectrum amplitude-decorrelation angiography. Lasers Surg Med. 2016;48(7):660–7.
37. Araki S, Miki A, Goto K, Yamashita T, Takizawa G, Haruishi K, et al. Macular retinal and choroidal thickness in unilateral amblyopia using swept source optical coherence tomography. BMC Ophthalmol. 2017;17(1):167.
38. Aslan Bayhan S, Bayhan HA. Effect of amblyopia treatment on choroidal thickness in children with hyperopic anisometropic amblyopia. Curr Eye Res. 2017;42(9):1254–9.
39. Lonngi M, Velez FG, Tsui I, Davila JP, Rahimi M, Chan C, et al. Spectral-domain optical coherence tomography angiography in children with amblyopia. JAMA Ophthalmol. 2017;135(10):1086–91.
40. Repka MX, Kraker RT, Tamkins SM, Suh DW, Sala NA, Beck RW, Pediatric Eye Disease Investigator Group. Retinal nerve fiber layer thickness in amblyopic eyes. Am J Ophthalmol. 2009;148(1):143–7.

41. Borrelli E, Lonngi M, Balasubramanian S, Tepelus TC, Baghdasaryan E, Pineles SL, et al. Increased choriocapillaris vessel density in amblyopic children: a case-control study. J AAPOS. 2018;pii: S1091-8531(18)30118-6.
42. Sobral I, Rodrigues TM, Soares M, Seara M, Monteiro M, Paiva C, et al. OCT angiography findings in children with amblyopia. J AAPOS. 2018;pii: S1091-8531(18)30121-6.
43. Yilmaz I, Ocak OB, Yilmaz BS, Inal A, Gokyigit B, Taskapili M. Comparison of quantitative measurement of foveal avascular zone and macular vessel density in eyes of children with amblyopia and healthy controls: an optical coherence tomography angiography study. J AAPOS. 2017;21:224–8.
44. Kim YW, Kim SJ, Yu YS. Spectral-domain optical coherence tomography analysis in deprivational amblyopia: a pilot study with unilateral pediatric cataract patients. Graefes Arch Clin Exp Ophthalmol. 2013;251(12):2811–9.
45. Bansal P, Ram J, Sukhija J, Singh R, Gupta A. Retinal nerve fiber layer and macular thickness measurements in children after cataract surgery compared with age-matched controls. Am J Ophthalmol. 2016;166:126–32.
46. Al-Haddad C, Mehanna CJ, Ismail K. High-definition optical coherence tomography of the macula in deprivational amblyopia. Ophthalmic Surg Lasers Imaging Retina. 2018;49(3):198–204.
47. Bowering ER, Maurer D, Lewis TL, Brent HP. Sensitivity in the nasal and temporal hemifields in children treated for cataract. Invest Ophthalmol Vis Sci. 1993;34(13):3501–9.
48. Kanamori A, Naka M, Nagai-Kusuhara A, Yamada Y, Nakamura M, Negi A. Regional relationship between retinal nerve fiber layer thickness and corresponding visual field sensitivity in glaucomatous eyes. Arch Ophthalmol. 2008;126(11):1500–6.

Pediatric Neuro-Ophthalmology and OCT

22

Maja Kostic, Gábor Márk Somfai, Edmund Arthur, and Delia Cabrera DeBuc

22.1 Introduction

Eyes are one of the vital organs that provide more than 80% of all information we received and that help us to grow and develop.

Embryology and early development of eyes as part of the brain can help us to better understand developmental, degenerative and ocular pathology in ophthalmology. The changes of the retinal structure and microvasculature are seemingly correlated with neurodegenerative and cerebrovascular lesions, which in turn supports the view that the retina may serve as a window to the brain.

The changes of the retinal structure and microvasculature are seemingly correlated with neurodegenerative and cerebrovascular lesions, which in turn supports the view that the retina may serve as a window to the brain. It can be postulated that retinal microvascular structure could be mirroring that of the brain while the substructure of the retina may be like the structure of the brain.

Many diagnostic methods for diagnostics of the central nervous system in childhood period needs general anesthesia of kids, which are very stressful for kids, time-consuming and high costly depending. However, discovering low-cost diagnostic instruments whereas retinal imaging could provide a meaningful surrogate marker for disease detection and disease management that could be available not only for institutions and big clinic, and also for all doctors in primary care.

In this chapter, we will give an overview of embryology and ocular and neurological development, as well as overview of Optical Coherence Tomography (OCT)

M. Kostic · E. Arthur · D. C. DeBuc (✉)
Bascom Palmer Eye Institute, University of Miami Miller School of Medicine, Miami, FL, USA
e-mail: mkostic@miami.edu; exa647@med.miami.edu; dcabrera2@med.miami.edu

G. M. Somfai
Augenzentrum, Pallas Kliniken, Olten, Switzerland

A. Grzybowski, P. Barboni (eds.), *OCT and Imaging in Central Nervous System Diseases*, https://doi.org/10.1007/978-3-030-26269-3_22

in neonatology and pediatric neuro-ophthalmology as an emerging technology in neurology applications and express our view about how retinal imaging could serve the above goals and open a window, which could serve as a direct view to the brain in the earlier ages.

22.2 Ocular and Neurological Development

The eye is a very complex organ from the embryogenic standpoint since its development involves diencephalic neuroectoderm, surface ectoderm and extraocular mesenchyme (Fig. 22.1) [1]. During the development, the retina, trabecular meshwork, the epithelium of the ciliary body and the iris, as well as the optic nerve shall form from the neuroectoderm. The lens, anterior surface of the cornea, eyelids, and skin shall emerge from surface ectoderm. Ectomesenchyme originates from the neural crest, and it is involved in the genesis of the sclera, part of the cornea, choroid, ciliary body, blood vessels and the muscles of the eye [2].

In the human embryo, the structures of the eye start appearing around the 22nd day of development, before the closing of neural folds into the neural tube (Fig. 22.2). Early in the 4th week of gestation, the optic recesses start appearing within the diencephalon [1, 2]. After closing of the rostral neuropore (anterior opening), around the 24th day of gestation, the primordial eye can be observed, in the form of an evagination being shaped as a vesicle, known as an optic vesicle [2]. The optic vesicle is connected to the diencephalon through a thin, hollow optic stem, the future optic nerve (Fig. 22.3). The distal anterior part of the optic vesicle grows externally, approaching the ectoderm, from which, during this phase of development, it is separated by a thin layer of ectomesenchyme. Upon approaching the ectoderm, the optic vesicle initially flattens and later, around the 32nd day of gestation, the distal anterior part of the optic vesicle creates an invagination, and the

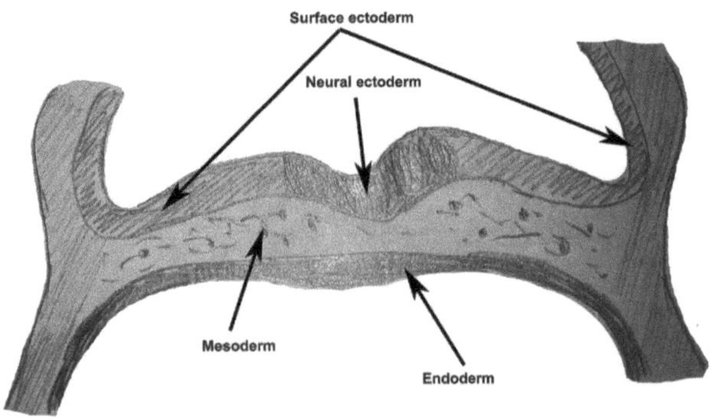

Fig. 22.1 Drawing of an about 16-day-old embryo. Note that ectoderm is differentiated into surface ectoderm on the lateral part (light gray part) and neural ectoderm in the middle (dark gray part) (*Image courtesy of Maja Kostic, M.D., Ph.D.; drawing inspired from images in "Pediatric Ophthalmology and Strabismus", K. Wright and P. Spiegel* [3], *second edition,* ISBN 978-0-387-21753-6)

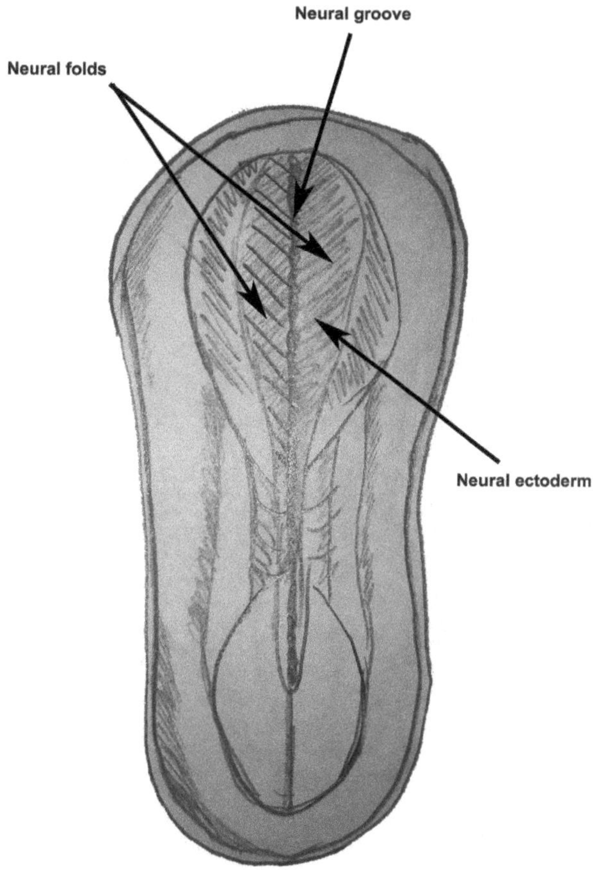

Fig. 22.2 Drawing of human embryo about 20 days' gestation. Neural groove originates from the neural plate, represent neural ectoderm (black line), and on each side of the groove are neural folds and represents surface ectoderm (*Image courtesy of Maja Kostic, M.D., Ph.D.; drawing inspired from images in "Pediatric Ophthalmology and Strabismus", K. Wright and P. Spiegel* [3], *second edition,* ISBN 978-0-387-21753-6)

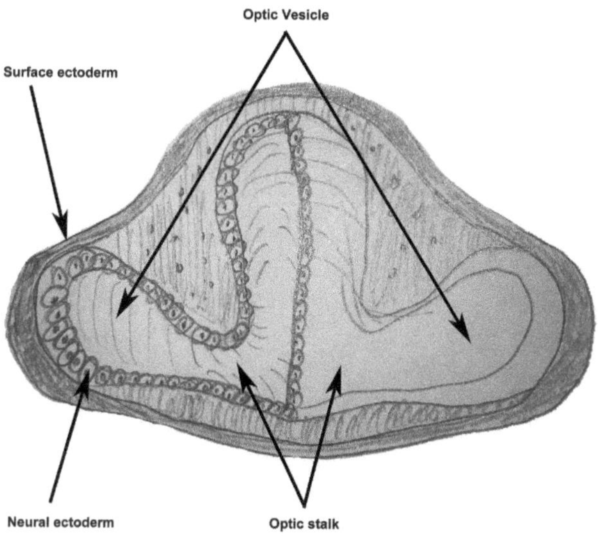

Fig. 22.3 Drawing of the optical vesicle of the about 25-day-old embryo. Optic vesicles and optic stalk are formed. Lens placode is formed from surface ectoderm (*Image courtesy of Maja Kostic, M.D., Ph.D.; drawing inspired from images in "Pediatric Ophthalmology and Strabismus", K. Wright and P. Spiegel* [3], *second edition,* ISBN 978-0-387-21753-6)

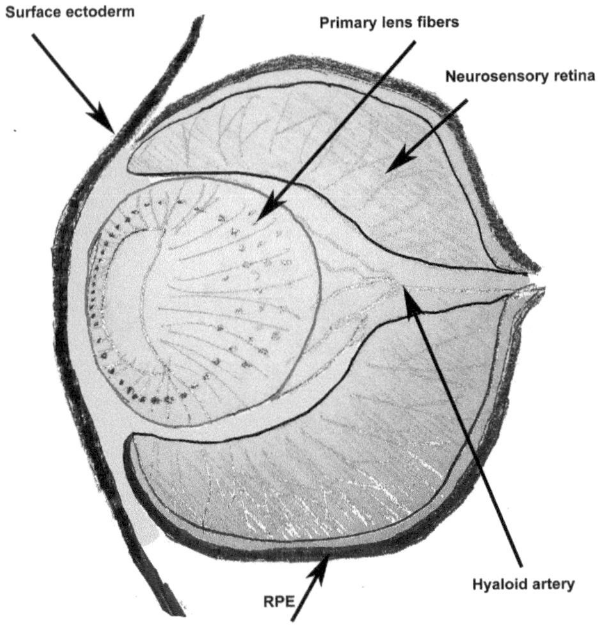

Fig. 22.4 Drawing of the embryonic eye in about 45 days. The hyaloid artery is seen in the posterior part of the eye between the lens and neurosensory retina. The posterior fibers (cells) of lens elongate from posterior towards anterior and make future lens (*Image courtesy of Maja Kostic, M.D., Ph.D.; drawing inspired from images in "Pediatric Ophthalmology and Strabismus", K. Wright and P. Spiegel* [3], *second edition,* ISBN 978-0-387-21753-6)

vesicle transforms into the optic cup. During its development, the optic cup takes the shape of an asymmetric invagination. On the ventral, inferior side of the optic stalk, before the complete adhesion of its walls, the choroidal or retinal fissure is created [2, 3]. Through this fissure, the hyaloid artery reaches the optic cup (Fig. 22.4). Due to these changes, the optic vesicle transforms into a two-layer optic cup. The tissue invagination increases, and the cavity of the optic vesicle decrease during the development. The cavity of the vesicle finally changes into the fissure separating the outer pigmented layer of the retina from the inner neural layer. All layers of the optical part of retina shall develop from the posterior internal layers of the optic cup.

The blind part of the retina, covering internal surfaces of ciliary body and iris, shall form from the ridges of the optic cup [2, 3]. The external epithelial part of the ciliary body derives from the pigmented layer of the optic cup and the internal one, from the neural retina, as was mentioned previously. The ciliary body stroma originates from ectomesenchyme, as well as the muscle cells of the ciliary muscle. The iris stroma also originates from ectomesenchyme, whereas the muscle cells arise from the neuroectoderm of the optic cup. The external part of ectomesenchyme, surrounding the optic vesicle, shall transform into the external tunic of the bulb of the eye and its components, cornea, and sclera, while the internal part shall form the choroid. Hyaloid blood vessels passing through the choroid fissure and vitreous chamber and reaching the lens shall form from the ectomesenchyme as well [3, 4].

Lens genesis starts around the 30th day in the form of superficial ectoderm thickening in the region of the optic cup. Thickened surface ectoderm shall transform into the lens placode during differentiation. Invagination of the lens placode shall create the fovea of the lens, which will completely separate from surface ectoderm and shall become the lens vesicle during growth [4]. In this stage, the lens vesicle is confined within the optic cup, practically in mesenchyme. Differentiation of mesenchyme on its internal side shall create the gelatinous structure from which the primary vitreous shall emerge. Primary vitreous is located between the lens and the internal layer of the optic cup.

Ectodermal cells covering the optic cup surface shall create its capsule. By the end of the 7th week of gestation, the lens turns into a solid structure, vascularized in the beginning by the branches of the hyaloid artery. Later, during fetal growth, it becomes avascular. Initially, the lens fills the optic cup almost completely, while later it takes only the smaller part of it with the vitreous body occupying most of it [5, 6].

The vitreous body originates from the cells of the internal layer of the optic cup and the base of the optic vesicle. The lens capsule is formed from the cells of the lens epithelium [6]. Differentiation of the retina starts at the end of 6th weeks when the two layers of the optic cup when the outer retinal pigment epithelium (RPE) and the inner neural retina began to form. Bruch's membrane which is a basal lamina of the RPE forms a functional unit with RPE and choriocapillaris [7]. Ganglion cells, horizontal cells, and cone photoreceptors are born first, followed by amacrine and bipolar cells. Rod photoreceptors and Muller cells are last retinal cells to differentiate [8]. A foveal region started to develop at about 10–11 weeks' gestation when in the central region of retina only cone photoreceptors are detected. According to primate retinal studies, the fovea is the initiation point for most developmental events in the retina, including mitosis, apoptosis, opsin expression, and synaptogenesis [9] and development of retina radiates from this region across the retina. In week 34, cones and rods near the cone area of fovea have outer segments and forming elongated axons which terminate in the OPL [9].

Optic nerve develops from the edge of the optic fissure that is divided into two parts: the optic groove that originates from the optic stalk and the retinal fissure originates from the ventral optic vesicle. The optic disc will form at the transition between the optic groove and retinal fissure [10]. Type I astrocytes arise from neuroepithelial cells of the optic stalk and migrate onto the retinal surface where they associate with the surface vasculature to form blood/retinal barrier [10]. Retinal ganglion cells axons grow in close contact with Muller glial cells and with vitreal basal lamina [2, 11]. In the 29 gestational weeks, there is about 1.1 million retinal ganglion cell axons that entering the optic nerve.

All cranial nerves are formed by the seventh week of gestation. The cranial motor neurons are organized within individual or pairs rhombomeres (neuromeres of the rhombencephalon). The oculomotor (III) nucleus is located in the posterior midbrain, the trochlear (IV) nucleus in the anterior part of rhombomere 1, trigeminal

(V) in rhombomeres 2 and 3, the abducens (VI) nucleus in rhombomere 4 and 5, the facial in 5 and 6 [12]. Normal development of efferent cranial nerves is critical for normal development of extraocular muscles [13]. Extraocular muscles develop from unsegmented prechordal and paraxial mesoderm form craniofacial muscles. Eye movement depends on the unique way of connectivity between cranial motor axons and the extraocular muscles [14]. The development of the eye bulb doesn't finish with birth. The axial length (AL) of the child's eye is around 17 mm and around 24 mm in adults. The growth of the eye is generally completed by age 5–8.

22.2.1 Embryonic Development of the Retinal Blood Vessels

The vascular system originates from mesoderm and appears in very early stages of development. At the basis of the vascular system development is the processes of vasculogenesis and angiogenesis [15], the apoptosis of blood vessels and their maturation [16]. In the early stages of retinal development, the necessary amount of oxygen is provided by the choroidal and hyaloid vascular systems, and later by the retinal ones.

22.2.1.1 Choroidal Vascular Plexus

Up to the 6th week of gestation, the retina is nourished exclusively through the choroid by diffusion [17]. In the 5 mm long human embryo, the primitive dorsal ophthalmic and primitive ventral ophthalmic arteries are separated from the internal carotid artery. The hyaloid artery originates from the primitive dorsal ophthalmic artery, passes through the embryonal fissure and reaches the indent in the region of the future optic nerve head.

The choroidal vascular plexus is observed in the human embryo of 4–5 mm in length. Its occurrence corresponds to the time of optic vesical genesis. It develops from the mesoderm and cranial part of the neural fold. Endothelial cells originate from mesoderm, while melanocytes, pericytes, and stromal cells originate from the neural fold [18]. The choroidal vascular plexus is composed of large primitive blood vessels that originate from the vascular system surrounding the neural tube and spreading up to the superficial layers of the optical cupulas. In the 13 mm long human embryo, choroidal capillaries surround the optical cupulas. They are separated from the retina by the membrane of the retinal pigmented layer. The complex vascular plexus connecting with the posterior ciliary arteries, forming varicose veins and choriocapillary layer originates from the primitive vascular plexus during the 2nd and 3rd month of intrauterine growth [15]. The choroidal vascular plexus is of greatest importance for normal retinal function. It nourishes the retinal pigmented layer and photoreceptors [18].

22.2.1.2 Hyaloid Plexus

During the eye's development, the multiplication of retina cells causes an increase in its metabolic needs, which then leads to a demand that choroidal circulation cannot meet. As a result, a temporary hyaloid plexus which exists only during the first

4 months of intrauterine development, start developing [17]. The hyaloid plexus or the hyaloid artery starts developing at the beginning of the 4th gestation week off the dorsal ophthalmic artery. The development of the hyaloid artery is induced by retinal hypoxia.

As the hyaloid artery develops and reaches the cup of the future optic disc, it creates a vascular network which carries nutrients to the eye structures. When the embryo grows to 7 mm, the hyaloid artery has already made its way through the vitreous body and reaches the lens' back end. Once the embryo is 8–9 mm long, a dense capillary plexus can be observed, and it connects to the choroid plexus at the level of the front edge of the optic cup. This dense capillary plexus is called tunica vasculosa lentis, and through anastomosis, it is connected to the choroid plexus.

The hyaloid plexus has no veins, meaning the hyaloid system is solely made of arteries, whereas the vein part of the system is made of choroid veins. During its development, the hyaloid artery reaches the front side of the lens and builds the pupil membrane. In the 9th gestation week, or when the embryo is 60–80 mm long, the hyaloid plexus is fully developed and supplies the eye with needed nutrients. Parallel with the full development of the hyaloid network, the early start of the retinal plexus can be seen, as well as the beginning of the regression of the hyaloid vascular system [15].

The regression of the hyaloid vascular system starts around the 2nd month of intrauterine development, which is followed by the macrophage capillary occlusion. As the vascular structures start regrading, the primary vitreous body retracts. During the 5th month of intrauterine development, the back part of the eye is filled with the secondary vitreous body, while the primary vitreous body is S-shaped and positioned horizontally in the center [19].

22.2.2 The Retinal Vasculature

Further complexity of retinal growth and development is followed by the increased metabolic needs, which choroid and hyaloid vasculature cannot satisfy, so at the beginning of the 14th gestation week, a network of individual retinal blood vessels starts developing, which eventually creates the retinal vasculature [20]. The development of the retinal blood vessels begins with the occurrence of astrocytes, which play the active role in directing the blood vessels' endothelial cells during the 16th gestation week. It is the first time that the astrocytes can be seen in proximity of the hyaloid artery and around the optic nerve papilla. There, they are organized into a four-lobe formation, of which the two larger ones are temporal, and the two smaller ones are nasal. They all mark the pathways for the future main arteries and veins.

The early retina is made of only one undifferentiated layer. At the same time as the retina layers evolve and mature, the retinas' complex or network starts forming. The formation of the early vessel network of the central two-thirds of the retina is formed by vasculogenesis. The remainder of the vessels is formed by angiogenesis—by the creation of new blood vessels and sprouting of endothelial cells from the existing vessels, or by splitting of an existing blood vessel. Research indicates that both mentioned processes, vasculogenesis as well as angiogenesis, are essential for the development of the nerve/vessel network [21].

22.2.2.1 Vasculogenesis and Angiogenesis

Retinal blood vessels are created by the process of vascular and angiogenesis. This dual way of creation of the retinal vessel network, indicates its uniqueness, complexity, high differentness and dynamics of its development. The development of the retinal cells, primarily photoreceptors, and ganglion cells requires fast and extensive metabolic processes [16]. Retina's high demand for energy during its evolution/development/growth also requires an adequate blood vessel network, which can meet these needs [16].

The process of vasculogenesis in the embryo starts on the 17th day of its life. Chorion mesenchymal cells, yolk sac, mesenchymal stems, form blood islands. From the superficial mesenchymal cells of the angioblast blood islands, primitive angioblasts will develop [1]. Vasculogenesis is the process of "*de novo*" blood vessel formation. In the process of vasculogenesis, the differentiation of primitive angioblasts leads to the creation of a primitive blood vessel network responsible for the formation of large blood vessels, like the central retinal artery and its branches due to the positioning of the end part of the central retinal artery and the optic disc, nasal retinal blood vessels reach the ora serrata on the 36th week of gestation, whereas temporal retinal blood vessels reach it on the 40th week of gestation [16, 22].

Angiogenesis is the formation and growth of the new blood vessels from pre-existing vasculature. During this process, new blood vessels are formed by the sprouting of endothelial cells of the existing vessels, or by splitting angiogenesis, the process where a new blood vessel is created by splitting of an existing blood vessel (*intussusceptive growth*). This process represents proliferation and migration of vascular endothelial cells, as well as the processes that enable growth and blood vessel remodeling [15, 16]. As a physiological process, angiogenesis is typical in the areas with swift capillary growth [23]. The main inducer of the process of angiogenesis is hypoxia [24]. Angiogenesis is initiated by the VEGF via retinal Muller glia cells and astrocytes growth [24]. By this process of angiogenesis, perifoveal regions and blood vessels of deep retinal layers are formed.

As astrocytes lead the way for the direction and growth of endothelial cells into the retinal tissue, they play the crucial role in the development of retinal blood vessels. Along with the maturity of retinal cells, which occurs in the period of 14–15 gestation week, the development of the superficial, deep and radial peripapillary capillary plexus that originate from a central retinal artery [23]. Superficial blood plexus is made of arterioles, capillaries, and post-capillary venules. This plexus is located in the layer of nerve fibers and the ganglion cell layer. Deep blood plexus is located between the inner nuclear layer (INL) and the OPL. It is mostly made of capillary size blood vessels. Superficial and deep blood plexus stretch to the FAZ area where the retina is extremely thin and where all the needs are satisfied by the choroid plexus.

Radial peripapillary plexus forms a tiny ring-shaped area, which is surrounded by the optic disc. Same as the superficial blood plexus, it is also located in the layer of nerve fibers. Radial peripapillary plexus is developed into a capillary network on the 21st week of gestation. In the 26–27-week-old embryo, it is located in the superficial layers of the nerve fibers and from the optic disc, it stretches radially in all directions. It is created by the process of angiogenesis [23].

Retinal capillaries are made of endothelial cells, basement membranes and intramural pericytes. Endothelial capillary cells are connected by strong protein links, which represent a hemato-retinal barrier known as adherents' junctions. The hemato-retinal barrier is a highly selective functional barrier. The inner hemato-retinal barrier operates at the level of endothelial capillaries and represents a circulation barrier. Outer hemato-retinal barrier operates at the level of RPE and is a barrier to choroid circulation. Pigment epithelial cells are connected by occluding junctions, which are strong connections based on protein. High concentrations of VEGF lead to destabilization of intercellular connections, the breakdown of the hemato-retinal barrier, and cause a wide range of retinal diseases, which include retinopathy of prematurity (ROP) [24, 25]. Pericytes are contractile cells on the capillary endothelium of retina, which play an essential role in the stabilization of the vascular retina.

22.3 OCT in Neonatology and Pediatric Neuro-Ophthalmology

Extremely preterm neonates who develop severe ROP are more likely than their equals unaffected by ROP to have evidence of brain damage, including severe disability, developmental delay, cerebral palsy, and lower scores on measures of verbal and performance IQ, general conceptual ability, and spatial ability [26–29]. OCT as a diagnostic tool for different neuro-ophthalmological diseases, it is in everyday practice in adults. However, neonates and small children were excluded, until a new handheld spectral-domain OCT (HH-SDOCT) was developed and optimized in neonatology and pediatric ophthalmology [30–33]. Nowadays, there are multiple applications in prematurity and neonatology in ROP, retinal dystrophies and dysplasia, optic nerve pathology, nystagmus, different injuries or trauma and in diagnosis and monitoring ocular tumors [34–36].

The natural development of the retina and foveal region is a complicated procedure, comprising centripetal migration of the cone photoreceptors into the central fovea and elongation of the outer retinal layers (ORLs), outer nuclear layer (ONL), and photoreceptor inner and outer segments (IS, OS), as well as centrifugal migration of the inner retinal layers (IRLs), RNFL, GCL, IPL, inner nuclear layer (INL), and OPL away from the central fovea with increasing age [34, 37–39].

22.3.1 Retinopathy of Prematurity

ROP is an abnormal development of retinal blood vessels in premature infants that can potentially lead to blindness [40–43]. Early diagnosis, an area where the application of OCT has been most investigated, is the key for detection, follow-up, and decision-making regarding the need for treatment.

There are many characteristic features of the infant's eye compared with the adult eye. All those characteristics are challenging factors for OCT application in neonatology. Premature babies and neonates have greater astigmatism and higher refractive errors, predominantly myopia, and between 40–52 weeks they shift to hyperopia [30, 44, 45]. The AL is shorter; investigations with ocular echography have estimated the ocular AL of the premature infant as 15 mm at 31 weeks' postmenstrual age (PMA) and reported the fastest growth to take place from 32 to 52 weeks PMA [46]. The cornea is steeper than the adult cornea, decreasing to adult values by 3 months [43, 47–51].

The typical features observed in the retina of babies with ROP are the persistence of the IRLs, reduction of foveal pit depth, reduction in the diameter of the foveal avascular zone (FAZ), with global decreases and segmental (temporal) increases in RNFL thickness measurements [52–55], increase in central macular thickness (CMT) measurements, thinning of the GCC, delay in photoreceptor development, and thinning of the photoreceptor layers [56–60]. Also, choroidal thickness is reduced in preterm children [61–63]. According to Maldonado et al. increased central foveal, IRL and foveal to parafoveal retinal thickness are associated with a higher risk of developing plus disease or ROP stage 3 [64]. Moreover, a new handheld SDOCT (HH-SDOCT) has played a very important role in detecting pre-retinal tissue, epiretinal membranes, cystoid macular edema (CME), retinal layer schisis, vascular abnormalities, and foveal architectural abnormalities not visible on conventional clinical examination. Interestingly, CME is reported in all stages in ROP with an incidence of more than 87.5% in stage three of ROP [65, 66]. The macular or foveal involvement in ROP, that can be detected by OCT has been very helpful as part of the decision-making process and in predicting visual and neurodevelopmental outcome in babies with ROP [67–69].

22.3.2 Infantile Nystagmus, Retinal Dystrophies and Dysplasia

Except induced by trauma or disease, nystagmus practically always is instigated by neurological complications in most people with nystagmus which usually are born with the condition or develop it early in life. Retinal dystrophies are chronic and progressive diseases characterized by defective color vision and night blindness due to neuronal death and consequent loss of functional connections. Retinal dysplasia is a congenital malformation of the retina, with the formation of folds or rosettes that appear clinically as retinal folds or larger areas of geographic dysplasia.

Congenital (infantile) nystagmus is characterized by involuntary rhythmic eye movements. The waveform, amplitude, and frequency of the oscillations, which are typically horizontal in direction but may be primarily vertical, torsional, or any combination of these three, can vary with changes in focal distance, the direction of gaze, and under monocular or binocular viewing conditions. Often, infantile nystagmus is associated with other ocular conditions (e.g., bilateral congenital cataracts) that impair visual acuity and sometimes can create life-threatening conditions [70]. OCT can be very helpful in identifying the etiology of infantile nystagmus syndrome (INS), a heterogeneous group of disorders, with multiple causes and different prognoses [71].

Lee et al. [71] recommended dividing INS into four diagnostic categories: typical foveal hypoplasia, atypical foveal hypoplasia, abnormal foveal morphology, and normal foveal morphology. The etiology of nystagmus can be anticipated, and diagnostic exams can be designated to confirm the diagnosis based on the presence or absence of foveal hypoplasia or the presence or absence of other abnormal macular morphology as visualized by OCT. If there is a typical foveal hypoplasia, it is most likely associated with albinism and PAX6 mutations. Retinal development is ongoing in early childhood, characterized by foveal hypoplasia and a reduction in ORL thickness measurements *as demonstrated by* longitudinal OCT imaging studies in albinism [72].

Also, achromatopsia (ACHM) is characterized by atypical foveal hypoplasia which is the foveal hypoplasia associated with photoreceptor disruption and/or the presence of a hyporeflective zone located between the external limiting membrane (ELM) and RPE at the fovea. OCT imaging has also demonstrated that there is evidence that retinal development is not arrested but is ongoing in ACHM, at a reduced rate and magnitude in comparison to controls [73]. This expresses as foveal hypoplasia, and reductions in total retinal thickness, ORL thickness and parafoveal IRL, IPL, and OPL thickness measurements [73]. Intriguingly, there is a primary decrease in CMT in early infancy in albinism because of ongoing regression of the IRLs from the fovea, which can indicate that there is a period of retinal developmental plasticity in childhood in both ACHM and albinism, that might help normalize retinal development and optimize vision. Abnormal morphology of fovea (category 3) is characteristic of retinal dystrophies, which are typically associated with abnormal lamination of the IRLs and ORLs, loss or disruption of photoreceptor integrity, and thinning of the ONL and RPE [67]. The fourth category in this group is idiopathic manifest latent nystagmus, characterized by normal foveal morphology.

22.3.3 Optic Nerve Pathology

OCT has also been used as a diagnostic and monitoring tool in wide pediatric optic nerve pathology like glaucoma, optic nerve atrophy or hypoplasia, and pseudotumor cerebri.

Hypoplasia of the optic nerve is the most usual hereditary disorder of the optic nerve which can be diagnosed by OCT with the following features: significantly smaller discs, horizontal cup diameter, thinning of the RNFL, GCL, IPL, ONL with increasing grade of glaucoma damage [74]. HH-SDOCT can be used as a marker of visual function to differentiate measurements between RNFL, GCL, and IPL in children with and without vision loss [74, 75].

Pseudotumor cerebri is idiopathic intracranial hypertension, which is a condition characterized by increased ICP without a detectable cause [76]. The main symptoms are headache, vision disturbances, pulsatile ringing in the ears, and shoulder pain [76, 77]. Complications may include vision loss [77]. OCT characteristics in pseudotumor cerebri are an increased central macular, temporal, and superior RNFL thickness. Moreover, optic atrophy and photoreceptor loss in OCT are findings associated with irreversible visual loss [78, 79]. Likewise, OCT can be used to diagnose and monitor pediatric pseudotumor cerebri and is potentially useful as a visual prognostic tool in this condition [78, 79].

22.3.4 Non-accidental Injury or Trauma

Abusive head trauma known as shaken baby syndrome (SBS) is characterized by many body injuries including broken bones, skull fractures, brain hemorrhage and retinal hemorrhages [80, 81]. SBS occurs when a baby is shaken repeatedly, often by a frustrated caretaker trying to quiet an inconsolable baby [82, 83]. The eyes of babies are more vulnerable to bleeding due to shaking because of a disproportionally large head and fragile blood vessels [83]. Symptoms may range from subtle to obvious that can lead to death [84]. However, very often there are no detectable signs of trauma with many complications in later life that include epileptic seizures, changes in visual acuity, or permanent visual loss, changes in cognitive functions as well as cerebral palsy [82, 83]. OCT has been reported to be helpful as a diagnostic tool in SBS with posterior vitreous separation and multilayered retinoschisis [84]. Also, it can be used to guide treatment in infants with shaken baby syndrome by providing additional morphologic information [85].

22.3.5 Pediatric Neuro-Oncology

In early childhood, the incidence of tumors is around 1 in 12,000 to 1 in 27,500 babies [86, 87]. Most ocular and orbital tumors of childhood are distinct from tumors that occur in adults. Many are congenital with early presentations. Most pediatric orbital tumors are benign like a dermoid cyst and capillary hemangiomas. A dermoid cyst is characterized by a sac that contains fluid and tissue that is not part of the eye or its surrounding area. The benign growth of tiny blood vessels, capillary hemangiomas along with a dermoid cyst are the most common benign lesions in the first months of life. The most common orbital malignancy is rhabdomyosarcoma, a cancerous tumor that develops in muscle or connective tissue. Also, a cancerous tumor that grows inside the retina of the eye known as retinoblastoma, is the most common intraocular malignant lesion.

Signs of orbital and ocular tumors differ depending on their location and whether they are benign or malignant. These symptoms may include bulging or crossed eye, redness or swelling near the eye, a bright red birthmark on or near the eye, and white pupillary reflex, mydriasis, or a red painful eye.

The role of OCT in neuro-oncology is a differentiation between types of tumors of the retina and RPE, to detect the degree of involvement of individual retinal layers and differentiate between abnormal and normal retina [88–90]. OCT images reveals the retinoblastoma lesions as isodense or hyperdense features, which are associated with patches of calcification, and usually have an abrupt transition toward uninvolved retina (Fig. 22.5) [89, 90].

In smaller tumors, depending on the lesion size, there is a different degree of retinal layer involvement from the inner nuclear and middle retinal layers. In larger tumors, there is involvement of the full thickness of the retina [36]. Also, small lesions- the pre-retinal seeds are located superficial to the retina, appear isodense and smooth, and are associated with shadowing of the underlying structures on OCT [36].

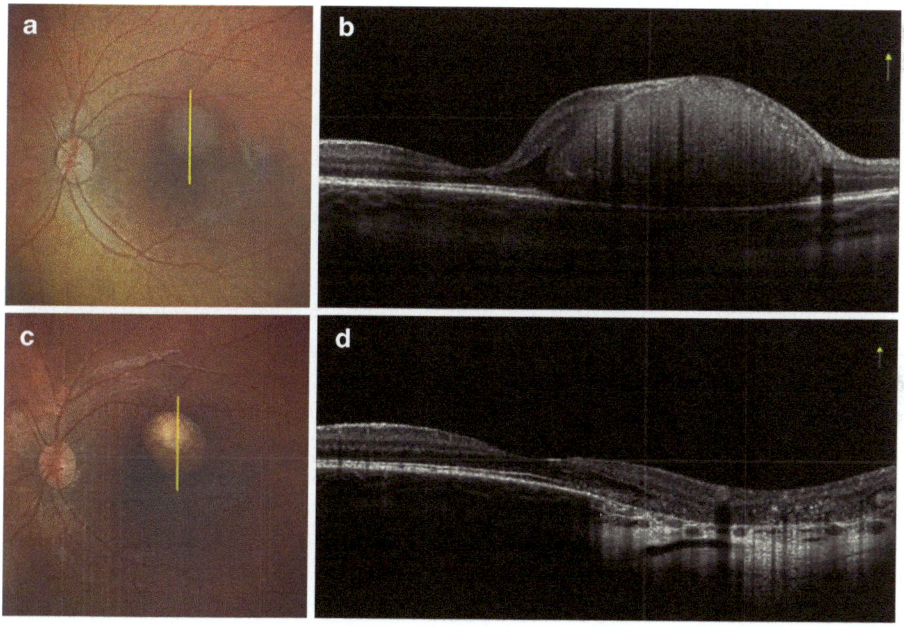

Fig. 22.5 Clinical case demonstrating the application of the Spectral domain hand-held optical coherence tomography (HH-OCT) system in a retinoblastoma patient (3-week-old girl), with a family history of maternal unilateral retinoblastoma [89]. (**a**) The left eye demonstrated a small dome-shaped, outer retinal tumor recurrence of (**b**) 2750 μm in basal dimension and 792 μm thickness in the para-foveolar region following 6 cycles of intravenous chemotherapy for bilateral retinoblastoma; and with adjacent shallow sub-retinal fluid. The mass was 615 μm from the foveola. (**c**) The tumor showed complete regression following 1 cycle of intra-arterial chemotherapy, (**d**) A concave scar of 120 μm in thickness and located 663 μm from foveolar documented by the HH-OCT. There was OCT light transmission through atrophic retinal pigment epithelial accentuating the underlying thin choroid. The foveola remained intact (*Image taken from Yarovaya* et al. *Int J Retin Vitr (2017) 3:43*)

OCT has been demonstrated to be useful for monitoring tumor progression, identifying new lesions and recurrences, monitoring treatment response, and guiding further management of ocular and orbital tumor complications [36, 91, 92].

22.4 Controversies and Challenges in Neonatology and Pediatric Neuro-Ophthalmology

Although, the OCT can be very helpful for diagnosing retinal and optic nerve diseases in infants and young children, there are many neuro-ophthalmological conditions that are very difficult to diagnose in early childhood due to the limited ability of this age group to cooperate with standard adult diagnostic and monitoring tools. Some challenges for the use of OCT still exist in pediatric ophthalmology. For example, the OCT scan of the retina works by rotating the OCT beam in the iris plane, but because of the shorter AL in children's eyes, the scanning procedure should be corrected by shortening the OCT reference [30]. Maldonado et al. suggested that to correct for any refractive errors, the image should be further optimized by adjusting the focus of the handheld probe (range, 10–12 diopters) [30]. Also, to facilitate comparisons at specific locations across different age groups, the lateral scales for the OCT data need to be adjusted based on age-specific AL estimates [30]. Gerth and Chong, in their research, suggested that images obtained using the handheld probe may also contain movement artifacts caused by the examiner and/or the child [34, 93]. Moreover, the HH-SDOCT imaging is limited by its lack of automatic registration for serial measurements.

In addition, it is important to adjust OCT to the age of the child when assessing foveal morphology, because of age-related variations in measurements of each retinal layer due to ongoing foveal development [38]. Another very important technique to consider in testing the youngest kids is to prepare a friendly decorated environment for the performance of OCT testing and keep the area controlled from noise and light [94]. Besides the OCT challenges and controversies in children, the emerging applications of the OCT technology in neonatology and pediatric neuro-ophthalmology can be, potentially, an objective and noninvasive diagnostic and monitoring tool helpful in providing additional information that can assist in management decisions.

22.5 Final Remarks

Development of the human visual system is a complex process. Over the past decade, considerable progress has been made in our understanding of the developmental, degenerative and ocular pathology in the childhood period. OCT is a valuable diagnostic tool that can be very helpful in everyday practice to improve our understanding of all physiological and pathological changes in disorders commonly observed in pediatric neuro-ophthalmology and pediatric ophthalmic-oncology assessments. With that understanding, our knowledge of the eye defects that cause neuro-ophthalmic disease has significantly expanded. Continuous improvement of non-invasive, easy-applicable OCT technology can widely enable application in youngest ages. There is no doubt that the upcoming years offer great promise for the further characterization of neurodevelopmental disorders of the visual system.

References

1. Fuhrmann S. Eye morphogenesis and patterning of the optic vesicle. Curr Top Dev Biol. 2010;93:61–84. https://doi.org/10.1016/B978-0-12-385044-7.00003-5.
2. Fitzpatrick DR, van Heyningen V. Developmental eye disorders. Curr Opin Genet Dev. 2005;15:348–53. https://doi.org/10.1016/j.gde.2005.04.013.
3. Wright K, Spiegel P. Pediatric ophthalmology and strabismus. 2nd ed. New York: Springer; 2003.
4. Lovicu F, McAvoy J, de Iongh R. Understanding the role of growth factors in embryonic development: insights from the lens. Philos Trans R Soc Lond Ser B Biol Sci. 2011;366:1204–18. https://doi.org/10.1098/rstb.2010.0339.
5. Ponsioen TL, Hooymans JM, Los LI. Remodeling of the human vitreous and vitreoretinal interface – a dynamic process. Prog Retin Eye Res. 2010;29:580–95. https://doi.org/10.1016/j.preteyeres.2010.07.001.
6. Gunhaga L. The lens: a classical model of embryonic induction providing new insights into cell determination in early development. Philos Trans R Soc Lond Ser B Biol Sci. 2011;366:1193–203. https://doi.org/10.1098/rstb.2010.0175.
7. Booij JC, Baas DC, Beisekeeva J, Gorgel TG, Bergem AA. The dynamic nature of Bruch's membrane. Prog Retin Eye Res. 2010;29:1–18. https://doi.org/10.1016/j.preteyeres.2009.08.003.
8. Provis M, Penfold PL, Cornish EE, Sandercoe TM, Madigan MC. Anatomy and development of the macula: specialization and the vulnerability to macular degeneration. Clin Exp Optom. 2005;88:269–81.
9. Hendrickson A, Bumsted-O'Brien K, Natoli R, Ramamurthy V, Possin D, Provis J. Rod photoreceptor differentiation in fetal and infant human retina. Exp Eye Res. 2008;87:415–26. https://doi.org/10.1016/j.exer.2008.07.016.
10. Morcillo J, Martínez-Morales JR, Trousse F, Fermin Y, Sowden JC, Bovolenta P. Proper patterning of the optic fissure requires the sequential activity of BMP7 and SHH. Development. 2006;133:3179–90. https://doi.org/10.1242/dev.02493.
11. Mann F, Harris WA, Holt CE. New views on retinal axon development: a navigation guide. Int J Dev Biol. 2004;48:957–64. https://doi.org/10.1387/ijdb.041899fm.
12. Irving C, Malhas A, Guthrie S, Mason I. Establishing the trochlear motor axon trajectory: role of the isthmic organizer and Fgf8. Development. 2002;129:5389–98.
13. Nugent AA, Kolpak AL, Engle EC. Human disorders of axon guidance. Curr Opin Neurobiol. 2012;22:837–43. https://doi.org/10.1016/j.conb.2012.02.006.
14. Zacharias AL, Lewandoski M, Rudnicki MA, Gage PJ. Pitx2 is an upstream activator of extraocular myogenesis and survival. Dev Biol. 2011;349:395–405. https://doi.org/10.1016/j.ydbio.2010.10.028.
15. Saint-Geniez M, D'Amore PA. Development and pathology of the hyaloid, choroidal and retinal vasculature. Int J Dev Biol. 2004;48:1045–58. https://doi.org/10.1387/ijdb.041895ms.
16. Hughes S, Yang H, Ling C. Vascularisation of the human fetal retina: roles of vasculogenesis and angiogenesis. Invest Ophthalmol Vis Sci. 2000;41:1217–28.
17. Das A, McGuire PG. Retinal and choroidal angiogenesis: pathophysiology and strategies for inhibition. Prog Retin Eye Res. 2003;22:721–48.
18. Zhao S, Overbeek PA. Regulation of choroid development by retinal pigment epithelium. Mol Vis. 2001;7:277–82.

19. Anand-Apte B, Hollyfield JG. Developmental anatomy of the retinal and choroidal vasculature. Cleveland: Elsevier; 2010.
20. Jakobiec FA. Ocular anatomy, embryology, and teratology. Philadelphia: Harper and Row; 1982.
21. Provis JM, Hendrickson AE. The foveal avascular region of developing human retina. Arch Ophthalmol. 2008;126:507–11. https://doi.org/10.1001/archopht.126.4.507.
22. Fruttiger M. Development of the retinal vasculature. Angiogenesis. 2007;10:77–88. https://doi.org/10.1007/s10456-007-9065-1.
23. Penn J, editor. Retinal and choroidal angiogenesis. Dordrecht: Springer; 2008.
24. Chan-Ling T, McLeod DS, Hughes S, Baxter L, Chu Y, Hasegawa T, et al. Astrocyte/endothelial cell relationships during human retinal vascular development. Invest Ophthalmol Vis Sci. 2004;45:2020–32.
25. Jonssen AM, Gardner TW, Kirchof B, Ryan SJ. Retinal vascular disease. Cambridge: Cambridge University Press; 2006.
26. Hungerford J, Stewart A, Hope P. Ocular sequelae of preterm birth and their relation to ultrasound evidence of cerebral damage. Br J Ophthalmol. 1986;70:463–8.
27. Msall ME, Phelps DL, DiGaudio KM, Dobson V, Tung B, McClead RE, et al. Severity of neonatal retinopathy of prematurity is predictive of neurodevelopmental functional outcome at age 5.5 years. Behalf of the Cryotherapy for Retinopathy of Prematurity Cooperative Group. Pediatrics. 2000;106:998–1005.
28. Cooke RW, Foulder-Hughes L, Newsham D, Clarke D. Ophthalmic impairment at 7 years of age in children born very preterm. Arch Dis Child Fetal Neonatal Ed. 2004;89:F249–53.
29. Stephenson T, Wright S, O'Connor A, Fielder A, Johnson A, Ratib S, et al. Children born weighing less than 1701 g: visual and cognitive outcomes at 11–14 years. Arch Dis Child Fetal Neonatal Ed. 2007;92:F265–70. https://doi.org/10.1136/adc.2006.104000.
30. Maldonado RS, Izatt JA, Sarin N, Wallace DK, Freedman S, Cotten CM, et al. Optimizing hand-held spectral domain optical coherence tomography imaging for neonates, infants, and children. Invest Ophthalmol Vis Sci. 2010;51:2678–85. https://doi.org/10.1167/iovs.09-4403.
31. Maldonado RS, O'Connell RV, Sarin N, Freedman SF, Wallace DK, Cotten CM, et al. Dynamics of human foveal development after premature birth. Ophthalmology. 2011;118:2315–25. https://doi.org/10.1016/j.ophtha.2011.05.028.
32. Lee H, Proudlock F, Gottlob I. Is handheld optical coherence tomography reliable in infants and young children with and without nystagmus? Invest Ophthalmol Vis Sci. 2013;54:8152–9. https://doi.org/10.1167/iovs.13-13230.
33. Avery RA, Cnaan A, Schuman JS, Chen CL, Glaug NC, Packer RJ, et al. Intra- and intervisit reproducibility of ganglion cell-inner plexiform layer measurements using handheld optical coherence tomography in children with optic pathway gliomas. Am J Ophthalmol. 2014;158:916–23. https://doi.org/10.1016/j.ajo.2014.07.029.
34. Gerth C, Zawadzki RJ, Héon E, Werner JS. High-resolution retinal imaging in young children using a handheld scanner and Fourier-domain optical coherence tomography. J AAPOS. 2009;13:72–4. https://doi.org/10.1016/j.jaapos.2008.09.001.
35. Maldonado RS, Toth CA. Optical coherence tomography in retinopathy of prematurity: looking beyond the vessels. Clin Perinatol. 2013;40:271–96. https://doi.org/10.1016/j.clp.2013.02.007.
36. Rootman DB, Gonzalez E, Mallipatna A, Vandenhoven C, Hampton L, Dimaras H, et al. Handheld high-resolution spectral domain optical coherence tomography in retinoblastoma: clinical and morphologic considerations. Br J Ophthalmol. 2013;97:59–65. https://doi.org/10.1136/bjophthalmol-2012-302133.
37. Vajzovic L, Hendrickson AE, O'Connell RV, Clark LA, Tran-Viet D, Possin D, et al. Maturation of the human fovea: correlation of spectral-domain optical coherence tomography findings with histology. Am J Ophthalmol. 2012;154:779–89.e2. https://doi.org/10.1016/j.ajo.2012.05.004
38. Lee H, Purohit R, Patel A, Papageorgiou E, Sheth V, Maconachie G, et al. In vivo foveal development using optical coherence tomography. Invest Ophthalmol Vis Sci. 2015;56:4537–45. https://doi.org/10.1167/iovs.15-16542.

39. Hendrickson AE, Yuodelis C. The morphological development of the human fovea. Ophthalmology. 1984;91:603–12.
40. Oros A. Retinopathy of prematurity. Belgrade: Endowment Andrejevic; 2003.
41. Phelps DL. Retinopathy of prematurity: history, classification, and pathophysiology. NeoReviews. 2001;2:e153–66. https://doi.org/10.1542/neo.2-7-e153.
42. Terry TL. Extreme prematurity and fibroblastic overgrowth of persistent vascular sheath behind each crystalline lens. Preliminary report. Am J Ophthalmol. 1942;25:203–4.
43. Friling R, Weinberger D, Kremer I, Avisar R, Sirota L, Snir M. Keratometry measurements in preterm and full-term newborn infants. Br J Ophthalmol. 2004;88:8–10.
44. Cook A, White S, Batterbury M, Clark D. Ocular growth and refractive error development in premature infants with or without retinopathy of prematurity. Invest Ophthalmol Vis Sci. 2008;49:5199–207. https://doi.org/10.1167/iovs.06-0114.
45. Gordon RA, Donzis PB. Refractive development of the human eye. Arch Ophthalmol. 1985;103:785–9. https://doi.org/10.1001/archopht.1985.01050060045020.
46. Harvey PS, King RA, Summers CG. Spectrum of foveal development in albinism detected with optical coherence tomography. J AAPOS. 2006;10:237–42. https://doi.org/10.1016/j.jaapos.2006.01.008.
47. Wallman J, Winawer J. Homeostasis of eye growth and the question of myopia. Neuron. 2004;43(4):447–68. https://doi.org/10.1016/j.neuron.2004.08.008.
48. Isenberg S, Del Signore M, Chen A, Wei J, Christenson P. Corneal topography of neonates and infants. Arch Ophthalmol. 2004;122:1767–71. https://doi.org/10.1001/archopht.122.12.1767.
49. Inagaki Y. The rapid change of corneal curvature in the neonatal period and infancy. Arch Ophthalmol. 1986;104:1026–7.
50. Mohindra I, Held R, Gwiazda J, Brill S. Astigmatism in infants. Science. 1978;202:329–31.
51. Howland HC, Atkinson J, Braddock O, French J. Infant astigmatism measured by photorefraction. Science. 1978;202:331–3.
52. Wang J, Spencer R, Leffler JN, Birch EE. Characteristics of peripapillary retinal nerve fiber layer in preterm children. Am J Ophthalmol. 2012;153:850–855.e1. https://doi.org/10.1016/j.ajo.2011.10.028.
53. Pueyo V, González I, Altemir I, Pérez T, Gómez G, Prieto E, et al. Microstructural changes in the retina related to prematurity. Am J Ophthalmol. 2015;159:797–802. https://doi.org/10.1016/j.ajo.2014.12.015.
54. Åkerblom H, Holmström G, Eriksson U, Larsson E. Retinal nerve fibre layer thickness in school-aged prematurely-born children compared to children born at term. Br J Ophthalmol. 2012;96:956–60. https://doi.org/10.1136/bjophthalmol-2011-301010.
55. Park KA, Oh SY. Retinal nerve fiber layer thickness in prematurity is correlated with stage of retinopathy of prematurity. Eye (Lond). 2015;9:1594–602. https://doi.org/10.1038/eye.2015.166.
56. Ecsedy M, Szamosi A, Karkó C, Zubovics L, Varsányi B, Németh J, et al. A comparison of macular structure imaged by optical coherence tomography in preterm and full-term children. Invest Ophthalmol Vis Sci. 2007;48:5207–11.
57. Lago AD, Matieli L, Gomes M, Baba NT, Farah ME, Belfort Junior R, et al. Stratus optical coherence tomography findings in patients with retinopathy of prematurity. Arq Bras Oftalmol. 2007;70:19–21.
58. Hammer DX, Iftimia NV, Ferguson RD, Bigelow CE, Ustun TE, Barnaby AM, et al. Foveal fine structure in retinopathy of prematurity: an adaptive optics Fourier domain optical coherence tomography study. Invest Ophthalmol Vis Sci. 2008;49:2061–70. https://doi.org/10.1167/iovs.07-1228.
59. Akerblom H, Larsson E, Eriksson U, Holmström G. Central macular thickness is correlated with gestational age at birth in prematurely born children. Br J Ophthalmol. 2011;95:799–803. https://doi.org/10.1136/bjo.2010.184747.
60. Wu WC, Lin RI, Shih CP, Wang NK, Chen YP, Chao AN, et al. Visual acuity, optical components, and macular abnormalities in patients with a history of retinopathy of prematurity. Ophthalmology. 2012;119:1907–16. https://doi.org/10.1016/j.ophtha.2012.02.040.

61. Park KA, Oh SY. Analysis of spectral-domain optical coherence tomography in preterm children: retinal layer thickness and choroidal thickness profiles. Invest Ophthalmol Vis Sci. 2012;53:7201–7. https://doi.org/10.1167/iovs.12-10599.
62. Chrzanowska B, Szumiński M, Oziebło-Kupczyk M, Bakunowicz-Łazarczyk A. Macular morphology and peripapillary retinal nerve fiber layer thickness in children with regressed retinopathy of prematurity [in Polish]. Klin Ocz. 2013;115:280–4.
63. Moreno TA, O'Connell RV, Chiu SJ, Farsiu S, Cabrera MT, Maldonado RS, et al. Choroid development and feasibility of choroidal imaging in the preterm and term infants utilizing SD-OCT. Invest Ophthalmol Vis Sci. 2013;54:4140–7. https://doi.org/10.1167/iovs.12-11471.
64. Maldonado RS, O'Connell R, Ascher SB, Sarin N, Freedman SF, Wallace DK, et al. Spectral-domain optical coherence tomographic assessment of severity of cystoid macular edema in retinopathy of prematurity. Arch Ophthalmol. 2012;130:569–78. https://doi.org/10.1001/archopthalmol.2011.1846.
65. Scott AW, Farsiu S, Enyedi LB, Wallace DK, Toth CA. Imaging the infant retina with a hand-held spectral-domain optical coherence tomography device. Am J Ophthalmol. 2009;147:364–73.e2. https://doi.org/10.1016/j.ajo.2008.08.010.
66. Erol MK, Ozdemir O, Turgut Coban D, Bilgin AB, Dogan B, Sogutlu Sari E, et al. Macular findings obtained by spectral domain optical coherence tomography in retinopathy of prematurity. J Ophthalmol. 2014;2014:468653. https://doi.org/10.1155/2014/468653.
67. Lee AC, Maldonado RS, Sarin N, O'Connell RV, Wallace DK, Freedman SF, et al. Macular features from spectral-domain optical coherence tomography as an adjunct to indirect ophthalmoscopy in retinopathy of prematurity. Retina. 2011;31:1470–82. https://doi.org/10.1097/IAE.0b013e31821dfa6d.
68. Joshi MM, Trese MT, Capone A Jr. Optical coherence tomography finding in stage 4A retinopathy of prematurity: a theory for visual variability. Ophthalmology. 2006;113:657–60. https://doi.org/10.1016/j.ophtha.2006.01.007.
69. Patel CK. Optical coherence tomography in the management of acute retinopathy of prematurity. Am J Ophthalmol. 2006;141:582–4. https://doi.org/10.1016/j.ajo.2005.10.002.
70. Ehrt O. Infantile and acquired nystagmus in childhood. Eur J Pediatr Neurol. 2012;16:567–72. https://doi.org/10.1016/j.ejpn.2012.02.010.
71. Lee H, Sheth V, Bibi M, Maconachie G, Patel A, McLean RJ, et al. Potential of handheld optical coherence tomography to determine cause of infantile nystagmus in children by using foveal morphology. Ophthalmology. 2013;120:2714–24. https://doi.org/10.1016/j.ophtha.2013.07.018.
72. Lee H, Purohit R, Sheth V, Papageorgiou E, Maconachie G, McLean RJ, et al. Retinal development in albinism: a prospective study using optical coherence tomography in infants and young children. Lancet. 2015;385(Suppl 1):S14. https://doi.org/10.1016/S0140-6736(15)60329-4.
73. Lee H, Purohit R, Sheth V, McLean RJ, Kohl S, Leroy BP, et al. Retinal development in infants and young children with achromatopsia. Ophthalmology. 2015;122:2145–7. https://doi.org/10.1016/j.ophtha.2015.03.033.
74. Pilat A, Sibley D, McLean RJ, Proudlock FA, Gottlob I. High-resolution imaging of the optic nerve and retina in optic nerve hypoplasia. Ophthalmology. 2015;122:1330–9. https://doi.org/10.1016/j.ophtha.2015.03.020.
75. Gu S, Glaug N, Cnaan A, Packer RJ, Avery RA. Ganglion cell layer-inner plexiform layer thickness and vision loss in young children with optic pathway gliomas. Invest Ophthalmol Vis Sci. 2014;55:1402–8. https://doi.org/10.1167/iovs.13-13119.
76. Wall M. Update on idiopathic intracranial hypertension. Neurol Clin. 2017;35:45–57. https://doi.org/10.1016/j.ncl.2016.08.004.
77. National Eye Institute. Idiopathic intracranial hypertension. 2018. https://nei.nih.gov/health/iih/intracranial. Accessed 12 Dec 2018.
78. Gospe SM 3rd, Bhatti MT, El-Dairi MA. Anatomic and visual function outcomes in paediatric idiopathic intracranial hypertension. Br J Ophthalmol. 2015;100:505–9. https://doi.org/10.1136/bjophthalmol-2015-307043.

79. El-Dairi MA, Holgado S, O'Donnell T, Buckley EG, Asrani S, Freedman SF. Optical coherence tomography as a tool for monitoring pediatric pseudotumor cerebri. J AAPOS. 2007;11:564–70.
80. Shaahinfar A, Whitelaw KD, Mansour KM. Update on abusive head trauma. Curr Opin Pediatr. 2015;27:308–14. https://doi.org/10.1097/MOP.0000000000000207.
81. Chiocca E. Advanced pediatric assessment. 2nd ed. New York: Springer; 2014. p. 484.
82. Barr RG. Preventing abusive head trauma resulting from a failure of normal interaction between infants and their caregivers. Proc Natl Acad Sci. 2012;109(Suppl 2):17294–301. https://doi.org/10.1073/pnas.1121267109.
83. Christian CW, Block R, Committee on Child Abuse and Neglect, American Academy of Pediatrics. Abusive head trauma in infants and children. Pediatrics. 2009;123:1409–11. https://doi.org/10.1542/peds.2009-0408.
84. Muni RH, Kohly RP, Sohn EH, Lee TC. Hand-held spectral domain optical coherence tomography finding in shaken-baby syndrome. Retina. 2010;30:S45–50. https://doi.org/10.1097/IAE.0b013e3181dc048c.
85. Scott AW, Farsiu S, Enyedi LB, Wallace DK, Toth CA. Imaging the infant retina with a hand-held spectral-domain optical coherence tomography device. Am J Ophthalmol. 2009;147:364–373.e2. https://doi.org/10.1016/j.ajo.2008.08.010.
86. Isaacs H Jr. Tumors of the fetus and newborn. Philadelphia: WB Saunders; 1997.
87. Moore SW, Satge D, Sasco AJ, Zimmermann A, Plaschkes J. The epidemiology of neonatal tumours. Report of an international working group. Pediatr Surg Int. 2003;19:509–19. https://doi.org/10.1007/s00383-003-1048-8.
88. Huot CS, Desai KB, Shah VA. Spectral domain optical coherence tomography of combined hamartoma of the retina and retinal pigment epithelium. Ophthalmic Surg Lasers Imaging. 2009;40:322–4.
89. Yarovaya V, Sioufi K, Shields CL. Parafoveolar retinoblastoma regression with foveal preservation following intraarterial chemotherapy documented on hand-held optical coherence tomography in a newborn. Int J Retin Vitr. 2017;3:43.
90. Goel N, Pangtey B, Bhushan G, Raina UK, Ghosh B. Spectral-domain optical coherence tomography of astrocytic hamartomas in tuberous sclerosis. Int Ophthalmol. 2012;32:491–3. https://doi.org/10.1007/s10792-012-9586-5.
91. Takahashi A, Otto S, Yoshimura N. High-penetration optical coherence tomography and enhanced depth imaging in presumed retinal pigment epithelial hamartoma. Retin Cases Brief Rep. 2013;7:179–82. https://doi.org/10.1097/ICB.0b013e31827aee75.
92. Yousef YA, Shroff M, Halliday W, Gallie BL, Héon E. Detection of optic nerve disease in retinoblastoma by use of spectral domain optical coherence tomography. J AAPOS. 2012;16:481–3. https://doi.org/10.1016/j.jaapos.2012.05.010.
93. Chong GT, Farsiu S, Freedman SF, Sarin N, Koreishi AF, Izatt JA, et al. Abnormal foveal morphology in ocular albinism imaged with spectral-domain optical coherence tomography. Arch Ophthalmol. 2009;127:37–44.
94. Lambert V, Coad J, Hicks P, Glacken M. Young children's perspectives of ideal physical design features for hospital-built environments. J Child Health Care. 2013;18:57–71. https://doi.org/10.1177/1367493512473852.

Machine Learning Approaches in OCT: Application to Neurodegenerative Disorders

23

Rui Bernardes, Lília Jorge, Ana Nunes, and Miguel Castelo-Branco

23.1 The Classical Approach: Univariate Comparisons of Thickness Measures and Potential Sources of Bias

Studying the visual system in neurodegenerative disorders both at the retinal and cortical level has been justified by the fact that visual impairments are among the initial symptoms of Alzheimer's disease, especially in which concerns the loss of contrast sensitivity and motion perception [1–5]. Furthermore, the pathological mechanisms underlying the neurodegenerative process appear to be consistent across the retina and the brain [6].

If the tenet that the retina is a mirror for cortical neurodegeneration holds, then it might be feasible to use it in the diagnosis of Alzheimer's disease or Parkinson's disease [7–12]. Moreover, published data suggesting the retinal structure itself might be altered in Alzheimer's disease and Parkinson's disease patients [13–20], further supports the used of the retina towards the establishment of image-based biomarkers for these neurodegenerative disorders.

R. Bernardes · M. Castelo-Branco (✉)
CIBIT - Coimbra Institute for Biomedical Imaging and Translational Research, Coimbra, Portugal

ICNAS - Institute of Nuclear Sciences Applied to Health, Coimbra, Portugal

Faculty of Medicine, University of Coimbra, Coimbra, Portugal
e-mail: mcbranco@ibili.uc.pt

L. Jorge · A. Nunes
CIBIT - Coimbra Institute for Biomedical Imaging and Translational Research, Coimbra, Portugal

ICNAS - Institute of Nuclear Sciences Applied to Health, Coimbra, Portugal

A. Grzybowski, P. Barboni (eds.), *OCT and Imaging in Central Nervous System Diseases*, https://doi.org/10.1007/978-3-030-26269-3_23

Optical coherence tomography (OCT) represents an inexpensive tool to assess neural changes at the retinal level. However, simple univariate approaches based on the traditionally performed thickness measurements remain problematic. There are three main reasons for this:

1. Results are not consistent across the literature. While several studies do not report retinal thickness differences between Alzheimer's disease or Parkinson's disease patients and healthy subjects [13, 21, 22], others have found significant thinning of different retinal layers [14, 23–25];
2. Information about degeneration may be distributed across the tissue and not captured by simple thickness measurements;
3. There are still issues of reproducibility across sites.

We first review some of the reported findings in the literature. Peripapillary retinal nerve fiber layer (RNFL) thickness has been claimed to be reduced in patients with Alzheimer's disease and mild cognitive impairment [26]. If this holds, then changes would occur even before conversion to Alzheimer's disease. Similar promising findings have been reported by Cheung and colleagues concerning the reduced combined thickness of the ganglion cell layer (GCL) and inner plexiform layer (IPL) in mild cognitive impairment patients [27].

Overall, OCT studies in Alzheimer's disease do in general indicate a significant decline in peripapillary (not macular) RNFL in all quadrants [14, 28] and overall macular thickness [14], while [27] reports macular GCL-IPL reduction. However, explicitly segmented retinal layers have been little investigated so far. The authors of [15, 29] found a decline of peripapillary and macular RNFL thickness in an Alzheimer's disease sample with mild-to-moderate dementia.

Concerning the macular RFNL thickness, significant differences between patients and controls were found in [30] as well. Haan et al. [31] did not find significant differences in any of the 7 segmented sublayers (RNFL, GCL, IPL, inner nuclear layer (INL), outer plexiform layer (OPL), outer nuclear layer (ONL), and retinal pigment epithelium (RPE)).

Some other studies using other techniques have also provided evidence against RNFL thinning in Alzheimer's disease [32–34]. For instance, resorting to scanning laser polarimetry, Kergoat et al. [33], have assessed the RNFL thickness near the optic nerve head center, in 30 individuals with mild-to-moderate Alzheimer's disease and respective controls, and found no significant differences between both groups. They suggested that this layer seems unlikely to be affected in the initial stages of the disease.

The significance of these findings would need to be reevaluated by studies assessing OCT measurements together with other biomarkers of neurodegeneration in Alzheimer's disease. However, these types of studies are still scarce [14].

With the notable exceptions mentioned above, most of these studies have been conducted in patients in later stages of the disease, in mild-to-moderate or severe Alzheimer's disease stages. A consensus remains therefore difficult to achieve. A sizable number of studies have reported a decrease in retinal layer thickness [15,

28, 29, 35–41], but others failed to report this difference [13, 14, 22–25, 29, 31–34].

Regarding the RNFL, inconsistencies may also derive from the fact that some studies have been conducted on the peripapillary RNFL while others were performed in the macular region. Moreover, inconsistencies are also present concerning histological work [42–45].

Sources of potential bias in aging populations also must be taken into account. For example, in [40], it was found that the thickness of both the RNFL + GCL complex and the manually segmented RNFL were reduced in the Alzheimer's disease sample, whereas the external layers did not show significant differences. Although their study population had mild-to-moderate dementia, with less than 3 years of diagnosis, they noted that their sample might include glaucoma patients. Such sources of bias are often not disclosed.

The fact that the primary visual cortex has been claimed to be spared in the early stages of the disease [46–53] does also not favor a direct imaging approach to the retina, at least in terms of the concept of a "window to the brain".

It is nevertheless still possible that a significant amount of information discriminating between multiple neurodegenerative states is conveyed by OCT imaging of the human retina, even when differences in average thickness are not yet present. In other words, approaches capturing multivariate information, which is just not possible with simple thickness-based univariate comparisons, may still detect early changes.

In [32], it was suggested that fluorescence lifetime imaging ophthalmoscopy (FLIO) may reveal retinal changes earlier than OCT, in a wide range of mild-to-moderate forms of Alzheimer's disease, possibly because of earlier disease-specific changes in cellular metabolism. Even though OCT cannot directly capture these, potentially associated changes in the local biological environment may induce changes in the medium that are measurable.

It remains a question whether the detailed assessment of separate retinal layers will help identify earlier changes in OCT data. Most studies exploring Alzheimer's disease macular integrity have focused on the RNFL, occasionally extending to the RNFL + GCL and GCL + IPL complexes. A notable exception is the work described in [31], which analyzed 7 sublayers.

Given all the discrepancies and sources of bias mentioned above, it remains a fundamental question of whether data-driven machine learning approaches would allow identifying biomarkers of brain neurodegeneration.

23.2 Machine Learning

In a recent paper [54], regarding the use of machine learning on neuroimaging modalities towards dementia diagnosis, it is clear the recent focus on using this type of applications in medicine in general and in clinical neurosciences in particular, with 16 of the referenced papers been published from 2013 to 2018 [54]. Magnetic Resonance Imaging (MRI) is the preferred imaging modality by far, with 14 out of the 16 studies using it.

Machine learning can broadly be defined by the famous quote attributed to Arthur Samuel, in 1959 [55], as "Field of study that gives computers the ability to learn without being explicitly programmed," even though the exact quote is "Programming computers to learn from experience should eventually eliminate the need for much of this detailed programming effort." Actual and more accurate definitions exist now.

Two major approaches can be thought of, the unsupervised and the supervised learning methods. For both types of algorithms, a set of examples that algorithms can learn from are required.

In unsupervised learning, the algorithm looks for structure in the data and aggregates similar cases in clusters. The measure of similarity plays a fundamental role, and distinct similarity metrics may lead to significantly different clustering results.

The supervised learning algorithm, on the other hand, requires a set of labeled examples. The algorithm will look, at the training phase, for the best way to split the set of cases according to the provided data for each one and the respective label. After that, new cases, to which the labels are unknown, will be labeled, for a classification problem, according to its data and the decision boundary established at the training phase. The above algorithm does not require the explicit definition of how to proceed. It will come to the best decision based on the provided examples only (Fig. 23.1).

It is important to bear in mind that machine learning can only provide answers to a specific question and according to the metric used to measure the success in classifying the examples provided for the training (learning) phase.

A good insight on machine learning and its use in medical imaging can be found in [56].

One of the widely used methods in machine learning applied in the field of dementia diagnosis is the support vector machines (SVM) approach. Vapnik and Chervonenkis [57, 58] proposed the SVM method, which is based on the linear separation between two classes (binary classification). The SVM algorithm consists

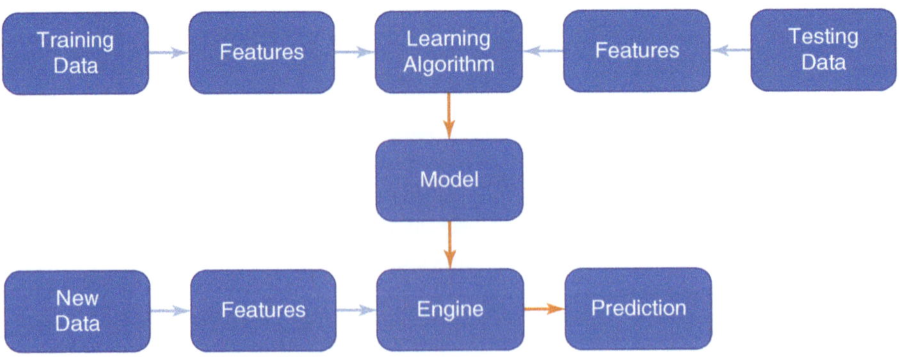

Fig. 23.1 Schematic of a machine learning model

of the identification of the hyperplane that makes most of the cases of one class lay in one side of it and the majority of the cases of the other class in the other side, while maximizing the distance between the hyperplane and the cases closer to it.

The characterization of individual cases is made by a set of values (features) that convey pertinent information on the case regarding the classification of interest. For example, the height and weight of a person would make sense for the classification of people in normal and overweight classes, while the iris color would not. Henceforth, it is required to compute/gather information thought to be relevant to the aimed classification.

Different machine learning approaches, like convolution neural networks (CNN) [59, 60], are possible and are based on a different rationale. The number of training cases is typically higher when compared to the SVM approach, where the rule of thumb to avoid overtraining is to have the number of training cases equal to ten times the number of classes times the number of features.

The application of machine learning is vast and can range from image segmentation and gene expression inference [61] to drug name recognition [62].

Using the retina as a window into the brain means to use the retina as a source of information that may convey the status of the brain concerning some aspect of interest, like the presence of signs of Alzheimer's disease, Parkinson's disease or any other neurodegenerative disorder of interest for a particular study. The rationale supporting this approach is that the retina is the visible part of the central nervous system (CNS) readily available to optical imaging. OCT is of particular interest for these studies because of its ability to detect changes in the refractive index, within the retina, with high sensitivity.

The traditional way to visualize OCT data from the ocular fundus is the direct visualization of B-scans, a way of presenting a set of A-scans taken side-by-side in the retina along a line, allowing for direct inspection of the structure of the retina (Fig. 23.2).

In addition to the structure, we postulate that information not perceivable to the user, by direct inspection of OCT data from the retina, may be present and may turn

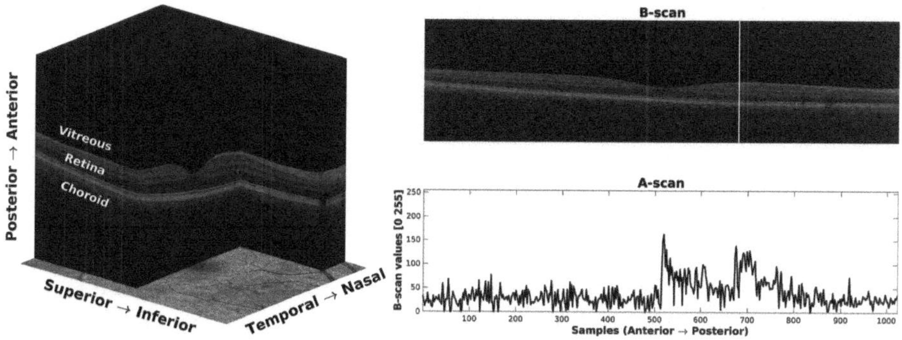

Fig. 23.2 Optical coherence tomography (OCT). Left: volumetric OCT data shown over an eye fundus reference computed from the inner limiting membrane (ILM) to the retinal pigment epithelium (RPE). Right: a B-scan (top) from the volume on the left, and an A-scan profile (bottom) from the B-scan

possible to identify differences from two different status based on the statistics of backscattered light. One possible way to compute information on the appearance of an image is through the use of texture.

Texture analysis methods [63, 64] may provide additional insights on such changes. Image texture relates to the relative distribution of the image's intensity values [65], which can be quantified using several different metrics (often called "textural features"). In brief, texture analysis allows determining how values of pixel intensity aggregate in an image or regions of an image, and compute metrics conveying information on the distinct ways pixels intensity aggregate. Two types of texture exist, the texture pattern and the random pattern. The former is the one where it is possible to visually identify a pattern, like squares, diamond shapes or the like. On the other hand, a random pattern is the one where it is not possible to visually identify a pattern, the typical case of a fundus image for an individual layer computed from an OCT retinal scan.

The use of texture-based methods has recently trespassed into the field of OCT imaging. In his doctoral thesis, Gao [66] has explored some of these features in addition to thickness measurements and other metrics on optical properties and reported that his combination of different methods yields additional insights into the macular pathology of diabetic retinopathy (DR) patients. González et al. [67] used co-occurrence [63] texture analysis methods to automatically detect cysts in OCT retinal images, having achieved a classification accuracy of 80%. In another classification study [68] based on the SVM algorithm, the different texture-based methods explored confirmed that texture carries useful information that can be used in addition to thickness measurements to detect changes caused by glaucoma. Subsequent studies by Varga et al. [69] and Morgan et al. [70] made use of texture analysis in OCT data to derive changes in the retinal tissue in multiple sclerosis and for the detection of retinal ganglion cell damage, respectively.

Besides the traditional OCT images, B-scans, fundus images can be computed for each retinal layer. Through image processing techniques, it is possible to determine the interfaces between consecutive retinal layers, like the RNFL-GCL and the GLC-IPL. The region between these two interfaces is, therefore, the GCL, meaning that it is possible to isolate a layer of interest from the rest of the gathered data. Imaging the retina, e.g., the macular region, by performing a series of B-scans side-by-side, and isolating the same a layer in each B-scan, allows collecting information on the retinal tissue of interest across the imaged region. Averaging the values of this layer along each A-scan allows computing a mean fundus image [71] of a particular layer, the GCL in the current example. The same principle can be applied to any of the layers of interest (Fig. 23.3) and allows analyzing each of these images using image analysis techniques, like texture analysis.

Other possibilities for texture analysis, besides the co-occurrence-based texture analysis, are the use of image transforms, like the wavelet transform, as in [72], or the well-known Fourier transform.

The use of specific texture metrics from mean fundus image images of individual retinal layers is utterly distinct from the approach of using a convolutional neural network, where the entire image is used, and no explicit computation of parameters from the image are pre-defined, as in [73].

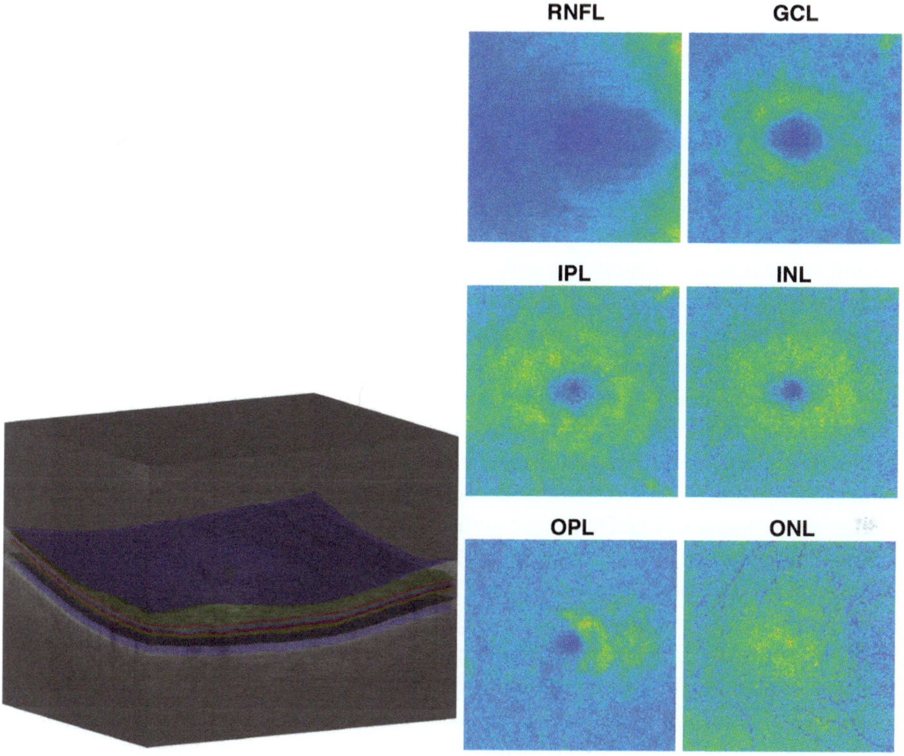

Fig. 23.3 An OCT volume (left) is shown with interfaces displayed in color, e.g., the interface vitreous-retina in blue. Pseudo-color fundus images (right) shown for retinal layers composing the neuroretina. Pseudo-color is used for the ease of visualization only

Exploratory studies performed on the retinas of mouse models of Alzheimer's disease, using the techniques already mentioned, hint at the hypothesis that early changes associated to this disorder can be identified in specific layers of the retina [74, 75]. Naturally, studies performed on animal models of disease have the advantages of allowing OCT data to be collected in the early stages of the disease, on the one hand, and making it possible, on the other hand, for the neurodegenerative process to be tracked at regular intervals of the disease's course. The key to identifying biomarkers of neurodegeneration in OCT human data may thus be found by leveraging the information contained in the corresponding animal data and comparing both species' datasets.

We have been using OCT and machine learning techniques to assess different health conditions through the retina. Our earliest work in this field aimed to assess retinal changes in OCT and distinguish between healthy controls (HC), patients diagnosed with diabetes and with no signs of DR (Early Treatment Diabetic Retinopathy Study level 10 eyes), and eyes diagnosed with diabetic macular edema (DME) [76].

In this preliminary work, using OCT from the whole retina (from the inner limiting membrane (ILM) to the RPE) within the macular region, and SVM for the classification of cases into one of the three possible classes (HC, DR and DME), it was possible to demonstrate that the retina may hold relevant information with respect to different statuses, even though that is not apparent from the traditional visual inspection, and that machine learning techniques may be helpful in gathering this information embedded in OCT data.

A subsequent work [77], following the same rationale and the same way of computing data to be used by the SVM classification algorithm, allowed to demonstrate, for the first time, the possibility to assess healthy ageing from OCT data, with the system being able to correctly classify healthy controls into one of two possible age groups with an overall accuracy of 70%.

Recently, we focused on using these techniques and approaches to assess changes in the retina associated with neurodegenerative disorders. To get an insight on which layer of the retina changes are predominant, we applied the methodology developed in [71] to compute a mean fundus image per retinal layer (Fig. 23.3).

In exploratory work, using OCT data from healthy controls' retinas, and OCT data from patients diagnosed with multiple sclerosis, we applied texture analysis to mean fundus image images [71]. Data were gathered by a Cirrus SD-OCT 5000 (Carl Zeiss Meditec, Dublin, CA, USA) using the 512 × 128 macular cube protocol and the layer segmentation was performed using the OCT Explorer software (Retinal Image Analysis Lab, Iowa Institute for Biomedical Imaging, Iowa City, IA, USA) [78–80].

For texture description, we applied the grey-level co-occurrence matrix (GLCM) [63] and computed 20 texture features from each GLCM [63, 81, 82] (Fig. 23.4).

We made use of SVM with radial basis function (RBF) kernel [83, 84], and each variable was z-score transformed at the pre-processing stage to eliminate

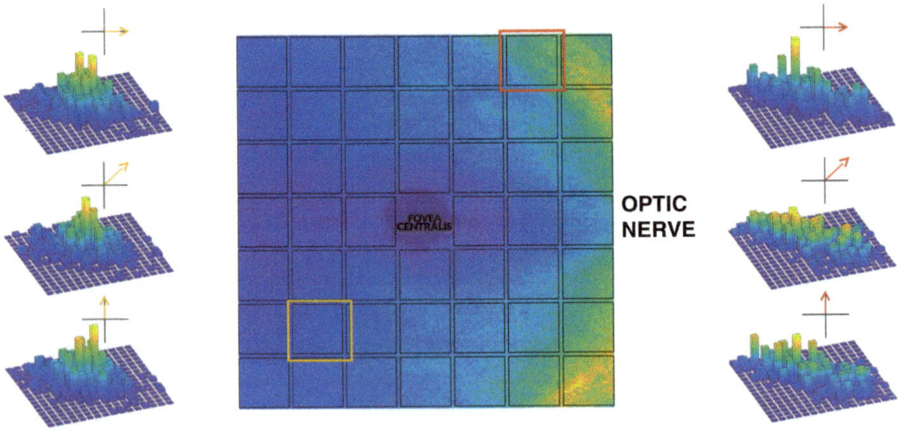

Fig. 23.4 The image in the center shows a pseudo-color fundus image from the retinal nerve fiber layer (RNFL). The grid delimits individual regions for texture analysis over the fundus image. Gray level co-occurrence matrices are plotted (left and right) for the two marked regions, respectively the marker region in the 6th row, and the marked region in row one. The arrows indicate the direction of analysis of texture using the grey-level co-occurrence matrix (GLCM) [63]. As shown, pixels' intensities aggregate differently in different regions conveying different texture characteristics

differences in scale that may interfere with the system performance. A twofold cross-validation (50% of the cases being used for training and 50% for testing) was used to assess the performance of the system in the classification of unknown cases.

The accuracy of the discrimination was over 75% for the GCL and under 72% for any of the remaining layers, when using only features of the layer under analysis. These results allowed to put forward the possibility to identify changes present in the retina of patients diagnosed with neurodegenerative disorders, on the one hand, and, on the other hand, that changes do not spread equally across the retina.

The approach we have been following is significantly distinct from the approaches that have been pursued, where the thickness of the retina or the thickness of specific layers of the retina is used to help the diagnosis of neurodegenerative disorders. Multiple sclerosis-related damage in the retina has been addressed by measuring the thickness of distinct layers [85, 86], with particular focus on the thickness of the RNFL that have been correlated to measures of brain atrophy in MRI [87, 88]. In a recent study [89], we show that texture-based metrics are not a surrogate for thickness measurements. In this study [89], we showed that 16 out of the 20 texture features present statistically significant differences (p-value $\leq$0.05) between the healthy controls and multiple sclerosis groups in at least one of the retinal quadrants (Fig. 23.5). Fourteen of the 16 texture features present highly statistically significant differences (p-value $\leq$0.01) and 5 of the 14 even higher (p-value $\leq$0.001), while the correlation between texture metrics and RNFL thickness is moderate, ranging from 0.50 to 0.62, for two features in the multiple sclerosis group and seven features in the healthy controls group.

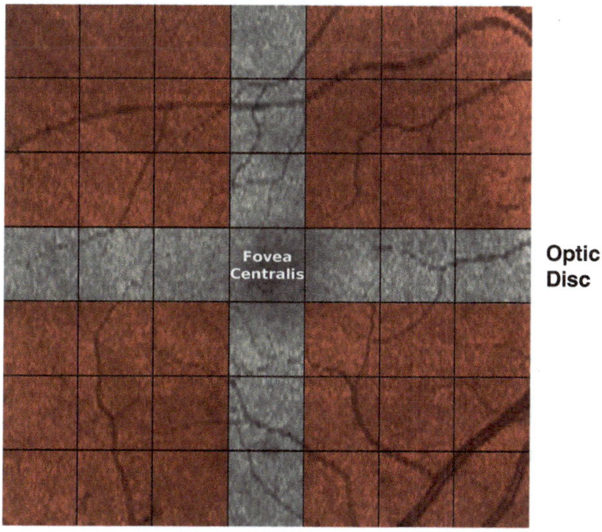

Fig. 23.5 Texture metrics are aggregated into retinal quadrants as shown by the reddish areas over the computed fundus image from the volumetric macular cube OCT scan of the right eye of a healthy control subject. Each of the 7 × 7 blocks shows the individual analyzed areas. Image axes are: x-axis (horizontal)—temporal (left) to nasal (right) and y-axis (vertical) superior (top) to inferior (bottom)

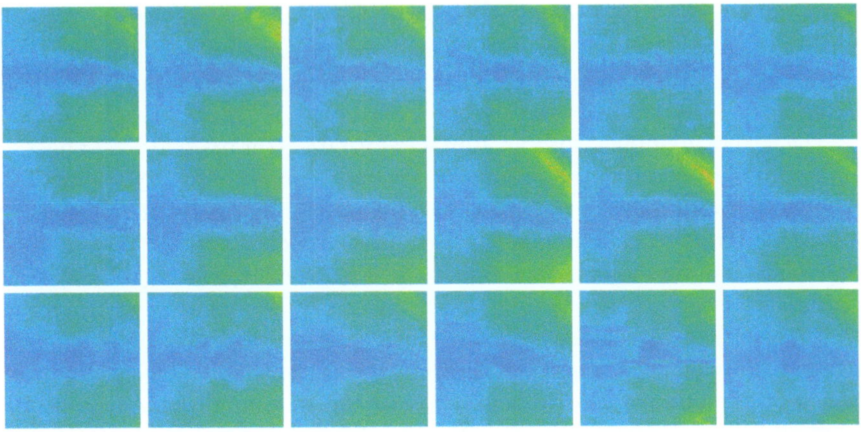

Fig. 23.6 Pseudo-color retinal nerve fiber layer (RNFL) fundus images of six eyes of healthy controls (HC) (top), six eyes of patients diagnosed with Alzheimer's disease (AD) (middle), and six eyes of patients diagnosed with Parkinson's disease (PD) (bottom) are shown. Through visual inspection, it would not be possible to identify characteristics distinguishing these groups. All cases are age-matched

Feeding machine learning techniques with data and class labels means that it is required to have a prior classification of known cases using currently accepted diagnosis methods. However, these can only provide a probable diagnosis at a particular disease stage, which for Alzheimer's disease is thought to be 10–15 years after disease onset [90]. Hence, we may be teaching the system to detect what is currently known instead of trying to teach it to detect early signs of disease.

Pushing the limits, we put forward a study aiming to simultaneously discriminate between healthy controls, Alzheimer's disease, and Parkinson's disease patients (Fig. 23.6). The analysis of texture from the mean fundus image images of the neuroretina, comprising layers from the RNFL to the ONL, allowed the classification system to identify eyes of healthy controls with a sensitivity (SEN) of 87.7% and specificity (SPE) of 83.9%, eyes of Alzheimer's disease patients with 79.5% (SEN) and 92.5% (SPE), and eyes of Parkinson's disease patients with 75.9% (SEN) and 97.8% (SPE). Of utmost importance, though, is the fact that 74.6% of the subjects have received the same classification in both eyes and that 92.8% of these people were classified in the correct group.

These findings suggest that information conveyed by texture analysis of OCT data from the human retina is specific for the neurodegenerative disorder, instead of merely signaling a difference from the health status.

To address the possibility of identifying early signs of Alzheimer's disease based on texture metrics from OCT data, we set a study using wild-type and mice models of Alzheimer's disease and imaged those every 4 months starting at the age of 4 months. The system used in this study to image mice's retinas is the Micron IV OCT (Phoenix Research Labs, Pleasanton, CA, USA), which is tailored to image mouse and rat retinas and allows scanning the posterior pole of the eye gathering

512 × 512 × 1024 voxels over 50° field of view. Because mice do not possess a macula, all scans were performed at the same retinal location, above the optic disc and horizontally centered in it.

After the acquisition, images were processed as in [76]. Features computed from the histograms of OCT intensity distribution fed an SVM algorithm to find the possibility to classify mice into the wild-type and Alzheimer's disease groups. This classifier achieved a median accuracy of 83% at the age of 4 months and 94% at the age of 8 months. We further tested texture information to find differences between groups, even using a gross split of the mouse retina into 3 layers. These findings paved the way for further ongoing studies.

Because of the suggested parallel between changes in the mice retina of the Alzheimer's disease model and those occurring in the human retina, we put forward a study to determine which retinal layers and which texture metrics match between the differences to the respective control population. Our preliminary results show that the RNFL and the IPL are the ones presenting the least overlap in terms of features showing statistically significant differences to the health status. On the other hand, the OPL is the layer presenting the higher number of statistically significant differences and those with the more considerable extent in the human retina: 8 features showing differences in 3 of the 4 retinal quadrants (the whole macular region except the inferior-temporal quadrant), with 7 of these presenting statistically significant differences between the wild-type and the transgenic mice model of Alzheimer's disease at the 8, 12 and 16 months of age. This overlap strongly suggests that a similar process is occurring in both human and mice retina.

Following the above results, we put forward a new study where mice models of Alzheimer's disease (born transgenic) are being imaged every month since the age of 1 month up to the age of 4 months, and every 4 months after that to identify biomarkers of Alzheimer's disease onset and progression.

Such biomarkers are of paramount importance as they will turn possible to identify patients at risk of developing Alzheimer's disease before they can be diagnosed using currently available methods and using an imaging technique which is widely available, inexpensive and non-invasive.

References

1. Gilmore GC, Groth KE, Thomas CW. Stimulus contrast and word reading speed in Alzheimer's disease. Exp Aging Res. 2005;31(1):15–33.
2. Graewe B, Lemos R, Ferreira C, Santana I, Farivar R, Weerd PD, Castelo-Branco M. Impaired processing of 3D motion-defined faces in mild cognitive impairment and healthy ageing: an fMRI study. Cereb Cortex. 2013;23(10):2489–99.
3. Javaid FZ, Brenton J, Guo L, Cordeiro MF. Visual and ocular manifestations of Alzheimer's disease and their use as biomarkers for diagnosis and progression. Front Neurol. 2016;7:55.
4. Lemos R, Figueiredo P, Santana I, Simões MR, Castelo-Branco M. Temporal integration of 3D coherent motion cues defining visual objects of unknown orientation is impaired in amnestic mild cognitive impairment and Alzheimer's disease. J Alzheimers Dis. 2012;28(4):885–96.

5. Risacher SL, Wudunn D, Pepin SM, McGee TR, McDonald BC, Flashman LA, Saykin AJ. Visual contrast sensitivity in Alzheimer's disease, mild cognitive impairment, and older adults with cognitive complaints. Neurobiol Aging. 2013;34(4):1133–44.
6. Masland RH. The neurological organization of the retina. Neuron. 2012;76(2):266–80.
7. Archibald NK, Clarke MP, Mosimann UP, Burn DJ. The retina in Parkinson's disease. Brain. 2009;132:1128–45.
8. Calabresi PA, Balcer LJ, Frohman EM. Retinal pathology in multiple scleroris: insights into the mechanisms of neuronal pathology. Brain. 2010;133(6):1575–7.
9. Cordeiro MF. Eyeing the brain. Acta Neuropathol. 2016;132(6):765–6.
10. London A, Benhar I, Schwartz M. The retina as a window to the brain - from eye research to CNS disorders. Nat Rev Neurol. 2013;9(1):44–53.
11. Svetozarskiy SN, Kopishinskaya SV. Retinal optical coherence tomography in neurodegenerative diseases (review). Sovremennye technologii v medicine. 2015;7(1):116–23.
12. Cheung CY, Ikram MK, Chen C, Wong TY. Imaging retina to study dementia and stroke. Prog Retin Eye Res. 2017;57:89–107.
13. Archibald NK, Clarke MP, Mosimann UP, Burn DJ. Retinal thickness in Parkinson's disease. Parkinsonism Relat Disord. 2011;17:431–136.
14. Haan JD, Verbraakb FD, Vissera PJ, Bouwmana FH. Retinal thickness in Alzheimer's disease: a systematic review and meta-analysis. Alzheimers Dement. 2017;6:162–70.
15. Ascaso FJ, Cruz N, Modrego PJ, Lopez-Anton R, Santabárbara J, Pascual LF, Lobo A, Cristóbal JA. Retinal alterations in mild cognitive impairment and Alzheimer's disease: an optical coherence tomography study. J Neurol. 2014;261:1566–30.
16. Hart NJ, Koronyo Y, Black KL, Koronyo-Hamaoui M. Ocular indicators of Alzheimer's: exploring disease in the retina. Acta Neuropathol. 2016;132:767–87.
17. Tian T, Zhu XH, Liu YH. Potential role of the retina as a biomarker for progression of Parkinson's disease. Int J Ophthalmol. 2011;4(4):433–8.
18. Cheung CY, Ong YT, Ikram MK, Ong SY, Li X, Hilal S, Catindig JAS, Venketasubramanian N, Yap P, Seow D, Chen CP, Wong TY. Microvascular network alterations in the retina of patients with Alzheimer's disease. Alzheimers Dement. 2014;10(2):135–42.
19. Garcia-Martin E, Larrosa JJM, Polo V, Satue M, Marques MLM, Alarcia R, Seral M, Fuertes I, Otin S, Pablo LEL. Distribution of retinal layer atrophy in patients with Parkinson disease and association with disease severity and duration. Am J Ophthalmol. 2014;157(2):470–8.
20. Chorostecki J, Seraji-Bozogard N, Shah A, Bao F, Bao G, George E, Gorden V, Caon C, Frohman E, Bhatti M, Khan O. Characterization of retinal architecture in Parkinson's disease. J Neurol Sci. 2015;355:44–8.
21. Lad EM, Mukherjee D, Stinnett SS, Cousins SW, Potter GG, Farsiu S, Whitson HE. Evaluation of inner retinal layers as biomarkers in mild cognitive impairment to moderate Alzheimer's disease. PLoS One. 2018;13(2):e0192646.
22. Aaker GD, Myung JS, Ehrlich JR, Mohammed M, Henchcliffe C, Kiss S. Detection of retinal changes in Parkinson's disease with spectral-domain optical coherence tomography. Clin Ophthalmol. 2010;4:1427–32.
23. Garcia-Martin E, Bambo MP, Marques ML, Satue M, Otin S, Larrosa JM, Polo V, Pablo LE. Ganglion cell layer measurements correlate with disease severity in patients with Alzheimer's disease. Acta Ophthalmol. 2016;94:e454–9.
24. Hajee ME, March WF, Lazzaro DR, Wolintz AH, Shrier EM, Glazman S, Bodis-Wollner IG. Inner retinal layer thinning in Parkinson disease. Arch Ophthalmol. 2009;127(6):737–41.
25. Altintaş Ö, Işeri P, Berna Ö, Yusuf Ç. Correlation between retinal morphological and functional findings and clinical severity in Parkinson's disease. Documenta Opthhalmologica. 2008;116:137–46.
26. Thomson KL, Yeo JM, Briony W, Cameron JR, Pal S. A systematic review and meta-analysis of retinal nerve fiber layer change in dementia, using optical coherence tomography. Alzheimers Dement. 2015;1:136–43.
27. Cheung CY, Ong YT, Hilai S, Ikram MK, Low S, Ong YL, Wong TY. Retinal ganglion cell analysis using high-definition optical coherence tomography in patients with mild cognitive impairment and Alzheimer's disease. J Alzheimers Dis. 2015;45(1):45–6.

28. Coppola G, Renzo AD, Ziccardi L, Martelli F, Fadda A, Manni G, Barboni P, Pierelli F, Sadun AA, Parisi V. Optical coherence tomography in Alzheimer's disease: a meta-analysis. PLoS One. 2015;10(8):e0134750.
29. Iseri PK, Altinas Z, Tokay T, Yüksel N. Relationship between cognitive impairment and retinal morphological and visual functional abnormalities in Alzheimer disease. J Neuroophthalmol. 2006;26:18–24.
30. Larrosa JM, Garcia-Martin E, Bambo MP, Pinilla J, Polo V, Otin S, Pablo LE. Potential new diagnostic tool for Alzheimer's disease using a linear discriminant function of Fourier domain optical coherence tomography. Invest Ophthalmol Vis Sci. 2014;55(5):3043.
31. Haan JD, Janssen SF, Kreeke JAVD, Scheltens P, Verbraak FD, Bouwman FH. Retinal thickness correlates with parietal cortical atrophy in early-onset Alzheimer's disease and controls. Alzheimers Dement. 2018;10:49–55.
32. Jentsch S, Schweitzer D, Schmidtke KU, Peters S, Dawczynski J, Bär KJ, Hammer M. Retinal fluorescence lifetime imaging ophthalmoscopy measures depend on the severity of Alzheimer's disease. Acta Ophthalmol. 2015;93(4):e241–7.
33. Kergoat H, Kergoat MJ, Justino L, Chertkow H, Robillard A, Bergman H. An evaluation of the retinal nerve fiver layer thickness by scanning laser polarimetry in individuals with dementia of the Alzheimer type. Acta Ophthalmol Scand. 2001;79(2):187–91.
34. Kurna SA, Akar G, Altun A, Agirman Y, Gozke E, Sengor T. Confocal laser tomography of the optic nerve head on the patients with Alzheimer's disease compared to glaucoma and control. Int Ophthalmol. 2014;34(6):1203–11.
35. Berisha F, Feke GT, Trempe CL, McMeel JW, Schepens CL. Retinal abnormalities in early Alzheimer's disease. Invest Ophthalmol Vis Sci. 2007;48(5):2285–9.
36. Gao L, Liu Y, Li X, Bai Q, Liu P. Abnormal retinal nerve fiber layer thickness and macula lutea in patients with mild cognitive impairment and Alzheimer's disease. Arch Gerontol Geriatr. 2015;60(1):162–7.
37. Kesler A, Vakhapova V, Korczyn AD, Naftaliev E, Neudorfer M. Retinal thickness in patients with mild cognitive impairment and Alzheimer's disease. Clin Neurol Neurosurg. 2011;113(7):523–6.
38. Kirbas S, Turkyilmaz K, Anlar O, Tufekci A, Durmus M. Retinal nerve fiber layer thickness in patients with Alzheimer's disease. J Neuroophthalmol. 2013;33(1):58–61.
39. Liu J, Harris A, Kanwisher N. Perception of faces parts and faces configurations: an fMRI study. J Cogn Neurosci. 2010;22(1):203–11.
40. Marziani E, Pomati S, Ramolfo P, Cigada M, Giani A, Mariani C, Staurenghi G. Evaluation of retinal nerve fiber layer and ganglion cell layer thickness in Alzheimer's disease using spectral-domain optical coherence tomography. Invest Opthalmol Vis Sci. 2013;54:5953–8.
41. Paquet C, Boissonnot M, Roger F, Dighiero P, Gil R, Hugon J. Abnormal retinal thickness in patients with mild cognitive impairment and Alzheimer's disease. Neurosci Lett. 2017;420(2):97–9.
42. Blanks JC, Torigoe Y, Hinton DR, Blanks RH. Retinal pathology in Alzheimer's disease: I. Ganglion cell loss in foveal/parafoveal retina. Neurobiol Ageing. 1996;17(3):377–84.
43. Blanks JC, Schimdt SY, Torigoe Y, Porrello KV, Hinton DR, Blanks RH. Retinal pathology in Alzheimer's disease: II. Regional neuron loss and glial changes in GCL. Neurobiol Aging. 1996;17(3):385–95.
44. Curcio CA, Drucker DN. Retinal ganglion cells in Alzheimer's disease and aging. Ann Neurol. 1993;33(3):248–57.
45. Davies DC, McCoubrie P, McDonald B, Jobst KA. Myelinated axon number in the optic nerve is unaffected by Alzheimer's disease. Br J Ophthalmol. 1995;79(6):596–600.
46. Benson D. The use of positron emission scanning techniques in the diagnosis of Alzheimer's disease. In: Corkin K, David J, Growdon E, Usdin E, Wurtman E, editors. Alzheimer's disease: a report of progress in research. New York: Raven Press; 1982. p. 79–82.
47. Brun A, Gustafson L. Distribution of cerebral degeneration in Alzheimer's disease. Eur Arch Psychiatry Clin Neurosci. 1976;233(1):15–33.
48. Buckner LR, Snyder AZ, Sanders AL, Raichle ME, Morris JC. Functional brain imaging of young, nondemented and demented older adults. J Cogn Neurosci. 2018;12(2):24–34.

49. Busatto GF, Diniz BS, Zanetti MV. Voxel-based morphometry in Alzheimer's disease. Expert Rev Neurother. 2008;8(11):1691–702.
50. Lerch JP, Pruessner JC, Zidenhos A, Hampel H, Teipel SJ, Evans AC. Focal decline of cortical thickness in Alzheimer's disease identified by computational neuroanatomy. Cereb Cortex. 2005;15(7):995–1001.
51. Orwin A, Wright CE, Harding GF, Rowan DC, Rolfe EB. Serial visual evoked potential recordings in Alzheimer's disease. Br Med J (Clin Res Ed). 1986;293(6538):9–10.
52. Prvulovic DHD, Sack AT, Melillo L, Maurer K, Frölich, Dierks T. Functional imaging of visuospatial processing in Alzheimer's disease. NeuroImage. 2002;17(3):1403–14.
53. Rizzo M, Anderson SW, Dawson J, Nawrot M. Vision and cognition in Alzheimer's disease. Neuropsychologia. 2000;38(8):1157–69.
54. Ahmed R, Zhang Y, Feng Z, Lo B, Inan OT, Liao H. Neuroimaging and machine learning for dementia diagnosis: recent advancements and future prospects. IEEE Rev Biomed Eng. 2018;12:19–33.
55. Samuel AL. Some studies in machine learning using the game of checkers. IBM J Res Dev. 1959;3(3):211–29.
56. Erickson BJ, Korfiatis P, Akkus Z, Kline TL. Machine learning for medical analysis. Radiographics. 2017;37:505–15.
57. Vapnik N. Theory of pattern recognition (in Russian) (German translation: WN Vapnik and AJ Chervonenkis, Theorie der Zeichenerkennung. Berlin: Akademia-Verlag 353, 1979). Moscow: Nauka; 1974.
58. Vapnik VN. An overview of statistical learning theory. IEEE Trans Neural Netw. 1999;10(5):988–99.
59. Anwar SM, Majid M, Qayyum A, Awais M, Alnowami M. Medical image analysis using convolutional neural networks: a review. J Med Syst. 2018;42:226.
60. Bakator M, Radosav D. Deep learning and medical diagnosis: a review of literature. Multimodal Technol Interact. 2018;2:47.
61. Cao C, Liu F, Tan H, Song D, Shu W, Li W, Zhou Y, Bo X, Xie Z. Deep learning and its applications in biomedicine. Genomics Proteomics Bioinformatics. 2018;16:17–32.
62. Chalapathy R, Borzeshi EZ, Piccardi M. An investigation of recurrent neural architectures for drug name recognition. In: 7th international workshop on health text mining and information analysis, 2016.
63. Haralick RM, Shanmugam K, DInstein I. Textural features for image classification. IEEE Trans Syst Man Cybern. 1973;3(6):610–21.
64. Kassner A, Thornhill RE. Texture analysis: a review of neurologic MR imaging applications. Am J Neuroradiol. 2010;31:809–16.
65. Meyer-Bäse A. Pattern recognition for medical imaging. San Diego: Elsevier; 2004.
66. Gao W. Improving the quantitative assessment of intraretinal features by determining both structural and optical properties of the retinal tissue with optical coherence tomography. Doctoral thesis; 2012.
67. González A, Remeseiro B, Ortega MPMG. Automatic cyst detection in OCT retinal images combining region flooding and texture analysis. In: IEEE symposium on computer-based medical systems, 2013.
68. Anantrasirichai N, Achim A, Morgan JE, Erchovay I, Nicholson L. SVM-based texture classification in optical coherence tomography. In: 2013 IEEE 10th international symposium on biomedical imaging: from nano to macro, 2013.
69. Varga B, Gao W, Laurik K, et al. Investigating tissue optical properties and texture descriptors of the retina in patients with multiple sclerosis. PLoS One. 2015;10(1):e0143711.
70. Morgan JE, Tribble J, Fergusson J, White N, Erchova I. The optical detection of retinal ganglion cell damage. Eye. 2017;31(2):199–205.
71. Guimarães P, Rodrigues P, Lobo C, Leal S, Figueira J, Serranho P, Bernardes R. Ocular fundus reference images from optical coherence tomography. Comput Med Imaging Graph. 2014;38:381–9.

72. Dermihan A. Neuroimage-based clinical prediction using machine learning tools. Wiley Periodics; 2017.
73. Choi SH, Park SJ, Kim NR. Macular ganglion cell-inner plexiform layer thickness is associated with clinical progression in mild cognitive impairment and Alzheimer's disease. PLoS One. 2017;11(9):e0162202.
74. Bernardes R, Silva G, Chiquita S, Serranho P, Ambrósio AF. Retinal biomarkers of Alzheimer's disease: insights from transgenic mouse models. In: 14th International Conference on Image Analysis and Recognition (ICIAR), 2017.
75. Nunes A, Ambrósio AF, Castelo-Branco M, Bernardes R. Texture biomarkers of Alzheimer's disease and disease progression in the mouse retina. In: International conference on Biological Information and Biomedical Engineering (BIBE), 2018.
76. Bernardes R. Optical coherence tomography: health information embedded on OCT signal statistics. In: 33rd annual international conference of the IEEE EMBS, 2011.
77. Bernardes R, Serranho P, Santos T, Gonçalves V, Cunha-Vaz J. Optical coherence tomography – automatic retina classification through support vector machines. Eur Ophthalmic Rev. 2012;6(4):200–3.
78. Garvin MK, Abràmoff MD, Wu X, Russell SR, Burns TL, Sonka M. Automated 3D intraretinal layer segmentation of macular spectral-domain optical coherence tomography images. IEEE Trans Med Imaging. 2009;28:1436–47.
79. Abràmoff MD, Garvin MK, Sonka M. Retinal imaging and image analysis. IEEE Rev Biomed Eng. 2010;3:169–208.
80. Li K, Wu X, Chen D, Sonka M. Optimal surface segmentation in volumetric images - a graph-theoretic approach. IEEE Trans Pattern Anal Mach Intell. 2006;28(1):119–34.
81. Soh L-K, Tsatsoulis C. Texture representation of SAR sea ice imagery using multi-displacement co-occurrence matrices. In: International geoscience and remote sensing symposium, 1996.
82. Clausi DA. An analysis of co-occurrence texture statistics as a function of grey-level quantization. Can J Remote Sens. 2002;8(1):45–62.
83. Duda RO, Hart PE, Stork DG. Pattern classification. 2nd ed. New York: Wiley; 2000.
84. Chang C-C, Lin C-J. LIBSVM: a library for support vector machines. ACM Trans Intell Syst Technol. 2011;2(3):27.
85. Britze J, Phil-Jensen G, Frederiksen JL. Retinal ganglion cell analysis in multiple sclerosis and optic neuritis: a systematic review and meta-analysis. J Neurol. 2017;264:1837–53.
86. Saidha S, Syc SB, Ibrahim MA, Eckstein C, Warner CV, Farrell SK, Oakley JD, Durbin MK, Meyer SA, Balcer LJ, Frohman EM, Rosenzweig JM, Newsome SDEA. Primary retinal pathology in multiple sclerosis as detected by optical coherence tomography. Brain. 2011;134:518–33.
87. Petzhold A, Boer JFD, Schippling S, Vermersch P, Kardon R, Green A, Calabresis PA, Polman C. Optical coherence tomography in multiple sclerosis: a systematic review and meta-analysis. Lancet Neurol. 2010;9:921–32.
88. Henderson AP, Trip SA, Schlottmann PG, Altmann DR, Garway-Heath DF, Plant GT, Miller DH. An investigation of the retinal nerve fibre layer in progressive multiple sclerosis using optical coherence tomography. Brain. 2008;131:277–87.
89. Nunes A, Silva G, Alves C, Batista S, Sousa L, Castelo-Branco M, Bernardes R. Textural information from the retinal nerve fibre layer in multiple sclerosis. In: IEEE Portuguese Meeting in Bioengineering (ENBENG), 2019.
90. Krantic S, Torriglia A. Retina: source of the earliest biomarkers for Alzheimer's disease? J Alzheimers Dis. 2014;40:237–43.

Optical Coherence Tomography Angiography in Neurology and Neuro-Ophthalmology

24

Alexander Pinhas, Valerie I. Elmalem, Maria Castanos Toral, Davis B. Zhou, Jorge S. Andrade Romo, Alexander Barash, and Richard B. Rosen

24.1 Introduction

Alterations to blood circulation in the central nervous system and optic nerve in neurological and neuro-ophthalmological disease have been well documented by CT, MRI and Doppler in vivo, and histology ex vivo. It is unclear, however, whether the vascular alterations are secondary to neuronal loss from decreased metabolic demand and neurovascular coupling, or a pathogenic step preceding neurodegeneration. Studies using new tools and biomarkers involving the vasculature can help elucidate the relationship between the neuronal and vascular tissues in these diseases, as well as help diagnose disease earlier and monitor treatment efficacy.

Given the similarities between brain and retinal tissues, retinal imaging offers a readily accessible, non-invasive window into the vascular changes that accompany the pathophysiologic developments of neurological and neuro-ophthalmological diseases. Classical retinal vascular features including vascular attenuation, tortuosity and foveal avascular zone (FAZ) alterations, as well as structural optical coherence tomography (OCT) changes in retinal and choroidal layer thickness have received increasing attention in the setting of neurological and neuro-ophthalmological diseases.

A. Pinhas (✉)
Department of Ophthalmology, New York Eye and Ear Infirmary of Mount Sinai, New York, NY, USA

Department of Ophthalmology, State University of New York Downstate Medical Center, Brooklyn, NY, USA

V. I. Elmalem · M. Castanos Toral · D. B. Zhou · J. S. Andrade Romo · A. Barash
R. B. Rosen
Department of Ophthalmology, New York Eye and Ear Infirmary of Mount Sinai, New York, NY, USA

A. Grzybowski, P. Barboni (eds.), *OCT and Imaging in Central Nervous System Diseases*, https://doi.org/10.1007/978-3-030-26269-3_24

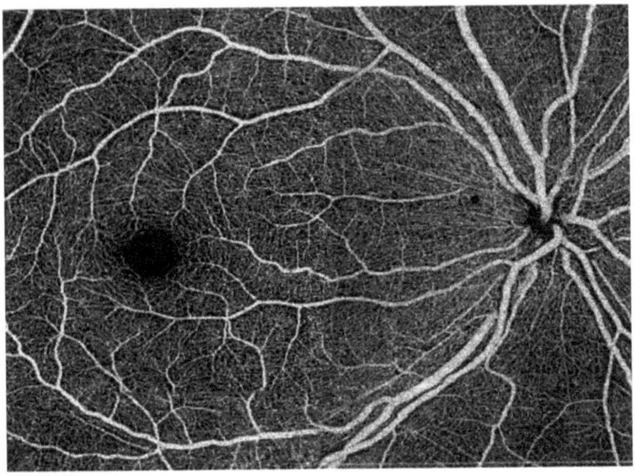

Fig. 24.1 OCT-A montage of the superficial capillary circulation of the macular and peripapillary retina in a healthy individual. Reproduced with permission from Elsevier, Spaide et al. [1]

OCT angiography (OCT-A) is a recent advancement in retinal imaging that uses high-speed OCT and advanced processing algorithms to generate *en face* angiographic images of the retinal and choroidal microcirculation utilizing the non-invasive motion-contrast of intra-luminal erythrocyte flow [1]. OCT-A images have enabled the *in vivo* study of retinal arterioles, venules and capillary beds at resolution rivaling the histologist's microscope (Fig. 24.1). This technology opens up a new world of possibilities for *in situ* analysis of the retinal microvasculature and correlation to ocular and systemic disease.

This chapter offers a review of the recent translational and clinical applications of OCT-A in the fields of neurology and neuro-ophthalmology, focusing on non-glaucomatous optic neuropathies and other human neurological disorders.

24.2 Neurology

24.2.1 Alzheimer's Dementia

Alzheimer's dementia (AD) is a chronic progressive neurodegenerative disease resulting in cognitive impairment. It is the most common cause of dementia (60–70%), with a prevalence of 5.4 million among US residents, affecting 1 in every 5 individuals at age 85 worldwide. AD is characterized by deep brain atrophy due to accumulation of misfolded protein, namely extracellular amyloid-beta plaques and intracellular tau neurofibrillary tangles.

The presence of a vasculopathy in AD has been supported by a growing body of evidence. A number of cardiovascular risk factors have been associated with AD, including increasing age, diabetes, hypertension, stroke, atherosclerosis, smoking, physical inactivity and obesity, in addition to genetic predisposition, depression and cognitive inactivity. AD has been associated with cerebral hypoperfusion, decreased cerebral vascular density and increased tortuosity. The term cerebral amyloid angiopathy has been used to describe the presence of amyloid-beta deposits in vessel walls of AD cerebral tissue.

Visual problems in AD, including color vision deficits, depth misperception, visual field defects, and reduced contrast sensitivity have traditionally been attributed to cortical lesions. The retina, however, may be more directly involved in the pathogenic process. Studies have shown presence of amyloid-beta plaques and tau proteins, decreased angiogenesis, activated microglia and proinflammatory molecules and decreased neuronal activity in the retinas of AD patients. Morphological changes to the retina in AD patients have been well documented, including the presence of optic disc pallor and neuroretinal rim thinning, arteriolar narrowing, venular widening, as well as OCT evidence of choroidal, retinal nerve fiber layer (RNFL) and ganglion cell-inner plexiform layer (GC-IPL) thinning.

OCT-A evaluation of AD patients demonstrated significantly lower macular microvascular densities and choroidal thicknesses, and larger FAZ sizes, compared to controls [2]. Mini Mental State Examination (MMSE) scores correlated significantly with these changes. Preclinical AD is a period prior to symptom onset but with measureable amyloid burden. O'Bryhim et al. imaged 30 asymptomatic participants ranging in age from 62 to 92 years using OCT-A, along with PET scans and/or cerebrospinal fluid (CSF) testing to determine presence of amyloid (Fig. 24.2) [3]. Fourteen of 30 asymptomatic participants had biomarkers positive for AD. OCT-A revealed increases in FAZ size and decreases in inner foveal thickness in these preclinical AD patients (Figs. 24.2 and 24.3). However, no significant differences in vascular density were detected between the two groups.

Pathological changes at the tissue level prior to symptom onset is a consistent finding in many AD studies. Microvascular compromise due to age and/or cardiovascular disease has been proposed as the cause of impaired autophagy and accumulation of amyloid deposits. Lumen stenosis, vessel dropout, and blood-brain barrier compromise are the result of accumulation of deposits in internal vessel walls. Binding and confining of trophic factors such as VEGF within the deposits may lead to decreased angiogenesis.

Mild cognitive impairment (MCI) is a clinical entity that describes patients prior to AD onset that have mild cognitive function decline but are still able to perform their activities of daily living. Using OCT-A, a statistically significant trend of decreasing capillary densities from healthy controls to MCI patients to AD patients was found [4]. Interestingly, MCI macular capillary density decreases were positively related to lower MMSE scores, but were not reflected in structural GC-IPL changes. In contrast, AD capillary density decreases were related to GC-IPL thinning. Prior longitudinal studies have demonstrated that decreased cerebral perfusion in MCI can predict progression to AD. Retinal microvascular loss in MCI as revealed by OCT-A may be a sensitive indicator of progressive vascular impairment that precedes neuronal death, and may be a useful tool in predicting the risk of potential conversion from MCI to AD.

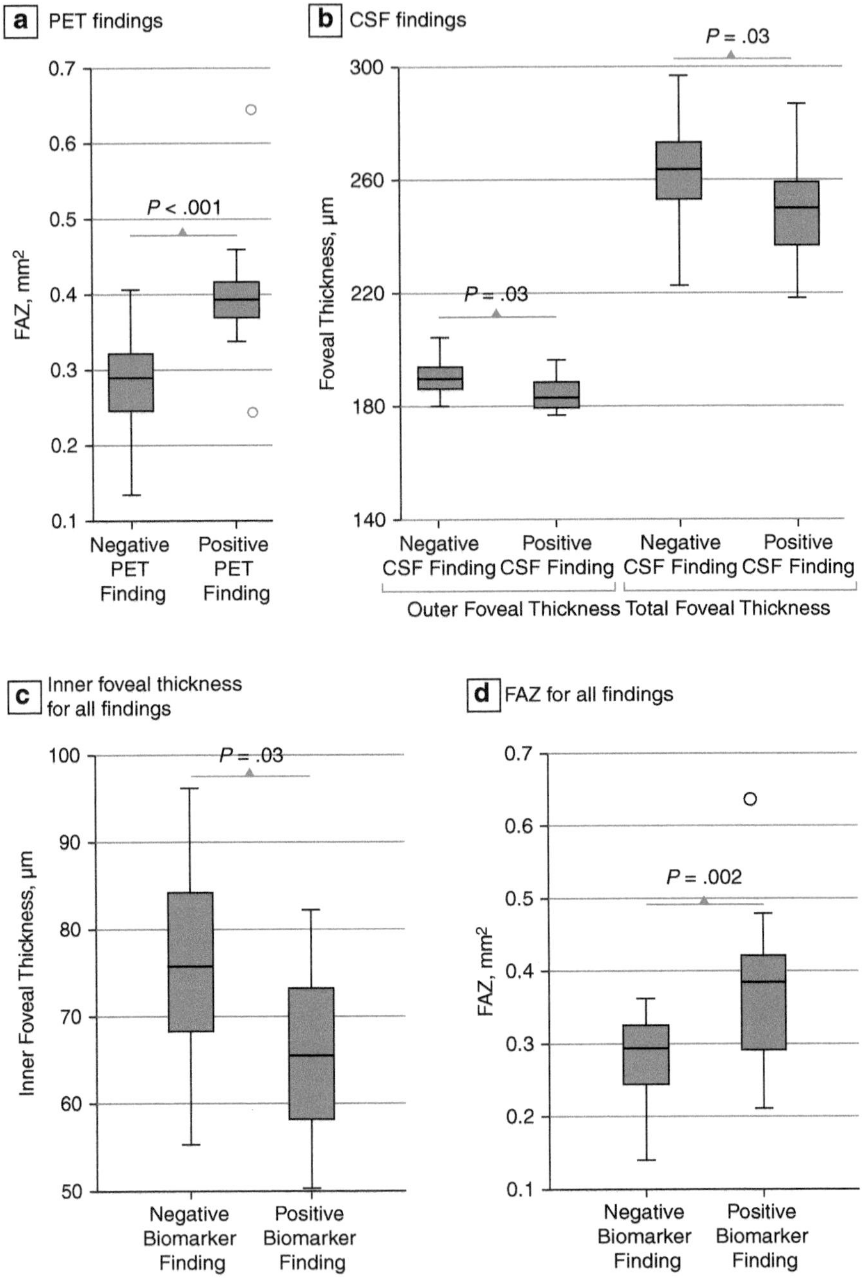

Fig. 24.2 Data are shown as box and whisker plots, where whiskers represent 1.5 times the interquartile range. (**a**) Positron emission tomography (PET) imaging results are shown for fluorine 18–labeled florbetapir compound testing. Open circles indicate outliers. (**b**) CSF analysis results are shown for β-amyloid 42 and τ protein biomarkers. (**c**, **d**) Participants with negative findings for all biomarkers (PET and/or CSF) were compared with those with positive findings for at least 1 test. Reproduced with permission from American Medical Association, O'Bryhim et al. [3]

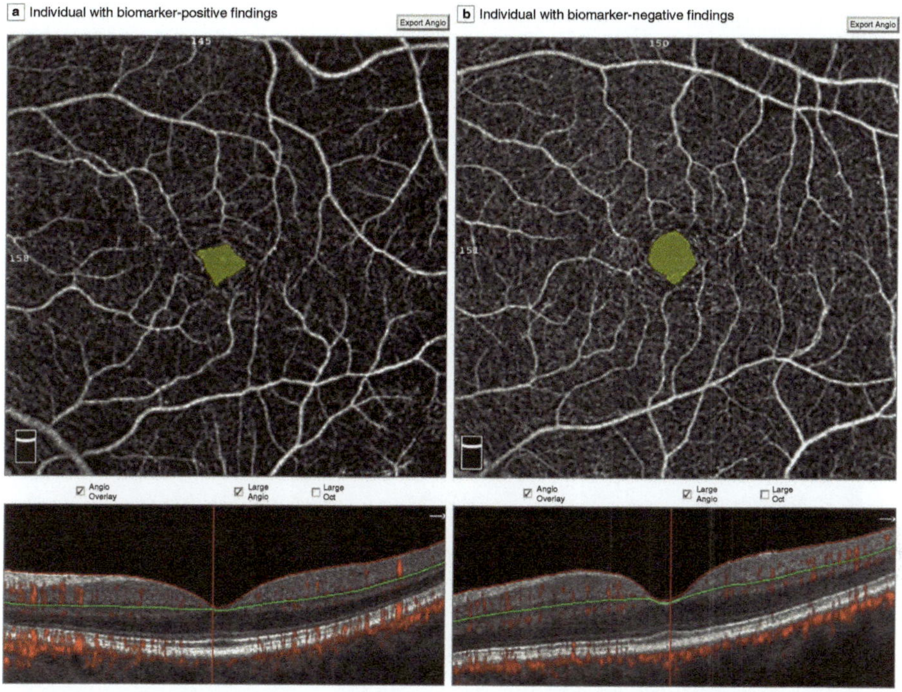

Fig. 24.3 Top images depict macular OCT-As with FAZ areas of (**a**) 0.212 mm^2 in an individual with biomarker-positive findings in preclinical AD, and (**b**) 0.311 mm^2 in an individual with biomarker negative findings. Bottom images depict their respective OCT scans. Reproduced with permission from American Medical Association, O'Bryhim et al. [3]

24.2.2 Parkinson's Disease

Parkinson's disease (PD) is a chronic progressive neurodegenerative disease resulting in cognitive impairment. It is the second most common neurodegenerative condition in the aging human population, with a prevalence of 1 million persons in the United States. PD is characterized by the loss of dopaminergic neurons in the central nervous system, leading to brain atrophy and irreversible deterioration in cognitive function. Risk factors for PD include male gender, increased age, genetic predisposition, Hispanic and non-Hispanic white races, and history of head trauma.

Visual problems such as decreased visual acuity, visual hallucinations, and deficits in visuospatial orientation have been associated with PD. As in AD, these problems have traditionally been considered to be of central origin. Recent studies have shown that retinal dopamine, which serves a vital role in retinal visual processing, is deficient in PD patients. Furthermore, OCT studies have shown inner retinal thinning in PD patients.

OCT-A images of early PD patients were recently shown to have a significantly lower macular superficial capillary plexus density compared to controls, showing a positive correlation with GC-IPL thinning (Figs. 24.4 and 24.5) [5]. A major

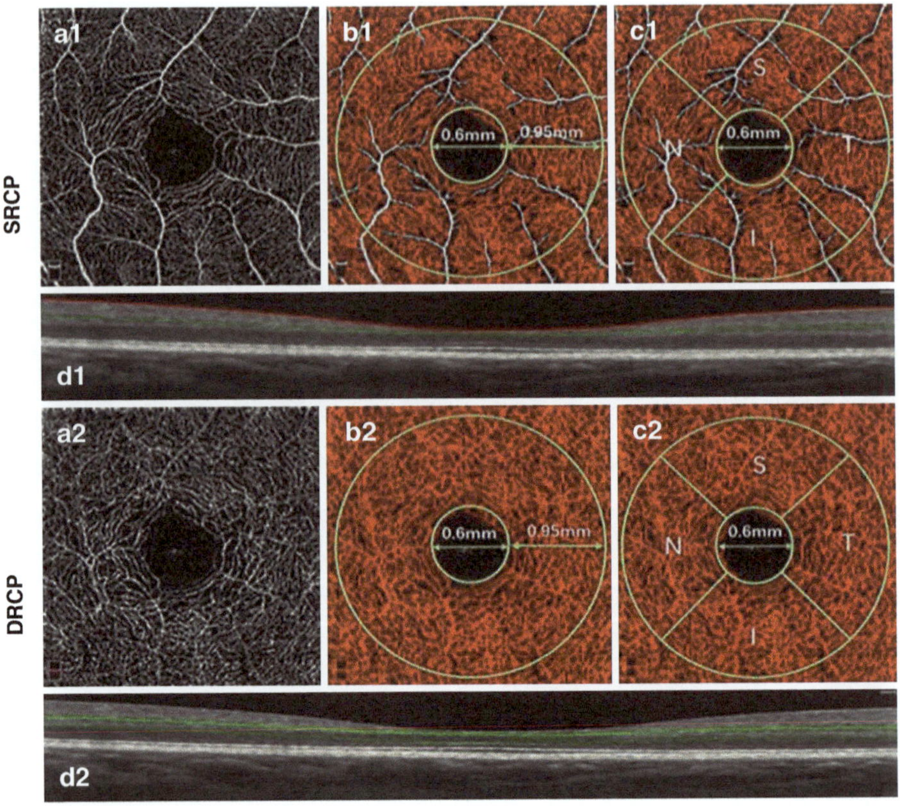

Fig. 24.4 Representative OCT-A images and diagrammatic sketch showing the microvascular density analysis of the superficial retinal capillary plexus (SRCP) and deep retinal capillary plexus (DRCP) in patients with PD. Original OCT-A images of both the SRCP (**A1**) and DRCP (**A2**). Binary images of the microvascular network after removing the large vessels with a width ≥25 μm and background noise in the SRCP (**B1**) and DRCP (**B2**). Microvascular density was performed on the total annulus zone with a diameter of 2.50 mm after excluding the FAZ (diameter 1/4 0.60 mm) in both the SRCP (**B2**) and DRCP (**B2**). Images of the capillaries are shown with microvascular density performed in the parafoveal four quadrant sectors, S, T, I, and N, of a circular zone with a diameter of 2.50 mm after excluding the FAZ in the SRCP (**C1**) and DRCP (**C2**). Reproduced with permission from IOVS, Kwapong et al. [5]

limitation of the study was that all PD patients were already on levodopa therapy at the time of imaging. The local impact of levodopa on microvascular density measures is not well understood.

Microvascular compromise may contribute to the pathophysiology of PD. The mechanism may involve alpha-synuclein deposits in vessel walls, leading to lumen stenosis, vessel dropout, and blood-brain barrier compromise. It is yet unclear from this single cross-sectional OCT-A study whether microvascular changes precede neuronal loss, or are secondary to the neuronal loss.

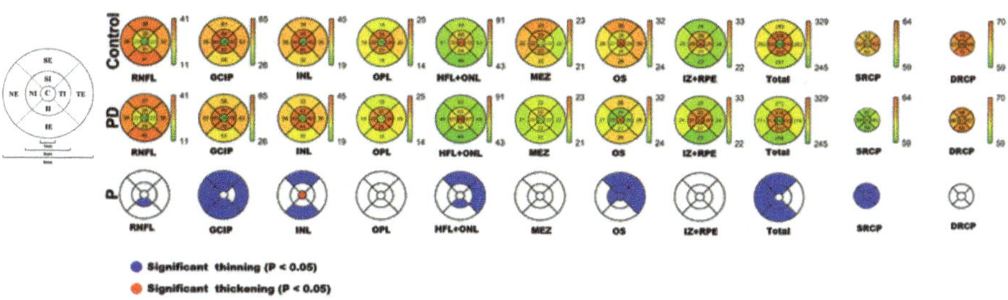

Fig. 24.5 Comparison of the microvascular density and retinal thickness between patients with PD and healthy controls. The first two rows represent the retinal thickness maps and microvascular density of healthy controls and PD patients, respectively. The retinal thickness and microvascular density are indicated by the colors shown in the color bar for each row. The third row shows the corresponding parameters between the healthy controls and the PD patients; blue represents significant thinning ($P < 0.05$), red represents significant thickening ($P < 0.05$). Reproduced with permission from IOVS, Kwapong et al. [5]

24.2.3 Multiple Sclerosis

Multiple sclerosis (MS) is an inflammatory demyelinating disorder of the CNS associated with progressive neurodegeneration. An estimated 1 million individuals in the US and 2.5 million worldwide have MS. Optic neuritis is the initial manifestation of MS in approximately 25% of patients, and occurs in approximately 50% of patients at some point in the disease course. Other ocular findings include ocular motility dysfunction, peripheral vasculitis, retinitis and pars planitis.

Patients with MS have decreased cerebral perfusion, and increased ischemic risk. Comorbid vascular risk factors result in more rapid progression of neurodegeneration and disability in MS. In the retina, OCT has been used to show decreased total blood vessel diameter and number in MS, with associated ganglion cell loss. It is unclear whether the vasculopathy present in MS plays a causative role in progressive neurodegeneration, or whether it is secondary.

A number of recent OCT-A studies attempted to elucidate the relationship between retinal vasculopathy, neuronal death and disease burden in MS. Figure 24.6 shows representative examples of optic nerve head (ONH) and macular OCTA images in a healthy control, a patient with multiple sclerosis without optic neuropathy, and a patient with multiple sclerosis with a history of optic neuropathy. Compared to healthy controls, MS patients with a mean disease duration of 11 years, with or without history of optic neuritis, had significantly decreased parafoveal vessel densities as measured by OCT-A, along with RNFL and ganglion cell complex (GCC) thinning as measured by SD-OCT, compared to healthy controls [6]. The study found that OCT-A parafoveal vessel density was inversely correlated with the Expanded Disability State Scale (EDSS), while RNFL and GCC thicknesses were inversely correlated with the Multiple Sclerosis Severity Score.

At 1-year follow up, a small but significant increase in parafoveal vessel density occurred in the MS patients on average, which the authors postulated may have been

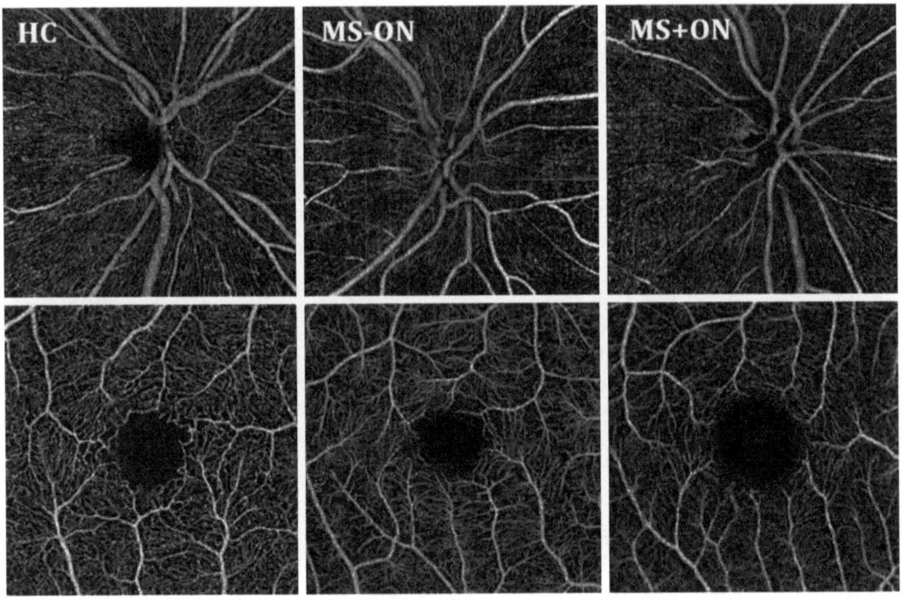

Fig. 24.6 Representative en face ONH and macular OCT-As of a 45 year old healthy control male (HC), a 34 year old male with multiple sclerosis without optic neuritis (MS-ON) and a 47 year old male with multiple sclerosis with history of optic neuritis (MS+ON)

due to therapy [7]. Patients with decreased parafoveal vessel density also demonstrated higher accrual of disability, as measured by EDSS. Despite the observed vessel density variations at 1-year follow up, no significant structural changes were seen, as indicated by stable RNFL thickness measurements. Thus, the authors concluded that reduced retinal vessel density correlated well with progressive disability. Additionally, microcirculation may improve with treatment and over time, without structural changes to the inner retina, indicating that blood flow and neuronal death may reflect different aspects of MS pathology.

At a shorter mean disease duration of 2 years, MS or clinically isolated syndrome (CIS) patients with history of optic neuritis were shown to have reduced deep and superficial vessel densities, correlating with inner retinal layer thinning, while those without a history of optic neuritis did not show such changes [8]. Two studies, at a mean disease duration of 14 years [9] and 14.5 years [10], showed that MS patients with a history of optic neuritis had more significant reductions in their ONH flow index and inner retina layer thickness compared to MS patients without history of optic neuritis. These results indicate that in longstanding MS, both cellular layer and vasculature of the retina seem to show alterations regardless of optic neuritis history. Optic neuritis might cause a more rapid and more significant decrease in vessel density.

Higher choriocapillary vessel densities have been associated with ongoing inflammatory disease activity within 24 months of imaging [8]. It is postulated that this may be a consequence of inflammation-induced microvascular dilatation, and/

or endothelial pro-angiogenetic factor upregulation occurring during MS activity. This evidence suggests a possible mechanism of the progressive neurodegeneration seen in MS, where inflammation-induced endothelial cell dysfunction causes vascular alteration and attenuation, leading to poor blood flow and ischemia of the neural tissue. Regardless of which occurs first in MS—vascular attenuation or neuronal death—combination indices of retinal angiographic and structural parameters have been shown to significantly improve the diagnostic accuracy of detecting prior history of optic neuritis in MS patients when compared to separate flow and structural indices [9].

24.2.4 Migraine

Migraine is a primary headache disorder characterized by recurrent, pulsating, moderate to severe headaches that typically include one half of the head. Migraines may be associated with nausea, vomiting, and sensitivity to light, sound or smell. Migraines affect about 15% of the world's population, and are approximately twice as prevalent in women as they are in men.

The pathophysiology of migraines is poorly understood, but may involve a vascular ischemic component. About one-third of migraine patients experience auras that immediately precede the migraines. Auras are focal neurological disturbances that are typically visual, and are thought to be secondary to cerebral transient focal ischemia. Migraine is furthermore associated with ischemic events such as stroke and myocardial infarction, as well as retinal vascular occlusion, ischemic optic neuropathy, normal tension glaucoma and paracentral acute middle maculopathy. Stroke and myocardial infarction associations are stronger for migraine with aura than without. Studies have also found a higher incidence of retinopathy in migraine patients compared to those without migraine.

OCT-A has the potential to reveal ocular perfusion changes in migraine patients, which may explain the predisposition of these patients to ischemic complications. Female migraine patients with aura, in a recent OCT-A study, had significantly lower superficial parafoveal and peripapillary vessel densities, and significantly enlarged FAZs, compared to female migraine patients without aura and female controls [11]. No significant differences were found between female migraine patients without aura and female controls, between male participants across the groups, or in structural OCT parameters including RNFL and GCC thicknesses across the groups. A major limitation of the study was that 7 out of 15 migraine with aura and 6 out of 12 migraine without aura patients were taking triptans, which is a class of migraine medications associated with vasoconstriction. The authors of the study concluded that the pathophysiology of the relationship between gender and ischemia in migraine may be related to the effect of estrogen and progesterone on endothelial cells. This may possibly mediate increased risk of ocular and systemic vascular complications in these patients.

Following 3 migraine patients at their baseline without migraine, and then during visual aura and post-aural migraine with 6 × 6 mm OCT-A macular scans, Barash

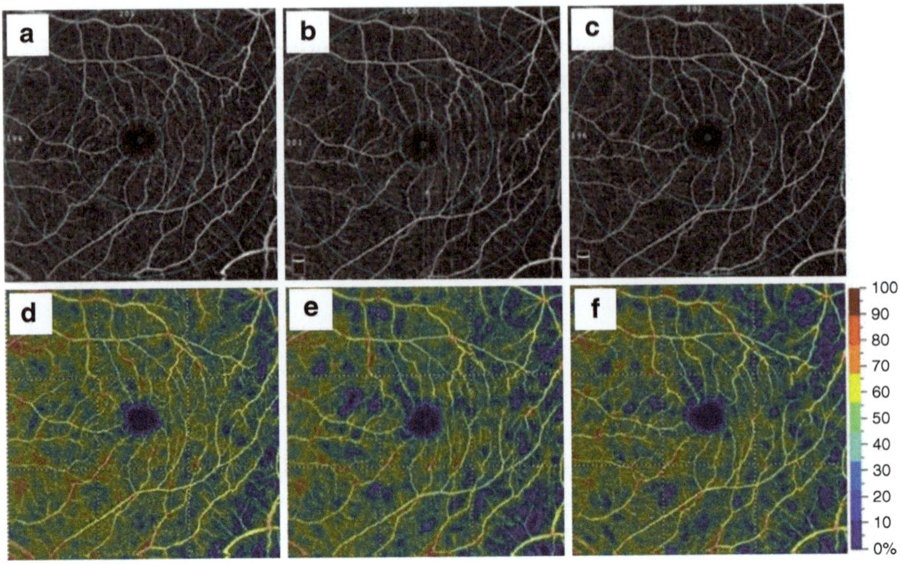

Fig. 24.7 OCT-A 6 × 6 mm superficial macular scans of a 32-year-old male with ocular migraine during (**a**) baseline, (**b**) visual aura, and (**c**) post-aural migraine, with respective (**d–f**) perfusion density color maps

et al. recently found that macular perfusion density was bilaterally and significantly decreased during post-aural migraine when compared to baseline and during visual aura (Fig. 24.7) [12]. Although the pathophysiology that may explain these changes remains unclear, these results imply systemic vascular involvement in migraine with aura patients and may explain their increased risk for cardiovascular disease. More studies using OCT-A are needed to confirm and expand on these results.

24.2.5 Amblyopia

Amblyopia represents an insult to the visual system during a critical period of neuronal plasticity and development, resulting in decreased visual acuity, color vision, contrast sensitivity and motion perception in one or both eyes. It affects approximately 3–5% of children, making it the most common cause of visual loss in children.

Although an ocular pathology such as strabismus, anisometropia, ptosis or cataract may cause the incongruence of visual information received by the eyes, amblyopia has classically been understood as a central nervous system disorder, involving neuronal structural and functional alterations in the lateral geniculate body as well as the visual cortex. More recent studies however implicate a larger role of the retina and choroid in the development of amblyopia.

Studies on amblyopic eyes have demonstrated an increased number of amacrine synapses and reduced number of bipolar synapses in the inner plexiform layer, as well as thinning of the RNFL, inner plexiform layer and outer nuclear layer, and a diminished Mueller fiber density. Amblyopic eyes have also been shown to have subfoveal choroidal thickening as compared to nonamblyopic eyes. Some studies have conversely reported an increased thickness of the outer nuclear layer in amblyopic eyes. Furthermore, amblyopic eyes have been shown to have abnormally orientated photoreceptors.

Recent studies using OCT-A have shown that superficial and deep capillary plexus densities of amblyopic eyes were lower than those in their nonamblyopic fellow eyes and age-matched control eyes (Figs. 24.8 and 24.9) [13–15]. Amblyopic eyes were found to have atrophic choroidal capillary perfusion with increased subfoveal choroidal thickness compared to their nonamblyopic fellow eyes [16]. The subfoveal choroidal thickening was found to be moderately and negatively correlated with visual acuity.

The decreased retinal and choroidal microvascular density in amblyopic eyes may be a secondary change due to neuronal atrophy and underuse. Choroidal capillary atrophy may induce malfunction of the outer retina, which may explain the observed increase in subfoveal choroidal thickness as a compensatory mechanism.

With growing evidence of retinal involvement in amblyogenesis, continued studies with OCT-A may shed light on the involvement of retinal and choroidal vessels. OCT-A may become a useful ancillary tool to help diagnose and monitor progression of amblyopia. A conflicting OCT-A study found no statistically significant

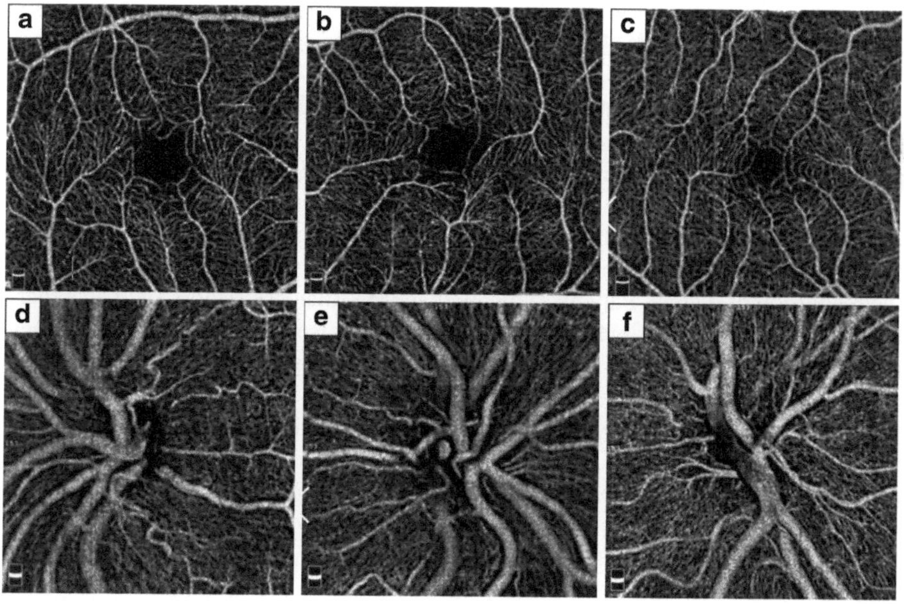

Fig. 24.8 Examples of central 3 × 3 mm macular superficial capillary plexus scans (top row) and optic nerve scans (bottom row) from children studied: amblyopic eye (**a**, **d**), contralateral eye (**b**, **e**), control eye (**c**, **f**). Reproduced with permission from Elsevier, Sobral et al. [15]

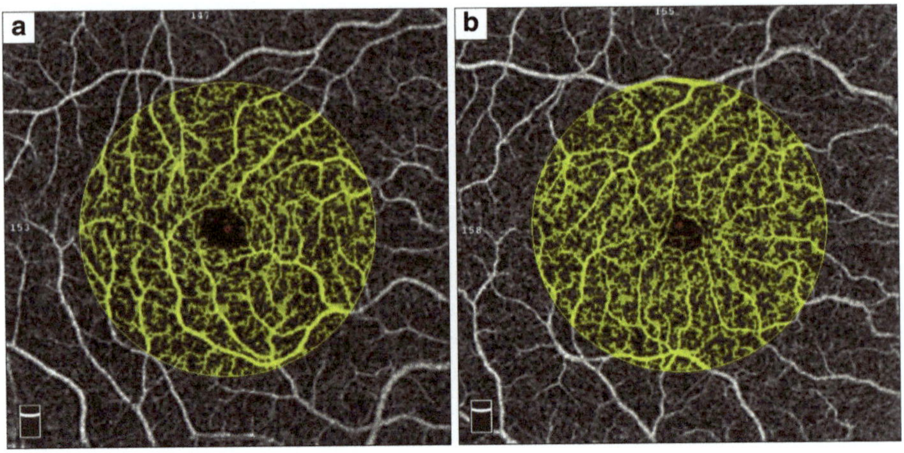

Fig. 24.9 2 mm diameter vessel density of superficial capillary plexus of an amblyopic eye (**a**) and a control eye (**b**). Vessel density is lower in the amblyopic eye, 6.059 mm^2 vs 6.617 mm^2. Reproduced with permission from Elsevier, Yilmaz et al. [13]

differences in FAZ areas or retinal microvascular densities between amblyopic and nonamblyopic eyes [17]. Further prospective studies are needed to follow amblyopic eyes through time and treatment, with a larger sample size.

24.3 Neuro-Ophthalmology

24.3.1 Non-arteritic Anterior Ischemic Optic Neuropathy

Non-arteritic anterior ischemic optic neuropathy (NAION) is the most common acute optic neuropathy over 50 years of age, affecting approximately 6 per 100,000 individuals per year. It is characterized by acute, painless unilateral vision loss or visual field loss in the presence optic disc edema. Optic disc pallor usually follows the resolution of edema. Patients typically have vascular risk factors such as hypertension, diabetes, hyperlipidemia, hypercoagulable disorders, anemia, sleep apnea and nocturnal hypotension. Other risk factors include optic disc drusen, and medications such as interferons and PDE-5 inhibitors.

The specific location of vasculopathy and pathophysiology of NAION is poorly understood. NAION usually occurs in a structurally crowded optic disc. It is believed to involve a transient hypoperfusion of the anterior optic disc microvasculature, which is chiefly contributed by the short posterior ciliary arteries. Histopathological studies have suggested that the probable location of the initial insult is the posterior laminar and retrolaminar optic nerve.

Doppler ultrasound, intravenous fluorescein angiography (FA) and indocyanine green angiography (ICGA) are limited in their ability to visualize the microcirculation in and surrounding the anterior optic nerve. Conventional OCT has shown choroidal thinning in NAION, indicating that the choroidal circulation may be involved in its pathogenesis. OCT-A, as a technology that is able to discern between different layers of microvasculature in and surrounding the anterior optic nerve, despite the possible presence of edema, may provide further insight on NAION.

Using OCT-A, non-acute NAION eyes were found to have significantly decreased perfusion through the optic disc, which was closely correlated with both central (best-corrected visual acuity) and peripheral (visual field) vision [18]. Additionally, in some NAION eyes, OCT-A revealed a significant decrease in perfusion through the optic disc without alteration of visual acuity or visual fields, suggesting that OCT-A changes in NAION may be at times subclinical and more sensitive in its diagnosis and monitoring.

Acute and non-acute NAION (range 1 week to 10 years, average 23 months since diagnosis) have been shown to have peripapillary perfusion deficits in both retinal and choroidal capillary beds, which correlate well with retinal structural (RNFL and GCC) and visual field defects [19]. Retinal peripapillary perfusion deficits in acute and non-acute NAION have been shown to be significantly correlated to decreased visual acuity as well [20]. Furthermore, fellow eyes and healthy control eyes were shown to have no significant differences in retinal peripapillary or optic disc microvasculature.

Acute NAION imaged within 7 days of symptom onset was shown to have the presence of peripapillary retinal and choroidal perfusion deficits [21]. A prospective subset of these acute NAION patients was re-imaged after resolution of optic disc edema and shown to have a partial spontaneous recovery of the retinal and choroidal microcirculations. Atrophic NAION (at least 3 months after symptom onset) was shown to have significant retinal peripapillary capillary rarefaction that was strongly correlated with visual acuity, RNFL thickness and visual field parameters (Fig. 24.10) [22], and macular retinal capillary rarefaction that correlated with visual acuity [23]. Importantly, no differences in either peripapillary or macular choriocapillaris densities were detected at this time interval.

Gandhi et al. compared the peripapillary choroidal microvascular network and visual fields of unilateral acute NAION (with disc edema present at time of imaging) with their normal fellow eyes and non-ischemic papilledema eyes, in order to rule out the possible contribution of microvascular alterations by disc edema itself [24]. Compared to normal eyes, the authors found that both NAION and papilledema eyes showed diffuse loss of the microvasculature cuff surrounding the optic disc at the choroidal level. These changes were not related to visual field changes. The authors concluded that this pattern of microvascular loss was likely a result of disc edema itself, which could cause mechanical compression of blood vessels or affect scan acquisition. NAION eyes showed an additional area of sectoral loss of choroidal vasculature extending from the disc. These changes were not seen in papilledema eyes, and were strongly correlated with visual field defects (91.6% of the time). The authors concluded that this focal pattern of choroidal microvascular loss was more likely to represent true hypoperfusion.

The short posterior ciliary arteries supplying the posterior laminar and retrolaminar optic nerve are likely involved in the initial ischemic insult in NAION. Recent

OCT-A studies show a decreased peripapillary choroidal perfusion in acute NAION, which may be the tributary circulation from the involved short posterior ciliary arteries. After the acute presentation resolves, the involved peripapillary choroidal perfusion seems to recover at least in part.

The OCT-A studies also showed rarefaction of the peripapillary retinal microcirculation. Since retinal capillaries depend on the central retinal artery and therefore should not be affected by abnormal posterior ciliary arteries, the mechanism by which they are altered must be different. Augstburger et al. propose that the resultant optic nerve edema due to swelling of ischemic axons from a transient ischemic insult in the short posterior ciliary arteries propagates anteriorly, compressing the retinal vessels and capillaries and aggravating tissue ischemia in a vicious cycle. This mechanism may explain findings that peripapillary capillary density in the temporal sector significantly decreased over 3 months following NAION, correlating with development of temporal nerve pallor and GC-IPL thinning [25].

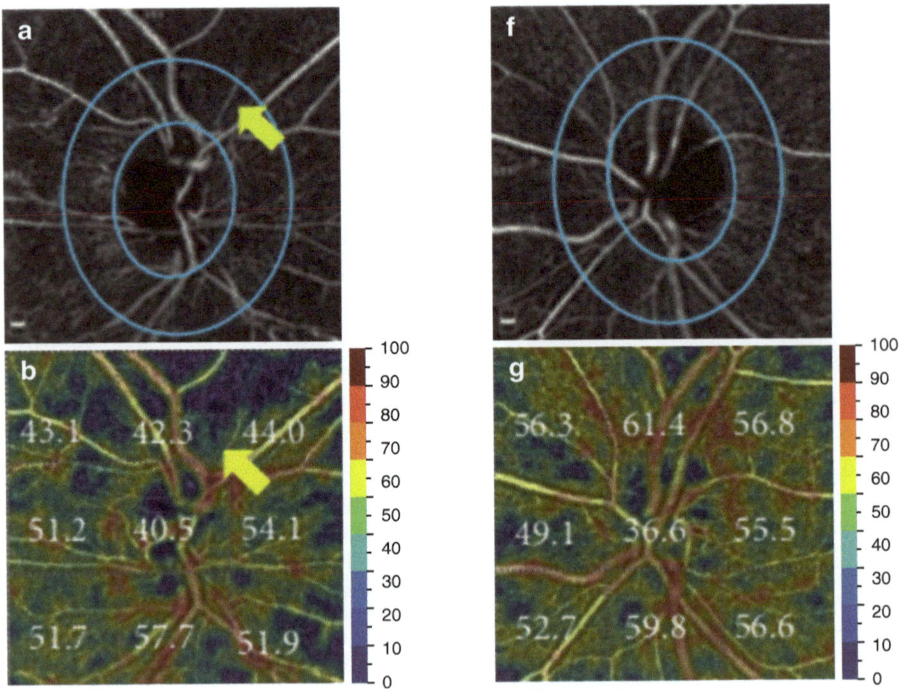

Fig. 24.10 Comparison of the peripapillary and parafoveal retinal angiograms: (**a**, **f**) en face OCT-A in the RPC layer (**b**, **g**), vessel density (%) of RPCs with a color-coded map (**c**, **h**), OCT-A in the parafoveal area (**d**, **i**), vessel density (%) in the parafoveal area with a color-coded map, and (**e**, **j**) total deviation of the visual field in a representative NAION eye and the normal fellow eye. In the NAION eye (**a**–**e**), the microvascular network of the RPC layer was attenuated (arrow) compared with that of the normal fellow eye (**f**–**j**). The parafoveal microvascular networks in these examples showed no clear differences. The circles indicate the measured area for circumpapillary and parafoveal vessel density. Reproduced with permission from Hindawi, Liu et al. [22]

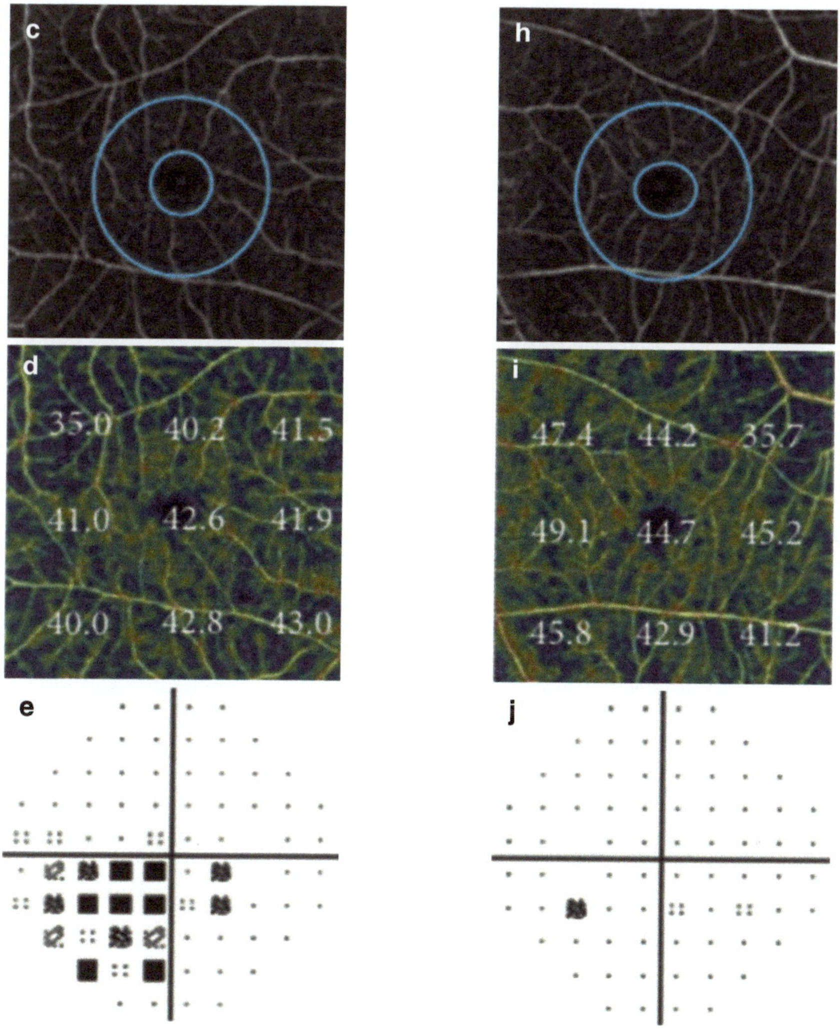

Fig. 24.10 (continued)

Importantly, the OCT-A studies demonstrated that vessel density measurements correlate well with visual acuity and visual field parameters, suggesting that OCT-A could be of prognostic value in the assessment of ischemic severity in NAION patients.

24.3.2 Leber's Hereditary Optic Neuropathy

Leber's Hereditary Optic Neuropathy (LHON) is the most common inherited mitochondrial disorder. Males are more likely to be affected than females, and age of onset is typically between 15–30 years. Mitochondrial DNA point mutations cause dysfunction in the mitochondrial respiratory chain, increasing reactive oxygen species (ROS) production. Given mitochondrial heteroplasmy, some individuals termed unaffected carriers remain asymptomatic throughout life. In individuals with a high enough mutation load, the increased ROS are thought to cause retinal ganglion cell and axonal injury and apoptosis, leading to a progressive optic neuropathy with initial optic disc swelling and subsequent RNFL thinning and optic nerve atrophy. Vision may worsen to less than 20/200, but rarely progresses to no light perception. There is no established medical therapy for LHON, and gene therapy studies are underway.

The optic disc microangiopathy in LHON is present with optic disc swelling and is characterized by an increase in tortuosity and size of the capillaries. The pathogenesis of the microangiopathy is unclear. It may be secondary to optic disc swelling and retinal ganglion cell damage, and may be involved in causing further RGC damage. OCT-A has been used to show that parafoveal vessel density is decreased in LHON patients compared to controls, at both superficial and deep levels (Fig. 24.11) [26]. Furthermore, microvascular density, as opposed to OCT-detectable structural changes, correlated well with visual acuity.

Several stages of LHON are recognized. The sub-acute stage involves a progressive evolution of optic disc and RNFL swelling for 3 months followed by thinning, resulting in a central scotoma that enlarges for a few months, becoming a stable defect within 6 months. The dynamic stage involves minor RNFL thinning after 6 months. Transition to the chronic stage occurs within 12 months of initial onset. OCT-A has recently been used to show that retinal peripapillary capillary density

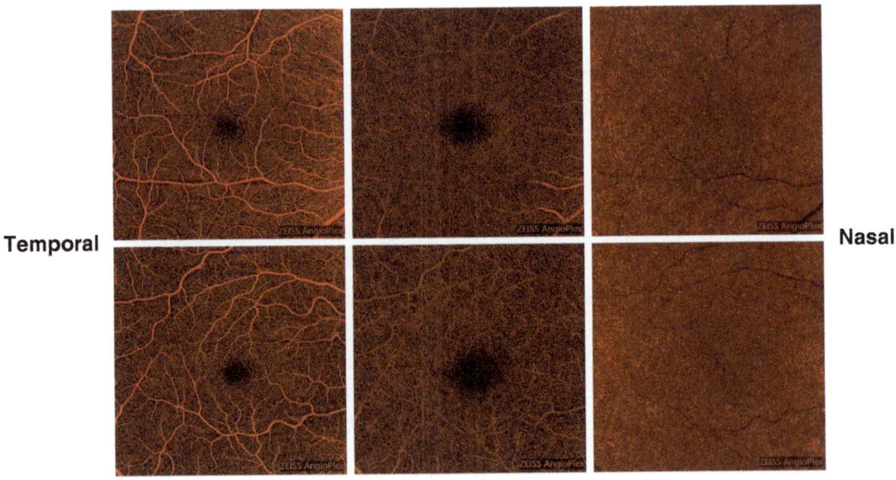

Fig. 24.11 Representation of LHON and healthy patients. Representative OCTA 6 × 6-mm scans segmented at the level of the superficial capillary plexus (SCP; Left images), deep capillary plexus (DCP; Middle images), and choriocapillaris (CC, Right images) from a healthy subject (Above) and an LHON patient (Below). A reduced flow was demonstrated at the level of the SCP and DCP, especially in the nasal and inferior parafoveal sectors, in LHON patients. Reproduced with permission from Elsevier, Borrelli et al. [26]

incrementally worsens over progressive stages of LHON [27]. Importantly, microvascular changes in the temporal sector were shown to precede RNFL changes, and mirrored GC-IPL changes.

Microvascular density appears to correlate with visual acuity better than structural changes, pointing to a microvascular dysfunction in LHON preceding neuronal dysfunction. This suggests that microvascular dysfunction may be an important contributor to retinal ganglion cell dysfunction and loss. One proposed mechanism includes mitochondrial dysfunction influencing endothelial cell and vascular smooth muscle viability, similar to its effect on retinal ganglion cells and their axons. OCT-A studies on LHON indicate that microvascular dysfunction may play a more important part than previously realized in the pathogenesis of LHON.

24.3.3 Optic Disc Swelling

Optic disc swelling is most commonly due to non-arteritic ischemic optic neuropathy (NAION), optic neuritis, or papilledema (swelling from elevated intracranial pressure). Clinically, optic disc swelling may appear similar across the three entities, while having different risk factor profiles, associated systemic diseases, prognosis and treatment. Bilateral NAION or optic neuritis may be mistaken for papilledema. Vice versa, papilledema may be mistaken for bilateral NAION or optic neuritis.

Using OCT-A, NAION and optic neuritis eyes have been shown to have a significantly lower retinal peripapillary vessel density compared to papilledema eyes and healthy control eyes (Fig. 24.12) [28]. No significant differences were found between NAION and optic neuritis eyes, or between papilledema and healthy control eyes. These results indicate that OCT-A can be employed, together with other imaging modalities and standard work up, in a clinical situation where it is otherwise difficult to differentiate NAION or optic neuritis from papilledema.

24.3.4 Optic Nerve Head Drusen

Optic nerve head drusen (ONHD) are calcium and phosphorus deposits within a filamentous protein matrix that accumulate in the optic nerve. ONHD occur in approximately 2% of the population, are usually asymptomatic, and are bilateral in 75% of cases. They can be buried or superficial. Superficial drusen can be directly visualized, while deeper drusen may need ultrasound for visualization, and can alter the contour of the optic nerve giving it an elevated, congested and swollen appearance. There are contradictory reports regarding which type of ONHD is more likely to cause visual field deficits with associated RNFL loss.

ONHD are associated with small and crowded optic discs. They are associated with optic nerve pallor and choroidal neovascularization, as well as vascular alterations and vascular occlusive disease such as NAION, central retinal artery occlusion

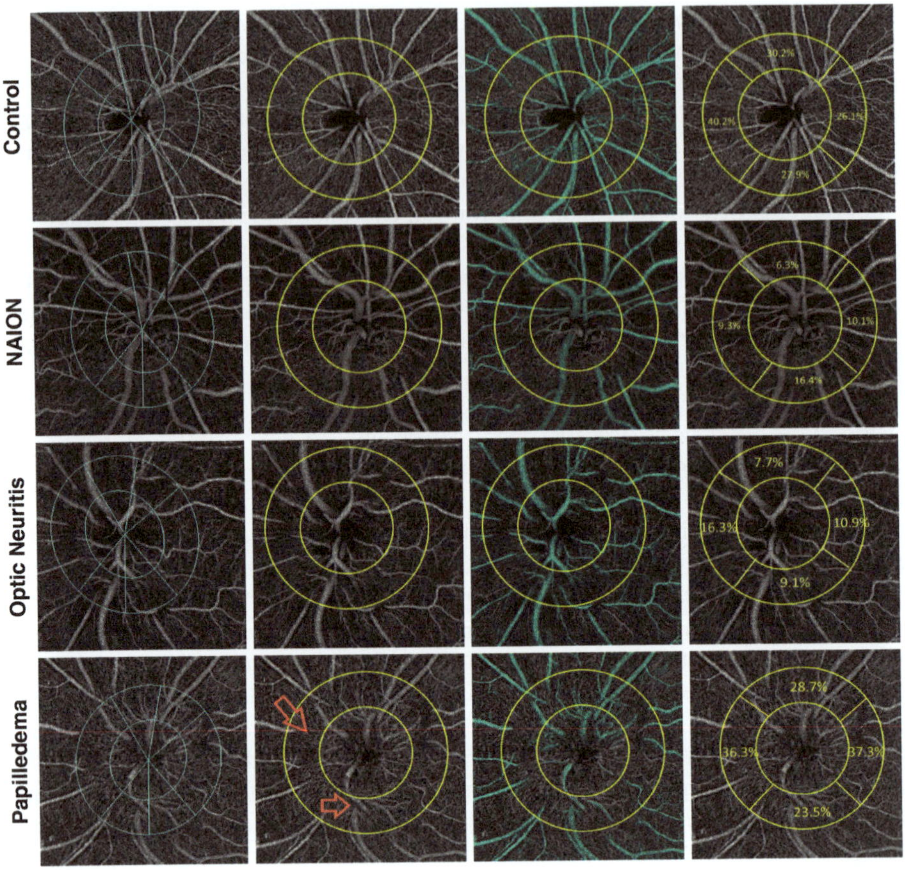

Fig. 24.12 OCT-A of peripapillary total vasculature and capillaries in eyes with optic disc swelling. (Left column) OCT-A sectors of peripapillary vasculature. (Second column) OCT-A images with 2 concentric circles with 3.45 mm and 1.95 mm diameter with customized software. (Third column) Major vessel (in cyan) removal using customized software. (Fourth column) Peripapillary capillary density (%) in each sector. Capillary density in NAION eyes is lower than papilledema and control eyes. OCT-A images of papilledema eyes show large vessel distortions and obscurations (arrows) compared to other disc swellings. Reproduced with permission from Elsevier, Fard et al. [28]

and central retinal vein occlusion. ONHD can mimic several pathologies such as optic disc edema and glaucoma as signs and symptoms are similar.

The pathogenesis of ONHD is unclear. Some postulate that the deposits originate from extruded mitochondria, while others postulate that the primary pathology is an inherited dysplasia of the optic disc and its blood supply leading to abnormal transudation of plasma proteins and other extracellular materials.

The mechanisms by which ONHD cause visual damage are also poorly understood. It is unclear whether ONHD cause retinal nerve fiber injury directly through axonal compression or indirectly through vascular compression and resultant nerve fiber ischemia. Conventional microvasculature imaging modalities such as intravenous FA have not been successful in answering this question due to limitations in resolution of the retinal peripapillary capillary network. Doppler ultrasound has been used to show lower systolic and diastolic flow velocities in the central retinal artery and short posterior ciliary arteries, but not the ophthalmic artery, in eyes with ONHD, which correlated with visual field loss.

OCT-A has revealed that ONHD are associated with focal decreases in vessel density within their localization [29]. OCT-A was recently used to image a patient who developed decreased vision in the right eye and was then found to have a heavy burden of superficial ONHD [30]. In this patient, superficial microvascular attenuation was associated with most but not all drusen, while RNFL thinning corresponded to some but not all areas of microvascular attenuation. The authors concluded that superficial ONHD may cause focal areas of poor superficial retinal perfusion that may in turn lead to nerve fiber ischemia and rarefaction, causing visual acuity loss and visual field deficits. These results indicate that OCT-A may be more sensitive than traditional peripapillary RNFL and visual field analysis for the earlier detection and monitoring of optic nerve and retinal injury from ONHD.

24.3.5 Thyroid Eye Disease and Dysthyroid Optic Neuropathy

Thyroid eye disease (TED) is an orbitopathy associated with thyroid dysfunction and a complex immunologic process. Treatment is aimed at ameliorating the resulting orbital congestion and inflammation. The most serious although infrequent (8–10%) vision-threatening complication of TED is dysthyroid optic neuropathy (DON). Clinical scoring systems such as the Clinical Activity Score have been used as assessment tools for guiding evaluation and treatment of TED, however no system prevails as the gold standard. Furthermore, none of the clinical scoring systems were designed to grade effectiveness of treatment of DON.

A number of studies using a variety of modalities have concluded that an important component of the pathophysiology of TED and DON is changes in blood flow in the orbit and optic nerve in the setting of compression and congestion/inflammation. Some have reported an increased blood flow through the ophthalmic artery and central retinal artery, while others have reported decreased chorioretinal perfusion, as well as congestion of the retinal veins and superior ophthalmic vein.

OCT-A may help shed light onto the perfusion status of the optic nerve head and retina in TED, and onto the early pathogenesis of DON. Using OCT-A, eyes with active TED were found to have an increased retinal microvascular density compared to healthy controls [31]. The increase in density was moderately negatively correlated with visual acuity. Another study using OCT-A performed a prospective case series in a cohort of TED patients with and without DON who underwent bilateral orbital decompression [32]. The authors found that eyes with TED generally showed reduction in peripapillary microvascular density following decompression surgery, more so in eyes with DON (Fig. 24.13).

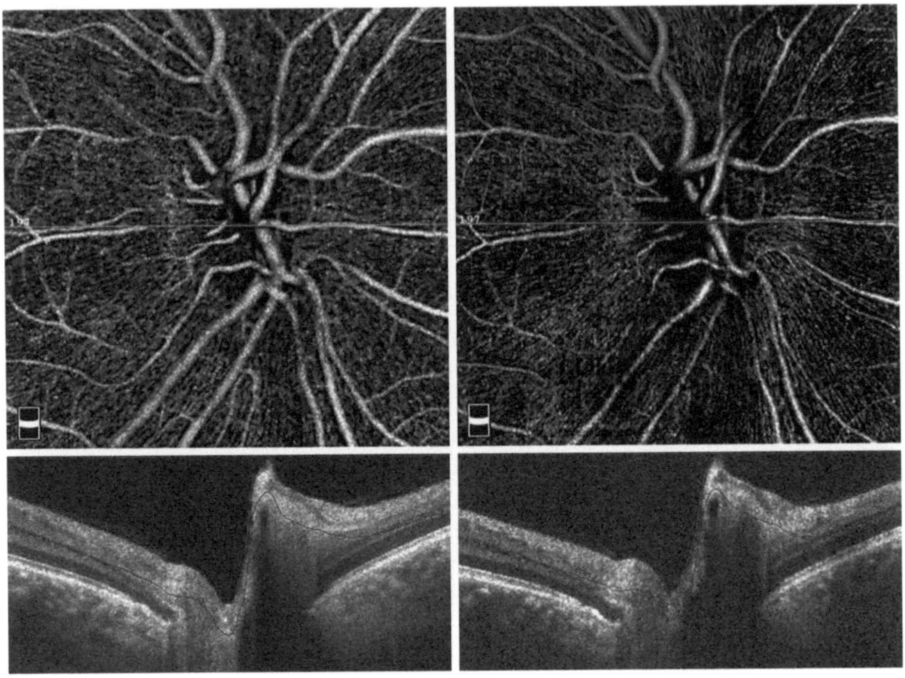

Fig. 24.13 Preoperative (left) and postoperative (right) OCT-A of the right eye in a patient with dysthyroid optic neuropathy. A significant reduction in blood vessel density was found after decompression (−2.45 within the peripapillary ring and −7.11 over the optic disk). Reproduced with permission from Taylor & Francis, Lewis et al. [32]

These studies demonstrate that OCT-A has potential to be a more sensitive and quantitative tool in grading clinical activity of TED, diagnosing DON earlier, and offering clinicians a tool to monitor response to treatment.

24.4 Summary

The early studies using OCT-A reviewed here demonstrate its potential for sorting out the interplay of vascular and neuronal changes in the pathophysiology of common neurological and neuro-ophthalmological disorders. OCT-A shows promise in becoming an important tool for researchers and clinicians in their multimodal approach in detecting pathological changes, monitoring disease progression and evaluating response to treatment in these disorders.

References

1. Spaide RF, Fujimoto JG, Waheed NK, Sadda SR, Staurenghi G. Optical coherence tomography angiography. Prog Retin Eye Res. 2018;64:1–55.
2. Bulut M, Kurtuluş F, Gözkaya O, Erol MK, Cengiz A, Akıdan M, et al. Evaluation of optical coherence tomography angiographic findings in Alzheimer's type dementia. Br J Ophthalmol. 2018;102(2):233–7.

3. O'Bryhim BE, Apte RS, Kung N, Coble D, Van Stavern GP. Association of preclinical Alzheimer disease with optical coherence tomographic angiography findings. JAMA Ophthalmol. 2018;136(11):1242–8.
4. Jiang H, Wei Y, Shi Y, Wright CB, Sun X, Gregori G, et al. Altered macular microvasculature in mild cognitive impairment and Alzheimer disease. J Neuroophthalmol. 2018;38(3):292–8.
5. Kwapong WR, Ye H, Peng C, Zhuang X, Wang J, Shen M, et al. Retinal microvascular impairment in the early stages of Parkinson's disease. Invest Ophthalmol Vis Sci. 2018;59(10):4115–22.
6. Lanzillo R, Cennamo G, Criscuolo C, Carotenuto A, Velotti N, Sparnelli F, et al. Optical coherence tomography angiography retinal vascular network assessment in multiple sclerosis. Mult Scler. 2018;24(13):1706–14.
7. Lanzillo R, Cennamo G, Moccia M, Criscuolo C, Carotenuto A, Frattaruolo N, et al. Retinal vascular density in multiple sclerosis: a 1-year follow-up. Eur J Neurol. 2019;26:198–201.
8. Feucht N, Maier M, Lepennetier G, Pettenkofer M, Wetzlmair C, Daltrozzo T, et al. Optical coherence tomography angiography indicates associations of the retinal vascular network and disease activity in multiple sclerosis. Mult Scler. 2018:1352458517750009.
9. Spain RI, Liu L, Zhang X, Jia Y, Tan O, Bourdette D, et al. Optical coherence tomography angiography enhances the detection of optic nerve damage in multiple sclerosis. Br J Ophthalmol. 2018;102(4):520–4.
10. Wang X, Jia Y, Spain R, Potsaid B, Liu JJ, Baumann B, et al. Optical coherence tomography angiography of optic nerve head and parafovea in multiple sclerosis. Br J Ophthalmol. 2014;98(10):1368–73.
11. Chang MY, Phasukkijwatana N, Garrity S, Pineles SL, Rahimi M, Sarraf D, et al. Foveal and peripapillary vascular decrement in migraine with aura demonstrated by optical coherence tomography angiography. Invest Ophthalmol Vis Sci. 2017;58(12):5477–84.
12. Barash AT, Pinhas MJ, Rosen A, Richard B. Macular and peripapillary retinal perfusion changes during migraine with aura detected by optical coherence tomography angiography. Paper presentation at the American Society of Retina Specialists, Chicago, July 2019.
13. Yilmaz I, Ocak OB, Yilmaz BS, Inal A, Gokyigit B, Taskapili M. Comparison of quantitative measurement of foveal avascular zone and macular vessel density in eyes of children with amblyopia and healthy controls: an optical coherence tomography angiography study. J AAPOS. 2017;21(3):224–8.
14. Lonngi M, Velez FG, Tsui I, Davila JP, Rahimi M, Chan C, et al. Spectral-domain optical coherence tomographic angiography in children with amblyopia. JAMA Ophthalmol. 2017;135(10):1086–91.
15. Sobral I, Rodrigues TM, Soares M, Seara M, Monteiro M, Paiva C, et al. OCT angiography findings in children with amblyopia. J AAPOS. 2018;22(4):286–9.e2.
16. Guo L, Tao J, Xia F, Yang Z, Ma X, Hua R. In vivo optical imaging of amblyopia: digital subtraction autofluorescence and split-spectrum amplitude-decorrelation angiography. Lasers Surg Med. 2016;48(7):660–7.
17. Demirayak B, Vural A, Onur IU, Kaya FS, Yigit FU. Analysis of macular vessel density and foveal avascular zone using spectral-domain optical coherence tomography angiography in children with amblyopia. J Pediatr Ophthalmol Strabismus. 2018;56:1–5.
18. Ling JW, Yin X, Lu QY, Chen YY, Lu PR. Optical coherence tomography angiography of optic disc perfusion in non-arteritic anterior ischemic optic neuropathy. Int J Ophthalmol. 2017;10(9):1402–6.
19. Wright Mayes E, Cole ED, Dang S, Novais EA, Vuong L, Mendoza-Santiesteban C, et al. Optical coherence tomography angiography in nonarteritic anterior ischemic optic neuropathy. J Neuroophthalmol. 2017;37:358–64.
20. Song Y, Min JY, Mao L, Gong YY. Microvasculature dropout detected by the optical coherence tomography angiography in nonarteritic anterior ischemic optic neuropathy. Lasers Surg Med. 2018;50(3):194–201.
21. Sharma S, Ang M, Najjar RP, Sng C, Cheung CY, Rukmini AV, et al. Optical coherence tomography angiography in acute non-arteritic anterior ischaemic optic neuropathy. Br J Ophthalmol. 2017;101(8):1045–51.

22. Liu CH, Kao LY, Sun MH, Wu WC, Chen HS. Retinal vessel density in optical coherence tomography angiography in optic atrophy after nonarteritic anterior ischemic optic neuropathy. J Ophthalmol. 2017;2017:9632647.
23. Augstburger E, Zéboulon P, Keilani C, Baudouin C, Labbé A. Retinal and choroidal microvasculature in nonarteritic anterior ischemic optic neuropathy: an optical coherence tomography angiography study. Invest Ophthalmol Vis Sci. 2018;59(2):870–7.
24. Gandhi U, Chhablani J, Badakere A, Kekunnaya R, Rasheed MA, Goud A, et al. Optical coherence tomography angiography in acute unilateral nonarteritic anterior ischemic optic neuropathy: a comparison with the fellow eye and with eyes with papilledema. Indian J Ophthalmol. 2018;66(8):1144–8.
25. Rebolleda G, Díez-Álvarez L, García Marín Y, de Juan V, Muñoz-Negrete FJ. Reduction of peripapillary vessel density by optical coherence tomography angiography from the acute to the atrophic stage in non-arteritic anterior ischaemic optic neuropathy. Ophthalmologica. 2018;240(4):191–9.
26. Borrelli E, Balasubramanian S, Triolo G, Barboni P, Sadda SR, Sadun AA. Topographic macular microvascular changes and correlation with visual loss in chronic Leber hereditary optic neuropathy. Am J Ophthalmol. 2018;192:217–28.
27. Balducci N, Cascavilla ML, Ciardella A, La Morgia C, Triolo G, Parisi V, et al. Peripapillary vessel density changes in Leber's hereditary optic neuropathy: a new biomarker. Clin Exp Ophthalmol. 2018;46:1055–62.
28. Fard MA, Jalili J, Sahraiyan A, Khojasteh H, Hejazi M, Ritch R, et al. Optical coherence tomography angiography in optic disc swelling. Am J Ophthalmol. 2018;191:116–23.
29. Flores-Reyes E, Hoskens K, Mansouri K. Optic nerve head drusen: imaging using optical coherence tomography angiography. J Glaucoma. 2017;26(9):845–9.
30. Gaier ED, Rizzo JF, Miller JB, Cestari DM. Focal capillary dropout associated with optic disc drusen using optical coherence tomographic angiography. J Neuroophthalmol. 2017;37(4):405–10.
31. Ye L, Zhou SS, Yang WL, Bao J, Jiang N, Min YL, et al. Retinal microvasculature alteration in active thyroid-associated ophthalmopathy. Endocr Pract. 2018;24(7):658–67.
32. Lewis KT, Bullock JR, Drumright RT, Olsen MJ, Penman AD. Changes in peripapillary blood vessel density in Graves' orbitopathy after orbital decompression surgery as measured by optical coherence tomography angiography. Orbit. 2019;38:87–94.

Conclusion: The Exciting Future of OCT and New Imaging of Retina and Optic Nerve

25

Piero Barboni and Andrzej Grzybowski

The book aims to improve our knowledge of the wide spectrum of neurological diseases that can be investigated by OCT and new imaging techniques. We focused our attention on different pathologies that in the past were of exclusive interest to neurologists, like stroke or neurodegenerative diseases. Some ocular alteration detectable by OCT precede systemic manifestations of neurological diseases or are closely related to disease severity. From a clinical point of view, the information obtained by this technology improve the neurological diagnosis and provide useful parameters for therapeutic trials. Moreover, the development of hand-held or mobile and cost-effective OCT instruments could improve systematic screenings for neurological diseases [1, 2]. Thanks to the OCT accuracy and diffusion, we are accumulating more and more information about ocular tissues, regarding both anatomy and pathology.

The evolution of retinal imaging are moving toward different directions:

First, OCT technology is going to look for the best definition and resolution in order to be more similar to histology and to improve the reliability and the definition of pathological images. Today, many companies are moving toward Swept Source technology or other technologies focused on retinal or vascular layers segmentation in order to study the role of different structures in neurological diseases [3–5].

Second, physicians often ask to the machine a diagnostic role. This could be achieved if the normative database of each instrument will be improved by increasing the control group and stratifying it according to any confounding factor, or if a protocol analysis unaffected by anatomical variability will be developed.

P. Barboni (✉)
Studio Oculistico d'Azeglio, Bologna, Italy

Scientific Institute San Raffaele, Milan, Italy
e-mail: p.barboni@studiodazeglio.it

A. Grzybowski
University of Warmia and Mazury, Olsztyn, Poland

Institute for Research in Ophthalmology, Poznań, Poland

A. Grzybowski, P. Barboni (eds.), *OCT and Imaging in Central Nervous System Diseases*, https://doi.org/10.1007/978-3-030-26269-3_25

Moreover, a standardized protocol of images acquisition and of data analysis is needed in order to reduce the inter-studies variability and to improve the comprehension and comparability of published data [6].

Third, retinal imaging will hopefully be able to obtain data about ocular function too. OCT angiography (OCT-A), for example, is a new technology that can visualize retinal, optic nerve head and choriocapillary vessels. To date, information about vessel density are provided by different models of OCT-A and correlation between vessel density and retinal anatomy (such as ganglion cells and retinal nerve fiber layer thickness) has been demonstrated in different ocular and neurological diseases [7, 8]. In the next future, it is desiderable that also functional data about ocular blood flow will be analyzable, as they could be very useful for studying neurological pathophysiology and for monitoring therapeutic approcheas.

The combination of structural and functional technologies is desirable. At this moment, at least three new techniques are being developed in this area. Flavoprotein fluorescence methodology (OcuSciences, Inc., Ann Arbor, MI) is a kind of autofluorescence, which uses a very specific wavelength to excite natural fluorophores of the retina. This technology can potentially detects mitochondrial damage by measuring oxidized flavoproteins in the retina [9, 10]. In this way, retinal fibers swelling and ganglion cell atrophy due to mitochondrial structural damage can be potentially combined to functional information.

Another high-resolution optical imaging approach was developed to detect beta-amyloid plaques in the retina. The system is based on a specific marker (fluorescent curcumin) as an imaging agent to detect Alzheimer's disease-related plaques in the retinas. The technique, developed at Cedars-Sinai Medical Centers, is a tool for early Alzheimer's disease diagnosis as well as assessment of therapy [11].

DARC (detection of apoptosing retinal cells) technology uses confocal laser-scanning ophthalmoscopy to visualize single neural cell apoptosis in vivo. This fluorescent technique is effective in the identification of the protein annexin 5 that represents an early feature in the apoptotic process. This method is able to image changes occurring in nerve cell apoptosis over time and could provide the opportunity for detailed investigation of fundamental neurodegenerative disease mechanisms and the evaluation of interventions with potential clinical applications [12, 13].

Moreover, new emerging techniques are in progress, such as hyperspectral imaging, photoacustic ophthalmoscopy and molecular imaging [14, 15, 16]. From an experimental point of view OCT could give us important information that we could share with genetist, biochemist and clinicians in order to better define phenotype/genotype correlation and to study animal model.

In conclusion OCT and other retinal imaging gives us the opportunity to study brain diseases through the eye window in an objective and not invasive method.

References

1. Jung W, Kim J, Jeon M, et al. Handheld optical coherence tomography scanner for primary care diagnostics. IEEE Trans Biomed Eng. 2011;58:741–4.

2. Chen DL, Kraus M, Potsaid B. Handheld ultrahigh speed swept source optical coherence tomography instrument using a MEMS scanning mirror. Biomed Opt Express. 2014;5:293–311.
3. Tan O, Liu L, Liu L, Huang D. Nerve fiber flux analysis using wide-field swept-source optical coherence tomography. Transl Vis Sci Technol. 2018;7:16.
4. Jia Y, Simonett JM, Wang J, et al. Wide-field OCT angiography investigation of the relationship between radial peripapillary capillary plexus density and nerve fiber layer thickness. Invest Ophthalmol Vis Sci. 2017;58:5188–94.
5. Oberwahrenbrock T, Weinhold M, Mikolajczak J, et al. Reliability of intra-retinal layer thickness estimates. PLoS One. 2015;10:e0137316.
6. Pinhas A, Linderman R, Mo S, Krawitz BD, et al. A method for age-matched OCT angiography deviation mapping in the assessment of disease-related changes to the radial peripapillary capillaries. PLoS One. 2018;13:e0197062.
7. Makita S, Hong Y, Yamanari M, Yatagai T, Yasuno Y. Optical coherence angiography. Opt Express. 2006;14:7821–40.
8. Huang Y, Zhang Q, Thorell MR, An L, Durbin MK, Laron M, et al. Swept-source OCT angiography of the retinal vasculature using intensity differentiation-based optical microangiography algorithms. Ophthalmic Surg Lasers Imaging Retina. 2014;45:382–9.
9. Field MG, Elner VM, Puro DG, Feuerman JM, Musch DC, Pop-Busui R, et al. Rapid, non-invasive detection of diabetes-induced retinal metabolic stress. Arch Ophthalmol. 2008;126:934–8.
10. Field MG, Yang D, Bian ZM, Petty HR, Elner VM. Retinal flavoprotein fluorescence correlates with mitochondrial stress, apoptosis, and chemokine expression. Exp Eye Res. 2011;93:548–55.
11. Koronyo-Hamaoui M, Koronyo Y, Ljubimov AV, Miller CA, Ko MK, Black KL, et al. Identification of amyloid plaques in retinas from Alzheimer's patients and noninvasive in vivo optical imaging of retinal plaques in a mouse model. Neuroimage. 2011;54(Suppl 1):S204–17.
12. Guo L, Cordeiro MF. Assessment of neuroprotection in the retina with DARC. Prog Brain Res. 2008;173:437–50.
13. Normando EM, Dehabadi MH, Guo L, Turner LA, Pollorsi G, Cordeiro MF. Real-time imaging of retinal cell apoptosis by confocal scanning laser ophthalmoscopy. Methods Mol Biol. 2015;1254:227–37.
14. Mordant DJ, Al-Abboud I, Muyo G, et al. Spectral imaging of the retina. Eye (Lond). 2011;25:309–20.
15. Zhang HF, Puliafito CA, Jiao S. Photoacoustic ophthalmoscopy for in vivo retinal imaging: current status and prospects. Ophthalmic Surg Lasers Imaging. 2011;42:S106–15.
16. Jiao S, Jiang M, Hu J, et al. Photoacoustic ophthalmoscopy for in vivo retinal imaging. Opt Express. 2010;18:3967–72.

Index

A. Grzybowski, P. Barboni (eds.), *OCT and Imaging in Central Nervous System Diseases*, https://doi.org/10.1007/978-3-030-26269-3

B

C

Kolibri 360 GmbH
Ferdinand-Jühlke-Straße 7
99095 Erfurt, Deutschland
produktsicherheit@kolibri360.de